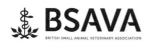

T0198311

Small Animal Formulary

11th Edition – Part A: Canine and Feline

Editor-in-chief:

Fergus Allerton BSc BVSc CertSAM DipECVIM-CA MRCVS
Willows Veterinary Centre and Referral Service,
Highlands Road, Shirley, Solihull, West Midlands B90 4NH

Published by:
British Small Animal Veterinary Association
Woodrow House, 1 Telford Way,
Waterwells Business Park, Quedgeley,
Gloucester GL2 2AB

A Company Limited by Guarantee in England
Registered Company No. 2837793
Registered as a Charity

Small Animal Formulary
First edition 1994, Second edition 1997, Third edition 1999, Fourth edition 2002,
Fifth edition 2005, Sixth edition 2008, Seventh edition 2011, Eighth edition 2014
Small Animal Formulary – Part A: Canine and Feline
Ninth edition 2017, Tenth edition 2020
Eleventh edition 2023
Small Animal Formulary – Part B: Exotic Pets
Ninth edition 2015, Tenth edition 2020
Eleventh edition 2023

ISBN 978-1-913859-07-7

The publishers, editors and contributors cannot take responsibility for information provided on
dosages and methods of application of drugs mentioned or referred to in this publication. Details
of this kind must be verified in each case by individual users from up to date literature published
by the manufacturers or suppliers of those drugs. Veterinary surgeons are reminded that in each
case they must follow all appropriate national legislation and regulations (for example, in the
United Kingdom, the prescribing cascade) from time to time in force.

Printed in the UK by Zenith Media, Pontypool NP4 0DQ.
Printed on ECF paper made from sustainable forests.

WORLD LAND TRUST™
www.carbonbalancedpaper.com
CBP016948

Carbon Balancing is delivered by World Land Trust, an
international conservation charity, who protects the
world's most biologically important and threatened
habitats acre by acre. Their Carbon Balanced
Programme offsets emissions through the purchase
and preservation of high conservation value forests.

17779PUBS23

Contents

Editorial panel

Fergus Allerton BSc BVSc CertSAM DipECVIM-CA MRCVS
Willows Veterinary Centre and Referral Service,
Highlands Road, Shirley, Solihull, West Midlands B90 4NH

Daniel Batchelor BVSc PhD DSAM DipECVIM-CA SFHEA MRCVS
Department of Small Animal Clinical Sciences, University of Liverpool,
Leahurst, Chester high road, Neston CH64 7TE

Nick Bexfield BVetMed PhD DSAM DipECVIM-CA PGDipMEdSci PGCHE
FHEA MRCVS
Department of Veterinary Medicine, University of Cambridge,
Madingley Road, Cambridge CB3 OES

Daniel L. Chan DVM DipACVECC DipECVECC DipACVIN(Nutrition) FHEA
MRCVS
The Royal Veterinary College, Hawkshead Lane,
North Mymms, Hatfield, Hertfordshire AL9 7TA

Polly Frowde MA VetMB DipECVIM-CA MRCVS
Davies Veterinary Specialists Limited, Manor Farm Business Park,
Higham Gobion, Hertfordshire SG5 3HR

Jenny Helm BVMS CertSAM DipECVIM-CA FHEA MRCVS
Vets-Now Emergency and Specialty Hospital,
123–145 North Street, Glasgow G3 7DA

Hannah Hodgkiss-Geere BVM&S MSc PhD DipECVIM-CA FHEA MRCVS
Institute of Veterinary Science, University of Liverpool,
Leahurst, Chester high road, Neston CH64 7TE

Hilary Jackson BVM&S DVD DipACVD DipECVD MRCVS
The Dermatology Referral Service,
528 Paisley Road West, Glasgow G51 1RN

Andrew Kent BVSc DipECVIM-CA MRCVS
Blaise Veterinary Referral Hospital, 1601 Bristol Road South,
Longbridge, Birmingham B45 9UA

David Killick BVetMed PgDip-AP PhD CertSAM DipECVIM-CA (Onc) FHEA
FRCVS
Institute of Infection, Veterinary and Ecological Science,
University of Liverpool, Leahurst, Chester high road, Neston CH64 7TE

Daniel S. Mills BVSc PhD CBiol FRSB FHEA CCAB DipECAWBM(BM) FRCVS
Joseph Banks Laboratories, Department of Life Sciences,
University of Lincoln, Lincoln LN6 7DL

Jo Murrell BVSc(Hons) PhD DipECVAA MRCVS
Highcroft Veterinary Referrals, 615 Wells Road,
Whitchurch, Bristol BS14 9BE

Mike Rhodes BVMS CertVOphthal DipECVO MRCVS
Focus Referrals Ltd, Sandpiper House,
Beaumont Close, Banbury, Oxfordshire OX16 1TG

Stephanie Sorrell BVetMed(Hons) MANZCVS DipECVIM-CA MRCVS
The Mindful Vet, 14 Victoria Square,
Droitwich Spa, Worcestershire WR9 8DS

Catherine Stalin MA VetMB DipECVN FHEA MRCVS
Small Animal Hospital, University of Glasgow,
Bearsden Road, Glasgow G61 1BD

James W. Swann MA VetMB DPhil DipACVIM DipECVIM-CA MRCVS
Columbia Stem Cell Initiative, Columbia University,
650 W 168th Street, New York, NY 10032, United States

Andrew Tanner BSc(Hons)
Willows Veterinary Centre and Referral Service,
Highlands Road, Shirley, Solihull, West Midlands B90 4NH

Angelika von Heimendahl MScAg BVM DipECAR MScVet (Cons) FRCVS
Veterinary Reproduction Service, Reed Veterinary Surgery,
London Road, Hertfordshire SG8 8BD

James Warland MA VetMB Dip-ECVIM-CA MRCVS
Wellcome – MRC Cambridge Stem Cell Institute,
Jeffrey Cheah Biomedical Centre, University of Cambridge,
Puddicombe Way, Cambridge CB2 0AW

Foreword

The *BSAVA Small Animal Formulary* has firmly secured its place as one of the most valued BSAVA publications, whether that be in print in practice pharmacies, via the BSAVA app or the BSAVA library. It is considered a 'must-have' by students, primary care clinicians and specialists alike, and is a key membership benefit.

The ability to rapidly obtain accurate, reviewed and current information on an extensive range of medications including available formulations, licensing data, action, uses, dose rates, contraindications, drug interactions and adverse reaction risks alongside safety and handling information in a simple alphabetical format makes this an incredibly user-friendly resource.

The 11th edition has been fully updated and sees an additional 20 new drug monographs added to the Formulary, with an indication of which species each drug is authorized in where relevant. There is a clearer indication of which drugs are available as reformulations from veterinary specials manufacturers. A new section detailing sedation for dogs with the *ABCB1* gene provides an important update for improved safety in sedation and anaesthesia for affected patients.

An important addition is a clear visual indicator on every antibiotic to clearly show its European Medicines Agency (EMA) category accompanied by expanded guidelines in the appendix explaining the EMA categories and promoting responsible use of antibiotics to protect public and animal health. In tandem with this there is a new appendix with guidance on the responsible use of parasiticides in companion animal practice.

Fergus Allerton and his team are to be congratulated on the valuable additions and updates to this 11th edition of the *BSAVA Small Animal Formulary – Part A: Canine and Feline*.

Alison Speakman BVMS Hons PhD CertAVP GPCert(VPS) MRCVS
BSAVA President 2022–2023

Preface

Welcome to Part A of the 11th edition of the *BSAVA Small Animal Formulary*, providing fully reviewed and up-to-date information about medications used for the treatment of cats and dogs. Alongside several new monographs readers will notice the introduction of a splash of colour for each antibiotic medication. Given the One Health importance of antimicrobial resistance, the editorial team remain committed to promoting rational and tiered antibiotic selection. The colour code reflects the European Medicines Agency's classification of antibiotics and reminds prescribers to seek an antibiotic that minimizes any danger to public health through the possible development of antimicrobial resistance.

Data relating to drug use, adverse reactions and drug interactions can change between print editions of the formulary; veterinary surgeons and nurses are reminded to also consult the online or app version of the Formulary and other reliable sources when confronted with a medication with which they are unfamiliar.

The Formulary provides information about many drugs not authorized for use in animals. Authorized products should be considered first but when such products are not available, are not clinically suitable, or are from a higher antibiotic tier, unauthorized medicines may be used in accordance with the cascade. In such cases, a clear clinical justification, made on an individual basis, should be recorded in the clinical notes or on the prescription.

I would like to thank the Editorial Panel members for their hard work in updating the monographs and developing a wealth of supplementary material for this edition. My sincere gratitude also goes to the editorial team members at BSAVA for driving this project forward with enthusiasm and good humour. Please do provide comments and feedback on this latest edition of the *BSAVA Small Animal Formulary* so that it can be further improved in the future.

Fergus Allerton
January 2023

Introduction

Notes on the monographs

- **Name.** The rINN generic name is used where this has been agreed. When a choice of names is available the more commonly used in the UK has been provided. The list of trade names is not necessarily comprehensive, and the mention or exclusion of any particular commercial product is not a recommendation or otherwise as to its value. Any omission of a product that is authorized for a particular canine or feline indication is purely accidental. All monographs were updated in the period March–September 2022. Products that are not marketed for use in animals (whether authorized by the Veterinary Medicines Directorate (VMD) or not) are marked with an asterisk. Products that are authorized for use in dogs or cats are marked with a superscript d or c. Note that an indication that a product is authorized does not necessarily mean that it is authorized for all species and indications listed in the monograph; users should check individual data sheets. You may also wish to refer to the VMD's Product Information Database (www.vmd.defra.gov.uk/ ProductInformationDatabase/).

- **Formulations.** Only medicines and formulations that are available in the UK have been included – many others are available outside the UK and some medicines in different formulations. Common trade names of human medicines are provided. In many cases they are available as generic formulations and may be cheaper. However, be careful of assuming that the bioavailability of one brand is the same as that of another. Avoid switching between brands unnecessarily.

- **Action** and **Use**. Veterinary surgeons using this publication are warned that **many of the drugs and doses listed are not currently authorized** by the VMD or the European Medicines Agency (EMA) (either at all or for a particular species), or manufacturers' recommendations may be limited to particular indications. **The decision, and therefore the responsibility, for prescribing any drug for an animal lies solely with the veterinary surgeon.** Expert assistance should be obtained when necessary. The 'cascade' and its implications are discussed below. For information on combination drugs, it is important to refer to all relevant monographs.

- **Safety and handling.** This section only outlines specific risks and precautions for a particular drug that are in addition to the general advice given below in the 'Health and safety in dispensing' section. A separate Appendix deals with chemotherapeutic drugs.

- **Contraindications** and **Adverse reactions.** The list of adverse reactions is not intended to be comprehensive and is limited to those effects that may be of clinical significance. The information for both of these sections is taken from published veterinary and human references and not just from product literature.

- **Drug interactions.** A listing of those interactions which may be of clinical significance.

- **Doses.** These are based on those recommended by the manufacturers in their data sheets and package inserts or are based on those given in published articles or textbooks or are based on clinical experience. **These recommendations should be used only as guidelines and should not be considered appropriate for every case.** Clinical judgement must take precedence. Doses for small mammals, birds, reptiles and other groups of animals should never be extrapolated from the doses provided in this book for dogs and cats. The *BSAVA Small Animal Formulary: Part B – Exotic Pets* and other sources should be consulted where such doses are required. The colour banding on the antibiotic drug monographs denotes their category as classified by the EMA (**see Appendix for Guidelines for responsible antibiotic use**).

- **References.** A listing of references and further reading to support the information in the monograph.

Distribution categories

Authorized small animal medicines within Great Britain now fall within the first four categories below and all packaging supplied by drug manufacturers and distributors was changed in 2008. Medical products not authorized for veterinary use retain their former classification (e.g. GSL, P, POM). Other laws apply in other jurisdictions. Some nutritional supplements (nutraceuticals) are not considered medicinal products and therefore are not classified. Where a product does not have a marketing authorization it is designated 'general sale'.

AVM-GSL: Authorized veterinary medicine – general sales list. This may be sold by anyone.

NFA-VPS: Non-food animal medicine – veterinarian, pharmacist, Suitably Qualified Person (SQP). These medicines for companion animals must be supplied by a veterinary surgeon, pharmacist or SQP. An SQP must be registered with the Animal Medicines Training Regulatory Authority (AMTRA). Veterinary nurses can become SQPs, but it is not automatic.

POM-VPS: Prescription-only medicine – veterinarian, pharmacist, SQP (formerly PML livestock products, MFSX products and a few P products). These medicines for food-producing animals (including horses) can only be supplied on an oral or written veterinary prescription from a veterinary surgeon, pharmacist or SQP and can only be supplied by one of those groups of people in accordance with the prescription.

POM-V: Prescription-only medicine – veterinarian. These medicines can only be supplied against a veterinary prescription that has been prepared (either orally or in writing) by a veterinary surgeon to animals under their care following a clinical assessment and can only be supplied by a veterinary surgeon or pharmacist in accordance with the prescription.

CD: Controlled Drug. A substance controlled by the Misuse of Drugs Act 1971 and Regulations. The CD is followed by (Schedule 1), (Schedule 2), (Schedule 3), (Schedule 4) or (Schedule 5) depending on the Schedule to The Misuse of Drugs Regulations 2001 (as amended) in which the preparation is included. You could be prosecuted for failure to comply with this act. Prescribers are reminded that there are additional requirements relating to the prescribing of Controlled Drugs. For more information see the *BSAVA Guide to the Use of Veterinary Medicines* at www.bsavalibrary.com/medicinesguide.

Schedule 1: Includes LSD, cannabis, lysergide and other drugs that are not used medicinally. Possession and supply are prohibited except in accordance with Home Office Authority.

Schedule 2: Includes etorphine, fentanyl, ketamine, morphine, methadone, papaveretum, pethidine, secobarbital (quinalbarbitone), diamorphine (heroin), cocaine and amphetamine. Record all purchases and each individual supply (within 24 hours). Registers must be kept for 2 calendar years after the last entry. Drugs must be kept under safe custody (locked secure cabinet), except secobarbital. There are specific requirements regarding the destruction of Schedule 2 Controlled Drugs, which may require an independent veterinary surgeon or person authorized by the Secretary of State to witness.

Schedule 3: Includes buprenorphine, pentazocine, the barbiturates (e.g. pentobarbital and phenobarbital but not secobarbital – which is Schedule 2), midazolam, tramadol, gabapentin and others. Buprenorphine, with some others (e.g. diethylpropion and temazepam), must be kept under safe custody (locked secure cabinet); it is advisable that all Schedule 3 drugs are locked away. Tramadol, gabapentin and pregabalin are exempt from safe custody requirements but must follow CD prescription writing requirements. Retention of invoices for 2 years is necessary.

Schedule 4: Includes most of the benzodiazepines except midazolam and temazepam (which are now Schedule 3), and androgenic and anabolic steroids (e.g. clenbuterol, nandralone). Exempted from control when used in normal veterinary practice.

Schedule 5: Includes preparations (such as several codeine products) which, because of their strength, are exempt from virtually all Controlled Drug requirements other than the retention of invoices for 2 years.

Extemporaneous preparations

Extemporaneous preparations (also known as 'veterinary specials' and denoted as **VSP** in the Formulations section of the monographs) are products that do not hold a marketing authorization. These products have not been assessed against the same standards of quality, safety (for the target animal, user, consumer and environment) and efficacy as authorized veterinary medicines. They can legally be prescribed, supplied and used under the last step of the cascade (see below). Extemporaneous preparations carry a higher risk than authorized medicines and this should be taken into consideration when prescribed. Manufacturers of extemporaneous products must be authorized (i.e. hold a ManSA) and comply with the general principles of Good Manufacturing Practice (GMP). Their facilities, equipment and procedures are regularly inspected to ensure they manufacture extemporaneous products to a set quality standard (**see Appendix for Useful websites**).

The prescribing cascade

Veterinary medicinal products (VMPs) must be administered in accordance with the prescribing cascade, as set out in The Veterinary Medicines Regulations (VMR) 2013. The current law starts from the principle that all VMPs must be authorized, and that use of an unauthorized medicine, or use of an authorized medicine in an unauthorized way, is an offence. However, the law recognizes that there are circumstances where the benefits of treatment of animals with unauthorized medicines outweigh the risks, particularly where there are not veterinary authorized medicines for a condition or for a species. As a result, the legislators have given veterinary surgeons an exemption from the legal requirement to use an authorized VMP for the species and condition that they are treating. This exemption is known as the prescribing cascade.

'Off-label' use of medicines

'Off-label' use is the use of medicines outside the terms of their marketing authorization (MA). It may include medicines authorized outside the UK or NI that are used in accordance with an import certificate issued by the VMD. A veterinary surgeon, with detailed knowledge of the medical history and clinical status of a patient, may reasonably prescribe a medicine 'off-label' in accordance with the prescribing cascade. Authorized medicines have been scientifically assessed against statutory criteria of safety, quality and efficacy when used in accordance with the authorized recommendations on the product literature. Use of an unauthorized medicine provides none of these safeguards and may, therefore, pose potential risks that the authorization process seeks to minimize.

Medicines may be used 'off-label' for a variety of reasons, including:

- No authorized product is suitable for the condition or specific subpopulation being treated
- Need to alter the duration of therapy, dosage, route of administration, etc., to treat the specific condition presented
- An authorized product has proved ineffective in the circumstances of a particular case (all cases of suspected lack of efficacy of authorized veterinary medicines should be reported to the VMD).

Responsibility for the use of a medicine 'off-label' lies solely with the prescribing veterinary surgeon. They should inform the owner of the reason why a medicine is to be used 'off-label' and record this reason in the patient's clinical notes. When electing to use a medicine 'off-label' always:

- Discuss all therapeutic options with the owner
- Use the cascade to determine your choice of medicine
- Obtain signed informed consent if an unauthorized product is to be used, ensuring that all potential problems are explained to the client
- Administer unauthorized medicines against a patient-specific prescription. Do not administer to a group of animals if at all possible.

An 'off-label' medicine must show a comparative clinical advantage to the authorized product in the specific circumstances presented (where applicable). Medicines may be used 'off-label' in the following ways (this is not an exhaustive list):

- Authorized product at an unauthorized dose
- Authorized product for an unauthorized indication
- Authorized product used outwith the authorized age range
- Authorized product administered by an unauthorized route
- Authorized product used to treat an animal in an unauthorized physiological state, e.g. pregnancy (i.e. an unauthorized indication)
- Product authorized for use in humans or a different animal species to that being treated.

Adverse effects may or may not be specific for a species, and idiosyncratic reactions are always a possibility. If no adverse effects are listed, consider data from different species. When using novel or unfamiliar drugs, consider pharmaceutical and pharmacological interactions. In some species, and with some diseases, the ability to metabolize/excrete a drug may be impaired/enhanced. Use the lowest dose that might be effective and the safest route of administration. Ensure that you are aware of the clinical signs that may suggest toxicity. Information on 'off-label' use may be available from a wide variety of sources (**see Appendix for Further reading and Useful websites**).

Marketing authorizations

Following the exit of the United Kingdom (UK) from the European Union (EU) there are now three MAs for veterinary medicines in the UK. The options that veterinary surgeons must consider under the prescribing cascade depend on whether they are working in Great Britain (GB) or Northern Ireland (NI). The Northern Ireland Protocol requires that the use of veterinary medicines in Northern Ireland be compliant with the regulations of the European veterinary medicines regulatory system. In practice, for the cascade this means that where no suitable NI-authorized veterinary medicine is available, veterinary surgeons in NI should consider using an EU authorized veterinary medicine before using an alternative medicine authorized elsewhere in the world. The three types of authorization are:

- UK MA – a product with a UK MA has been approved for marketing in England, Wales, Scotland and Northern Ireland. These MAs were issued pre-2021 and retain a UK-wide authorization
- GB MA – a product with a GB MA has been approved for marketing in England, Wales and Scotland. These authorizations have been assessed and issued by the VMD against the requirements set out within the UK VMR 2013, as amended
- NI MA – a product with an NI MA has been approved for marketing in Northern Ireland. There are four different routes to obtain an NI MA:
  - A national authorization (valid in NI only)
  - A centralized authorization issued by the European Commission (valid in all EU member states, including NI)
  - A mutual recognition procedure (valid in select EU member states where the product is already authorized on a national basis in one of them)
  - A decentralized procedure (valid in select EU member states).

Compliance with the cascade

The cascade differs depending on whether the prescribing veterinary surgeon is based in Great Britain or Northern Ireland.

Veterinary surgeons in Great Britain: The steps, in descending order of suitability, are:

- Veterinary medicine with an MA valid in GB or UK wide for the indicated species and condition
- Veterinary medicine with an MA valid in NI for the indicated species and condition
- Veterinary medicine with an MA valid in GB, NI or UK wide for a different species or condition
- Human medicine with an MA valid in GB, NI or UK wide OR an authorized veterinary medicine from outside the UK. In the case of a food-producing animal, the medicine must be authorized in a food-producing species

INTRODUCTION

- Extemporaneous preparation prepared by a veterinary surgeon, pharmacist or person holding an appropriate Manufacturer's Authorization, located in the UK
- In exceptional circumstances, a human medicine may be imported from outside of the UK.

NOTE: For products not authorized in GB or UK wide, a Special Import Certificate from the VMD is required.

Veterinary surgeons in Northern Ireland: The steps, in descending order of suitability, are:

- Veterinary medicine with an MA valid in NI or UK wide for the indicated species and condition
- Veterinary medicine with an MA valid in NI or UK wide for a different species or condition
- Human medicine with an MA valid in NI or UK wide or a veterinary medicine with an MA valid in an EU member state. In the case of a food-producing animal, the medicine must be authorized in a food-producing species
- Extemporaneous preparation prepared by a veterinary surgeon, pharmacist or person holding an appropriate Manufacturer's Authorization, located in the UK
- In exceptional circumstances, a veterinary medicine with an MA in GB or outside the EU may be imported, or a human medicine from outside NI may be imported.

NOTE: For products not authorized in NI or UK wide, a Special Import Certificate from the VMD is required.

Drug storage and dispensing

For further information on the storage and dispensing of medicines see the *BSAVA Guide to the Use of Veterinary Medicines* at www.bsavalibrary.com/medicinesguide. Note that veterinary surgeons may only supply a veterinary medicine from practice premises that are registered with the RCVS and that these premises must be inspected. It is recommended that, in general, medications are kept in and dispensed in the manufacturer's original packaging. Medicines can be adversely affected by adverse temperatures, excessive light, humidity and rough handling. Loose tablets or capsules that are repackaged from bulk containers should be dispensed in child-resistant containers and supplied with a package insert (if one exists). Tablets and capsules in foil strips should be sold in their original packaging or in a similar cardboard box for smaller quantities. Preparations for external application should be dispensed in coloured fluted bottles. Oral liquids should be dispensed in plain glass bottles with child-resistant closures.

All medicines should be labelled. The label should include:

- The owner's name and address
- Identification of the animal
- Date of supply (and, if applicable, the expiry date)
- Product name (and strength)
- Total quantity of the product supplied in the container
- Instructions for dosage
- Practice name and address
- The name of the veterinary surgeon who prescribed the medication (if not an authorized use)

- Any specific pharmacy precautions (including storage, disposal, handling)
- The wording 'Keep out of reach of children' and 'For animal treatment only'
- Withdrawal period, if relevant
- Any other necessary warnings.

The words 'For external use only' should be included on labels for products for topical use. All labels should be typed. If this information will not fit on a single label then it is permissible to include the information on a separate sheet.

For medicines that are not authorized for veterinary use, and even for some that are, it is useful to add to the label or on a separate information sheet the likely adverse effects, drug interactions and the action to be taken in the event of inadvertent mis-dosing or incorrect administration written in plain English. Samples of such Client Information Leaflets (shown as **CIL** in the monographs) for many commonly used, but unauthorized, drugs are available for BSAVA members to download from www.bsavalibrary.com.

In order to comply with the current Veterinary Medicines Regulations, records of all products supplied on prescription must be kept for 5 years. When a batch is brought into use in a practice, the batch number and date should be recorded. It is not necessary to record the batch number of each medication used for a given animal.

Owners should be informed that any unused or left over medication should be returned to the practice for safe disposal.

Health and safety in dispensing

All drugs are potentially poisonous to humans as well as animals. Toxicity may be mild or severe and includes carcinogenic and teratogenic effects. Warnings are given in the monographs. However, risks to humans dispensing medicines are not always well characterized and idiosyncratic reactions may occur. **It is good practice for everyone to wear protective clothing (including gloves) when directly handling medicines, not to eat or drink (or store food or drink) near medicines**, and to wash their hands frequently when working with medicines. Gloves, masks and safety glasses should be worn if handling potentially toxic liquids, powders or broken tablets. Do not break tablets of antineoplastic cytotoxic drugs, and use laminar flow cabinets for the preparation and dispensing of these medications (**see Appendix for Safety and handling of chemotherapeutic agents**).

Many prescribers and users of medicines are not aware of the carcinogenic potential of the drugs they are handling. Below are lists of medicines included in the BSAVA Formulary that are known or potential carcinogens or teratogens. The lists are not all-inclusive: they include only those substances that have been evaluated. Most of the drugs are connected only with certain kinds of cancer. The relative carcinogenicity of the agents varies considerably and some do not cause cancer at all times or under all circumstances. Some may only be carcinogenic or teratogenic if a person is exposed in a certain way (for example, ingesting as opposed to touching the drug). For more detailed information refer to the International Agency for Research on Cancer (IARC) or the National Toxicology Program (NTP) (information is available on their respective websites).

Examples of drugs known or suspected to be human carcinogens (c) or teratogens (t):

- ACE inhibitors (t), e.g. benazepril, enalapril
- Androgenic (anabolic) steroids (t, c)
- Antibiotics (c), e.g. metronidazole, chloramphenicol
- Antibiotics (t) e.g. aminoglycosides, doxycycline, trimethoprim, sulphonamides
- Antifungals (c), e.g. fluconazole, itraconazole
- Antineoplastic drugs (c, t) – all
- Antithyroid drugs (t), e.g. carbimazole/methimazole
- Beta-blockers (t)
- Deferoxamine (t)
- Diltiazem (t)
- Finasteride (t)
- Immunosuppressives (c), e.g. azathioprine, ciclosporin
- Methotrexate (t)
- Misoprostol (t)
- NSAIDs (t)
- Penicillamine (t)
- Phenoxybenzamine (c)
- Progestagens (c) and some oestrogens (c)
- Vitamin A (t)

Note that most carcinogens are also likely to be teratogens.

Acepromazine (ACP)

(Acecare [c,d], ACP [c,d]) **POM-V**

Formulations: Injectable: 2 mg/ml solution. Oral: 10 mg tablets.

Action: Phenothiazine with depressant effect on the CNS, thereby causing sedation and a reduction in spontaneous activity.

Use:

- Sedation or pre-anaesthetic medication in dogs and cats.
- ACP raises the threshold for cardiac arrhythmias and has antiemetic properties.
- Sedation can be unreliable when ACP is used alone; combining ACP with an opioid drug improves sedation (neuroleptanalgesia) and the opioid provides analgesia.
- Also used for the management of thromboembolism in cats because of its peripheral vasodilatory action.

Depth of sedation is dose dependent up to a plateau (0.1 mg/kg); higher doses provide little benefit but increase the duration of action, and the risk and severity of adverse effects. The lower end of the dose range should be used for giant-breed dogs to allow for the effects of metabolic body size. Onset of sedation is 20–30 minutes after i.m. administration; clinical doses cause sedation for up to 6 hours. The oral dose required to produce sedation varies between individual animals and high doses can lead to very prolonged sedation. ACP is not recommended for the management of sound phobias, such as firework or thunder phobia, in dogs.

Safety and handling: Normal precautions should be observed

Contraindications: Hypotension due to shock, trauma or cardiovascular disease. Avoid in animals <3 months and animals with liver disease. Use cautiously in anaemic animals as it will exacerbate anaemia by sequestration of red blood cells in the spleen. In Boxers, spontaneous fainting and syncope can occur due to sinoatrial block caused by excessive vagal tone; use low doses or avoid.

Adverse reactions: Rarely, healthy animals may develop profound hypotension following administration of phenothiazines. Supportive therapy to maintain body temperature and fluid balance is indicated until the animal is fully recovered.

Drug interactions: Other CNS depressants (e.g. barbiturates, propofol, alfaxalone, volatile anaesthetics) will cause additive CNS depression if used with ACP. Doses of other anaesthetic drugs should be reduced when ACP has been used for premedication. Increased levels of both drugs may result if propranolol is administered with phenothiazines. As phenothiazines block alpha-adrenergic receptors, concomitant use with adrenaline may lead to unopposed beta activity, thereby causing vasodilation and tachycardia. Antidiarrhoeal mixtures (e.g. kaolin/pectin, bismuth salicylate) and antacids may cause reduced GI absorption of oral phenothiazines.

DOSES

When used for sedation and premedication is generally given as part of a combination with opioids. See Appendix for sedation protocols in cats and dogs.

Dogs (not Boxers), Cats: 0.01–0.02 mg/kg slowly i.v.; 0.01–0.05 mg/kg i.m., s.c.; 1–3 mg/kg p.o.

- Boxers: 0.005–0.01 mg/kg i.m.

Acetaminophen see **Paracetamol**

Acetazolamide
(Diamox*) **POM**

Formulations: Oral: 250 mg tablets, capsules.

Action: Systemic carbonic anhydrase inhibitor.

Use:
- Used as treatment for the management of episodic falling in the Cavalier King Charles Spaniel experiencing a high frequency of collapse episodes which are refractory to other treatments (clonazepam and diazepam). If there is no favourable response after 2 weeks of use q12h, then the drug should be stopped.
- May be beneficial for other paroxysmal dyskinesias.
- No longer used for canine glaucoma.

Safety and handling: Normal precautions should be observed.

Contraindications: Avoid in anorexic dogs, those with hepatic or renal dysfunction and those with sulphonamide hypersensitivity. Cats are particularly susceptible to the adverse effects of systemic carbonic anhydrase inhibitors; avoid in this species.

Adverse reactions: Weakness, GI disturbances (anorexia, vomiting, diarrhoea), panting, metabolic acidosis, diuresis, electrolyte disturbances (potassium depletion in particular).

Drug interactions: Acetazolamide alkalinizes urine; thus, excretion rate of weak bases may be decreased and of weak acids increased. Concomitant use of corticosteroids may exacerbate potassium depletion, causing hypokalaemia.

DOSES
Dogs: CKCS episodic falling syndrome: 4–8 mg/kg p.o. q8–12h.
Cats: Do not use.

References
Packer RA, Wachowiak I, Thomovsky SA *et al.* (2021) Phenotypic characterization of PIGN-associated paroxysmal dyskinesia in Soft-coated wheaten terriers and preliminary response to acetazolamide therapy. *The Veterinary Journal* **269**, 105606
Royaux E, Bhatti S, Harvey R *et al.* (2016) Acetazolamide-responsive paroxysmal dyskinesia in a 12-week-old female golden retriever dog. *Veterinary Quarterly* **36**, 45–49

Acetylcysteine CIL
(Stromease [c,d], Ilube*, Parvolex*) **POM-V, POM**

Formulations: Injectable: 200 mg/ml solution. Ophthalmic: 2.5% solution (Stromease); 5% acetylcysteine + 0.35% hypromellose drops in 10 ml bottle.

Action: Decreases the viscosity of bronchial secretions, maintains glutathione levels in the liver and has some anticollagenase activity.

Use: Reduces the extent of liver injury in cases of paracetamol poisoning and other forms of liver toxicity involving oxidative damage or impaired glutathione synthesis (e.g. xylitol poisoning).

- Has been used in non-specific acute hepatopathies of suspected toxic origin.
- Can also be used as a mucolytic in respiratory disease.
- Acetylcysteine may be useful in the treatment of keratoconjunctivitis sicca (KCS), or in 'melting' corneal ulcers although *in vivo* work to confirm this is limited.

Oral solution should be diluted to a 5% solution and given via a stomach tube as it tastes unpleasant. In the eye it may be used in conjunction with hypromellose.

Safety and handling: Normal precautions should be observed.

Contraindications: No information available.

Adverse reactions: Acetylcysteine has caused hypersensitivity and bronchospasm when used in the pulmonary tree (use with care in bronchospastic respiratory disease, e.g. feline asthma). When given orally for paracetamol poisoning it may cause GI effects (nausea, vomiting) and, rarely, urticaria.

Drug interactions: In cases of paracetamol poisoning, the concurrent administration of activated charcoal is controversial as it may also reduce acetylcysteine absorption.

DOSES

Dogs, Cats:
- **Mucolytic:** either nebulize 50 mg as a 2% solution (dilute with saline) over 30–60 min or instil 1–2 ml of a 20% solution directly into the trachea.
- **Paracetamol poisoning:** (after inducing emesis if appropriate, i.e. presented within 2 hours of ingestion) give 140–280 mg/kg diluted to a 5% solution using 5% dextrose by slow i.v. infusion over 15–20 min, followed by further slow infusions of 70 mg/kg (similarly diluted) q6h for at least 7 doses, depending on dose of paracetamol consumed (seek advice from a poisons information service). The intravenous solution can be administered orally but should be diluted to improve palatability; however, i.v. administration is preferred for serious intoxications as bioavailability is reduced with oral administration in cats.
- **KCS:** 1 drop of the ophthalmic solution topically q6–8h. Rarely used for this indication.
- **Melting corneal ulcers:** 2 drops of 2.5% ophthalmic solution q6–8h (Stromease); 1 drop of 5% ophthalmic solution q1–4h in the affected eye for 24–48 hours. Topical autologous serum is more effective for the treatment of a melting corneal ulcer and is preferred.

References
Dunayer EK (2006) New Findings on the effects of xylitol ingestion in dogs. *Veterinary Medicine* **101**, 791–796

Acetylsalicylic acid see Aspirin

Aciclovir

(Zovirax*) **POM**

Formulations: Ophthalmic: 3% ointment in 4.5 g tubes.

Action: Inhibits viral replication (viral DNA polymerase); depends on viral thymidine kinase for phosphorylation.

Use:
- Management of ocular feline herpesvirus-1 (FHV-1) infections.

The clinical efficacy of aciclovir is questionable but frequent application (0.5% ointment 5 times daily) may achieve adequate corneal concentrations. Aciclovir is virostatic and is unable to eradicate latent viral infection. Consider ganciclovir and famciclovir before aciclovir. In refractory and severe cases of FHV-1 ulceration, combined therapy including antiviral medication can be used.

Safety and handling: Normal precautions should be observed.

Contraindications: No information available for the ophthalmic preparation. Systemic aciclovir is toxic in cats.

Adverse reactions: Ocular irritation may occur and the frequency of application should be reduced if this develops. Treatment should not be continued for >3 weeks.

Drug interactions: No information available.

DOSES

Dogs: Not applicable.

Cats: Apply a small amount to affected eye 5 times daily for a maximum of 3 weeks.

References

Thomasy SM and Maggs DJ (2016) A review of antiviral drugs and other compounds with activity against feline herpesvirus type 1. *Veterinary Ophthalmology* **19**, 119–130

ACP see **Acepromazine**
ACTH see **Tetracosactide**
Actinomycin-D see **Dactinomycin**
Activated charcoal see **Charcoal**
ADH see **Desmopressin**

Adrenaline (Epinephrine)

(Adrenaline*, Epinephrine*) **POM**

Formulations: Injectable: Range of concentrations for injection: 0.1–10 mg/ml, equivalent to 1:10,000 to 1:100.

Action: Adrenaline exerts its effects via alpha-1 and -2 and beta-1 and -2 adrenoreceptors.

Use:
- Cardiac resuscitation, status asthmaticus and to offset the effects of histamine release in severe anaphylactoid reactions.
- The ophthalmic preparation is used in open-angle glaucoma.

The effects of adrenaline vary according to dose. Infusions of low doses mainly result in beta-adrenergic effects (increases in cardiac output, myocardial oxygen consumption, and a reduced threshold for arrhythmias with peripheral vasodilation and a fall in diastolic blood pressure). At high doses, alpha-1 effects predominate, causing a rise in systemic vascular resistance and diverting blood to the central organs; however, this may improve cardiac output and blood flow. Adrenaline is not a substitute for fluid replacement therapy. Respiratory effects include bronchodilation and an increase in pulmonary vascular resistance. Renal blood flow is moderately decreased. The duration of action of adrenaline is short (2–5 min).

Safety and handling: Overdosage can be fatal so check dose, particularly in small patients – do not confuse adrenaline vials of different concentrations. Adrenaline is sensitive to light and air: do not use if it is pink, brown or contains a precipitate. It is unstable in 5% dextrose.

Contraindications: Human adrenaline pen injections are not recommended for the treatment of suspected anaphylaxis; doses are usually too small to be effective and unlikely to have any effect on outcome by the time an animal has collapsed. If such pen injections are administered by owners, then, in common with medical practice, patients must be carefully monitored for at least 6 hours. Beware of use in animals with diabetes mellitus (monitor blood glucose concentration), hypertension or hyperthyroidism. Use with caution in hypovolaemic animals. Do not administer adrenaline directly into the myocardium because of the risk of arrhythmias. Intracardiac injection is not recommended.

Adverse reactions: Increases myocardial oxygen demand and produces arrhythmias, including ventricular fibrillation. These may be ameliorated by administering oxygen and slowing the heart rate with beta-2 antagonists. Other adverse effects include tachycardia, dry mouth and cold extremities. Repeated injections can cause necrosis at the injection site.

Drug interactions: Toxicity may occur if used with other sympathomimetic amines because of additive effects. The effects of adrenaline may be potentiated by antihistamines and thyroxine. Propranolol may block the beta effects of adrenaline, thus facilitating an increase in blood pressure. Alpha-blocking agents or diuretics may negate or diminish the pressor effects. When adrenaline is used with drugs that sensitize the myocardium (e.g. halothane, high doses of digoxin), monitor for signs of arrhythmias. Hypertension may result if adrenaline is used with oxytocic agents.

DOSES

Dogs, Cats:
- Cardiopulmonary arrest (CPA):
    - 10 µg (micrograms)/kg of a 1:1000 solution (1000 µg/ml) i.v. or intraosseously every 3–5 min. Peripheral administration into a vein should be followed by a fluid bolus to push the drug into the central circulation.
    - High-dose adrenaline (0.1 mg/kg i.v.) may be considered after prolonged CPA. Can be given intratracheally for resuscitation of intubated animals, but higher doses (0.2 mg/kg) may be required. A long catheter should be used to ensure the drug is delivered into the bronchi beyond the end of the endotracheal tube.

- **Bronchoconstriction and anaphylaxis:** 10 µg (micrograms)/kg of a 1:1000 solution (1000 µg/ml) i.v. or i.m. The i.v. route is preferred if hypotension accompanies an anaphylactoid reaction.

References
Fletcher DJ, Boller M, Brainard BM *et al.* (2012) RECOVER evidence and knowledge gap analysis on veterinary CPR. Part 7: Clinical guidelines. *Journal of Veterinary Emergency and Critical Care (San Antonio)* **22**, S102–S131

Afoxolaner

(Nexgard [d], Nexgard Spectra [d]) **POM-V**

Formulations: Oral: 11.3 mg, 28.3 mg, 68 mg, 136 mg tablets (Nexgard); also available in 5 tablet sizes with milbemycin oxime (Nexgard Spectra).

Action: Acts at ligand-gated chloride channels, in particular those gated by the neurotransmitter GABA, thereby blocking pre- and post-synaptic transfer of chloride ions across cell membranes.

Use:
- Used in the treatment of fleas and ticks in dogs. Kills fleas within 8 hours and ticks within 48 hours.
- Treatment of sarcoptic acariasis and demodicosis in dogs.

Safety and handling: Normal precautions should be observed. Tablets should not be divided.

Contraindications: Do not use in dogs <8 weeks or <2 kg.

Adverse reactions: Rare mild GI signs (vomiting, diarrhoea), lethargy, anorexia, pruritus and neurological signs (convulsions, ataxia).

Drug interactions: No information available.

DOSES
See Appendix for guidelines on responsible parasiticide use.
Dogs: Administer monthly. Tablet size should be chosen based on bodyweight, as per manufacturer's instructions. The tablets supply 2.5–6.9 mg/kg of afoxolaner.
Cats: Do not use.

References
Beugnet F, Halos L, Larsen D and de Vos C (2016) Efficacy of oral afoxolaner for the treatment of canine generalised demodicosis. *Parasite* **23**, 14

Aglepristone

(Alizin [d]) **POM-V**

Formulations: Injectable: 30 mg/ml solution.

Action: Progesterone receptor blockage leads to elimination of progesterone support for up to 7 days.

Use:
- Termination of pregnancy throughout pregnancy but preferably in the first two trimesters.
- Treatment of pyometra in dogs, although recurrence is not unusual especially in older bitches.
- Induction of parturition in cats and dogs.

- Treatment of progesterone-induced hypersomatotropism in dogs and progesterone-induced fibroadenomatous mammary hyperplasia in cats.

To induce abortion in bitches, wait until the end of oestrus (10–14 days post-mating). In queens, as induced ovulators, it can be used immediately after mating. May be unsuccessful when used in pro-oestrus and early oestrus in bitches as progesterone has not yet risen or sperm survival may be longer than activity of aglepristone. In bitches confirmed as pregnant, a partial abortion may occur in up to 5% of cases. In late abortions, clinical examination (ultrasound) is recommended 10 days after treatment in order to confirm termination. If the abortion is unsuccessful, treatment can be repeated 10 days later, up to day 45 of pregnancy. After induced abortion, an early return to oestrus is frequently observed (the oestrus-to-oestrus interval may be shortened by 1–3 months). Bitches will usually be able to carry subsequent pregnancies successfully.

Safety and handling: Use with care. People who are or may become pregnant should not handle this drug.

Contraindications: Consider avoiding in dogs with diagnosed or suspected hypoadrenocorticism.

Adverse reactions: Transient pain at the injection site; any local inflammation produced resolves uneventfully. In bitches/queens treated beyond the 20th day of gestation, abortion may be accompanied by the physiological signs of parturition, i.e. fetal expulsion, anorexia, mammary congestion.

Drug interactions: Aglepristone binds to glucocorticoid receptors and may therefore interfere with the actions of glucocorticoids; however, the clinical significance of this is unclear.

DOSES

Dogs: Maximum of 5 ml injected at any one site.
- **Pregnancy termination:** 10 mg/kg s.c. within 24 hours for 2 doses.
- **Progesterone-induced hypersomatotropism:** 10 mg/kg s.c. q24h for 2 doses and then q7d for 3 more doses.
- **Pyometra:** 10 mg/kg s.c. on days 1, 2 and 7. Additional doses may be given on days 14 and 21 if response is inadequate.

Cats: Maximum of 5 ml injected at any one site.
- **Pregnancy termination:** 15 mg/kg s.c. within q24h for 2 doses.
- **Fibroadenomatous hyperplasia:** 20 mg/kg s.c. q7d (also consider atenolol if cat is tachycardic with heart rate >200 bpm).
- **Pyometra:** 15 mg/kg s.c. on days 1, 2 and 7. Additional doses may be given on days 14 and 21 if response is inadequate.

References
Gogny A and Fiéni F (2016) Aglepristone: a review on its clinical use in animals. *Theriogenology* **85**, 555–566

A
B
C
D
E
F
G
H
I
J
K
L
M
N
O
P
Q
R
S
T
U
V
W
X
Y
Z

A

Alendronate (Alendronate sodium)   CIL

(Fosamax*) **POM**

Formulations: Oral: 10 mg, 70 mg tablets; 0.7 mg/ml solution.

Action: Primary action is to inhibit osteoclastic bone reabsorption (through inhibiting osteoclast function). Also promotes apoptosis, inhibits angiogenesis, cancer cell division and osteoclastogenesis.

Use:
- Treatment of idiopathic hypercalcaemia
- To reduce pain associated with osteolytic conditions (e.g. bone tumours).

There is limited information in the literature regarding the use of alendronate in dogs. Poor absorption after oral administration limits efficacy in this species.

Safety and handling: Store at room temperature.

Contraindications: Alendronate is contraindicated in humans with oesophageal disease; however, it is unknown if this is the case for dogs and cats. Use with caution in patients with renal insufficiency and avoid in patients with renal failure. Avoid in patients with a history of hypersensitivity to bisphosphonates.

Adverse reactions: Alendronate is thought to cause oesophageal irritation (oesophagitis) and upper GI ulcers. There are limited reports of vomiting and inappetence in dogs. Pathological fractures have been reported in cats after prolonged use (5–9 years). Other potential adverse effects include osteonecrosis and musculoskeletal pain. Hypocalcaemia is also possible.

Drug interactions: Do not use in combination with aspirin (increased risk of upper GI adverse events) and use with caution with other NSAIDs. Avoid drugs/supplements/diets that contain calcium as this is likely to decrease the bioavailability of alendronate.

DOSES

Dogs: Hypercalcaemia and/or to reduce bone pain: 0.5–1 mg/kg p.o. q24h on an empty stomach.

Cats: Hypercalcaemia: 5–10 mg/cat p.o. once per week on an empty stomach (avoid splitting tablets if possible). Follow with a syringe of water (at least 6 ml). Ionized calcium levels should be monitored after 3–4 weeks, and dose adjusted. If tolerated well, the dose can be increased (stepwise) to 30 mg/cat p.o. per week.

References
Council N, Dyce J, Drost WT *et al.* (2017) Bilateral patellar fractures and increased cortical bone thickness associated with long-term oral alendronate treatment in a cat. *Journal of Feline Medicine and Surgery Open Reports* **3**, 1–6
Hardy BT, de Brito Galvao JF, Green TA *et al.* (2015) Treatment of ionized hypercalcemia in 12 cats (2006–2008) using PO-administered alendronate. *Journal of Veterinary Internal Medicine* **29**, 200–206

B C D E F G H I J K L M N O P Q R S T U V W X Y Z

Alfaxalone

(Alfaxan [c,d]) **POM-V**

Formulations: Injectable: 10 mg/ml solution; the alfaxalone is solubilized in a cyclodextrin.

Action: Anaesthesia induced by the CNS depressant effect of the alfaxalone.

Use:

* Induction agent used before inhalational anaesthesia, or as a sole anaesthetic agent for examination or surgical procedures.

As with all i.v. anaesthetic drugs, premedication will reduce the dose required for induction and maintenance of anaesthesia. The drug should be given slowly and to effect in order to prevent inadvertent overdose. The dose recommended by the manufacturer for induction of anaesthesia can usually be reduced. Analgesia is insufficient for surgery: other analgesic drugs such as opioids should be incorporated into the anaesthetic protocol. Alfaxalone can be given i.m. or s.c. to provide sedation in cats and small dogs although it is not authorized for these routes. Do not use in combination with other i.v. anaesthetic agents. Although not authorized for use in animals <12 weeks of age, safety in dogs between 6 and 12 weeks old has been demonstrated using a similar dose for induction of anaesthesia as used in adult dogs.

Safety and handling: One preparation of alfaxalone does not contain an antimicrobial preservative; thus it is recommended that the remainder of an opened bottle is discarded after a single use. A multidose preparation of alfaxalone is also available with a shelf life of 28 days once the vial has been broached.

Contraindications: No information available.

Adverse reactions: An increase in heart rate can occur immediately after i.v. injection as a compensatory response to maintain blood pressure in the face of mild hypotension. This effect can be minimized by slow i.v. injection. As with all anaesthetic drugs, respiratory depression can occur with overdoses.

Drug interactions: No information available.

DOSES

See Appendix for sedation protocols in cats and dogs.

Dogs:

* **Induction of anaesthesia:** 3 mg/kg i.v. in unpremedicated dogs; 2 mg/kg i.v. in premedicated dogs, although lower doses can commonly be used.
* **Maintenance:** 6–9 mg/kg/h is recommended as a CRI or top-up boluses of 1–1.5 mg/kg q10min. A maximum period of one hour is recommended for maintenance of anaesthesia using alfaxalone.
* **Intramuscular sedation (unauthorized):** 1–2 mg/kg i.m. Volume precludes use in medium to large breed dogs. Duration of sedation is short (5–10 minutes).

Cats:

* **Induction of anaesthesia:** 2–5 mg/kg i.v.; the lower end of the dose range is often adequate.
* **Maintenance:** 7–10 mg/kg/h is recommended as a CRI or top-up boluses of 1–1.5 mg/kg q10min.

- Intramuscular sedation (unauthorized): 1–2 mg/kg i.m. Duration of sedation is short (5–10 minutes).

References

Ramoo S, Bradbury LA, Anderson GA and Abraham LA (2013) Sedation of hyperthyroid cats with subcutaneous administration of a combination of alfaxalone and butorphanol. *Australian Veterinary Journal* **91**, 131–136

Ribas T, Bublot I, Junot S *et al.* (2015) Effects of intramuscular sedation with alfaxalone and butorphanol on echocardiographic measurements in healthy cats. *Journal of Feline and Medicine Surgery* **17**, 530–536

Alfentanil

(Rapifen*) **POM CD SCHEDULE 2**

Formulations: Injectable: 0.5 mg/ml solution, available in 2 ml or 10 ml vials.

Action: Pure mu agonist of the phenylpiperidine series.

Use:
- Very potent opioid analgesic (10–20 times more potent than morphine) used to provide intraoperative analgesia during anaesthesia in dogs and cats.

Use of such potent opioids contributes to balanced anaesthesia but they must be administered accurately. It has a rapid onset (15–30 seconds) and short duration of action. It is best given using CRI. The drug is not suited to provision of analgesia in the postoperative period.

Safety and handling: Normal precautions should be observed.

Contraindications: No information available.

Adverse reactions: A reduction in heart rate is likely whenever alfentanil is given; atropine or glycopyrrolate can be administered to counter bradycardia if necessary. Respiratory depression leading to cessation of spontaneous respiration is likely following administration. Do not use unless facilities for positive pressure ventilation are available (either manual or automatic). Rapid i.v. injection can cause a severe bradycardia, even asystole.

Drug interactions: Alfentanil reduces the dose requirements of concurrently administered anaesthetics, including inhaled anaesthetics, by at least 50%. In humans it is currently recommended to avoid giving alfentanil to patients receiving monoamine oxidase inhibitors due to the risk of serotonin toxicity.

DOSES

Dogs: 0.001–0.005 mg/kg i.v. as a single bolus or 0.001–0.0025 mg/kg/min CRI.

Cats: 0.001 mg/kg i.v. as a single bolus or 0.001 mg/kg/min CRI.

References

Padilha ST, Steagall PVM, Monteiro BP *et al.* (2011) A clinical comparison of remifentanil or alfentanil in propofol-anaethetised cats undergoing ovariohysterectomy. *Journal of Feline Medicine and Surgery* **13**, 738–743

Allopurinol

(Zyloric*) **POM**   CIL

Formulations: Oral: 100 mg, 300 mg tablets.

Action: Xanthine oxidase inhibition decreases formation of uric acid by blocking the conversion of hypoxanthine to xanthine, and of xanthine to uric acid.

Use:
- Treatment and prevention of recurrent uric acid uroliths and hyperuricosuric calcium oxalate urolithiasis in dogs.
- To treat leishmaniosis in combination with meglumine antimoniate or miltefosine.

Safety and handling: Normal precautions should be observed.

Contraindications: Use with caution in patients with impaired renal function.

Adverse reactions: May predispose to xanthine urolithiasis, especially if used for several months and not fed a purine-restricted diet.

Drug interactions: In humans, allopurinol may enhance the effects of azathioprine and theophylline.

DOSES
See Appendix for guidelines on responsible parasiticide use.
Dogs:
- Uric acid urolithiasis:
  - Dissolution: 10 mg/kg p.o. q8h or 15 mg/kg p.o. q12h for up to 4 weeks.
  - Prevention: 10–15 mg/kg p.o. q24h (or divided q12h).
- Leishmaniosis: 10 mg/kg p.o. q12h for at least 6–12 months with meglumine antimoniate for 1–2 months, or miltefosine for 1 month (NB: this does not result in complete parasitological cure).
Cats: Leishmaniosis: 10–20 mg/kg p.o. q12–24h has been shown to be effective (although experience is limited in this species).

References
Reguera RM, Moran M, Perez-Perteio Y, García-Estrada C and Balaña-Fouce R (2016) Current status on prevention and treatment of canine leishmaniasis. *Veterinary Parasitology* **227**, 98–114

Alphaxalone see Alfaxalone

Alprazolam

(Alprazolam*, Xanax*) **POM**   CIL

Formulations: Oral: 0.25 mg, 0.5 mg, 1 mg, 2 mg tablets.

Action: Increases GABA activity within the CNS, resulting in anxiolysis and a range of cognitive effects including the inhibition of memory.

Use:
- Treatment of anxiety and fear-related disorders in dogs and cats, especially where there are signs of panic.
- As an adjunct to clomipramine or specific serotonin reuptake inhibitors (e.g fluoxetine) for the management of phobic responses.

- It can also be used for the management of urine spraying in cats but a high relapse rate upon withdrawal should be expected.

Best if used approximately 30 minutes before a fear-inducing event although absorption characteristics have not been described for cats or dogs. Its short half-life and rapid onset of action make it useful for the management of acute episodes, with treatment given as needed within the dosing limits described. However, dosing limits and responses are very variable, with some animals showing no measurable effect at the recommended doses. Its anterograde and retrograde amnesic properties, especially on subjective memory, mean it can be used before (<1 hour), during or immediately following an aversive experience to minimize emotional impact. This may be necessary during a long-term behavioural therapy programme to avoid relapses due to exposure to an intense fear-inducing stimulus during treatment. In experimental circumstances, single higher range doses (>0.25 mg/kg) have been found to block memory significantly and may be useful in companion animals, but may result in temporary sedation. As imepitoin is now authorized for the treatment of fears in dogs, if a benzodiazepine is indicated, it is preferable to use this.

Safety and handling: Normal precautions should be observed.

Contraindications: Hypersensitivity to benzodiazepines, glaucoma, significant liver or kidney disease (although alprazolam appears to be less hepatotoxic than diazepam or clorazepate). Not recommended in pregnant or lactating animals. There is concern over its use with anxiously aggressive animals due to the theoretical potential for disinhibition.

Adverse reactions: Drowsiness and mild transient incoordination may develop. Disinhibition and the subsequent emergence of aggression is a general concern with benzodiazepines. Idiosyncratic hepatotoxicity associated with benzodiazepines (largely diazepam, but not alprazolam) has been reported in the cat.

Drug interactions: Caution is advised if used in association with antifungals such as itraconazole, which inhibit its metabolism.

DOSES

Dogs: Anxiolysis: initial dose of 0.01–0.1 mg/kg p.o. as needed up to 4 times a day; the dose can be titrated up or down to the minimum effective dose, which may be below this level.

Cats: Anxiolysis: initial dose of 0.125–0.25 mg/kg p.o. as needed up to twice a day is suggested, but doses as low as 0.25 mg/cat p.o. q8–12h and as high as 0.6 mg/kg p.o. have been reported. After initial medication, the dose should be titrated down to the minimum effective dose.

References

Crowell-Davis SL, Seibert LM, Sung W, Parthasarathy V and Curtis TM (2003) Use of clomipramine, alprazolam, and behavior modification for treatment of storm phobia in dogs. *Journal of the American Veterinary Medical Association* **222**, 744–748

Dale AR, Walker JK, Farnworth MJ, Morrissey SV and Waran NK (2010) A survey of owners' perceptions of fear of fireworks in a sample of dogs and cats in New Zealand. *New Zealand Veterinary Journal* **58**, 286–291

Pineda S, Anzola B, Ruso V, Ibáñez M and Olivares Á (2018) Pharmacological therapy with a combination of alprazolam and fluoxetine and use of the trace element lithium gluconate for treating anxiety disorders and aggression in dogs. *Journal of Veterinary Behavior* **28**, 30–34

Aluminium antacids (Aluminium hydroxide)

(Alu-cap*, Acidex*, Gastrocote*, Gaviscon Advance*, Peptac*, Asilone*, Maalox*, Mucogel*) **P, GSL**

Formulations: Oral: Aluminium hydroxide is available as a dried gel (Alu-cap). Other products are composite preparations containing a variety of other compounds including magnesium oxide, hydroxide or trisilicate, potassium bicarbonate, sodium carbonate and bicarbonate, alginates and dimeticone. Aluminium hydroxide content varies.

Action: Neutralizes gastric acid. May also bind bile acids and pepsin and stimulate local prostaglandin (PGE-1) production. Also binds inorganic phosphate in the GI tract, making it unavailable for absorption.

Use:
- Management of gastritis and gastric ulceration. Frequent administration is necessary to prevent rebound acid secretion.
- In kidney disease, to lower serum phosphate in cats and dogs with serum phosphate above recommended target according to IRIS stage. Phosphate binding agents are usually only used if low-phosphate diets are unsuccessful. Monitor serum phosphate levels at 14–28 day intervals and adjust dosage accordingly. Discontinue if serum phosphate is <0.9 mmol/l.
- Thoroughly mix the drug with food to disperse it and to increase its palatability.

Safety and handling: Normal precautions.

Contraindications: No information available.

Adverse reactions: Constipation may occur. This is an effect of the aluminium compound and is counteracted by inclusion of a magnesium salt. Hypophosphataemia can develop. Long-term use (many years) of oral aluminium products in humans has been associated with aluminium toxicity and possible neurotoxicity. This is rarely a problem in veterinary medicine but is reported – monitor for signs of ataxia, altered peripheral reflexes or decreased menace response.

Drug interactions: Do not administer allopurinol, digoxin, fluoroquinolones, gabapentin, H2 antagonists, iron salts, itraconazole, mycophenolate, tetracyclines or thyroid hormones orally within 2 hours of aluminium salts as their absorption may be impaired.

DOSES

Dogs, Cats: All uses: Initially 10–30 mg/kg p.o. q6–8h (tablets) or 0.5–1.0 ml/kg (2–30 ml) p.o. q6–8h (gel) with or immediately after meals. Dosages are empirical; none have been properly defined. The daily dosage of aluminium hydroxide should not exceed 100 mg/kg.

References

Marks SL, Kook PH, Papich MG, Tolbert MK and Willard MD (2018) ACVIM consensus statement: support for rational administration of gastrointestinal protectants to dogs and cats. *Journal of Veterinary Internal Medicine* **32**, 1823–1840

Aluminium hydroxide see Aluminium antacids

Amantadine

(Lysovir*, Symmetrel*) **POM**

`CIL`

Formulations: Oral: 25 mg, 50 mg, 75 mg, 100 mg capsules; 10 mg/ml syrup.

Action: Provides analgesia through N-methyl-D-aspartate antagonist action which may potentiate the effects of other analgesics.

Use:
- Adjunctive analgesic in animals that are unresponsive to NSAIDs, or that require chronic pain relief in a home environment (e.g. osteoarthritis or cancer pain).
- Physical activity was improved in dogs with osteoarthritis that were refractory to an NSAID, suggesting that amantadine might be a useful adjunct in the clinical management of canine osteoarthritic pain.
- In a small study in cats with osteoarthritis, amantadine caused sedation but increased owner reported quality of life and decreased pain scores.

Safety and handling: Normal precautions should be observed.

Contraindications: No information available.

Adverse reactions: In humans, minor GI and CNS effects have been reported, although these have not been reported in animals. Amantadine is renally excreted and should be used cautiously in animals with renal dysfunction.

Drug interactions: No information available.

DOSES

Dogs: 3.0–5.0 mg/kg p.o. q24h. Pharmacokinetic studies in Greyhounds suggest that twice daily dosing may be necessary in some animals. Note that there is a limited evidence base for the currently recommended dose range.

Cats: 3.0–5.0 mg/kg p.o. q24h; start at the lowest dose and increase slowly. Higher doses (5.0 mg/kg) may be associated with sedation. Note that there is a limited evidence base for the currently recommended dose range.

References

Lascelles BD, Gaynor JS, Smith ES et al. (2008) Amantadine in a multimodal analgesic regimen for alleviation of refractory osteoarthritis pain in dogs. *Journal of Veterinary Internal Medicine* **22**, 53–59

Shipley H, Flynn K, Tucker L et al. (2021) Owner evaluation of quality of life and mobility in osteoarthritic cats treated with amantadine or placebo. *Journal of Feline Medicine and Surgery* **23**, 568–574

Amethocaine see Tetracaine

Amikacin

(Amikacin*, Amikin*) **POM**

Formulations: Injectable: 50 mg/ml, 250 mg/ml solutions.

Action: Aminoglycosides inhibit bacterial protein synthesis with a concentration-dependent mechanism of killing, leading to a marked post antibiotic effect, allowing prolonged dosing intervals (which may reduce toxicity).

Use:
- Active against many Gram-negative bacteria, *Staphylococcus aureus* and *Nocardia* spp., including some that may be resistant to gentamicin.

Streptococci and anaerobes are usually resistant. Amikacin is only indicated for organisms shown to be resistant to other aminoglycosides, such as gentamicin, after sensitivity testing. Activity at low-oxygen sites may be limited. Movement across biological membranes may also be limited, hence systemic levels require parenteral administration, and access to sites such as the CNS and ocular fluids is very limited. Consider monitoring serum amikacin to ensure therapeutic levels and minimize toxicity, particularly in neonates, geriatric patients and those with reduced renal function. Monitor renal function during treatment of any animal. Intravenous doses should be given slowly, generally over 30–60 minutes. Concurrent fluid therapy is advised.

Safety and handling: Normal precautions should be observed.

Contraindications: If possible, avoid use in animals with reduced renal function.

Adverse reactions: Nephrotoxic and ototoxic.

Drug interactions: Synergism may occur *in vivo* when aminoglycosides are combined with beta-lactam antimicrobials. Avoid the concurrent use of other nephrotoxic, ototoxic or neurotoxic agents (e.g. amphotericin B, furosemide). Aminoglycosides may be inactivated *in vitro* by beta-lactam antibiotics (e.g. penicillins, cephalosporins) or heparin; do not give these drugs in the same syringe. Can potentiate neuromuscular blockade, so avoid use in combination with neuromuscular blocking agents.

DOSES

Classified as category C (Caution) by the EMA.

See Appendix for guidelines on responsible antibiotic use.

Dogs: 15–30 mg/kg i.v., i.m., s.c. q24h. Due to a lower volume of distribution in Greyhounds, a lower dose of 12 mg/kg is recommended in this breed and other sighthounds.

Cats: 10–15 mg/kg i.v., i.m., s.c. q24h.

Dogs, Cats: Higher doses are recommended by some authors for managing sepsis, although these increase the risk of adverse effects. Local use may be considered, especially if the site of infection is easily accessible for direct delivery of the drug and if the animal is showing signs of nephrotoxicity. For example, amikacin has been used locally in joints and the bladder.

Amiloride

(Amiloride Hydrochloride*, Amilamont*) **POM**

Formulations: Oral: 5 mg tablets; 1 mg/ml solution (Amilamont). Also present in compound preparations with hydrochlorothiazide (Moduret, Moduretic, Co-amilozide) and furosemide (Co-amilofruse, Frumil, Frumil LS).

Action: Potassium-sparing diuretic which inhibits sodium absorption in the cells of the distal tubule and collecting duct, leading to less available sodium for exchange with potassium. This leads to a failure of the normal renal concentration gradient and results in sodium loss and potassium retention. It is a weak diuretic when used alone, so is almost always used in combination with a thiazide or furosemide.

Use:
- Treatment of oedema or ascites due to liver or heart failure.

Often added to more potent diuretics such as furosemide or weaker diuretics such as hydrochlorothiazide in cases of refractory heart failure to achieve sequential nephron blockade. Doses have not been widely reported in the veterinary literature. Monitor urea, creatinine, electrolytes and blood pressure before and after dose adjustments.

Safety and handling: Normal precautions should be observed.

Contraindications: No information available.

Adverse reactions: Hypotension, hyperkalaemia, acidosis and hyponatraemia may develop.

Drug interactions: Avoid the concomitant administration of potassium.

DOSES
Dogs, Cats: 0.1 mg/kg p.o. q12h is used in humans and has been suggested for dogs and cats. In combination with hydrochlorothiazide: 0.05–0.4 mg/kg p.o. (dogs); 0.1–0.4 mg/kg p.o. (cats); start at low dose and titrate upwards cautiously.

Amino acid solutions

(Duphalyte [c,d], Aminoplasmal*, Aminoven*, Clinimix*, Glamin*, Hyperamine*, Intrafusin*, Kabiven*, Kabiven Peripheral*, Nutriflex*) **POM, POM-V**

Formulations: Injectable: synthetic crystalline l-amino acid solutions for i.v. use only (Duphalyte). Numerous human products are available, varying in concentrations of amino acids. Most products also contain electrolytes (e.g. potassium). Some products contain varying concentrations of glucose and lipid emulsions.

Action: Supports protein anabolism, arrests protein and muscle wasting and maintains intermediary metabolism.

Use:
- Used parenterally in patients requiring nutritional support but unable to receive enteral support. Amino acid solutions supply essential and non-essential amino acids for protein production.
- Infusions of amino acid solutions have also been used in the treatment of superficial necrolytic dermatitis in dogs.

The authorized veterinary preparation (Duphalyte) contains insufficient amino acids to meet basal requirements for protein production and is intended as an aid for i.v. fluid support. None of the human formulations contain taurine, which is essential for cats and for specific conditions in dogs. All products are hyperosmolar. **NB:** the use of concentrated amino acid solutions for parenteral nutrition support should not be undertaken without specific training and requires central venous access and intensive care monitoring. Parenteral nutrition may also be able to meet the patient's requirements for fluids, essential electrolytes (sodium, potassium, magnesium) and phosphate. Additionally, if treatment is prolonged, vitamins and trace elements may need to be given. Intravenous lines for parenteral nutrition should be dedicated for that use alone and not used for other medications. Maximal acceptable rates of infusion will depend on the potassium content of the amino acid preparation.

Safety and handling: Normal precautions should be observed.

Contraindications: Dehydration, hepatic encephalopathy, severe azotaemia, shock, congestive heart failure and electrolyte imbalances.

Adverse reactions: The main complications of parenteral nutrition are metabolic, including hyperglycaemia, hyperlipidaemia, hypercapnia, acid–base disturbances and electrolyte disturbances. Other complications include catheter-associated thrombophlebitis, bacterial colonization of the catheter and resulting bacteraemia and septicaemia. Potentially life-threatening electrolyte imbalances including hypophosphataemia may also be seen (also referred to as refeeding syndrome). As with other hyperosmolar solutions, severe tissue damage could occur if extravasated, although this has not been reported.

Drug interactions: Consult specific product data sheet(s).

DOSES
Dogs:
- **Aid to i.v. fluid therapy:** up to 10 ml/kg (Duphalyte).
- **Parenteral nutritional support:** 4–6 g protein/100 kcal (418 kJ) energy requirements.
- **Superficial necrolytic dermatitis:** 3 ml/kg/h i.v. for 24 hours (Aminoven 25).

Cats:
- **Aid to i.v. fluid therapy:** up to 10 ml/kg (Duphalyte).
- **Parenteral nutritional support:** 6–8 g protein/100 kcal (418 kJ) energy requirements.

References
Chan DL, Freeman LM, Labato MA *et al.* (2002) Retrospective evaluation of partial parenteral nutrition in dogs and cats. *Journal of Veterinary Internal Medicine* **16**, 440–445
Olan NV and Prittie J (2015) Retrospective evaluation of ProcalAmine administration in a population of hospitalized ICU dogs: 36 cases (2010–2013) *Journal of Emergency and Critical Care* **25**, 405–441

Aminophylline
(Aminophylline*) **POM**

Formulations: Injectable: 25 mg/ml solution. Oral: 225 mg tablets. For modified-release preparations **see Theophylline** (100 mg of aminophylline is equivalent to 79 mg of theophylline).

Action: Aminophylline is a stable mixture of theophylline and ethylenediamine. Causes inhibition of phosphodiesterase, alteration of intracellular calcium, release of catecholamine, and antagonism of adenosine and prostaglandin, leading to bronchodilation and other effects. Spasmolytic agent and has a mild diuretic action.

Use:
- Treatment of lower airway disease.

Beneficial effects include bronchodilation, enhanced mucociliary clearance, stimulation of the respiratory centre, increased sensitivity to P_aCO_2, increased diaphragmatic contractility, stabilization of mast cells and a mild inotropic effect. Aminophylline has a low therapeutic index and should be dosed on a lean bodyweight basis. Therapeutic plasma aminophylline values are 5–20 µg (micrograms)/ml.

Safety and handling: Do not mix aminophylline in a syringe with other drugs.

Contraindications: Patients with known history of arrhythmias or seizures. Administer with caution in patients with severe cardiac disease, gastric ulcers, hyperthyroidism, renal or hepatic disease, severe hypoxia or severe hypertension.

Adverse reactions: Vomiting, diarrhoea, polydipsia, polyuria, reduced appetite, tachycardia, arrhythmias, nausea, twitching, restlessness, agitation, excitement and convulsions. Hyperaesthesia is seen in cats. Most adverse effects are related to serum level and may be symptomatic of toxic serum concentrations. The severity of these effects may be decreased by the use of modified-release preparations. They are more likely to be seen with more frequent administration. Aminophylline causes intense local pain when given i.m. and is very rarely used or recommended via this route.

Drug interactions: Agents that may increase the serum levels of aminophylline include cimetidine, diltiazem, erythromycin, fluoro-quinolones and allopurinol. Phenobarbital may decrease the serum concentration of aminophylline. Aminophylline may decrease the effects of pancuronium. Aminophylline and beta-adrenergic blockers (e.g. propranolol) may antagonize each other's effects. Aminophylline administration with halothane may cause an increased incidence of cardiac dysrhythmias and with ketamine an increased incidence of seizures.

DOSES

Dogs: Emergency bronchodilation: 10 mg/kg p.o. q8h or slowly i.v. (diluted).
Cats: Emergency bronchodilation: 5 mg/kg p.o. q12h or 2–5 mg/kg slowly i.v. (diluted).

References

Hirota K, Yoshioka H, Kabara S et al. (2001) A comparison of the relaxant effects of olprinone and aminophylline on methacholine-induced bronchoconstriction in dogs. *Anaesthesia and Analgesia* **93**, 230–233

Amiodarone

CIL

(Amiodarone*, Cordarone*) **POM**

Formulations: Oral: 100 mg, 200 mg tablets. Injectable: 50 mg/ml for dilution and use as an infusion.

Action: Antiarrhythmic agent with primarily class 3 (potassium-channel blocker), but also potent class 1 (sodium-channel blocker) and ancillary class 2 (beta-blocker) and class 4 (calcium-channel blocker) actions. Prolongs action potential duration and therefore effective refractory period in all cardiac tissues, including bypass tracts (class 3 action), inhibits sodium channels (class 1 action), blocks alpha- and beta-adrenergic receptors (class 2 action), slows the sinus rate, prolongs sinus node recovery time, and inhibits AV node conduction.

Use:
- To treat ventricular arrhythmias and supraventricular arrhythmias in dogs.

- May be useful in ventricular pre-excitation syndromes because it can prolong AV nodal and bypass tract effective refractory periods.
- Used successfully for rate control or conversion to sinus rhythm in some dogs with atrial fibrillation and as an adjunct to electrical cardioversion. Use as an i.v. infusion in dogs with recent onset atrial fibrillation has been reported, with a variable efficacy for restoring sinus rhythm but high frequency of severe adverse effects.

It has slow and variable GI absorption, a slow onset of action and a long elimination half-life (up to 3.2 days after repeated dosing). Because numerous side effects have been documented in humans and dogs, its use is advised for patients in which other antiarrhythmic agents have not been effective or are not tolerated. Owing to the risks of thyroid dysfunction and hepatotoxicity, it is advisable to evaluate hepatic enzyme activities and thyroid function prior to starting therapy and at 1–3 monthly intervals during maintenance therapy.

Safety and handling: Normal precautions should be observed.

Contraindications: Avoid in dogs with sinus bradycardia, AV block or thyroid dysfunction.

Adverse reactions: Amiodarone can cause bradycardia, AV block and prolongation of the QT interval. It is a negative inotrope and can cause hypotension. Systemic side effects described in dogs include anorexia, GI disturbances, hepatotoxicity, keratopathy and positive Coombs' test. Pulmonary fibrosis and thyroid dysfunction have also been reported in humans. In dogs, I4 level decreases with amiodarone administration, but clinically apparent hypothyroidism is less common. Adverse effects associated with i.v. administration include pain at injection site, hypo-tension, hypersalivation and hypersensitivity reactions, which may be a reaction to the carrier solvent. Should i.v. preparations be considered, prior treatment with dexamethasone should be considered to reduce risk of anaphylactic reactions.

Drug interactions: Amiodarone may significantly increase serum levels and/or pharmacological effects of anticoagulants, beta-blockers, calcium-channel blockers, ciclosporin, digoxin, lidocaine, methotrexate, quinidine and theophylline. Cimetidine may increase serum levels of amiodarone.

DOSES
Dogs:
- **Oral:** 10–15 mg/kg p.o. q12h for 7 days, then 5–7.5 mg/kg p.o. q12h for 14 days; thereafter, 5–7.5 mg/kg p.o. q24h (loading dose leading to steady state doses). Serum amiodarone levels should be assessed 3 weeks after starting therapy.
- **Intravenous:** not well defined. Doses of 0.03–0.05 mg/kg/min have been administered as a CRI for cardioversion of atrial fibrillation and sustained supraventricular tachycardia non-responsive to other antiarrhythmics. Bolus administration of 2.5–5 mg/kg given very slowly i.v. has been used in ventricular tachycardia but is not recommended due to high risk of adverse event. Prior administration of dexamethasone/antihistamines for anaphylaxis prophylaxis could be considered in both scenarios.

Cats: No information available.

References

Bicer S, Nakayama T and Hamlin RL (2002) Effects of chronic oral amiodarone on left ventricular function, ECGs, serum chemistries, and exercise tolerance in healthy dogs. *Journal of Veterinary Internal Medicine* **3**, 247

Pedro B, López-Alvarez J, Fonfara S et al. (2012) Retrospective evaluation of the use of amiodarone in dogs with arrhythmias (from 2003 to 2010). *Journal of Small Animal Practice* **53**, 19–26

Amitriptyline

(Amitriptyline*) **POM**

Formulations: Oral: 10 mg, 25 mg, 50 mg tablets; 5 mg/ml, 10 mg/ml solutions.

Action: Blocks noradrenaline and serotonin reuptake in the brain, resulting in antidepressive activity. Also stabilizes mast cells so can reduce impact of inflammatory irritation.

Use:

- Management of chronic anxiety problems, including compulsive disorders and potentially separation anxiety in dogs (note authorized medications are available for the latter indication).
- Management of psychogenic alopecia, hypervocalization and idiopathic cystitis in cats.

The non-specific serotonergic reuptake inhibitor clomipramine and specific serotonin reuptake inhibitor fluoxteine are both authorized preparations for use in dogs. It is claimed that clomipramine may have better anticompulsive properties. Amitriptyline is bitter and can be very distasteful to cats. Some caution and careful monitoring is warranted in patients with cardiac or renal disease. Its antipruritic properties may make it useful in anxiety-related conditions featuring inflammation, such as certain acral lick lesions and idiopathic cystitis.

Safety and handling: Normal precautions should be observed.

Contraindications: Hypersensitivity to tricyclic antidepressants, glaucoma, history of seizures or urinary retention, severe liver disease.

Adverse reactions: Sedation, dry mouth, vomiting, excitability, arrhythmias, hypotension, syncope, increased appetite, weight gain and, less commonly, seizures and bone marrow disorders have been reported in humans. The bitter taste can cause ptyalism in cats.

Drug interactions: Should not be used with monoamine oxidase inhibitors or drugs metabolized by cytochrome P450 2D6 (e.g. chlorphenamine, cimetidine). If changing medication from one of these compounds, a minimal washout period of 2 weeks is recommended (the washout period may be longer if the drug has been used for a prolonged period of time). Should not be used alongside serotonin reuptake inhibitors (e.g. clompramine, fluoxetine) and caution is warranted if using alongside tramadol due to risk of serotonin syndrome. Concomitant use with diazepam may increase blood levels of amitriptyline.

DOSES

Dogs: 1–2 mg/kg p.o. q12–24h.

Cats: 0.5–1 mg/kg p.o. q24h.

References

Takeuchi Y, Houpt KA and Scarlett JM (2000) Evaluation of treatments for separation anxiety in dogs. *Journal of the American Veterinary Medical Association* **217**, 342–345

Amlodipine

(Amodip^c, Amlodipine*, Istin*) **POM-V, POM**

`CIL` A

Formulations: Oral: 1.25 mg chewable tablets (Amodip); 5 mg, 10 mg tablets; 1 mg/ml, 2 mg/ml sugar-free solutions. **Special reformulations available:** 0.3125 mg tablets; 12.5 mg/ml transdermal gel. **VSP**

Action: Calcium-channel antagonist, with predominant action affecting peripheral arteriolar vasculature, causing vasodilation and reducing afterload. Has mild negative inotropic and chronotropic effects, which are negligible at therapeutic doses.

Use:
- Treatment of systemic hypertension in cats (appears to be safe even with concurrent renal failure).
- Treatment of systemic hypertension in dogs (evidence for efficacy is not well established).
- It has also been shown to decrease proteinuria in cats with systemic hypertension.

When used as a single agent in dogs, may increase renin–angiotensin–aldosterone system activity – concurrent use of an ACE inhibitor should be considered. Amlodipine is metabolized in the liver and dosage should be reduced in animals with hepatic dysfunction.

Safety and handling: Normal precautions should be observed.

Contraindications: Avoid in cardiogenic shock, severe hepatic failure and pregnancy.

Adverse reactions: Lethargy, hypotension or inappetence are rare side effects. Gingival hyperplasia has been reported in cats and dogs.

Drug interactions: Little is known in animals. Hepatic metabolism may be impaired by drugs such as cimetidine, ciclosporin, ketoconazole and itraconazole, which may increase circulating doses. CYP3A4 inducers (such as rifampin) may reduce circulating amlodipine levels. Hypotension is a risk if combined with other antihypertensives (e.g. ACE inhibitors, diuretics, beta-blockers).

DOSES

Dogs: Initial dose 0.05–0.1 mg/kg p.o. q12–24h. The dose may be titrated upwards weekly as required, up to 0.5 mg/kg, monitoring blood pressure regularly.

Cats: 0.625–1.25 mg/cat p.o. q24h. The dose may be increased slowly or the frequency increased to q12h if necessary. Blood pressure monitoring is essential.

References

Huhtinen M, Derré G, Renoldi HJ et al. (2015) Randomized placebo-controlled clinical trial of a chewable formulation of amlodipine for the treatment of hypertension in client-owned cats. *Journal of Veterinary Internal Medicine* **3**, 786–793

Taylor SS, Sparkes AH, Briscoe K et al. (2017) ISFM consensus guidelines on the diagnosis and management of hypertension in cats. *Journal of Feline Medicine and Surgery* **19**, 288–303

Amoxicillin (Amoxycillin)

(Amoxibactin ^{c,d}, Amoxycare ^{c,d}, Amoxypen ^{c,d}, Betamox ^{c,d}, Bimoxyl ^d, Clamoxyl ^{c,d}, Trymox LA ^{c,d}) **POM-V**

Formulations: Injectable: 150 mg/ml suspension. **Oral:** 40 mg, 50 mg, 200 mg, 250 mg, 500 mg tablets; suspension that provides 50 mg/ml when reconstituted.

Action: Binds to penicillin-binding proteins involved in bacterial cell wall synthesis, thereby decreasing cell wall strength and rigidity, affecting cell division, growth and septum formation. Acts in a time-dependent fashion.

Use:
- Active against certain Gram-positive and Gram-negative aerobic organisms and many obligate anaerobes.

Resistance is possible due to bacterial production of penicillinases (beta-lactamases), e.g. some *Escherichia coli*, *Staphylococcus aureus*. Gram-negative organisms (*Pseudomonas*, *Proteus*, *Klebsiella*) are usually resistant. Amoxicillin is excreted well in bile and urine, achieving high concentrations in urine. Oral amoxicillin may be given with or without food. It is important to maintain levels above the MIC for a high percentage of the time by ensuring regular dosing; missing doses can seriously compromise efficacy.

Safety and handling: Refrigerate oral suspension after reconstitution; discard if solution becomes dark or after 7 days.

Contraindications: Avoid oral antibiotics in critically ill patients, as absorption from the GI tract may be unreliable.

Adverse reactions: Nausea, diarrhoea and skin rashes (type 1 (Ig-E mediated) reaction) are the commonest adverse effects.

Drug interactions: Do not mix in the same syringe as aminoglycosides. A synergistic effect is seen when beta-lactam and aminoglycoside antimicrobials are used concurrently.

DOSES

Classified as category D (Prudence) by the EMA.
See Appendix for guidelines on responsible antibiotic use.
Dogs, Cats:
- Parenteral: 7 mg/kg i.m. q24h; 15 mg/kg i.m. q48h for depot preparations.
- Oral:
  - 10 mg/kg p.o. q8–12h.
  - 11–15 mg/kg p.o. q8h for bacterial cystitis. Evidence of a need for clavulanic acid is lacking even in infections with beta-lactamase producing bacteria.

Dose chosen will depend on site of infection, causal organism and severity of the disease. (Doses of 16–33 mg/kg i.v. q8h are used in humans to treat serious infections.)

References
Weese JS, Blondeau J, Boothe D *et al.* (2019) International Society for Companion Animal Infectious Diseases (ISCAID) guidelines for the diagnosis and management of bacterial urinary tract infections in dogs and cats. *The Veterinary Journal* **247**, 8–25

Amoxicillin/Clavulanate see Co-amoxiclav
Amoxycillin see Amoxicillin

Amphotericin B
(Abelcet*, AmBisome*, Amphocil*, Fungizone*) **POM**

Formulations: Injectable: 50 mg/vial powder for reconstitution.

Action: Binds to sterols in fungal cell membrane creating pores and allowing leakage of contents.

Use:
- Management of systemic fungal infections and leishmaniosis.

Given the risk of severe toxicity, it is advisable to reserve use for severe/potentially fatal fungal infections only. Abelcet, AmBisome and Amphocil are lipid formulations that are less toxic. Physically incompatible with electrolyte solutions. Lipid formulations are far less toxic than conventional formulations for i.v. use because the drug is targeted to macrophages, but these preparations are far more expensive. Usually given i.v. but if regular venous catheterization is problematic then an s.c. alternative has been used for cryptococcosis and could potentially be used for other systemic mycoses. Renal values and electrolytes should be monitored pre- and post- each treatment; urinalysis and liver function tests weekly. If considering use in patients with pre-existing renal insufficiency (where other treatment options have failed and benefits outweigh risks), consider lipid formulations, concurrent saline administration and dose reduction.

Safety and handling: Keep in the dark, although loss of drug activity is negligible for at least 8 hours in room light. After initial reconstitution (but not further dilution), the drug is stable for 1 week if refrigerated and stored in the dark. Do not dilute in saline. Pre-treatment heating of the reconstituted concentrated solution to 70°C for 20 minutes produces superaggregates which are less nephrotoxic. To produce a lipid-formulated product if not commercially available, mix 40 ml sterile saline, 10 ml of lipid infusion (q.v.) and 50 mg of the reconstituted concentrated solution.

Contraindications: Do not use in renal or hepatic failure.

Adverse reactions: Include hypokalaemia, leading to cardiac arrhythmias, phlebitis, hepatic failure, renal failure, vomiting, diarrhoea, pyrexia, muscle and joint pain, anorexia and anaphylactoid reactions. Nephrotoxicity is a major concern; do not use other nephrotoxic drugs concurrently. Nephrotoxicity may be reduced by saline or lactated Ringer's infusion (5 ml/kg/hr) for 30 minutes prior to and 120 minutes following administration of amphotericin B (taking care to flush i.v. line thoroughly with 5% dextrose in between). Fever and vomiting may be decreased by pre-treating with aspirin, diphenhydramine or an antiemetic.

Drug interactions: Amphotericin B may increase the toxic effects of fluorouracil, doxorubicin and methotrexate. Flucytosine is synergistic with amphotericin B *in vitro* against *Candida*, *Cryptococcus* and *Aspergillus*.

DOSES
Dogs:
- Systemic mycoses (conventional amphotericin): 0.25–1 mg/kg i.v. q48h. Administer slowly over 4–6 hours. Reconstitute vial with 10 ml

water to produce 5 mg/ml solution; dilute required volume further 1:50 with 5% dextrose to give 0.1 mg/ml solution. Alternatively, 0.25–1 mg/kg may be dissolved in 10–60 ml 5% dextrose and given i.v. over 10 min 3 times a week. Start at the lower end of the dose range and increase gradually as the patient tolerates therapy. Several months of therapy are often necessary. A total cumulative dose of 4–8 mg/kg is recommended by some authors.

- **Cryptococcosis (conventional amphotericin, subcutaneous alternative):** 0.5–0.8 mg/kg added to 400–500 ml of 0.45% saline/2.5% dextrose. This total volume is then administered s.c. 2–3 times a week to a cumulative level of 8–26 mg/kg. Do not inject solutions more concentrated than 20 mg/l as they will cause subcutaneous abscesses. Intralesional injections may also be performed in this condition at a dose of 1 mg/kg q7d in combination with oral itraconazole.
- **Irrigation of bladder (conventional amphotericin):** 30–50 mg in 50–100 ml of sterile water infused at a rate of 5–10 ml/kg into the bladder lumen daily for 5–15 days.
- **Systemic mycoses (lipid formulations, general guidelines):** 1 mg/kg q48h to cumulative dose of 12 mg/kg. Higher doses are tolerated (e.g. 1–2.5 mg/kg i.v. q48h for 4 weeks/to cumulative dose of 24–30 mg/kg). Reconstitute to 5 mg/ml with sterile water, then dilute required volume to 1 mg/ml with 5% dextrose water.
- **Leishmaniosis (lipid formulations):** 1–2.5 mg/kg i.v. twice weekly for 8 injections. Increase dose rate gradually. A total cumulative dose of at least 10 mg/kg is required but treatment may be continued long term depending on clinical response. Use in this context is discouraged to avoid resistance developing to therapy for humans.

Cats:
- **Systemic mycoses (conventional amphotericin):** 0.1–0.25 i.v. q48h. For details on administration, see doses for dogs.
- **Cryptococcosis (conventional amphotericin, subcutaneous alternative):** 0.5–0.8 mg/kg added to 400–500 ml of 0.45% saline/2.5% dextrose. This total volume is then administered s.c. 2–3 times a week to a cumulative level of 10–15 mg/kg. Do not inject solutions more concentrated than 20 mg/l as they will cause subcutaneous abscesses. Intralesional injections may also be performed in this condition at a dose of 1 mg/kg q7d in combination with oral itraconazole.
- **Systemic mycoses (lipid formulations, general guidelines):** 1 mg/kg q48h to cumulative dose of 12 mg/kg. Higher doses are tolerated (e.g. 1–2.5 mg/kg i.v. q48h for 4 weeks/to cumulative dose of 24–30 mg/kg).

References

Foy DS and Trepanier LA (2010) Antifungal treatment of small animal veterinary patients. *Veterinary Clinics of North America: Small Animal Practice* **40**, 1171–1188

Pennisi MG, Hartmann K, Lloret A *et al.* (2013) Cryptococcosis in cats: ABCD guidelines on prevention and management. *Journal of Feline Medicine and Surgery* **15**, 611–618

Ampicillin

(Amfipen [c,d], Ampicare [d]) **POM-V**

Formulations: Injectable: Ampicillin sodium 250 mg, 500 mg powders for reconstitution (human licensed product only); 100 mg/ml long-acting preparation. **Oral:** 250 mg capsules.

Action: Binds to penicillin-binding proteins involved in bacterial cell wall synthesis, thereby decreasing cell wall strength and rigidity, affecting cell division, growth and septum formation. It acts in a time-dependent fashion.

Use:
- Active against many Gram-positive and Gram-negative aerobic organisms and obligate anaerobes, but not against those that produce penicillinases (beta-lactamases), e.g. *Escherichia coli*, *Staphylococcus aureus*.

The difficult Gram-negative organisms such as *Pseudomonas aeruginosa* and *Klebsiella* are usually resistant. Ampicillin is excreted well in bile and urine. Maintaining levels above the MIC is critical for efficacy; prolonged dosage intervals or missed doses can compromise therapeutic response. Dose and dosing interval is determined by infection site, severity and organism. Oral bioavailability is reduced in the presence of food.

Safety and handling: After reconstitution, the sodium salt will retain adequate potency for up to 8 hours if refrigerated. Use within 2 hours if kept at room temperature.

Contraindications: Avoid the use of oral antibiotic agents in critically ill patients, as absorption from the GI tract may be unreliable. Do not use in animals with hypersensitivity to penicillins.

Adverse reactions: Nausea, diarrhoea and skin rashes are the commonest adverse effects.

Drug interactions: Avoid the concurrent use of ampicillin with bacterio-static antibiotics (e.g. tetracycline, erythromycin, chloramphenicol). Do not mix in the same syringe as aminoglycosides. A synergistic effect is seen when beta-lactam and aminoglycoside antimicrobials are used concurrently.

DOSES

Classified as category D (Prudence) by the EMA.
See Appendix for guidelines on responsible antibiotic use.
Dogs:
- 10–20 mg/kg i.v., i.m., s.c., p.o. q6–8h.
- **CNS or serious bacterial infections:** up to 40 mg/kg i.v. q6h has been recommended.
Cats: 10–20 mg/kg i.v., i.m., s.c., p.o. q6–8h.

Amprolium

(Harkers Pigeon Coccidiosis Treatment) **AVM-GSL**

Formulations: Oral: 3.84% solution for dilution in water.
Action: Thiamine analogue that disrupts protozoal metabolism.
Use: Treatment of coccidiosis in dogs and cats.
Safety and handling: Normal precautions should be observed.

Contraindications: Do not use for more than 2 weeks to minimize risk of thiamine deficiency in the host animal.

Adverse reactions: Anorexia, diarrhoea and depression in dogs. Prolonged high doses can cause thiamine deficiency and may result in neurological signs.

Drug interactions: Exogenously administered thiamine may reduce efficacy.

DOSES
See Appendix for guidelines on responsible parasiticide use.

Dogs: 200–300 mg/dog p.o. q24h for 7–12 days; **small puppies:** reduce to 60–100 mg/dog p.o. q24h; **larger puppies:** use 200 mg/dog p.o. q24h.

Cats: 60–100 mg/cat p.o. q24h for 7 days or 110–220 mg/kg on food q24h for 7–12 days.

Antivenom (European Adder)
POM

Formulations: Injectable: 10 ml vial for injection (100 mg/ml).

Action: Immunoglobulin raised against venom inhibits toxic effects.

Use:
- Used in the management of snake bites by the European Adder (Viper).

Current approved suppliers can be found on the VMD website and a special dispensation from the VMD can enable supply, purchase and use prior to special treatment certificate approval in urgent cases (contact the VMD). Before submitting an application, contact the relevant manufacturer to ensure they are able to supply the quantity of product you wish to import. Urgent provision may also be possible via the VPIS ToxBox service. The value of antivenom decreases with time following the bite (benefits to local swelling are limited to administration within 24 hours post bite; however, benefits towards systemic signs, when present, continue even with administration >24 hours post bite). There are no published studies conclusively supporting improved recovery time in small animals. This antivenom is unlikely to work for other snake bites and specialist help should be urgently sought for such bites.

Safety and handling: Normal precautions should be observed.

Contraindications: No information available.

Adverse reactions: Anaphylactic reactions may develop. Milder reactions reported include facial swelling unrelated to snake bite, profound panting and unproductive cough.

Drug interactions: No information available.

DOSES
Dogs, Cats: 10 ml/animal slow i.v. (regardless of size). Consider giving 0.5 ml i.v. first and waiting 20 min to test for anaphylaxis.

References
Hodgson L, Brambilla G (2017) In dogs with a European adder bite, does the use of antivenom with supportive treatment compared to supportive treatment alone improve time to recovery? *Veterinary Evidence* **2**, 1–11

Lund HS, Kristiansen V, Eggertsdóttir AV *et al.* (2013) Adverse reactions to equine-derived F(ab')2 -antivenin in 54 dogs envenomated by *Vipera berus berus*. *Journal of Veterinary Emergency and Critical Care* **23**, 532–553

Apomorphine

(Apometic) **POM-V**

A

Formulations: Injectable: 10 mg/ml solution in 2 ml ampoules. Other non-authorized formulations available.

Action: Stimulates emesis through D2 dopamine receptors in the chemoreceptor trigger zone.

Use:
- Induction of self-limiting emesis within a few minutes of administration in dogs where vomiting is desirable, e.g. following the ingestion of a toxic, non-caustic substance.

Emesis generally occurs rapidly and within a maximum of 10 minutes. If emesis is not induced following a single injection, repeated injections will also prove ineffective and should not be given.

Safety and handling: Normal precautions should be observed.

Contraindications: Induction of emesis is contraindicated if strong acid or alkali has been ingested, due to the risk of further damage to the oesophagus. Do not use in cases of gastric foreign bodies. Do not use in cases of poisoning due to pyrethroids. Induction of vomiting is contraindicated if the dog is unconscious, fitting or has a reduced cough reflex, if it has been >2 hours since ingestion, or if the ingesta contains paraffin, petroleum products or other oily or volatile organic products, due to the risk of inhalation.

Adverse reactions: Apomorphine may induce excessive vomiting, respiratory depression and sedation. Dose-dependent hypotension can be seen. Ivermectin-sensitive (*ABCB1* mutation) collies may be more susceptible to the effects of apomorphine and for this reason the drug should be avoided if possible in such animals. If use is unavoidable, then the dose should be reduced.

Drug interactions: In the absence of compatibility studies, apomorphine must not be mixed with other products. Antiemetic drugs, particularly antidopaminergics (e.g. phenothiazines) may reduce the emetic effects of apomorphine. Additive CNS or respiratory depression may occur when apomorphine is used with opiates or other CNS or respiratory depressants.

DOSES

Dogs: 0.1 mg/kg s.c. (authorized dose), 40 µg (micrograms)/kg i.v. (non-authorized dose and route but some evidence to suggest is at least as effective).

Cats: Not recommended; xylazine is a potent emetic in cats and at least as safe.

References

Khan SA, McLean MK, Slater M *et al.* (2012) Effectiveness and adverse effects of the use of apomorphine and 3% hydrogen peroxide solution to induce emesis in dogs. *Journal of the American Veterinary Medical Association* **241**, 1179–1184

Apraclonidine

(Iopidine*) **POM**

Formulations: Ophthalmic: 0.5% solution (5 ml bottle); preservative-free 1% solution (single-dose vials).

Action: Topical alpha-2-selective agonist that decreases aqueous humour production by inhibition of adenylate cyclase activity in the ciliary body.

Use:
- Reducing intraocular pressure in glaucoma; however, effect in dogs is inconsistent and it is unlikely to be effective as a sole agent in most forms of canine glaucoma.
- It may be most useful in alleviating pressure rises after intraocular surgery.

It is prudent to monitor heart rate before and after topical application of apraclonidine, particularly with initial use and in small dogs. To limit systemic absorption, raise head and compress lower nasolacrimal punctum for topical administration.

Safety and handling: Normal precautions should be observed.

Contraindications: Commercial preparations are considered too toxic for use in cats. Do not use in dogs with uncontrolled cardiac disease.

Adverse reactions: Causes blanching of conjunctival vessels and bradycardia in dogs and cats. Causes mydriasis in dogs, miosis and severe vomiting in cats.

Drug interactions: No information available.

DOSES

Dogs: 1 drop per eye q8–12h for short-term use only.
Cats: Do not use.

Ara-C see Cytarabine

Asparaginase (L-Asparginase, Crisantaspase)

(Asparginase*, Elspar*, Erwinase*) **POM**

Formulations: Injectable: 5,000 IU, 10,000 IU vials of powder for reconstitution.

Action: Lymphoid tumour cells are not able to synthesize asparagine and are dependent upon supply from the extracellular fluid. Asparaginase deprives malignant cells of this amino acid, which results in cessation of protein synthesis and cell death.

Use: Management of lymphoid malignancies.

Safety and handling: Cytotoxic drug; see Appendix and specialist texts for further advice on chemotherapeutic agents. Store in a refrigerator.

Contraindications: Patients with active pancreatitis or a history of pancreatitis. History of anaphylaxis associated with previous administration. Use with caution in patients with pre-existing liver dysfunction and/or thrombosis, haemorrhagic events. i.v. administration is not recommended.

Adverse reactions: Anaphylaxis may follow administration, especially if repeated. Premedication with an antihistamine is recommended 30 minutes before administration. Haemorrhagic pancreatitis has been reported in dogs. GI disturbances, hepatotoxicity including acute hyperammonaemia (presenting with encephalopathy) and coagulation deficits may also be observed. Bone marrow depression is very rare.

Drug interactions: Administration with or before vincristine may reduce clearance of vincristine and increase toxicity; thus, if used in combination, some oncologists recommend that vincristine should be given 12–24 hours before the enzyme.

DOSES
See Appendix for chemotherapy protocols and conversion of bodyweight to body surface area.
Dogs, Cats: 10,000 IU/m^2 or 400 IU/kg i.m. or s.c. q7d or less frequently, depending on the protocol being used.

References
MacDonald VS, Thamm DH, Kurzman ID *et al.* (2005) Does L-Asparaginase influence efficacy or toxicity when added to a standard CHOP protocol for dogs with lymphoma? *Journal of Veterinary Internal Medicine* **19**, 732–736

Saba CF, Thamm DH and Vail DM (2007) Combination chemotherapy with L-asparaginase, lomustine, and prednisone for relapsed or refractory canine lymphoma. *Journal of Veterinary Internal Medicine* **21**, 127–132

Aspirin (Acetylsalicylic acid) `CIL`
(Aspirin BP* and component of many others) **P**

Formulations: Oral: 75 mg, 300 mg tablets.

Action: Produces irreversible inhibition of cyclo-oxygenase (COX-1, prostaglandin synthetase) by acetylation, thereby preventing the production of both prostaglandins and thromboxanes from membrane phospholipids.

Use:
- Prevention of arterial thromboembolism. Recent evidence suggests that clopidogrel may be superior to aspirin in cats for prevention of recurrence of cardiogenic thromboembolic events if used as a single agent.
- Can be used to control mild to moderate pain, although NSAIDs that are more selective for the COX-2 enzyme have a better safety profile; not an NSAID of choice for analgesia in dogs or cats.
- In one study, the use of ultra low dose aspirin (0.5 mg/kg q12h) may have improved short-term and long-term survival in dogs with immune-mediated haemolytic anaemia (IMHA) when combined with glucocorticoid and azathioprine therapy.

Administration of aspirin to animals with renal disease must be carefully evaluated. It is advisable to stop aspirin before surgery (at least 2 weeks) to allow recovery of normal platelet function and prevent excessive bleeding.

Safety and handling: Normal precautions should be observed.

Contraindications: Do not give aspirin to dehydrated, hypovolaemic or hypotensive patients, or those with GI disease. Do not give to pregnant animals or animals <6 weeks old.

Adverse reactions: GI ulceration and irritation are common side effects of all NSAIDs. It is advisable to stop therapy if diarrhoea or nausea persists beyond 1–2 days. Stop therapy immediately and begin symptomatic treatment if GI bleeding is suspected. There is a small risk that NSAIDs may precipitate cardiac failure in humans and this risk in animals is unknown. All NSAIDs carry a risk of renal papillary necrosis due to reduced renal perfusion caused by a reduction in the production of renal prostaglandins. This risk is greatest when NSAIDs are given to animals that are hypotensive or animals with pre-existing renal disease.

Drug interactions: Do not administer concurrently or within 24 hours of other NSAIDs and glucocorticoids. Do not administer with other potentially nephrotoxic agents, e.g. aminoglycosides.

DOSES

Dogs: Doses are anecdotal and the ideal doses are unknown.
- **Reduction of platelet aggregation (e.g. IMHA):** 0.5–1 mg/kg p.o. q24h or 0.5 mg/kg p.o. q12h.
- **Analgesia, pyrexia, inflammation:** 10–20 mg/kg p.o. q12h; the safety and efficacy of this dose has not been established.

Cats: Reduction of platelet aggregation: 18.75 mg/cat p.o. 3 days a week (low dose) or 75 mg/cat p.o. 3 days a week (high dose); this dose may be associated with a higher risk of GI side effects. Some authors suggest a very low dose (0.5 mg/kg p.o. q24h) to inhibit platelet COX without preventing the beneficial effects of prostacyclin production. The safety and efficacy of these doses have not been evaluated in clinical or experimental studies.

References

Hogan DF, Fox PR, Jacob K *et al.* (2015) Secondary prevention of cardiogenic arterial thromboembolism in the cat: The double-blind, randomized, positive-controlled feline arterial thromboembolism; clopidogrel versus aspirin trial (FAT CAT). *Journal of Veterinary Cardiology* **17**, s306–s317

Stiller A (2013) Effect of low-dose aspirin or heparin on platelet-derived urinary thromboxane metabolite in dogs with immune-mediated hemolytic anemia (IMHA). *ACVIM Proceedings 2013, Washington*

Atenolol

(Atenolol*, Tenormin*) **POM**

Formulations: Oral: 25 mg, 50 mg, 100 mg tablets; 5 mg/ml sugar-free syrup. Injectable: 0.5 mg/ml. Special reformulations available: 6.25 mg tablets. **VSP**

Action: Cardioselective beta-adrenergic blocker. It is relatively specific for beta-1 adrenergic receptors but can antagonize beta-2 receptors at high doses. Blocks the chronotropic and inotropic effects of beta-1 adrenergic stimulation on the heart, thereby reducing myocardial oxygen demand. Bronchoconstrictor, vasodilatory and hypoglycaemic effects are less marked due to its cardioselective nature.

Use:
- Treatment of cardiac tachyarrhythmias (including those associated with feline hyperthyroidism).
- Treatment of hypertrophic obstructive cardiomyopathy (cats) or obstructive cardiac disease (severe aortic or pulmonic stenosis).
- Treatment of systemic hypertension.

- Can be used following introduction of alpha blockade in management of phaeochromocytoma.
- It is recommended to withdraw therapy gradually in patients who have been receiving the drug chronically.

Safety and handling: Normal precautions should be observed.

Contraindications: Patients with bradyarrhythmias, acute or decompensated congestive heart failure. Poorly tolerated in animals with medically controlled congestive heart failure.

Adverse reactions: Most frequently seen in geriatric patients with chronic heart disease or in patients with acute or decompensated heart failure. Include bradycardia, AV block, myocardial depression, heart failure, syncope, hypotension, hypoglycaemia, bronchospasm and diarrhoea. Depression and lethargy may occur as a result of atenolol's high lipid solubility and its penetration into the CNS.

Drug interactions: Do not administer concurrently with alpha-adrenergic agonists (e.g. phenylpropanolamine) unless specifically indicated (phaeochromocytoma). The hypotensive effect of atenolol is enhanced by many agents that depress myocardial activity including anaesthetic agents, phenothiazines, antihypertensive drugs, diuretics and diazepam. There is an increased risk of bradycardia, severe hypotension, heart failure and AV block if atenolol is used concurrently with calcium-channel blockers. Concurrent digoxin administration potentiates bradycardia. The metabolism of atenolol is accelerated by thyroid hormones; thus, the dose of atenolol may need to be decreased when initiating carbimazole therapy. Atenolol enhances the effects of muscle relaxants (e.g. suxamethonium, tubocurarine). Hepatic enzyme induction by phenobarbital may increase the rate of metabolism of atenolol. The bronchodilatory effects of theophylline may be blocked by atenolol. Atenolol may enhance the hypoglycaemic effect of insulin.

DOSES

Dogs: 0.2–2 mg/kg p.o. q12h; a lower dose is often used initially with gradual titration upwards if necessary.

Cats: 6.25–12.5 mg/cat p.o. q12–24h; a lower dose is often used initially with gradual titration upwards if necessary. If using the oral liquid, doses of 0.2–2 mg/kg p.o. q12h can be used, with gradual titration upwards as necessary.

References

Schober KE, Zientek J, Li X *et al.* (2013) Effect of treatment with atenolol on 5-year survival in cats with preclinical (asymptomatic) hypertrophic cardiomyopathy. *Journal of Veterinary Cardiology* **15**, 93–104

Atipamezole

(Alzane [c,d], Antisedan [c,d], Atipam [c,d], Atipazole [c,d], Revertor [c,d], Sedastop [c,d], Tipafar [c,d]) **POM-V**

Formulations: Injectable: 5 mg/ml solution.

Action: Selective alpha-2 adrenoreceptor antagonist.

Use:
- Reverses the sedative effects of medetomidine or dexmedetomidine.
- Will also reverse other alpha-2 agonists to provide a quick recovery from anaesthesia and sedation.

Atipamezole also reverses other effects such as the analgesic, cardiovascular and respiratory effects of alpha-2 agonists. It does not alter the metabolism of medetomidine or dexmedetomidine but occupies the alpha-2 receptor, preventing binding of the drug. The duration of action of atipamezole and medetomidine or dexmedetomidine are similar, so resedation is uncommon. Atipamezole should not be administered until at least 30 minutes after medetomidine/ketamine combinations have been given, to avoid CNS excitation in recovery. Routine administration of atipamezole i.v. is not recommended because the rapid recovery from sedation is usually associated with excitation, although i.v. administration may be indicated in an emergency (e.g. excessive sedation from medetomidine or dexmedetomidine, cardiovascular complications).

Safety and handling: Normal precautions should be observed. In particular, skin contact with atipamezole should be avoided and impervious gloves should be worn during administration.

Contraindications: Atipamezole has been administered to a limited number of pregnant dogs and cats and therefore cannot be recommended in pregnancy.

Adverse reactions: Transient over-alertness and tachycardia may be observed after overdosage. This is best handled by minimizing external stimuli and allowing the animal to recover quietly.

Drug interactions: No information available.

DOSES

Dogs: 5 times the previous medetomidine or 10 times the previous dexmedetomidine (0.5 mg/ml) dose i.m. (i.e. equal volume of solution to medetomidine or dexmedetomidine (0.5 mg/ml) given). When medetomidine or dexmedetomidine has been administered at least an hour before, the dose of atipamezole can be reduced by half and repeated if recovery is slow.
* **Amitraz toxicity:** 25 µg (micrograms)/kg i.m. but if there is no benefit within 30 minutes this can be repeated or incrementally increased every 30 minutes up to 200 µg/kg.

Cats: 2.5 times the previous medetomidine or 5 times the previous dexmedetomidine (0.5 mg/ml) dose i.m. (i.e. half the volume of medetomidine or dexmedetomidine (0.5 mg/ml) solution given). When medetomidine or dexmedetomidine has been administered at least an hour before, the dose of atipamezole can be reduced by half and repeated if recovery is slow.

References

Ambrisko TD and Hikasa Y (2003) The antagonistic effects of atipamezole and yohimbine on stress-related neurohormonal and metabolic responses induced by medetomidine in dogs. *Canadian Journal of Veterinary Research* **67**, 64–67

Granholm M, McKusick BC, Westerholm FC *et al.* (2007) Evaluation of the clinical efficacy and safety of intramuscular and intravenous doses dexmedetomidine in dogs and their reversal with atipamezole. *Veterinary Record* **160**, 891–897

Atracurium

(Tracrium*) **POM**

Formulations: Injectable: 10 mg/ml solution.

Action: Inhibits the actions of acetylcholine at the neuromuscular junction by binding competitively to the nicotinic acetylcholine receptor on the post-junctional membrane.

Use:
- Neuromuscular blockade during anaesthesia.
- To improve surgical access through muscle relaxation, to facilitate positive pressure ventilation or for intraocular surgery.

Atracurium has an intermediate duration of action (15–35 min) and is non-cumulative due to non-enzymatic (Hofmann) elimination. It is therefore suitable for administration to animals with renal or hepatic disease. Monitoring (using a nerve stimulator) and reversal of the neuromuscular blockade is recommended to ensure complete recovery before the end of anaesthesia. Hypothermia, acidosis and hypokalaemia will prolong the duration of action of neuromuscular blockade. Use the low end of the dose range in patients with myasthenia gravis and ensure that neuromuscular function is monitored during the period of the blockade and recovery using standard techniques.

Safety and handling: Store in refrigerator.

Contraindications: Do not administer unless the animal is adequately anaesthetized and facilities to provide positive pressure ventilation are available.

Adverse reactions: Can precipitate the release of histamine after rapid i.v. administration, resulting in bronchospasm and hypotension. Diluting the drug in normal saline and giving slowly i.v. minimizes these effects.

Drug interactions: Neuromuscular blockade is more prolonged when atracurium is given in combination with volatile anaesthetics, aminoglycosides, clindamycin or lincomycin.

DOSES

Dogs, Cats: 0.2–0.5 mg/kg i.v. initially, followed by increments of 0.2 mg/kg i.v.

References
Kastrup MR, Marsico FF, Ascoli FO *et al.* (2005) Neuromuscular blocking properties of atracurium during sevoflurane or propofol anaesthesia in dogs. *Veterinary Anaesthesia and Analgesia* **32**, 222–227

Atropine

CIL

(Atrocare[c,d], Atropine) **POM-V**

Formulations: Injectable: 0.6 mg/ml. Ophthalmic: 1% solution in single-use vials, 10 ml bottle.

Action: Blocks the action of acetylcholine at muscarinic receptors at the terminal ends of the parasympathetic nervous system, reversing para-sympathetic effects and producing mydriasis, tachycardia, broncho-dilation and general inhibition of GI function.

Use:
- Prevent or correct bradycardia and bradyarrhythmias.

- Dilate pupils.
- Management of organophosphate and carbamate toxicities.
- In conjunction with anticholinesterase drugs during antagonism of neuromuscular blockade.

Routine administration prior to anaesthesia as part of premedication is no longer recommended; it is better to monitor heart rate and give atropine to manage a low heart rate if necessary. Atropine has a slow onset of action (10 min i.m., 2–3 min i.v.); therefore, it is important to wait for an adequate period of time for the desired effect before redosing. The ophthalmic solution tastes very bitter and can cause hypersalivation in cats (and in some dogs).

Safety and handling: The solution does not contain any antimicrobial preservative; therefore, any remaining solution in the vial should be discarded after use. The solution should be protected from light.

Contraindications: Glaucoma, lens luxation, keratoconjunctivitis sicca.

Adverse reactions: Include sinus tachycardia (usually of short duration after i.v. administration), blurred vision from mydriasis, which may worsen recovery from anaesthesia, and drying of bronchial secretions. Atropine increases intraocular pressure and reduces tear production. Ventricular arrhythmias may be treated with lidocaine if severe. Other GI side effects such as ileus and vomiting are rare in small animals.

Drug interactions: Atropine is compatible (for at least 15 min) mixed with various medications but not with bromides, iodides, sodium bicarbonate, other alkalis or noradrenaline. Antihistamines, quinidine, pethidine, benzodiazepines, phenothiazines, thiazide diuretics and sympatho-mimetics may enhance the activity of atropine. Combining atropine and alpha-2 agonists is not recommended. Atropine may aggravate some signs seen with amitraz toxicity, leading to hypertension and gut stasis.

DOSES

Dogs, Cats:
- **Ophthalmic:** 1 drop in the affected eye q12–24h to cause mydriasis, then q24–96h to maintain mydriasis.
- **Bradyarrhythmias:** 0.01–0.03 mg/kg i.v. Low doses may exacerbate bradycardia; repetition of the dose will usually promote an increase in heart rate. 0.03–0.04 mg/kg i.m. can be given to prevent development of bradycardia during administration of potent opioids such as fentanyl.
- **Organophosphate poisoning:** 0.2–0.5 mg/kg (¼ dose i.v., ¾ i.m., s.c.) to effect, repeat as necessary; or 0.1–0.2 mg/kg (½ i.v., ½ i.m.) then 0.1–0.2 mg/kg i.m. q6h.
- **Neuromuscular blockade antagonism:** 0.04 mg/kg i.v. with neostigmine (0.02–0.04 mg/kg).

Azathioprine

(Azathioprine*, Imuran*) **POM**

Formulations: Oral: 25 mg, 50 mg tablets.

Action: Inhibits purine synthesis, which is necessary for cell proliferation especially of leucocytes and lymphocytes. Although exact mechanism is unknown, it suppresses cell-mediated immunity, alters antibody production and inhibits cell growth.

Use:
- Management of immune-mediated diseases such as immune-mediated haemolytic anaemia and immune-mediated polyarthritis.
- Often used in conjunction with corticosteroids.

Routine haematology (including platelets) and biochemistry should be monitored closely: initially every 1–2 weeks; and every 1–2 months when on maintenance therapy. In animals with renal impairment, dosing interval should be extended. Clinical responses can take up to 6 weeks. Alternative immunosuppressants may be preferred if a more rapid response is required.

Safety and handling: Cytotoxic drug; see Appendix and specialist texts for further advice on chemotherapeutic agents. Azathioprine tablets should not be divided and should be stored at room temperature in well closed containers and protected from light.

Contraindications: Do not use in patients with bone marrow suppression, in those at high risk of infection or those with hepatic disease. Use with caution in patients with a history of pancreatic disease. Not recommended for use in cats.

Adverse reactions: Bone marrow suppression is the most serious adverse effect. This may be influenced by the activity of thiopurine s-methyltransferase, which is involved in the metabolism of the drug and which can vary between individuals due to genetic polymorphism. GI upset/anorexia, poor hair growth, acute pancreatitis and hepatotoxicity have been seen in dogs (the latter typically within 4 weeks of starting treatment). Cats in particular often develop a severe, non-responsive fatal leucopenia and thrombocytopenia. Avoid rapid withdrawal as this may cause a rebound hyperimmune response.

Drug interactions: Enhanced effects and increased azathioprine toxicity when used with allopurinol. Increased risk of azathioprine toxicity with aminosalicylates and corticosteroids, avoid with ACE inhibitors as this may increase potential for haematological adverse events.

DOSES
See Appendix for immunosuppression protocols.
Dogs: 2 mg/kg p.o. q24h for a maximum of 2–3 weeks, then 0.5–2 mg/kg p.o. q48h.
Cats: Not recommended.

References
Swann JW, Garden OA, Fellman CL *et al.* (2019) ACVIM consensus statement on the treatment of immune-mediated hemolytic anemia in dogs. *Journal of Veterinary Internal Medicine* **33**, 1–32
Wallisch K and Trepanier LA (2015) Incidence, timing, and risk Factors of azathioprine hepatotoxicosis in dogs. *Journal of Veterinary Internal Medicine* **29**, 513–518

Azidothymidine see Zidovudine

Azithromycin

(Azyter*, Clamelle*, Zedbac*, Zithromax*) **POM**

Formulations: Oral: 250 mg, 500 mg capsules and tablets; 200 mg/5 ml suspension (reconstitute with water); 30 mg azithromycin + 35 mg rifampicin capsules (veterinary special). Injectable: 500 mg powder for reconstitution. **VSP**

Action: Time-dependent macrolide antibacterial that binds to the 50S bacterial ribosome (like erythromycin), inhibiting peptide bond formation. Azithromycin has a longer tissue half-life than erythromycin, shows better oral absorption and is better tolerated in humans.

Use:
- Alternative to penicillin in allergic individuals as it has a similar, although not identical, antibacterial spectrum. It is active against Gram-positive cocci (some *Staphylococcus* species are resistant), Gram-positive bacilli, some Gram-negative bacilli (*Haemophilus*, *Pasteurella*), mycobacteria, obligate anaerobes, *Chlamydia*, *Mycoplasma* and *Toxoplasma*. Some strains of *Actinomyces*, *Nocardia* and *Rickettsia* are also inhibited. Most strains of the Enterobacteriaceae (*Pseudomonas*, *Escherichia coli*, *Klebsiella*) are resistant. Useful in the management of respiratory tract, mild to moderate skin and soft tissue, and non-tubercular mycobacterial infections. Is used to treat chlamydiosis in birds, but it has not proved possible to eliminate *Chlamydia felis* from chronically infected cats using azithromycin, even with once daily administration.
- Also reported for the treatment of small *Babesia* spp. (e.g *Babesia gibsoni*) and *Cytauxzoon felis*.
- In addition to its antimicrobial activity, it has been reported for use in reducing gingival hyperplasia secondary to ciclosporin administration in cases where cessation of treatment is not possible.
- Little information is available on the use of this drug in animals and drug pharmacokinetics have not been studied closely in the dog and cat. Doses are empirical and subject to change as experience with the drug is gained. More work is needed to optimize the clinically effective dose rate. Azithromycin activity is enhanced in an alkaline pH; administer on an empty stomach.

Safety and handling: Normal precautions should be observed.

Contraindications: Avoid in renal and hepatic failure in all species.

Adverse reactions: In humans, similar adverse effects to those of erythromycin are seen, i.e. vomiting, cholestatic hepatitis, stomatitis and glossitis, but the effects are generally less marked than with erythromycin.

Drug interactions: Azithromycin may increase the serum levels of methylprednisolone, theophylline and terfenadine. The absorption of digoxin may be enhanced.

DOSES

Classified as category C (Caution) by the EMA.
See Appendix for guidelines on responsible antibiotic use.

Dogs: 5–10 mg/kg p.o. q24h. May increase dosing interval to q48h after 3–5 days of treatment; for small *Babesia* spp.: 10mg/kg q24h for 10 days, in combination with atovaquone.

Cats: Various regimens are suggested: 5–10 mg/kg p.o. q24h for 3–5 days; 5 mg/kg p.o. q24h for 2 days then every 3–5 days up to a total of 5 doses; for upper respiratory tract disease: 5–10 mg/kg p.o. q24h for 5 days then q72h. Specialist texts should be consulted.

AZT see **Zidovudine**

Bedinvetmab

(Librela [d]) **POM-V**

Formulations: Injectable: 1 ml vials containing 5 mg, 10 mg, 15 mg, 20 mg, 30 mg bedinvetmab.

Action: Canine monoclonal antibody that targets nerve growth factor (NGF). The inhibition of NGF-mediated cell signalling has been demonstrated to provide relief from pain associated with osteoarthritis.

Use:
* Alleviation of pain associated with osteoarthritis in dogs.

If no or a limited response is observed within 1 month of initial dosing, an improvement may be observed after administration of a second dose 1 month later. If the dog does not show a better response after a second injection, then alternative analgesics should be considered.

Safety and handling: Store under refrigeration (2–8°C). Protect from light. Avoid shaking or excessive foaming of the solution. Due to the role of NGF in ensuring normal fetal nervous system development, people who are or may become pregnant, or who are breastfeeding should take extreme care to avoid accidental self injection. In the case of accidental self injection, seek medical advice immediately and take the package leaflet or label.

Contraindications: Do not use in dogs under 12 months of age. Do not use in animals intended for breeding or in pregnant or lactating animals.

Adverse reactions: Mild reactions at the injection site such as swelling and heat may be uncommonly observed.

Drug interactions: There are no safety data on the concurrent long term use of NSAIDs with bedinvetmab in dogs. In clinical trials in humans, rapidly progressive osteoarthritis has been reported in patients receiving anti-NGF monoclonal antibody therapy and NSAIDs for more than 90 days. Dogs have no reported equivalent of human rapidly progressive osteoarthritis. If vaccines are to be administered at the same time as treatment with bedinvetmab, they should be administered at a different site.

DOSES

Dogs: 0.5–1.0 mg/kg s.c. once a month. For dogs weighing less than 5 kg, aseptically withdraw 0.1 ml/kg from a single 5 mg vial and administer s.c. For dogs between 5 and 60 kg, administer the entire contents of one vial according to bodyweight.

Cats: Do not use.

References

Enomoto M, Mantyh PW, Murrell J, Innes JF and Lascelles BDX (2019) Anti-nerve growth factor monoclonal antibodies for control of pain in cats and dogs. *Veterinary Record* **184**, 23

Benazepril

(Benazecare Flavour [c,d], Benefortin [c,d], Cardalis [d], Fortekor [c,d], Fortekor-Plus [d], Kelapril [c,d], Nelio [c,d], Prilben [c,d], Vetpril)
POM-V

Formulations: Oral: 2.5 mg, 5 mg, 20 mg tablets; 2.5 mg benazepril + 20 mg spironolactone, 5 mg benazepril + 40 mg spironolactone, 10 mg benazepril + 80 mg spironolactone (Cardalis); 2.5 mg benazepril + 1.25 mg pimobendan, 10 mg benazepril + 5 mg pimobendan (Fortekor-Plus).

Action: Inhibits conversion of angiotensin I to angiotensin II and inhibits the breakdown of bradykinin. Overall effect is a reduction in preload and afterload via venodilation and arteriodilation, decreased salt and water retention via reduced aldosterone production and inhibition of the angiotensin–aldosterone-mediated cardiac and vascular remodelling. Efferent arteriolar dilation in the kidney can reduce intraglomerular pressure and therefore glomerular filtration. This may decrease proteinuria.

Use:
- Treatment of CHF in dogs and cats. Often used in conjunction with diuretics when heart failure is present. Can be used in combination with other drugs to treat heart failure (e.g. pimobendan, furosemide, spironolactone, digoxin).
- Management of proteinuria associated with chronic renal insufficiency, glomerular disorders and protein-losing nephropathies.
- May reduce blood pressure in hypertension and may be more potent in dogs. Less potent than amlodipine in reducing blood pressure in cats but sometimes used together.

Benazepril undergoes significant hepatic metabolism and may not need dose adjustment in renal failure. ACE inhibitors are more likely to cause or exacerbate prerenal azotaemia in hypotensive animals and those with poor renal perfusion (e.g. acute, oliguric renal failure). Use cautiously if hypotension, hyponatraemia or outflow tract obstruction are present. Regular monitoring of blood pressure, serum creatinine, urea and electrolytes is strongly recommended with ACE inhibitor treatment. The use of ACE inhibitors in cats with cardiac disease stems from extrapolation from theoretical benefits and studies showing a benefit in other species with heart failure and different cardiac diseases (mainly dogs and humans) and is not proven.

Safety and handling: Normal precautions should be observed.

Contraindications: Do not use in cases of cardiac output failure or hypotension.

Adverse reactions: Potential adverse effects include hypotension, hyperkalaemia and azotaemia. Monitor blood pressure, serum creatinine and electrolytes when used in cases of heart failure. Dosage should be reduced if there are signs of hypotension (weakness, disorientation). Anorexia, vomiting and diarrhoea are rare. In pre-clinical trials there were no serious reactions when the drug was given to normal dogs at 200 times the label dose. It is not recommended for breeding, or pregnant or lactating, dogs and cats, as safety has not been established. The safety of benazepril has not been established in cats <2.5 kg.

Drug interactions: Concomitant usage with potassium-sparing diuretics (e.g. spironolactone) or potassium supplements could result in hyperkalaemia. However, in practice, spironolactone and ACE inhibitors appear safe to use concurrently. There may be an increased risk of nephrotoxicity and decreased clinical efficacy when used with NSAIDs. There is a risk of hypotension with concomitant administration of diuretics, vasodilators (e.g. anaesthetic agents, antihypertensive agents) or negative inotropes (e.g. beta-blockers).

DOSES

Dogs:
- **Heart failure:** 0.25–0.5 mg/kg p.o. q12–24h. Additional benefit may be seen with twice daily dosing. Monitor blood pressure.
- **Adjunctive treatment of hypertension/proteinuria:** 0.25–0.5 mg/kg p.o. q12–24h. Increase by 0.25–0.5 mg/kg to a maximum daily dose of 2 mg/kg.

Cats:
- **Chronic renal insufficiency:** 0.5–1.0 mg/kg p.o. q24h.
- **Adjunctive therapy in heart failure:** 0.25–0.5 mg/kg p.o. q24h.

References
BENCH Study Group (1999) The effect of benazepril on survival times and clinical signs of dogs with congestive heart failure: results of a multicenter, prospective, randomized, double-blinded, placebo-controlled, long-term clinical trial. *Journal of Veterinary Cardiology* **1**, 7–18
Brown S, Elliott J, Francey T *et al.* (2013) Consensus recommendations for standard therapy of glomerular disease in dogs. *Journal of Veterinary Internal Medicine* **27**, S27–S43

Bentonite see Calcium aluminosilicate
Benzyl penicillin see Penicillin G

Betamethasone

(Isaderm[d], Osurnia[d], Otomax[d], Betnesol*, Maxidex*)
POM-V, POM

Formulations: Injectable: 4 mg/ml solution for i.v. or i.m. use. **Oral:** 0.25 mg tablets. **Topical:** 0.1% betamethasone + 0.5% fusidic acid cream. **Ophthalmic/Otic:** 0.1% solution; 0.88 mg/ml suspension with clotrimazole and gentamicin; 0.1% gel with florfenicol and terbinafine. Betamethasone is also present in varying concentrations in several topical preparations with or without antibacterials.

Action: Alters the transcription of DNA, leading to alterations in cellular metabolism which cause reduction in inflammatory responses. Has high glucocorticoid and virtually no mineralocorticoid activity. Betamethasone also antagonizes insulin and arginine vasopressin.

Use:
- Short-term relief of many inflammatory but non-infectious conditions.

Long duration of activity makes it unsuitable for long-term daily or alternate-day use. On a dose basis, 0.12 mg betamethasone is equivalent to 1 mg prednisolone. Prolonged use of glucocorticoids suppresses the hypothalamic–pituitary axis, resulting in adrenal atrophy. Animals on chronic corticosteroid therapy should be given tapered decreasing doses when discontinuing the drug. The use of long-acting steroids is of no benefit in most cases of shock, and may be detrimental. It is recommended to clean and dry the external ear canal before the first administration of the combination formulation with florfenicol and terbinafine. It is recommended not to repeat ear cleaning until 21 days after the second administration of the product.

Safety and handling: Wear gloves when applying cream.

Contraindications: Do not use in pregnant animals. Systemic corticosteroids are generally contraindicated in patients with renal disease and diabetes mellitus. Topical corticosteroids are contraindicated in ulcerative keratitis.

Adverse reactions: Catabolic effects of glucocorticoids lead to weight loss and cutaneous and muscle atrophy. Chronic therapy may lead to iatrogenic hypercortisolism. Vomiting, diarrhoea and GI ulceration may develop. Glucocorticoids may increase glucose levels and decrease serum triodothyronine (T3) and thyroxine (T4) values. Impaired wound healing and delayed recovery from infections may be seen.

Drug interactions: There is an increased risk of GI ulceration if used concurrently with NSAIDs. Glucocorticoids antagonize the effect of insulin. Phenobarbital may increase the metabolism of corticosteroids and antifungals (e.g. itraconazole) may decrease it. There is an increased risk of hypokalaemia when used concurrently with acetazolamide, amphotericin and potassium-depleting diuretics (furosemide, thiazides).

DOSES
Dogs:
- Otic: 4 drops of polypharmaceutical to affected ear q12h. If using combination formulation with florfenicol and terbinafine, administer into affected ear and repeat once after 7 days.
- Ocular: 1 drop of ophthalmic solution to affected eye q6–8h.
- Skin: apply cream to affected area q8–12h.
- Anti-inflammatory: 0.04 mg/kg i.v., i.m. q3w prn for up to 4 injections; 0.025 mg/kg p.o. q24h.

Cats:
- Ocular: dose as for dogs.
- Skin: dose as for dogs.
- Anti-inflammatory: 0.04 mg/kg i.v. q3w prn for up to 4 injections.

Betaxolol
(Betoptic*) **POM**

Formulations: Ophthalmic: 0.25% suspension in 5 ml bottle or single-use vials; 0.5% solution.

Action: Beta-1 selective beta-blocker that decreases aqueous humour production via beta-adrenoreceptor blockade in the ciliary body.

Use:
- Management of glaucoma.
- Used in the prophylactic management of glaucoma in the unaffected eye of dogs with unilateral primary closed-angle glaucoma.

It can be used alone or in combination with other topical glaucoma drugs, such as a topical carbonic anhydrase inhibitor.

Safety and handling: Normal precautions should be observed.

Contraindications: Avoid in uncontrolled heart failure and asthma.

Adverse reactions: Ocular adverse effects include miosis, conjunctival hyperaemia and local irritation.

Drug interactions: Additive adverse effects may develop if given concurrently with oral beta-blockers. Prolonged atrioventricular conduction times may result if used with calcium antagonists or digoxin.

DOSES

Dogs: 1 drop per eye q12h.

Cats: No information available.

References

Miller PE, Schmidt GM, Vainisi SJ *et al.* (2000) The efficacy of topical prophylactic anti-glaucoma therapy in primary closed-angle glaucoma in dogs: a multicenter clincial trial. *Journal of the American Animal Hospital Association* **36**, 431–438

Bethanecol

(Myotonine*) **POM**

Formulations: Oral: 10 mg, 25 mg tablets.

Action: A muscarinic agonist (cholinergic or parasympathomimetic) that increases urinary bladder detrusor muscle tone and contraction.

Use:
- Management of urinary retention with reduced detrusor tone. It does not initiate a detrusor reflex and is ineffective if the bladder is areflexic.
- Best given on an empty stomach to avoid GI distress.

Safety and handling: Normal precautions should be observed.

Contraindications: Do not use when urethral resistance is increased unless in combination with agents that reduce urethral outflow pressure (e.g. phenoxybenzamine).

Adverse reactions: Vomiting, diarrhoea, GI cramping, anorexia, salivation and bradycardia (with overdosage). Treat overdoses with atropine.

Drug interactions: No information available.

DOSES

Dogs: Detrusor atony: 2.5–15 mg/dog p.o. q8h. Titrate dose upwards to avoid side effects.

Cats: Detrusor atony: 1.25–5 mg/cat p.o. q8h. Titrate dose upwards to avoid side effects.

References

Byron JK (2015) Micturition disorders. *Veterinary Clinics of North America: Small Animal Practice* **45**, 769–782

Bezafibrate

(Bezalip*, Fibrazate XL*) **POM**

Formulations: Oral: 200 mg, 400 mg tablets.

Action: Mechanism of action is not fully understood. Effects are thought to be mediated by peroxisome proliferator-activated receptor (PPAR) alpha and include reduction in hepatic triglyceride synthesis and increased activity of lipoprotein lipase. Overall effect is to decrease serum lipids, with reduced fractions of low density lipoproteins (LDL, cholesterol rich) and very low density lipoproteins (VLDL, triglyceride-rich), as well as an increase in the high density lipoprotein (HDL) cholesterol fraction. Bezafibrate is highly protein bound and is excreted by the kidneys. May reduce blood glucose in diabetic animals.

Use:
- Effective in the management of hyperlipidaemia that is refractory to at least 1 month of dietary management (i.e. low fat diet; many authors additionally recommend omega-3 fatty acid supplements).

Primary disorders that can result in hyperlipidaemia (diabetes mellitus, hypercortisolism, hypothyroidism, pancreatitis, protein-losing nephropathy, high fat diet) must be identified and treated before bezafibrate is used. For dogs receivng treatment for hyperlipidaemia, aim to maintain serum triglycerides <5 mmol/l. Serum triglycerides normalized before 30 days in >90% of 46 dogs with primary or secondary hyperlipidaemia, and no adverse effects were observed in this time period.

Safety and handling: Normal precautions should be observed.

Contraindications: Do not use in pregnant or lactating animals. Contraindicated in severe liver or kidney disease.

Adverse reactions: Adverse effects have not been reported in dogs. Adverse effects in humans include muscle pain from myositis, and GI symptoms.

Drug interactions: Do not administer within 2 hours of cholestyramine (will reduce absorption of bezafibrate). Use with caution in diabetics as concurrent use with insulin may result in severe hypoglycaemia.

DOSES
Dogs: 4–10 mg/kg p.o. q24h. Dogs <12 kg: 50 mg q24h; Dogs 12–25 kg: 100 mg q24h; Dogs >25 kg: 200 mg q24h.
Cats: No information available.

References
De Marco V, Noronha KSM, Casado TC *et al.* (2017) Therapy of canine hyperlipidemia with bezafibrate. *Journal of Veterinary Internal Medicine* **31**, 717–722

Bisacodyl
(Dulcolax*, Entrolax*) **P**

Formulations: Oral: 5 mg yellow, enteric-coated tablets. Rectal: 5 mg, 10 mg suppositories.

Action: Mild stimulant laxative that increases intestinal motility, but inhibits absorption of water. It is locally active with <5% systemic absorption.

Use:
- Management of constipation.

Doses are empirical; none have been defined in the veterinary literature. Onset of action 6–10 hours (oral use) or 15–60 minutes (rectal use).

Safety and handling: Normal precautions should be observed. Do not crush or split the tablets (may lead to cramping).

Contraindications: Must not be used in patients with ileus, intestinal obstruction or dehydration. Not suitable for long-term use.

Adverse reactions: Abdominal discomfort and diarrhoea.

Drug interactions: No information available.

DOSES

Dogs: 5–15 mg/dog prn.
Cats: 2–5 mg/cat prn.

Bismuth salts (Bismuth carbonate, subnitrate and subsalicylate: tri-potassium di-citrato bismuthate (bismuth chelate))

(Pepto-Bismol*) **AVM-GSL, P**

Formulations: Oral: bismuth subsalicylate suspension in various forms, typically 17.5 mg/ml (1.75%); 30 mg bismuth subcarbonate + 240 mg calcium carbonate tablets.

Action: Bismuth is a gastric cytoprotectant with activity against spiral bacteria. Bismuth chelate is effective in healing gastric and duodenal ulcers in humans, through direct toxic effects on gastric *Helicobacter pylori* and by stimulating mucosal prostaglandin and bicarbonate secretion. Bismuth subsalicylate has a mild anti-inflammatory effect.

Use:
*   Management of gastric ulceration, diarrhoea, or as part of combination therapy for gastric *Helicobacter* infections.

It is often used in conjunction with an acid-blocking drug. Doses are empirical; none have been defined in dogs and cats.

Safety and handling: Normal precautions should be observed.

Contraindications: Use bismuth subsalicylate with caution in cats.

Adverse reactions: Avoid long-term use as absorbed bismuth is neurotoxic. Bismuth chelate is contraindicated in renal impairment. Nausea and vomiting reported in humans. Bismuth may cause grey/green/black discolouration of the faeces.

Drug interactions: Absorption of tetracyclines is reduced by bismuth.

DOSES

Dogs: 17.5 mg/ml suspension: 0.25–1 ml/kg p.o. q4–8h.
Cats: Doses as for dogs. Use with caution.

Bleomycin

(Bleomycin*) **POM**

Formulations: Injectable: 15 unit, 30 unit vials of lyophilized powder for reconstitution. 1 mg bleomycin is equivalent to 15 units or 15,000 IU.

Action: Bleomycin is an antibiotic; however its cytotoxicity prevents it from being a useful antimicrobial agent. Causes DNA cleavage and hence prevents cell replication.

Use:
*   Used rarely in canine and feline lymphoma, oral squamous carcinoma, teratomas and thyroid tumours. Single agent use of bleomycin resulted in minimal clinical response in a series of canine lymphoma patients.

- Used in veterinary electrochemotherapy and intralesionally in canine acanthomatous ameloblastoma and melanoma.

Low therapeutic index when used systemically, consult with a specialist before use.

Safety and handling: Potent cytotoxic drug that should only be prepared and administered by trained personnel. See Appendix and specialist texts for further advice on chemotherapeutic agents.

Contraindications: Patients with known hypersensitivity to bleomycin and patients with pre-existing pulmonary disease. Do not use in patients with pre-existing bone marrow suppression. Should be used with caution in patients with reduced renal function.

Adverse reactions: Dermatopathies, conjunctivitis, stomatitis, GI toxicity (e.g. anorexia, vomiting and diarrhoea), pyrexia, increased liver enzyme activities and nephrotoxicity are described. Pulmonary toxicity (pneumonitis or pulmonary fibrosis) is the most severe side effect in both veterinary and human patients (this can rarely progress to fatal pulmonary fibrosis). Unlike many other cytotoxic drugs, myelosuppression is rare but possible.

Drug interactions: General anaesthesia should be performed with extreme caution in patients previously exposed to bleomycin. Prior or concomitant use of radiotherapy or other chemotherapy drugs may lead to increased toxicity from bleomycin.

DOSES
See Appendix for chemotherapy protocols and conversion of bodyweight to body surface area.
Dogs, Cats: 300–500 IU/kg s.c. or i.m. once weekly (note there is a very narrow safety margin – use under the supervision of a veterinary specialist only). A total cumulative dose of 125–250 mg/m^2 should not be exceeded to reduce the risk of pulmonary toxicity.

References
Kelly JM, Belding BA and Schaefer AK (2010) Acanthomatous ameloblastoma in dogs treated with intralesional bleomycin. *Veterinary and Comparative Oncology* **2**, 81–86
Smith AA, Lejeune A, Kow K *et al.* (2017) Clinical response and adverse event profile of bleomycin chemotherapy for canine multicentric lymphoma. *Journal of the American Animal Hospital Association* **53**, 128–134
Stefanou A (2001) Rapid Response: Errors due to Bleomycin Nomenclature. *BMJ* **322**, 548

Bowel cleansing solutions (Macrogol, Polyethylene glycol)
(Klean-Prep*, Moviprep*) **P**

Formulations: Oral: powder for reconstitution.

Action: Bowel cleansing solutions contain polyethylene glycol as an osmotic laxative and balanced electrolytes to maintain isotonicity and prevent net fluid loss or gain.

Use:
- Bowel preparation before colonoscopy or radiographic examination; some authorities do not use in cats or small dogs before colonoscopy.
- May also be used for constipation.
- Powder may take several minutes to dissolve, and reconstitution is best performed by adding warm water to the powder. When administered orally, they should rapidly empty the bowel.

Safety and handling: Normal precautions should be observed.

Contraindications: GI obstruction or perforation. Do not administer to sedated patients or animals with a reduced gag reflex.

Adverse reactions: Diarrhoea is an expected outcome. Occasional vomiting is seen, especially if the maximum volume is administered. Inhalation can cause potentially fatal aspiration pneumonia.

Drug interactions: Oral medication should not be taken within 1 hour of administration as it may be flushed from the GI tract and not absorbed.

DOSES

Dogs: Prior to lower GI examination: 22–33 ml/kg p.o. via stomach tube, 2 or 3 times, at least 4 hours apart.

Cats: Prior to lower GI examination: 22–33 ml/kg p.o. via naso-oesophageal tube.

Brinzolamide CIL

(Azarga*, Azopt*) **POM**

Formulations: Ophthalmic: 10 mg/ml (1%) in 5 ml bottle (Azopt); 1% brinzolamide + 0.5% timolol in 5 ml bottle (Azarga).

Action: Carbonic anhydrase inhibitor; reduces intraocular pressure by reducing the rate of aqueous humour production by inhibition of the formation of bicarbonate ions within the ciliary body epithelium.

Use:
- In the control of all types of glaucoma in dogs, either alone or in combination with other topical drugs.

It may be better tolerated than dorzolamide because of its more physiological pH of 7.5. Brinzolamide is ineffective in normal cats but may reduce IOP in glaucomatous cats; by contrast, dorzolamide is effective in both dogs and cats.

Safety and handling: Normal precautions should be observed.

Contraindications: Severe hepatic or renal impairment. Timolol causes miosis and is therefore not the drug of choice in uveitis, anterior lens luxation or pupil block.

Adverse reactions: Local irritation, keratitis, blepharitis. Brinzolamide may cause less ocular irritation than dorzolamide. Timolol can cause bradycardia and hypotension. Rarely, carbonic anydrase inhibitors have been reported to cause hypokalaemia in cats, and metabolic acidosis in dogs, as a result of systemic absorption.

Drug interactions: No information available.

DOSES

Dogs, Cats: 1 drop per eye q8–12h.

References

Beckwith-Cohen B, Bentley E, Gasper DJ *et al.* (2015) Keratitis in six dogs after topical treatment with carbonic anhydrase inhibitors for glaucoma. *Journal of the American Veterinary Medical Association* **247**, 1419–1426

Thiessen CE, Tofflemire KL, Makielski KM *et al.* (2016) Hypokalemia and suspected renal tubular acidosis associated with topical carbonic anhydrase inhibitor therapy in a cat. *Journal of Veterinary Emergency and Critical Care* **26**, 870–874

British anti-lewisite see Dimercaprol

Bromhexine

(Bisolvon c,d) **POM-V**

Formulations: Oral: 10 mg/g powder.

Action: A bronchial secretolytic that disrupts the structure of acid mucopolysaccharide fibres in mucoid sputum and produces a less viscous mucus, which is easier to expectorate.

Use:
- Mucolytic activity could aid the management of respiratory disease.

Safety and handling: Normal precautions should be observed.

Contraindications: No information available.

Adverse reactions: No information available.

Drug interactions: No information available.

DOSES
Dogs: Mucolysis: 2 mg/kg p.o. q12h.
Cats: Mucolysis: 1 mg/kg p.o. q24h.

Budesonide

CIL

(Benacort*, Budelin*, Budenofalk*, Budenofalk Rectal Foam*, Cortiment*, Entocort*, Jorveza*, Pulmicort*, Rhinocort*) **P**

Formulations: Oral: 1 mg orodispersible tablets, 3 mg gastroresistant capsules, 3 mg capsules containing gastroresistant slow-release granules, 9 mg sustained-release gastrointestinal tablets, 9 mg sachet containing gastroresistant granules. **Rectal:** 2 mg (total dose) rectal foam, 0.02 mg/ml enema. **Inhaled powder:** 100–400 µg (micrograms) per dose. **Nasal spray:** 64–100 µg per dose.

Action: Anti-inflammatory and immunosuppressive steroid.

Use:
- Treatment of chronic enteropathy as a potent corticosteroid that is metabolized on its first pass through the liver in humans and therefore might be expected to have reduced systemic side effects. In a prospective study, dogs with inflammatory bowel disease received monotherapy with either pure powder budesonide (not the available enteric coated formulation) or prednisolone. Remission rates and frequency of adverse events were similar between groups. The dose of this drug is unclear and is extrapolated from use in humans. For enteric use, compounding may be required for small/medium dogs and cats.
- Inhaled formulations are used in humans for asthma or allergic rhinitis. Inhaled budesonide has been reported to improve clinical signs and pulmonary function tests in cats with bronchial disease. The uncoated powder for inhalant use in humans should not be used for oral administration because of hydrolysis by gastric acid.

Safety and handling: Normal precautions should be observed.

Contraindications: Intestinal perforation; severe hepatic impairment.

Adverse reactions: In theory, the rapid metabolism should give minimal systemic adverse effects. However, signs of iatrogenic hypercortisolism (hair loss, muscle wastage, increases in liver enzymes, hepatomegaly, lethargy, polyphagia and polyuria/polydipsia) may develop. Adrenal suppression has been documented in dogs and cats and iatrogenic hypocortisolaemia is a potential risk if budesonide is withdrawn rapidly following prolonged use. In theory, sudden transfer from other steroid therapy might result in signs related to reductions in steroid levels.

Drug interactions: Additive effect if given with other corticosteroids. The metabolism of corticosteroids may be decreased by antifungals. Avoid using with erythromycin, cimetidine, itraconazole and other drugs that inhibit the liver enzymes that metabolize budesonide. The dissolution of the drug's enteric coating depends on pH; do not administer at the same time as oral antacids.

DOSES
Dogs:
- **Intestinal diseases:** dose based on body size ranging from 1 mg/day p.o. q24h for small dogs to 3 mg/day p.o. q12–24h for large/giant dogs. The total dose should probably not exceed 3 mg p.o. q12h.
- **Inhaled:** no information available.

Cats:
- **Intestinal diseases:** Total oral dose should probably not exceed 1 mg p.o. q8h.
- **Inhaled:** 400 µg (micrograms) q12h reported.

References
Dye TL, Diehl KJ, Wheeler SL and Westfall DS (2013) Randomized, controlled trial of budesonide and prednisone for the treatment of idiopathic inflammatory bowel disease in dogs. *Journal of Veterinary Internal Medicine* **27**, 1385–1391
Galler A, Shibly S, Bilek A and Hirt RA (2013) Inhaled budesonide therapy in cats with naturally occurring chronic bronchial disease (feline asthma and chronic bronchitis). *Journal of Small Animal Practice* **54**, 531–536

Bupivacaine
(Marcain*, Sensorcaine*) **POM**

Formulations: Injectable: 2.5 mg/ml, 5.0 mg/ml, 7.5 mg/ml solutions; 2.5 mg/ml, 5.0 mg/ml solutions with 1:200,000 adrenaline.

Action: Reversible blockade of the sodium channel in nerve fibres produces local anaesthesia.

Use:
- Provision of analgesia by perineural nerve blocks, regional and epidural techniques.

Onset of action is significantly slower than lidocaine (20–30 minutes) but duration of action is relatively prolonged (6–8 hours). Lower doses should be used when systemic absorption is likely to be high (e.g. intrapleural analgesia). Small volumes of bupivacaine can be diluted with normal saline to enable wider distribution of the drug for perineural blockade. Doses of bupivacaine up to 2 mg/kg q8h are unlikely to be associated with systemic side effects if injected perineurally, epidurally or intrapleurally.

Safety and handling: Normal precautions should be observed.

Contraindications: Do not give i.v. or use for i.v. regional anaesthesia. Use of bupivacaine with adrenaline is not recommended when local vasoconstriction is undesirable (e.g. end arterial sites) or when a significant degree of systemic absorption is likely.

Adverse reactions: Inadvertent intravascular injection may precipitate severe cardiac arrhythmias that are refractory to treatment.

Drug interactions: All local anaesthetics share similar side effects, therefore the dose of bupivacaine should be reduced when used in combination with other local anaesthetics.

DOSES
Dogs:
- **Perineural:** volume of injection depends on the site of placement and size of the animal. As a guide: 0.1 ml/kg per injection site for femoral and sciatic nerve blocks; 0.1 ml/kg for each of the three injection sites for the combined radial, ulnar, musculocutaneous and median nerve blocks; 0.3 ml/kg for brachial plexus nerve block; 0.25–1 ml total volume for blockade of the infraorbital, mental, maxillary and mandibular nerves. Choose an appropriate concentration of bupivacaine to achieve a 1–2 mg/kg dose within these volume guidelines.
- **Epidural:** 1.6 mg/kg (analgesia to level of L4); 2.3 mg/kg (analgesia to level of T11–T13); 1 mg/kg bupivacaine combined with 0.1–0.2 mg/kg preservative-free morphine. Limit the total volume of solution injected into the epidural space to 1 ml/4.5 kg up to a maximum volume of 6 ml in order to limit the cranial distribution of drugs in the epidural space and prevent adverse pressure effects.
- **Interpleural:** 1 mg/kg diluted with normal saline to a total volume of 5–20 ml depending on the size of the animal. The solution can be instilled via a thoracotomy tube. Dilution reduces pain on injection due to the acidity of bupivacaine.

Cats: Doses as for dogs. Accurate dosing in cats is essential to prevent overdose.

References
Bernard F, Kudnig ST and Monnet E (2006) Hemodynamic effects of intrapleural lidocaine and bupivicaine combination in anaesthetized dogs with and without an open pericardium. *Veterinary Surgery* **35**, 252–258
Radlinsky MG, Mason DE, Roush JK *et al.* (2005) Use of a continuous local infusion of bupivicaine for postoperative analgesia in dogs undergoing total ear canal ablation. *Journal of the American Veterinary Medical Association* **227**, 414–419

Buprenorphine

`CIL`

(Bupaq [c,d], Buprecare [c,d], Buprenodale [c,d], Buprevet [c,d], Vetergesic [c,d], Bupredine [c,d]) **POM-V CD SCHEDULE 3**

Formulations: Injectable: 0.3 mg/ml solution; available in 1 ml vials that do not contain a preservative, or in 10 ml multidose bottle that contains chlorocresol as preservative.

Action: Analgesia through high affinity, low intrinsic activity and slow dissociation with the mu receptor.

Use:
- Relief of mild to moderate perioperative pain.
- It may antagonize the effects of full opioid agonists (e.g. methadone,

fentanyl), although the clinical relevance of interactions between full mu agonists and buprenorphine has been questioned.

It is not recommended to administer buprenorphine when the subsequent administration of full mu agonists is likely. If analgesia is inadequate after buprenorphine, a full mu agonist may be administered without delay. Buprenorphine may be mixed with acepromazine or dexmedetomidine to provide sedation for minor procedures or pre-anaesthetic medication. Response to all opioids is variable between individuals; therefore, assessment of pain after administration is imperative. Onset of action of buprenorphine may be slower than methadone (>15 min). Duration of effect is approximately 6 hours in cats and is likely to be similar in dogs. Buprenorphine is metabolized in the liver; some prolongation of effect may be seen with impaired liver function. The multidose preparation is unpalatable given sublingually due to the preservative. The analgesic efficacy of buprenorphine s.c. may be less than buprenorphine administered i.m. or i.v. to cats; this route is not recommended in cats or dogs.

Safety and handling: Normal precautions should be observed.

Contraindications: Combination with full mu agonists is not recommended for analgesia; therefore, do not use for premedication when administration of potent opioids during surgery is anticipated.

Adverse reactions: Side effects are rare after clinical doses. Buprenorphine crosses the placenta and may exert sedative effects in neonates born to bitches and queens treated prior to parturition. Pain on i.m. injection of the multidose preparation has been anecdotally reported.

Drug interactions: In common with other opioids, buprenorphine will reduce the doses of other drugs required for induction and maintenance of anaesthesia.

DOSES
When used for sedation is generally given as part of a combination. See Appendix for sedation protocols in cats and dogs.

Dogs: Analgesia: 0.02 mg/kg i.v., i.m., s.c. q6h.

Cats: Analgesia: 0.02–0.03 mg/kg i.v., i.m., s.c. q6h. Also well tolerated with some efficacy when given oral transmucosally.

References
Giordano T, Steagall PV, Ferreira TH et al. (2010) Postoperative analgesic effects of intravenous, intramuscular, subcutantous or oral transmucosal buprenorphine administered to cats undergoing ovariohysterectomy. Veterinary Anaesthesia and Analgesia **37**, 357–366
Goyenchea Jaramillo LA, Murrell JC and Hellebrekers LJ (2006) Investigation of the interaction between buprenorphine and sufentanil during anaesthesia for ovariectomy in dogs. Veterinary Anaesthesia and Analgesia **33**, 399–407

Butorphanol
(Alvegesic [c,d], Dolorex [c,d], Torbugesic [c,d], Torbutrol [c,d], Torphasol [c,d]) **POM-V**

Formulations: Injectable: 10 mg/ml solution.

Action: Analgesia resulting from affinity for the kappa opioid receptor. Also has mu receptor antagonist properties and an antitussive action resulting from central depression of the cough mechanism.

Use:
- Management of mild perioperative pain.

- Provision of sedation through combination with acepromazine or alpha-2 agonists.

Butorphanol has a very rapid and relatively short duration of action; in different models analgesia has been shown to last between 45 minutes and 4 hours. Butorphanol is metabolized in the liver and some prolongation of effect may be seen with impaired liver function. Butorphanol crosses the placenta and may exert sedative effects in neonates born to bitches and queens treated prior to parturition. Butorphanol is unlikely to be adequate for the management of severe pain. Higher doses of full mu agonists may be needed to provide additional analgesia after butorphanol but it is not necessary to wait 4 hours after butorphanol administration to give other opioids. Response to all opioids appears to be very variable between individuals; therefore, assessment of pain after administration is imperative.

Safety and handling: Protect from light.

Contraindications: Animals with diseases of the lower respiratory tract associated with copious mucus production. Premedication when administration of potent opioids during surgery is anticipated.

Adverse reactions: As a kappa agonist/mu antagonist, side effects such as respiratory depression, bradycardia and vomiting are rare after clinical doses.

Drug interactions: In common with other opioids, butorphanol will reduce the doses of other drugs required for induction and maintenance of anaesthesia. Combination with full mu agonists is not recommended for analgesia, addition of butorphanol will reduce analgesia produced from the full mu agonist.

DOSES
When used for sedation is generally given as part of a combination. See Appendix for sedation protocols in cats and dogs.
Dogs:
- **Analgesia:** 0.2–0.5 mg/kg i.v., i.m., s.c.
- **Antitussive:** 0.05–0.1 mg/kg i.v., i.m., s.c.

Cats: Analgesia: 0.2–0.5 mg/kg i.v., i.m., s.c.

References
Simon BT, Steagall PV, Monteiro BP *et al.* (2016) Antinociceptive effects of intravenous administration of hydromorphone hydrochloride alone or followed by buprenorphine hydrochloride or butorphanol tartrate to healthy conscious cats. *American Journal of Veterinary Research* **77**, 245–251

Butylscopolamine (Hyoscine)
(Buscopan [d], Spasmium [d], Spasmipur, Sympagesic [d])
POM-V, POM

Formulations: Injectable: 4 mg/ml butylscopolamine + 500 mg/ml metamizole in 100 ml multidose bottle; 20 mg/ml butylscopolamine only. Oral: 10 mg, 20 mg tablets.

Action: Inhibits M1 muscarinic acetylcholine receptors in the GI and urinary tracts causing smooth muscle relaxation but does not cross the blood–brain barrier.

Use:
- Part of supportive therapy for diarrhoea in dogs, particularly when pain or abdominal discomfort is present.
- Control of pain associated with urinary obstruction in dogs.

Should only be used in combination with investigations into the cause of abdominal pain or definitive relief of urinary obstruction.

Safety and handling: Avoid self-injection: metamizole can cause reversible but potentially serious agranulocytosis and skin allergies. Protect solution from light.

Contraindications: Intestinal obstruction.

Adverse reactions: Dry mouth, blurred vision, hesitant micturition and constipation at doses acting as gut neuromuscular relaxants. The i.m. route may cause a local reaction.

Drug interactions: Metamizole should not be given to dogs that have been treated with a phenothiazine, as hypothermia may result. Effects may be potentiated by concurrent use of other anticholinergic or analgesic drugs.

DOSES

Dogs: Control of diarrhoea and/or abdominal discomfort: 0.1 ml/kg i.v., i.m. q12h (Buscopan Compositum, Sympagesic); 0.5 mg/kg i.m., p.o. q12h (butylscopolamine only).

Cats: Do not use.

Cabergoline

(Galastop[d], Kelactin[c,d]) **POM-V**

Formulations: Oral: 50 μg (micrograms)/ml solution.

Action: Potent selective inhibition of prolactin, dopamine (D2) agonist.

Use:
- Induction of oestrus.
- Control of false pregnancy in the bitch, including associated behavioural problems.
- Treatment of galactostasis in lactating bitches.
- Also used to induce abortion in bitches and queens.

Safety and handling: Normal precautions should be observed.

Contraindications: Do not use in pregnant bitches unless abortion is desired. Should not be used in combination with hypotensive drugs or in animals in a hypotensive state.

Adverse reactions: Vomiting or anorexia may occur after the first one or two doses in a small proportion of cases; there is no need to discontinue treatment unless vomiting is severe or it persists beyond the second dose. A degree of drowsiness may be seen in the first two days of dosing. May induce transient hypotension.

Drug interactions: Metoclopramide antagonizes the effects on prolactin. Cabergoline may increase the hypotensive effects of other drugs.

DOSES

Dogs: 5 μg (micrograms)/kg p.o. q24h for 4–6 days. Control of aggression-related signs may require dosing for 2 weeks. **To induce abortion:** 15 μg/kg p.o. between days 30 and 42.

Cats: To induce abortion: 15 μg (micrograms)/kg p.o. between days 30 and 42.

References
Harvey MA, Dale MJ, Lindley S and Waterston MM (1999) A study of the aetiology of pseudopregnancy in the bitch and the effect of cabergoline therapy. *Veterinary Record* **144**, 433–436

CaEDTA see **Edetate calcium disodium**

Calcium acetate

(Phosex*, Renacet*) **POM**

Formulations: Oral: 475 mg (102.25 mg calcium), 950 mg (240.50 mg calcium) (Renacet), 1 g (Phosex) tablets.

Action: Binds phosphorus in GI tract, thus lowering serum phosphate levels over a wider range of pH than calcium carbonate.

Use:
- Phosphate reduction in chronic renal failure.

Phosphate-binding agents are usually only used if low phosphate diets are unsuccessful. Monitor serum phosphate levels at 4–6 week intervals and adjust dosage accordingly if trying to achieve target serum concentrations. Monitor for hypercalcaemia.

Safety and handling: Normal precautions should be observed.

Contraindications: Hypercalcaemia and calcium urolithiasis.

Adverse reactions: Risk of increasing the calcium:phosphate ratio and thus the incidence of soft tissue and vascular calcification.

Drug interactions: May affect absorption of tetracycline and fluoroquinolone antibiotics. Increased risk of hypercalcaemia with concurrent calcitriol administration.

DOSES

Dogs, Cats: Chronic kidney disease: 60–90 mg/kg p.o. q24h divided (give with each meal).

References
Polzin DJ (2013) Evidence-based step-wise approach to managing chronic kidney disease in dogs and cats. *Journal of Veterinary Emergency and Critical Care* **23**, 205–215

Calcium aluminosilicate (Bentonite, Hydrated calcium aluminosilicate, Smectite)
(VBS Clay) **AVM-GSL**

Formulations: Oral: Tub of 100 g powder. Each scoop contains 500 mg.

Action: Adsorbent antidiarrhoeal agent. May have other properties but the mechanism of action is not clearly understood.

Use:
• May be used as part of management of diarrhoea in dogs and cats.

In an open-label randomized clinical trial in dogs with chemotherapy-induced diarrhoea, the time to resolution of diarrhoea was shorter in the treated group compared with the control group.

Safety and handling: Normal precautions should be observed.

Contraindications: Intestinal obstruction or perforation.

Adverse reactions: No information available. Appears well tolerated and safe in human adults and children.

Drug interactions: May affect absorption of other drugs. It is suggested to administer these at least 2 hours apart.

DOSES

Dogs, Cats: Give one level scoop (500 mg, 1/8 teaspoon) p.o. for every 4.5 kg bodyweight, twice daily. Higher doses (500 mg/kg p.o. per day divided in two or three doses) were used in the above-mentioned trial.

References
Fournier Q, Serra JC, Williams C and Bavcar S (2021) Chemotherapy-induced diarrhoea in dogs and its management with smectite: Results of a monocentric open-label randomized clinical trial. *Veterinary and Comparative Oncology* **19**, 25–33

Calcium salts (Calcium borogluconate, Calcium carbonate, Calcium chloride, Calcium gluconate, Calcium lactate)

(Calcichew*, Many cattle preparations, e.g. Calcibor)
POM-V, POM

Formulations: There are many formulations available; a selection is given here.
- Injectable: 200 mg/ml calcium borogluconate solution equivalent to 15 mg/ml calcium formed from 168 mg/ml of calcium gluconate and 34 mg/ml boric acid (Calcibor 20); 100 mg/ml (10%) calcium chloride solution containing 27.3 mg/ml elemental calcium (1.36 mEq/ml, 680 μmol (micromoles)/ml); 100 mg/ml calcium gluconate solution in 10 ml ampoules containing 9 mg elemental calcium/ml (0.45 mEq/ml).
- Oral: 600 mg calcium gluconate tablets (53.4 mg elemental calcium); 1250 mg chewable calcium carbonate tablets (Calcichew) (500 mg elemental calcium).
- Note on other formulations: 11.2 mg calcium gluconate, 13.3 mg calcium borogluconate, 7.7 mg calcium lactate, 3.6 mg calcium chloride; each contains 1 mg (0.5 mEq) elemental calcium.
- Minor component of Aqupharm No.9 and No.11.

Action: Calcium is an essential element involved in maintenance of numerous homeostatic roles and key reactions including activation of enzymes, cell membrane potentials and nerve and musculoskeletal function.

Use:
- Management of hypocalcaemia.
- Management of hyperkalaemic cardiotoxicity associated with urinary obstruction.

Calcium gluconate and borogluconate are preferred. Serum calcium levels and renal function tests should be assessed before starting therapy. ECG monitoring during i.v. infusions is advised. Avoid mixed electrolyte solutions intended for cattle use if possible. Treatment of hyperkalaemic cardiotoxicity with calcium rapidly corrects arrhythmias but effects are short-lived (5–10 min to effect) and i.v. glucose 0.5–1 g/kg ± insulin may be needed to decrease serum potassium. Parenteral calcium should be used very cautiously in patients receiving digitalis glycosides or those with cardiac or renal disease.

Safety and handling: Normal precautions should be observed.

Contraindications: Ventricular fibrillation or hypercalcaemia. Calcium should be avoided in pregnancy unless there is a deficient state. Hyperkalaemia associated with hypoadrenocorticism is often associated with hypercalcaemia and therefore additional calcium is not recommended in those cases.

Adverse reactions: Hypercalcaemia can occur, especially in renal impairment or cardiac disease. Tissue irritation is common and can occur with injectable preparation regardless of route. Rapid injection may cause hypotension, cardiac arrhythmias and cardiac arrest. Perivascular administration is treated by stopping the infusion, infiltrating the tissue with normal saline and applying topical corticosteroids. Note that some chewable formulations of calcium (e.g. Calcichew) may contain xylitol and overdosage could produce hypoglycaemia.

Drug interactions: Animals receiving digitalis glycosides are more prone to develop arrhythmias if given i.v. calcium. All calcium salts may antagonize verapamil and other calcium-channel blockers. Calcium borogluconate is compatible with most i.v. fluids except those containing other divalent cations or phosphorus. Calcium borogluconate is reportedly compatible with lidocaine, adrenaline and hydrocortisone. Calcium chloride is incompatible with amphotericin B, cefalotin sodium and chlorphenamine. Calcium gluconate is incompatible with many drugs, including lipid emulsions, propofol, amphotericin B, cefamandole, naftate, cefalotin sodium, dobutamine, methylprednisolone sodium succinate and metoclopramide. Consult manufacturers' data sheets for incompatibilities with other solutions.

DOSES

Dogs:
- Parenteral treatment of hypocalcaemia or hyperkalaemic cardiotoxicity: 50–150 mg/kg calcium (boro)gluconate (3.8–11.4 mEq/kg of elemental calcium when borogluconate is used or 4.5–14 mg/kg of elemental calcium when gluconate is used). Alternatively, 5–10 mg/kg calcium chloride or 0.05–0.1 ml/kg of a 10% solution i.v. (equivalent to 0.068–0.136 mEq/kg). Additional doses to a maximum of 1–1.5 g/kg calcium (boro)gluconate may need to be administered i.v. over the next 24 hours. Adjust dose by monitoring serum calcium and phosphorus levels.
- Oral treatment of hypocalcaemia: 5–22 mg of elemental calcium/kg p.o. q8h; adjust dose by monitoring serum calcium and phosphorus levels.

Cats:
- Parenteral treatment of hypocalcaemia: 95–140 mg/kg calcium gluconate slowly i.v. to effect. Using 10% calcium gluconate, this is equivalent to 1–1.5 ml/kg slowly i.v. over 10–20 min. Monitor ECG if possible. If bradycardia or QT interval shortening occurs, slow rate or temporarily discontinue. Once life-threatening signs are resolved, add calcium gluconate to i.v. fluids and administer slowly at 60–90 mg/kg/day elemental calcium. This converts to 2.5 ml/kg of 10% calcium gluconate q6–8h or the equivalent as a constant rate infusion over 24 hours. Monitor serum calcium and adjust as needed.
- Oral treatment of hypocalcaemia: Begin oral therapy at 10–25 mg/kg elemental calcium q6–8h; adjust dose by monitoring serum calcium and phosphorus levels.

Cannabidiol (CBD oil)

(Epidiolex*, Sativex*) **POM, P, GSL**

Formulations: A variety of different forms of CBD oil are available over the counter at human pharmacies in the UK. Each formulation should come with a certificate of analysis providing information about the constituents of the drug, although commonly the actual cannabidiol content is lower than advertised. Only products containing <0.1% tetrahydrocannabinol (THC) are legal in the UK.

Action: Cannabidiols bind to cannabinoid receptors that form the endocannabinoid system in the body. Two main cannabinoid receptors have been identified, CB1 and CB2. CB1 receptors are widely distributed in the CNS and the periphery and are responsible for the psychoactive effects of THC. CB2 receptors principally modify homeostasis in the immune system, with marked upregulation of the CB2 receptor accompanying inflammation. Cannabidiols bind to CB1 and CB2 receptors. With respect to the pain pathway, cannabidiols reduce the release of excitatory neurotransmitters in the central nervous system, reducing onward transmission of noxious stimuli to higher brain centres. Use of multiple cannabinoid and terpene compounds together rather than pure isolates produces what is termed the 'entourage effect', whereby multiple receptors are targeted at once to increase efficacy.

Use:
- Cannabidiols have been used for the management of chronic pain, particularly pain associated with osteoarthritis.
- They have also been used for seizure control in epileptic patients.

The evidence base for both indications is very poor compared to that for authorized products.

Safety and handling: Normal precautions should be observed.

Contraindications: Avoid if there is marked liver dysfunction. The endocannabinoid system may be immature in neonates, along with immature liver function, so cannabinoids should be avoided in pregnant and nursing animals and animals less than 8 weeks of age.

Adverse reactions: Intoxication leading to CNS depression is common with THC. Cats find most formulations of cannabidiol aversive, showing signs of hypersalivation and headshaking.

Drug interactions: Cannabinoids are potent inhibitors of the cytochrome P450 enzymes, although clinical manifestations of this are rare in the animal and human literature. Caution should be used when combining cannabidiols with other drugs, and monitoring should be carried out to evaluate changes in liver enzymes, as for animals receiving chronic NSAIDs. There are also calcium channel effects seen with the cannabinoids, and drugs that work through calcium channels (such as gabapentin) will likely need to be modified when used concurrently.

DOSES
Dogs, Cats: 1–2 mg/kg p.o. q12h is normally recommended, although the evidence base for this dose range is limited. Start at the low end of the dose range and increase dose if no effect is seen within 7 days.

References
Brioschi FA, Di Cesare F, Gioeni D *et al.* (2020) Oral transmucosal cannabidiol oil formulation as part of a multimodal analgesic regimen: effects on pain relief and quality of life improvement in dogs affected by spontaneous osteoarthritis. *Animals* **10**, 1505
Gamble LJ, Boesch BJ, Frye CW *et al.* (2018) Pharmacokinetics, Safety, and Clinical, Efficacy of Cannabidiol Treatment in Osteoarthritic Dogs. *Frontiers in Veterinary Science* **5**, 165

Capromorelin (Capromorelin tartrate)
(Elura, Entyce) **POM**

Formulations: Oral: 20 mg/ml flavoured liquid for cats (Elura); 30 mg/ml flavoured liquid for dogs (Entyce).

Action: Selective ghrelin receptor agonist that stimulates appetite leading to weight gain and increasing concentrations of serum growth hormone (GH) and insulin-like growth factor-1 (IGF-1).

Use:
- Used to stimulate appetite in hyporexic dogs.
- Management of weight loss in cats with chronic kidney disease.

Safety and handling: Normal precautions should be observed.

Contraindications: Animals with hypersensitivity to capromorelin and those with hypersomatotropism. Avoid use in animals with significant liver dysfunction as primarily metabolized by the liver. Avoid use in animals predisposed to hypotension.

Adverse reactions: Appears to be well tolerated in dogs with only some GI side effects (e.g. vomiting, diarrhoea) at high dosages. In cats, vomiting, ptyalism, lip smacking and head shaking have been noted at high doses. Rarely, hypotension and bradycardia have been reported in cats, often necessitating fluid therapy.

Drug interactions: No information available.

DOSES

Dogs: 3 mg/kg p.o. q24h.

Cats: 1–3 mg/kg p.o. q24h.

References

Wofford JA, Zollers B, Rhodes L et al. (2018) Evaluation of the safety of daily administration of capromorelin in cats. *Journal of Veterinary Pharmacology and Therapeutics* **41**, 324–333

Zollers B, Huebner M, Armintrout G et al. (2017) Evaluation of the safety in dogs of long-term, daily oral administration of capromorelin, a novel drug for stimulation of appetite. *Journal of Veterinary Pharmacology and Therapeutics* **40**, 248–255

Carbimazole

(Vidalta [c]) **POM-V**

Formulations: Oral: 10 mg, 15 mg tablets in a sustained-release formulation.

Action: Carbimazole is metabolized to the active drug methimazole, which interferes with the synthesis of thyroid hormones in a dose-dependent fashion.

Use:
- Control of thyroid hormone levels in cats with hyperthyroidism.
- Carbimazole has also been used in canine hyperthyroidism but there are no data on the use of the sustained-release formulation in dogs.

Safety and handling: Normal precautions should be observed.

Contraindications: Animals that have an adverse reaction to methimazole are likely to also have an adverse reaction to carbimazole.

Adverse reactions: Vomiting and inappetence/anorexia may be seen but are often transient. Jaundice, cytopenias, immune-mediated diseases and dermatological changes (pruritus, alopecia and self-induced trauma) are reported but rare. Treatment of hyperthyroidism can decrease glomerular filtration rate, thereby increasing serum urea and creatinine values, and can occasionally unmask occult renal failure.

Drug interactions: Carbimazole should be discontinued before iodine-131 treatment. Do not use with low iodine prescription diets.

DOSES

Dogs, Cats: Hyperthyroidism: starting dose 15 mg/animal p.o. q24h unless total thyroxine concentrations are <100 nmol/l, in which case starting dose is 10 mg p.o. q24h. Adjust dose in 5 mg increments but do not break tablets.

References

Daminet S, Kooistra HS, Fracassi F et al. (2014) Best practice for the pharmacological management of hyperthyroid cats with antithyroid drugs. *Journal of Small Animal Practice* **55**, 4–13

Carbomer 980

(Lubrithal, Ocry-gel, OptixCare, Viscotears*) **P, general sale**

Formulations: Ophthalmic: 0.2% (10 g tube, single-use vial), 0.25% (10 g tube) gel. This formulation is marketed specifically for small animals. Other formulations are widely available for general sale.

Action: Linear polymer (polyacrylic acid). Replaces the aqueous and mucin layers of the trilaminar tear film (mucinomimetic).

Use:
- Tear replacement.
- Management of quantitative (keratoconjunctivitis sicca and qualitative tear film disorders.

It has longer corneal contact time than the aqueous tear substitutes (e.g. polyvinyl alcohol).

Safety and handling: Normal precautions should be observed.

Contraindications: No information available.

Adverse reactions: It is tolerated well and ocular irritation is unusual.

Drug interactions: No information available.

DOSES

Dogs, Cats: 1 drop per eye q4–6h.

Carboplatin

(Carboplatin*, Paraplatin*) **POM**

Formulations: Injectable: 10 mg/ml solution.

Action: Binds to DNA to form intra- and interstrand crosslinks and DNA-protein crosslinks, resulting in inhibition of DNA synthesis and function.

Use:
- May be of use in a number of neoplastic diseases including anal sac adenocarcinoma, squamous cell carcinoma, ovarian carcinoma, mediastinal carcinoma, pleural adenocarcinoma, nasal carcinoma and thyroid adenocarcinoma.
- Improves survival times when used as an adjunct to amputation in dogs with appendicular osteosarcoma.

The drug is highly irritant and must be administered via a preplaced i.v. catheter. Do not use needles or i.v. sets containing aluminium as precipitation of the drug may occur. This drug is generally now preferred over cisplatin due to reduced GI and renal toxicity. Use with caution in patients with abnormal renal function, active infections, hearing impairment or pre-existing hepatic disease.

Safety and handling: Potent cytotoxic drug that should only be prepared and administered by trained personnel. See Appendix and specialist texts for further advice on chemotherapeutic agents.

Contraindications: Contraindicated in patients with known hypersensitivity to platinum-containing compounds. Do not use in patients with pre-existing bone marrow suppression.

Adverse reactions: Include myelosuppression, nephrotoxicity, ototoxicity, nausea, vomiting, electrolyte abnormalities, neurotoxicity and anaphylactic reactions (including a delayed cutaneous hypersensitivity. However, produces fewer adverse reactions than cisplatin. Note that there may be delayed or unpredictable side effects in cats (thought to be due to changes in glomerular filtration rate in older cats).

Drug interactions: Concomitant use of aminoglycosides or other nephrotoxic agents may increase risk of nephrotoxicity. May adversely affect the safety and efficacy of vaccinations. Potential to act as a radiosensitizer for patients receiving concommitant radiotherapy.

DOSES

See Appendix for chemotherapy protocols and conversion of bodyweight to body surface area.

Dogs: 250–300 mg/m^2 i.v. q3–4wk injected into the side port of a freely running i.v. infusion of 0.9% NaCl over 10–15 min. Intrapleural/intraperitoneal dose: 225–300 mg/m^2 diluted in 0.9% NaCl or 5% dextrose water (in one text this is diluted to 10 mg/ml then again in 1 ml per 4.5 kg bodyweight) over 5–10 min (it is advised to consult a veterinary oncology specialist before administering via this route).

Cats: 200–260 mg/m^2 i.v. q3–4wk injected into the side port of a freely running i.v. infusion of 0.9% NaCl over 10–15 min. Intrapleural/intraperitoneal dose: 200–240 mg/m^2 diluted in 0.9% NaCl or 5% dextrose water over a 5–10 min period (it is advised to consult a veterinary oncology specialist before administering via this route).

References

Bailey DB, Rassnick KM, Erb HN *et al.* (2004) Effect of glomerular filtration rate on clearance and myelotoxicity of carboplatin in cats with tumors. *American Journal of Veterinary Research* **65**, 1502–1507

Skorupski KA, Uhl JM, Szivek A *et al.* (2016) Carboplatin *versus* alternating carboplatin and doxorubicin for the adjuvant treatment of canine appendicular osteosarcoma: a randomized, phase III trial. *Veterinary and Comparative Oncology* **14**, 81–87

Carprofen

(Canidryl [d], Carprieve [c,d], Carprodyl [d], Carprox Vet [d], Rimadyl [c,d], Rimifin [d], Rycarfa [c,d]) **POM-V**

Formulations: Injectable: 50 mg/ml. Oral: 20 mg, 50 mg, 100 mg, 120 mg tablets (in plain and palatable formulations).

Action: Preferentially inhibits COX-2 enzyme, thereby limiting the production of prostaglandins involved in inflammation. Other non-COX-mediated mechanisms are suspected to contribute to the anti-inflammatory effect but these have not yet been identified.

Use:
- Control of postoperative pain and inflammation following surgery.
- Reduction of chronic inflammation, e.g. degenerative joint disease, osteoarthritis.

In cats, carprofen is only authorized as a single perioperative dose for the control of postoperative pain. Carprofen also has antipyretic effects. All NSAIDs should be administered cautiously in the perioperative period. Although carprofen preferentially inhibits COX-2, it may still adversely affect renal perfusion during periods of hypotension. If hypotension during anaesthesia is anticipated, delay carprofen administration until the animal is fully recovered from anaesthesia and normotensive. Prolonged long-term treatment should be under veterinary supervision. In cats, due to the longer half-life and narrower therapeutic index, particular care should be taken not to exceed the recommended dose; use of a 1 ml graduated syringe is recommended to measure the dose accurately. Tablets are not authorized for use in cats.

Safety and handling: Formulations that use palatable tablets can be extremely palatable. Animals have been reported to eat tablets spontaneously, resulting in overdose. Ensure that tablets are stored out of reach of animals. Store injectable solution in the refrigerator; once broached the product is stable for use at temperatures up to 25°C for 28 days.

Contraindications: Do not give to dehydrated, hypovolaemic or hypotensive patients or those with GI disease or blood clotting abnormalities. Administration of carprofen to animals with renal disease must be carefully evaluated and is not advisable in the perioperative period. Do not give to pregnant animals or animals <6 weeks old. Liver disease prolongs the metabolism of carprofen, leading to the potential for drug accumulation and overdose with repeated dosing.

Adverse reactions: GI signs may occur in all animals after NSAID administration. Stop therapy if this persists beyond 1–2 days. Some animals develop signs with one NSAID and not another. A 3–5 day wash-out period should be allowed before starting another NSAID after cessation of therapy. Stop therapy immediately if GI bleeding is suspected. There is a small risk that NSAIDs may precipitate cardiac failure in humans and this risk in animals is unknown.

Drug interactions: Different NSAIDs should not be administered within 24 hours of each other. The optimal wash-out period between NSAID administration and glucocorticoid administration is unknown; allowing 3–5 days between the two classes of drugs is recommended. The nephrotoxic tendencies of all NSAIDs are significantly increased when administered concurrently with other nephrotoxic agents, e.g. aminoglycosides.

DOSES
Dogs: 4 mg/kg i.v., s.c. preoperatively or at time of anaesthetic induction; single dose should provide analgesia for up to 24 hours. Continued analgesia can be provided orally at 4 mg/kg/day in single or divided doses for up to 5 days after injection. In dogs started on oral medication, subject to clinical response, the dose may be reduced to 2 mg/kg/day as a single dose after 7 days.

Cats: 4 mg/kg i.v., s.c. preoperatively or at time of anaesthetic induction.

References
Mansa S, Palmer E, Grondahl C *et al.* (2007) Long term treatment with carprofen of 805 dogs with osteoarthritis. *Veterinary Record* **160**, 427–430

Carvedilol

(Carvedilol*) **POM**

Formulations: Oral: 3.125 mg, 6.25 mg, 12.5 mg, 25 mg tablets.

Action: Non-selective beta-adrenergic blocker with the afterload reduction properties of an alpha-1 adrenergic blocker. Additional antioxidant properties may decrease the oxidative stress associated with heart failure.

Use:
- Has been advocated for use as an adjunctive therapy in the management of chronic heart failure due to valvular disease or dilated cardiomyopathy.
- Potential antihypertensive drug in patients that do not respond to first-line therapy.

Veterinary experience is limited and benefit has not been established. Limited data on pharmacokinetics and pharmacodynamics in dogs. Treatment should not be started until congestive heart failure has been stabilized for at least 2 weeks initially. Since it undergoes extensive hepatic metabolism, caution should be exercised in patients with hepatic insufficiency.

Safety and handling: Normal precautions should be observed.

Contraindications: Patients with bradyarrhythmias, acute or decompensated heart failure and bronchial disease. Do not administer concurrently with alpha-adrenergic agonists (e.g. adrenaline).

Adverse reactions: Potential side effects include lethargy, diarrhoea, bradycardia, AV block, myocardial depression, exacerbation of heart failure, syncope, hypotension and bronchospasm. A reduction in the glomerular filtration rate may exacerbate pre-existing renal impairment.

Drug interactions: The hypotensive effect of carvedilol is enhanced by many agents that depress myocardial activity, including anaesthetic agents, phenothiazines, antihypertensive drugs, diuretics and diazepam. There is an increased risk of bradycardia, severe hypotension, heart failure and AV block if carvedilol is used concurrently with calcium-channel blockers. Hypotensive effect may be antagonized by NSAIDs. Concurrent digoxin administration potentiates bradycardia. Carvedilol may enhance the hypoglycaemic effect of insulin. Carvedilol increases plasma concentration of ciclosporin. Rifampin can decrease carvedilol plasma concentrations.

DOSES

Dogs: Start at 0.05–0.1 mg/kg p.o. q12h and gradually increase at 2-week intervals to target dose of 0.3–0.4 mg/kg p.o. q12h, if tolerated. Doses of 0.3 mg/kg p.o. q12h and then increased at intervals up to 1.1 mg/kg p.o. q12h have been reported in ACVIM stage B2 (cardiac remodelling, no signs on cardiac failure) degenerative mitral valve disease.

Cats: No information available.

References

Gordon SG, Saunders AB, Hariu CD *et al.* (2012) Retrospective review of carvedilol administration in 38 dogs with preclinical chronic valvular heart disease. *Journal of Veterinary Cardiology* **14**, 243–252

Oyama MA, Sisson D, Prosek R *et al.* (2007) Carvedilol in dogs with dilated cardiomyopathy. *Journal of Veterinary Internal Medicine* **21**, 1272–1279

α-**Casozepine** (Benzodiazepine-like decapeptide)

(Zylkene) **general sale**

Formulations: Oral: 75 mg, 225 mg, 450 mg capsules; also included in some other formulations including diets alongside other potentially calming nutraceuticals.

Action: GABA$_B$ agonist.

Use:
- Used to reduce the impact of a range of stressors, including unusual and unpredictable situations or before changes to the normal environment, such as kennelling or the arrival of a new baby.

It is suggested that dosing should start before exposure to the stressor; however, the value of the evidence in support of the use of α-casozepine for the management of anxiety is disputed.

Safety and handling: Normal precautions apply.

Contraindications: None.

Adverse reactions: Occasional anecdotal reports of diarrhoea noted.

Drug interactions: None.

DOSES
Dogs, Cats: 15 mg/kg p.o. q24h.

References
Buckley LA (2017) Is alpha-casozepine efficacious at reducing anxiety in dogs? *Veterinary Evidence* **2**, doi.org/10.18849/ve.v2i3.67

Cat appeasing pheromone

(Feliway Friends) **general sale**

Formulations: Diffuser. Feliway Optimum is an engineered pheromone variant, which claims to have properties of Feliway Classic and Cat Appeasing Pheromone.

Action: The mixture is based on derivatives of the dermal secretions produced by the queen after giving birth which help to keep kittens within the safety of the nest. The signal causes an innate emotional bias in the perception of the environment that does not require learning, but makes the cat feel more secure. This sense of safety and security appears to reduce antagonism between cats living in the same home.

Use:
- When there are signs of conflict between cats within the same household, including overt aggression, hissing, growling and chasing (not play related) and more subtle signs of social tension such as consistent blocking behaviour, and staring down or consistent avoidance.
- Also when a cat is stressed by the presence of another animal (e.g. dog) in the home.

In such circumstances some cats can also show repetitive minor medical ailments as a result of chronic stress, such as persistent vomiting, cystitis and overgrooming. In these cases, the animal should be carefully checked for medical causes before considering behaviour management. Should be used alongside a behaviour management plan that allows different cats access to their own core resources. Published reports show marginal effects and it is prefereable to use as a preventive if problems can be anticipated, e.g. when introducing a new cat.

In the case of tension between a cat and a dog, it seems that the use of dog appeasing pheromone may be preferable, as relaxing the dog reduces tension with the cat.

Safety and handling: Normal precautions apply.

Contraindications: None.

Adverse reactions: None reported; if no improvement within 1 month, reassess diagnosis.

Drug interactions: None.

DOSES

Cats: Plug-in diffuser which should be left running (not switched on and off), ideally where the cats rest; not where they come into conflict.

Dogs: Not applicable.

References

DePorter TL, Bledsoe DL, Beck A and Ollivier E (2019) Evaluation of the efficacy of an appeasing pheromone diffuser product *versus* placebo for management of feline aggression in multi-cat households: a pilot study. *Journal of feline medicine and surgery* **21**, 293–305

Prior M and Mills D (2020) Cats *versus* Dogs: the efficacy of Feliway FriendsTM and AdaptilTM products in multispecies homes. *Frontiers in Veterinary Science* **7**, 1–10

CBD oil see **Cannabidiol**
CCNU see **Lomustine**

Cefalexin (Cephalexin)

(Cefaseptin [c,d], Cephacare [c,d], Cephorum [d], Ceporex [c,d], Rilexine [c,d], Therios [c,d], Tsefalen [d]) **POM-V**

Formulations: Oral: 50 mg, 75 mg, 120 mg, 250 mg, 300 mg, 500 mg, 600 mg, 750 mg, 1000 mg tablets.

Action: 1st generation cephalosporin. Binds to penicillin-binding proteins involved in bacterial cell wall synthesis, decreasing cell wall strength and rigidity, and affecting cell division. Resistant to some penicillinases produced by *Staphylococcus* spp. but ineffective against methicillin-resistant staphylococci. Works in a time-dependent fashion.

Use:

- Active against most Gram-positive (not *Enterococcus*) and some Gram-negative organisms (*Pasteurella*, *Klebsiella* and *Escherichia coli*).

Pseudomonas and *Proteus* are often resistant. Maintaining levels above the MIC is critical for efficacy and prolonged dosage intervals or missed doses can compromise therapeutic response. Dose and dosing interval is determined by infection site, severity and organism. In severe or acute conditions, doses may be doubled or given at more frequent intervals.

Safety and handling: Normal precautions should be observed.

Contraindications: Avoid use in animals with hypersensitivity to other beta-lactam antimicrobials (cross-hypersensitivity in <10% of human patients).

Adverse reactions: Vomiting and diarrhoea most common; administration with food may reduce these reactions.

Drug interactions: May be an increased risk of nephrotoxicity if cephalosporins are used with aminoglycosides, amphotericin or loop diuretics (e.g. furosemide); monitor renal function.

DOSES

Classified as category C (Caution) by the EMA.

See Appendix for guidelines on responsible antibiotic use.

Dogs, Cats: 15–30 mg/kg p.o. q8–12h. Increased doses (20–30 mg/kg p.o. q8–12h) should be used for superficial pyoderma and to treat severe, Gram-negative or orthopaedic infections.

Cefazolin
POM

Formulations: Injectable: 1 g, 2 g powders for reconstitution (sodium salt).

Action: 1st generation cephalosporin. Binds to penicillin-binding proteins involved in bacterial cell wall synthesis, decreasing cell wall strength and rigidity, and affecting cell division. Resistant to some penicillinases produced by *Staphylococcus* spp. but ineffective against meticillin-resistant staphylococci. Works in a time-dependent fashion.

Use:
- Active against most Gram-positive (not *Enterococcus*) and some Gram-negative organisms (*Pasteurella*, *Klebsiella* and *Escherichia coli*). Highest activity against Gram-negative organisms of the 1st generation cephalosporins. Poor activity against anaerobic bacteria.
- Used for surgical prophylaxis (clean-contaminated or contaminated procedures).
- Treatment of respiratory tract, genitourinary tract, biliary tract, bone and joint infections.

Safety and handling: Normal precautions should be observed.

Contraindications: Avoid use in animals with hypersensitivity to other beta-lactam antimicrobials (cross-hypersensitivity in <10% of human patients).

Adverse reactions: Vomiting and diarrhoea most common.

Drug interactions: May be an increased risk of nephrotoxicity if cephalosporins are used with aminoglycosides, amphotericin or loop diuretics (e.g. furosemide); monitor renal function.

DOSES

Classified as category C (Caution) by the EMA.

See Appendix for guidelines on responsible antibiotic use.

Dogs, Cats:
- For surgical prophylaxis: 22 mg/kg i.v. slowly (over 5 min) 30–60 min prior to surgery and then repeat q2h during surgery.
- For susceptible infections: 20–30 mg/kg i.v. q8h.

Cefotaxime

(Cefotaxime*) **POM**

Formulations: Injectable: 500 mg, 1 g, 2 g powders for reconstitution.

Action: Binds to proteins involved in bacterial cell wall synthesis, thereby decreasing cell wall strength and rigidity and affecting cell division. Resistant to many bacterial beta-lactamases, particularly those produced by *Staphylococcus* spp. Works in a time-dependent fashion.

Use:
- Use should be based on antimicrobial susceptibility testing, wherever possible and where lower tier antimicrobials would not be effective.
- Good activity against many Gram-negative organisms, especially Enterobacteriaceae (not *Pseudomonas*) but lower activity against many Gram-positive organisms than 1st and 2nd generation cephalosporins.

It is important to maintain tissue concentrations above the MIC. Use should be reserved for patients with acute sepsis or serious infections where cultures are pending or culture and sensitivity testing shows sensitivity, or where other authorized preparations are not appropriate and the animal is not a good candidate for intensive aminoglycoside therapy (e.g. pre-existing renal dysfunction). Use with care in patients with renal disease and consider increasing dose interval. There are few published studies evaluating appropriate dosing rates and suggested dose rates are largely extrapolated from human pharmacokinetic information.

Safety and handling: The reconstituted solution is stable for 24 hours when refrigerated.

Contraindications: Patients hypersensitive to penicillins may also be sensitive to cephalosporins (cross-hypersensitivity in <10% of human patients); avoid use in animals with reported sensitivity to other beta-lactam antimicrobials.

Adverse reactions: May produce pain on injection. GI disturbance and superinfection with resistant microorganisms is a potential risk.

Drug interactions: The cephalosporins are synergistic with the aminoglycosides, but should not be mixed in the same syringe. May be increased risk of nephrotoxicity if cephalosporins are used with amphotericin or loop diuretics (e.g. furosemide); monitor renal function.

DOSES

Classified as category B (Restrict) by the EMA.

See Appendix for guidelines on responsible antibiotic use.

Dogs, Cats: Various doses have been suggested. 40–50 mg/kg i.v., i.m., s.c. q8h. Some authors have suggested that lower doses of 10–20 mg/kg q12h have good clinical efficacy in the dog.

References
Sumano H, Gutierrez I and Ocampo L (2004) Pharmacokinetics and clinical efficacy of cefotaxime for the treatment of septicaemia in dogs. *Acta Veterinaria Hungarica* **52**, 85–95

Cefovecin

(Convenia ^{c,d}) **POM-V**

Formulations: Injectable: lyophilized powder which, when reconstituted, contains 80 mg/ml cefovecin.

Action: 3rd generation cephalosporin that binds irreversibly to penicillin-binding proteins (enzymes involved in peptidoyglcan synthesis), weakening the bacterial cell wall and rendering bacteria susceptible to cell lysis and death. Greater activity against Gram-negative bacteria than 1st and 2nd generation cephalosporins; ineffective against meticillin-resistant *Staphylococcus* spp. Works in a time-dependent fashion.

Use:
- Use should be based on antimicrobial susceptibility testing, wherever possible.
- Indicated for the prolonged treatment of skin, soft tissue and urinary tract infections and as part of the management of severe periodontal disease.
- Cefovecin has an extremely long half-life and only requires administration every 14 days: cefovecin should not be considered if this length of cover would not ordinarily be required.

Safety and handling: Store in the refrigerator (2–8°C) prior to reconstitution; use reconstituted drug within 28 days.

Contraindications: Do not use in cats and dogs <8 weeks or in patients with known hypersensitivity to beta-lactam antibiotics. Avoid use during lactation and in pregnant animals, as safety has not been established

Adverse reactions: Reported adverse reactions include mild GI disturbance and transient swelling at the injection site, as well as type I, II and III hypersensitivity reactions.

Drug interactions: Highly bound to plasma proteins so may increase free concentrations of other highly protein-bound drugs such as furosemide, doxycycline, ketoconazole or NSAIDs.

DOSES

Classified as category B (Restrict) by the EMA.
See Appendix for guidelines on responsible antibiotic use.
Dogs, Cats: 8 mg/kg s.c., equivalent to 1 ml/10 kg of reconstituted drug. May be repeated after 14 days up to 3 times.

Ceftazidime

(Fortum*) **POM**

Formulations: Injectable: 500 mg, 1 g, 2 g, 3 g powders for reconstitution.

Action: 3rd generation cephalosporin. Binds to proteins involved in bacterial cell wall synthesis, thereby decreasing cell wall strength and rigidity and affecting cell division. Resistant to some bacterial beta-lactamases. It works in a time-dependent fashion.

Use:
- Use should be limited to cases with confirmed susceptibility and acute sepsis or serious infections where authorized preparations are found to be inappropriate.

Higher activity against many Gram-negative organisms but lower activity against many Gram-positive organisms when compared with 1st and 2nd generation cephalosporins. Very good activity against *Pseudomonas* in humans. Limited information on clinical pharmacokinetics in animal species and doses given below are empirical. Important to maintain tissue concentrations above the MIC with regular doses.

Safety and handling: Normal precautions should be observed.

Contraindications: Patients hypersensitive to penicillins may also be sensitive to cephalosporins (cross-hypersensitivity in <10% of human patients); avoid use in animals with reported sensitivity to other beta-lactam antimicrobials. Use with caution and consider dose adjustment in animals with significantly impaired renal function.

Adverse reactions: GI disturbances associated with drug use in humans. Pain may be noted following injection.

Drug interactions: May be an increased risk of nephrotoxicity if cephalosporins are used with amphotericin or loop diuretics (e.g. furosemide); monitor renal function. Do not mix in the same syringe as aminoglycosides. Ceftazidime is synergistic with the aminoglycoside antimicrobials *in vivo* (often used in humans for pseudomonal infection in neutropenic patients).

DOSES
Classified as category B (Restrict) by the EMA.
See Appendix for guidelines on responsible antibiotic use.
Dogs: Various doses suggested. **Susceptible infections:** 30 mg/kg i.v, i.m., s.c. q8h. Increased frequency for susceptible infections with *Pseudomonas aeruginosa* q4h or as CRI with a loading dose of 4.4 mg/kg followed by 4.1 mg/kg/h.
Cats: Various doses suggested. **Susceptible infections:** 30 mg/kg i.m. q8h. If *Pseudomonas*, more frequent dosing recommended q2–4h.

References
Albarellos GA, Ambros LA, Landoni MF *et al.* (2008) Pharmacokinetics of ceftazidime after intravenous and intramuscular administration to domestic cats. *Veterinary Journal* **178**, 238–243

Ceftiofur
(Cefenil) **POM-V**

Formulations: Injectable: 1 g, 4 g powder for reconstitution; 50 mg/ml suspension. Only authorized for use in large animals.

Action: 3rd generation cephalosporin. Binds to penicillin-binding proteins involved in bacterial cell wall synthesis, decreasing cell wall strength and rigidity and affecting cell division. Resistant to some penicillinases produced by *Staphylococcus* spp., but ineffective against meticillin-resistant staphylococci. Works in a time-dependent fashion. Uniquely among the cephalosporins, ceftiofur is metabolized to desfuroylceftiofur, which is an active metabolite.

Use: Should be reserved for patients suffering from acute sepsis or serious infections where cultures are pending, other authorized preparations are not appropriate and the animal is not a good candidate for intensive aminoglycoside therapy (pre-existing renal dysfunction). Important to maintain tissue concentrations above the MIC. Authorized for use in dogs in some countries where the main indication for use is in the treatment of urinary tract infections. Use with care in patients with renal disease and consider increasing dose interval.

Safety and handling: Store powder and diluent in the refrigerator; once reconstituted, store in the refrigerator and discard within 24 hours.

Contraindications: Avoid use in animals with hypersensitivity to other beta-lactam antimicrobials (cross-hypersensitivity in <10% of human patients).

Adverse reactions: May produce pain on injection. GI disturbance and superinfection with resistant microorganisms is a potential risk. Type I, II and III hypersensitivity reactions rarely reported. In dogs, a dose- and duration-dependent anaemia and thrombocytopenia has been recorded, although this should not occur with recommended doses.

Drug interactions: The cephalosporins are synergistic with the aminoglycosides, but should not be mixed in the same syringe. May be an increased risk of nephrotoxicity if cephalosporins are used with amphotericin or loop diuretics (e.g. furosemide); monitor renal function.

DOSES

Classified as category B (Restrict) by the EMA.
See Appendix for guidelines on responsible antibiotic use.
Dogs: For susceptible urinary tract infections: 2.2 mg/kg s.c. q24h.
Cats: Dose not established.
Higher (double) dose indicated to treat sepsis/bacteraemia.

References
Weese JS, Blondeau J, Boothe D *et al.* (2019) International Society for Companion Animal Infectious Diseases (ISCAID) guidelines for the diagnosis and management of bacterial urinary tract infections in dogs and cats. *The Veterinary Journal* **247**, 8–25

Cefuroxime

(Aprokam*, Zinacef*, Zinnat*) **POM**

Formulations: Injectable: 50 mg, 250 mg, 750 mg, 1.5 g powders for reconstitution (sodium salt). **Oral (as cefuroxime axetil):** 125 mg, 250 mg tablets; 125 mg/5 ml suspension.

Action: 2nd generation cephalosporin that binds to proteins involved in bacterial cell wall synthesis, thereby decreasing cell wall strength and rigidity and affecting cell division. Resistant to some bacterial beta-lactamases. Cefuroxime axetil is hydrolysed in intestinal mucosa and liver to yield active drug conferring oral bioavailability.

Use:
- Higher activity against many Gram-negative organisms when compared with 1st generation cephalosporins. Good activity against a wider spectrum of Enterobacteriaceae (not *Pseudomonas*). Many obligate anaerobes also susceptible.
- Used for surgical prophylaxis (clean-contaminated or contaminated procedures) and may be associated with fewer adverse effects than co-amoxiclav in this setting.

It is a time-dependent antimicrobial, so maintaining levels above the MIC is important for efficacy. Limited applications in veterinary species and limited pharmacokinetic data make appropriate dose selection problematic. Oral bioavailability in dogs reported to be low and erratic, with suspension appearing to have better absorption than tablets. Absorption is enhanced by giving with food. Short time above MIC of oral dosing means that expected efficacy is questionable.

Safety and handling: Normal precautions should be observed.

Contraindications: Patients hypersensitive to penicillins may also be sensitive to cephalosporins (cross-hypersensitivity in <10% of human patients); avoid use in animals with reported sensitivity to other beta-lactam antimicrobials.

Adverse reactions: May cause pain on i.m. and s.c. injection. GI disturbance has been reported in humans, particularly associated with the oral axetil formulation.

Drug interactions: May be an increased risk of nephrotoxicity if cephalosporins are used with amphotericin or loop diuretics (e.g. furosemide); monitor renal function. Synergistic with aminoglycosides, but do not mix in the same syringe.

DOSES

Classified as category C (Caution) by the EMA.
See Appendix for guidelines on responsible antibiotic use.
Dogs, Cats: For surgical prophylaxis: 20 mg/kg i.v. slowly (over 5 min) 30–60 min prior to surgery and then repeat q1.5–3h during surgery. For susceptible infections: 10–30 mg/kg i.v. q8–12h.

References

Albarellos GA, Montoya L, Lorenzini PM et al. (2016) Pharmacokinetics of cefuroxime after intravenous, intramuscular, and subcutaneous administration to dogs. *Journal of Veterinary Pharmacology and Therapeutics* **39**, 40–44

Cephalexin see Cefalexin

Cetirizine

(Piriteze*, Zirtec*) **GSL**

Formulations: Oral: 10 mg tablets; 5 mg/5 ml solution.

Action: Binds to H1 histamine receptors to prevent histamine from binding.

Use:
- Management of allergic disease.
- Prevention and early treatment of anaphylaxis.

Cetirizine is a metabolite of hydroxyzine. Less sedative effect in humans than chlorpheniramine.

Safety and handling: Normal precautions should be observed.

Contraindications: None reported.

Adverse reactions: May reduce seizure threshold.

Drug interactions: None reported.

DOSES
Dogs: 1 mg/kg p.o. q24h.
Cats: 5 mg/cat p.o. q24h.

References
Bizikova P, Papich MG and Olivry T (2008) Hydroxyzine and cetirizine pharmacokinetics and pharmacodynamics after oral and intravenous administration of hydroxyzine to healthy dogs. *Veterinary Dermatology* **19**, 348–357

Charcoal (Activated charcoal)

(Actidose-Aqua*, Carbomix*, Charcodote*, Liqui-Char*) **P**

Formulations: Oral: 50 g activated charcoal powder or premixed slurry (200 mg/ml available); 81.3% granules (containing 813 mg activated charcoal per gram).

Action: Absorbs toxins, fluids and gases in the GI tract. Activated charcoal has increased porosity and enhanced absorptive capacity.

Use:
- In acute poisoning with organophosphates, carbamates, chlorinated hydrocarbons, strychnine, ethylene glycol, inorganic and organic arsenical and mercurial compounds, polycyclic organic compounds (most pesticides), and dermal toxicants that may be ingested following grooming.

As a general rule, administer at a dose of at least 10 times the volume of intoxicant ingested. Repeat dosing as required if emesis or massive toxin ingestion occurs. Repeated dosing necessary if highly lipid-soluble toxins, which are likely to undergo enterohepatic recirculation, have been ingested. The addition of dog food to activated charcoal (up to 14 times the amount of charcoal used) slightly reduces its total adsorptive capacity for paracetamol but this effect is likely to be clinically insignificant.

Safety and handling: Activated charcoal powder floats, covering everything in the area; prepare very carefully as it will stain permanently.

Contraindications: Activated charcoal should not be used prior to the use of emetics.

Adverse reactions: Charcoal colours stools black, which is medically insignificant but may be alarming to the owner. GI obstruction (requiring surgery) has been reported following administration of multiple doses of activated charcoal to a dog.

Drug interactions: Activated charcoal reduces the absorption and therefore efficacy of orally administered drugs.

DOSES
Dogs, Cats: After toxin ingestion: 0.5–4 g/kg p.o. as a slurry in water.

References
Koenigshof AM, Beal MW, Poppenga RH *et al.* (2015) Effect of sorbitol, single, and multidose activated charcoal administration on carprofen absorption following experimental overdose in dogs. *Journal of Veterinary Emergency and Critical Care* **25**, 606–610

Chitosan

(Ipakitine) **general sale**

Formulations: Oral: powder containing 8% chitosan, 10% calcium carbonate and 82% lactose.

Action: Adsorbent for intestinal uraemic toxins, including phosphate.

Use:
- The combination product has been shown to reduce serum urea and phosphate in chronic kidney disease in cats.

Phosphate-binding agents are usually only used if low phosphate diets are unsuccessful. Monitor serum phosphate levels at 4–6 week intervals and adjust dosage accordingly if trying to achieve target serum concentrations. Monitor for hypercalcaemia. As formulation contains lactose, use with care in diabetic and lactose-intolerant animals.

Safety and handling: Normal precautions should be observed.

Contraindications: As formulation contains lactose, use with care in diabetic and lactose-intolerant animals.

Adverse reactions: Hypercalcaemia, possibly due to the calcium carbonate component.

Drug interactions: Increased risk of hypercalcaemia with concurrent calcitriol administration.

DOSES

Dogs, Cats: 200 mg/kg p.o. q12h (mixed with food).

Chlorambucil

(Leukeran*) **POM**

Formulations: Oral: 2 mg tablets.

Action: Alkylating agent that inhibits DNA synthesis and function through crosslinking with cellular DNA. Cell cycle non-specific.

Use:
- Management of some malignancies including in some metronomic chemotherapy protocols.
- May be useful in the treatment of feline pemphigus foliaceus and severe feline eosinophilic granuloma complex.
- Management of lymphoproliferative, myeloproliferative and immune-mediated diseases including protein-losing enteropathy.

Safety and handling: Cytotoxic drug; see Appendix and specialist texts for further advice on chemotherapeutic agents. Tablets should be stored in a closed, light-protected container under refrigeration (2–8°C).

Contraindications: Bone marrow suppression, factors predisposing to infection.

Adverse reactions: Anorexia, nausea, vomiting, leucopenia, thrombocytopenia, anaemia (rarely), neurotoxicity (one case reported in a cat), alopecia (rarely) and slow regrowth of clipped hair coat. Chlorambucil was suspected to have caused seizures in one dog.

Drug Interactions: Drugs that stimulate hepatic cytochrome P450 system increase cytotoxic effects. Prednisolone has a synergistic effect in the management of lymphoid neoplasia.

DOSES

See Appendix for chemotherapy protocols and conversion of bodyweight to body surface area.

Dogs: Give with food:

- **Chronic lymphocytic leukaemia:** 2–6 mg/m^2 p.o. q24h initially until remission achieved, then at reduced dosage/frequency as required to maintain remission; or 0.2 mg/kg q24h for 7 days then 0.1 mg/kg q24h for maintenance; or 20 mg/m^2 q1–2wk. Often used with prednisolone 40 mg/m^2 p.o. q24h for 7 days then 20 mg/m^2 q48h.
- **Lymphoma:** 15–20 mg/m^2 p.o. q2wk with prednisolone; or 2–6 mg/m^2 q24–48h. 1.4 mg/m^2 p.o. as single dose as substitute for cyclophosphamide in CHOP-type protocols.
- **Pemphigus complex (in combination with corticosteroids):** 0.1–0.2 mg/kg p.o. q24h initially until marked improvement of clinical signs; then alternate-day dosing, often for several weeks.
- **Protein-losing enteropathy and other immune-mediated diseases:** 2–6 mg/m^2 p.o. q24h until clinical remission, then tapered to the minimum effective dose.
- **For metronomic chemotherapy:** 4 mg/m^2 p.o. q24h.

Cats: Give with food:

- **Immune-mediated disease:** cats >4 kg: 2 mg (total dose) p.o. q48h for 2–4 weeks, then tapered to lowest effective dose; cats <4 kg: start at 2 mg (total dose) q72h.
- **Chronic lymphocytic leukaemia:** 2 mg/m^2 p.o. q48h or 20 mg/m^2 q14d, with or without prednisolone.
- **For low grade/small cell lymphoma:** 20 mg/m^2 p.o. q2wk with prednisolone or follow immune-mediated disease dosing.
- **As a substitute for cyclophosphamide in the CHOP protocol:** 1.4 mg/kg p.o. once.
- **Feline pemphigus foliaceus or severe feline eosinophilic granuloma complex (in combination with corticosteroids):** 0.1–0.2 mg/kg p.o. q24h until marked improvement of clinical signs; then alternate-day dosing, often for several weeks.

References

Dandrieux JRS, Noble PJM, Scase TJ *et al.* (2013) Comparison of a chlorambucil-prednisolone combination with an azathioprine-prednisolone combination for treatment of chronic enteropathy with concurrent protein-losing enteropathy in dogs: 27 cases (2007-2010). *Journal of the American Veterinary Medical Association* **242**, 1705–1714

Stein TJ, Pellin M, Steinberg H *et al.* (2010) Treatment of feline gastrointestinal small-cell lymphoma with chlorambucil and glucocorticoids. *Journal of the American Animal Hospital Association* **46**, 413–417

Chloramphenicol

(Chloramphenicol*, Chlorogen*, Chloromycetin Ophthalmic Ointment*, Chloromycetin Redidrops*, Kemicetine*, Minims*, Optrex*) **POM**

Formulations: Injectable: 1 g powder for reconstitution.
Ophthalmic: 1% ointment; 0.5% solution. Oral: 250 mg capsules.

Action: Time-dependent antimicrobial that acts by binding to the 50S ribosomal subunit of susceptible bacteria, preventing bacterial protein synthesis.

Use:
- Broad spectrum of activity against Gram-positive (e.g. Streptococcus, *Staphylococcus*), Gram-negative (e.g. *Brucella*, *Salmonella*, *Haemophilus*) and obligate anaerobic bacteria (e.g. *Clostridioides* spp., *Bacteroides fragilis*).
- Other sensitive organisms include *Chlamydia*, *Mycoplasma* (unreliable in treatment of ocular mycoplasmosis) and *Rickettsia*.

Resistant organisms include *Nocardia* and *Mycobacterium*. Acquired resistance may occur in Enterobacteriaceae. High lipid solubility makes it suitable for the treatment of intraocular infections. It will also access the CNS. However, due to concerns of resistance development and human toxicity, systemic use should be restricted to life-threatening infections resistant to other antimicrobials (e.g. meticillin-resistant staphylococci). Patients with hepatic or renal dysfunction may need adjustment to the dose. Use with caution or avoid in nursing bitches or queens as crosses into milk.

Safety and handling: Humans exposed to chloramphenicol may have an increased risk of developing a fatal aplastic anaemia. Products should be handled with care; use impervious gloves and avoid skin contact.

Contraindications: No information available.

Adverse reactions: Reversible dose-related bone marrow suppression can develop in all species. Unlike in humans, the development of irreversible aplastic anaemia in veterinary species does not appear to be a significant problem. Owing to a reduced capacity to metabolize chloramphenicol, cats are more susceptible to bone marrow suppression. Other adverse effects include nausea, vomiting, diarrhoea and anaphylaxis.

Drug interactions: Irreversible inhibition of hepatic cytochrome P450-dependent enzymes increases plasma levels of pentobarbital, phenobarbital, propofol and oral hypoglycaemic agents. Recovery requires synthesis of new liver enzymes and can take up to 3 weeks. Rifampin accelerates the metabolism of chloramphenicol, thus decreasing serum levels. Chloramphenicol may inhibit activity of aminoglycosides and beta-lactams. May also competitively inhibit macrolide or lincosamide antimicrobials.

DOSES

Classified as category C (Caution) by the EMA.
See Appendix for guidelines on responsible antibiotic use.
Dogs:
- **Ophthalmic:** 1 drop q4–8h; ointment q8–12h.
- **Systemic:** 40–50 mg/kg i.v., i.m., s.c., p.o. q8h.
- **CNS infections:** 10–15 mg/kg p.o. q4–6h is recommended in some texts.

Cats:
- **Ophthalmic:** 1 drop q4–8h; ointment q8–12h.
- **Systemic:** 10–20 mg/kg slow i.v., i.m., s.c., p.o. q12h.

Chlorhexidine

(Adaxio[d], Antisept, Clearium shampoo[d], Clorexyderm, CLX wipes, Douxo Pyo, Ermidra foam, Hibiscrub, Iryplus eye wipes, Malaseb[c,d], Microbex[d], Otodine, Stomidine F, Corsodyl*, Savlon*, TrizChlor*) **POM-V, GSL, general sale**

Formulations: Topical: 2% chlorhexidine + 2% miconazole (Malaseb); 31.2 mg/ml chlorhexidine (Microbex); 11.26 mg/ml chlorhexidine + 17.37 mg/ml miconazole (Adaxio); 3% chlorhexidine + ophytrion + phytosphingosine (Douxo Pyo shampoo/mousse/pads); 4% chlorhexidine (Clorexyderm 4% shampoo, spray, Ermidra foam); 3% chlorhexidine (Clearium shampoo); chlorhexidine digluconate + sodium acetate + acetic acid solution (Antisept spray); 4% chlorhexidine + Tris-EDTA + polyvinyl-pyrrolidone + lanolin + glycerine (Clorexyderm spot gel); 1.5% chlorhexidine + cetrimide (Savlon); 4% chlorhexidine + isopropyl alcohol solution (Hibiscrub); 0.12% chlorhexidine mouthwash (Chlorohex); chlorhexidine + Tris-EDTA + zinc gluconate + glycerine + climbazole + benzyl alcohol + propylene glycol (CLX wipes); 0.15% chlorhexidine + EDTA ear/wound cleaner (TrizChlor); chlorhexidine + Tris-EDTA + lactic acid ear cleaner (Otodine); 0.07% chlorhexidine + Tris-EDTA toothpaste (Stomidine F).

Action: Chemical antiseptic that disrupts bacterial cell membranes.

Use:
- Topical treatment of bacterial, dermatophyte and *Malassezia* skin infections in dogs as a shampoo. Concurrent systemic antibacterial therapy may be required when treating bacterial skin infections. Leave in contact with the skin for 5–10 minutes prior to washing off.
- Local infection can be treated with mousse, spray, gel or wipes.
- Ear flush for cleansing; Tris-EDTA and chlorhexidine have synergistic antimicrobial action. Chlorhexidine as a single agent is not consistently effective as a treatment for dermatophytosis.
- Washing surgical instruments, routine antisepsis for surgical operations and dental hygiene.

Safety and handling: Normal precautions should be observed.

Contraindications: Do not instil into ears where the integrity of the tympanum is unknown. Do not use on eyes.

Adverse reactions: Ototoxic. May irritate mucous membranes.

Drug interactions: Not known.

DOSES

Dogs, Cats:
- **Antispetic:** topical agents may be used daily to weekly.
- **Skin preparation before surgical procedure:** observe recommended solution concentrations and contact times. Do not use for ophthalmic surgical procedures or in combination with povidone–iodine.

References

Banovic F, Bozic F and Lemo N (2013) *In vitro* comparison of the effectiveness of polihexanide and chlorhexidine against canine isolates of *Staphylococcus pseudintermedius*, *Pseudomonas aeruginosa* and *Malassezia pachydermatis*. *Veterinary Dermatology* **24**, 409–413

Clark SM, Loeffler A and Bond R (2015) Susceptibility *in vitro* of canine methicillin-resistant and suceptible staphylococcal isolates to fusidic acid, chlorhexidine and miconazole: opportunities for topical therapy of canine superficial pyoderma. The *Journal of Antimicrobial Chemotherapy* **70**, 2048–2052

Chlorphenamine (Chlorpheniramine) `CIL`
(Piriton*) **POM, GSL**

Formulations: Injectable: 10 mg/ml solution. **Oral:** 4 mg tablets, 0.4 mg/ml syrup.

Action: Binds to H1 histamine receptors to prevent histamine binding.

Use:
- Management of allergic disease.
- Prevention and early treatment of anaphylaxis.
- Commonly used as premedication before transfusions and certain chemotherapeutic agents.

Specific doses for dogs and cats have not been determined by pharmacokinetic studies. Use with caution in cases with urinary retention, angle-closure glaucoma and pyloroduodenal obstruction.

Safety and handling: Normal precautions should be observed.

Contraindications: No information available.

Adverse reactions: May cause mild sedation. May reduce seizure threshold.

Drug interactions: No information available.

DOSES
Dogs: 4–8 mg/dog p.o. q8h; 2.5–10 mg/dog i.m. or slow i.v.
Cats: 2–4 mg/cat p.o. q8–12h; 2–5 mg/cat i.m. or slow i.v.

Chlortetracycline hydrochloride
(Ophtocycline c,d) **POM-V**

Formulations: Ophthalmic: 5 g tube (ointment).

Action: 1st generation time- and concentration-dependent antimicrobial that inhibits bacterial protein synthesis by binding to the 30S subunit of the bacterial ribosome.

Use:
- Treatment of feline chlamydial conjunctivitis (oral doxycycline is the treatment of choice).
- Treatment of mycoplasmal conjunctivitis and canine spontaneous chronic corneal epithelial defects (via an immunomodulatory mechanism).
- Chlortetracycline is authorized for treatment of keratitis, conjunctivitis and blepharitis caused by *Staphylococcus* spp., *Streptococcus* spp., *Proteus* spp. and/or *Pseudomonas* spp.

Tetracyclines have a broad spectrum including both aerobic and anaerobic Gram-positive and Gram-negative bacteria, mycoplasmas, *Chlamydia* spp. and rickettsiae. *Pseudomonas* spp. and *Staphylococci* spp. may be resistant.

Safety and handling: Normal precautions should be observed; avoid direct skin contact.

Contraindications: Safety during pregnancy and lactation unknown.

Adverse reactions: None known.

Drug interactions: No information specified.

DOSES

Classified as category D (Prudence) by the EMA.
See Appendix for guidelines on responsible antibiotic use.
Dogs, Cats: 0.5–2 cm of ointment to affected eye q6h for 5 days.

References

Chandler HL, Gemensky-Metzler AJ, Bras ID *et al.* (2010) *In vivo* effects of adjunctive tetracycline treatment on refractory corneal ulcers in dogs. *Journal of the American Veterinary Medical Association* **237**, 378–386

Hindley KE, Groth AD, King M *et al.* (2016) Bacterial isolates, antimicrobial susceptibility, and clinical characteristics of bacterial keratitis in dogs presenting to referral practice in Australia. *Veterinary Ophthalmology* **19**, 418–426

Kang MH, Chae MJ, Yoon JW *et al.* (2014) Antibiotic resistance and molecular characterization of ophthalmic *Staphylococcus pseudintermedius* isolates from dogs. *Journal of Veterinary Science* **15**, 409–415

Kimmitt BA, Moore GE and Stiles (2018) Comparison of the efficacy of various concentrations and combinations of serum, ethylenediaminetetraacetic acid, tetracycline, doxycycline, minocycline, and *N*-acetylcysteine for inhibition of collagenase activity in an *in vitro* corneal degradation model. *American Journal of Veterinary Research* **79**, 555–561

Sparkes AH, Caney SM, Sturgess CP *et al.* (1999) The clinical efficacy of topical and systemic therapy for the treatment of feline ocular chlamydiosis. *Journal of Feline Medicine and Surgery* **1**, 31–35

Cholestyramine see Colestyramine

Chorionic gonadotrophin (Human chorionic gonadotrophin, hCG)

(Chorulon [d]) **POM-V**

Formulations: Injectable: 1500 IU powder for reconstitution.

Action: Luteinizing hormone analogue.

Use:
- Induction of ovulation in the queen, especially during later part of oestrus (day 3–4).
- Although indicated for the treatment of delayed ovulation in the bitch, given the large variation in pro-oestrus time, timing and success are difficult.
- In males, short-term stimulation of testosterone secretion is possible, although this may increase aggression without improving libido.

Safety and handling: Reconstituted vials do not contain any preservative and so should be discarded within 24 hours.

Contraindications: No information available.

Adverse reactions: Anaphylactic reactions may occasionally occur.

Drug interactions: No information available.

DOSES

Dogs, Cats:
- **Delayed ovulation:** 22 IU/kg i.m. q24–48h or 44 IU/kg i.m. once; mate on behavioural oestrus.
- **Deficient male libido:** 100–500 IU/dog i.m. twice weekly for up to 6 weeks.

A
B
C
D
E
F
G
H
I
J
K
L
M
N
O
P
Q
R
S
T
U
V
W
X
Y
Z

Ciclosporin (Cyclosporin(e))

(Atopica [c,d], Cyclavance [c,d], Modulis [d], Optimmune [d], Sporimmune [c,d]) **POM-V**

Formulations: Ophthalmic: 0.2% ointment. **Oral:** 10 mg, 25 mg, 50 mg, 100 mg capsules; 50 mg/ml, 100 mg/ml solution. **Injectable:** 50 mg/ml solution.

Action: T-lymphocyte inhibition.

Use:
- Topical ophthalmic preparation for immune-mediated kerato-conjunctivitis sicca in dogs. May also be useful as an immuno-suppressant in chronic superficial keratoconjunctivitis (pannus).
- Oral preparation authorized for atopic dermatitis in dogs and cats.
- Used for perianal fistula, sebaceous adenitis and immune-mediated disease.

It is recommended that bacterial and fungal infections are treated before use. While the nephrotoxicity seen in human patients does not appear to be common in dogs, care should be taken in treating dogs with renal impairment, and creatinine levels should be monitored regularly. In dogs with atopic dermatitis, ciclosporin may reduce circulating levels of insulin and cause an increase in blood glucose and fructosamine. In dogs with diabetes mellitus, the effect of treatment on glycaemia must be carefully monitored.

Safety and handling: Use gloves to prevent cutaneous absorption.

Contraindications: The safety/efficacy of ciclosporin has not been evaluated in dogs and cats up to 6 months old or in dogs <2 kg or cats <2.3 kg. Do not use in progressive malignant disorders. Do not give live vaccines during treatment or within a 2-week interval before or after treatment. Ciclosporin may reduce the immune response to vaccines. The manufacturer does not recommend use in diabetic dogs or cats infected with FeLV or FIV.

Adverse reactions: Immediate discomfort on topical application (blepharospasm) has been reported in dogs. Transient vomiting and diarrhoea may follow systemic administration; these are usually mild and do not require cessation of treatment. Infrequently observed adverse effects include anorexia, mild to moderate gingival hyperplasia, hypertrichosis, papillomatous lesions of the skin, red and swollen pinnae, muscle weakness and muscle cramps. These effects resolve spontaneously after treatment is stopped. Systemic and topical treatment may be associated with an increased risk of malignancy. Cats that are seronegative for Toxoplasma gondii may be at risk of developing clinical toxoplasmosis if they become infected while undergoing treatment.

Drug interactions: The metabolism of ciclosporin is reduced, and thus serum levels increased, by various drugs that competitively inhibit or induce enzymes involved in its metabolism, particularly cytochrome P450, including diltiazem, doxycycline and imidazole antifungal drugs. Itraconazole and ketoconazole at 5–10 mg/kg are known to increase the blood concentration of ciclosporin in dogs up to five-fold, which is considered to be clinically relevant. During concomitant use of itraconazole and ciclosporin, consider halving the dose or doubling the treatment interval if the dog is receiving daily treatment. In humans, there is increased risk of nephrotoxicity if ciclosporin is administered with aminoglycosides, NSAIDs, quinolones or trimethoprim/sulphonamides; concomitant use of ciclosporin not recommended. Increased risk of hyperkalaemia if used with ACE inhibitors. As a substrate and inhibitor of the MDR 1 P-glycoprotein transporter, co-administration of ciclosporin with P-glycoprotein substrates such as macrocyclic lactones (e.g. ivermectin and milbemycin) could decrease the efflux of such drugs from blood–brain barrier cells, potentially resulting in signs of CNS toxicity.

DOSES
See Appendix for immunosuppression protocols.
Dogs:
- **Ocular disease:** apply approximately 0.5 cm of ointment to the affected eye q12h. It may take 2–4 weeks for improvement to occur (occasionally up to 12 weeks). Maintenance treatment should be continued with application q12h; in cases of excessive tear production, application can be reduced to q24h but only with caution and regular long-term monitoring of tear production.
- **Atopic dermatitis:** 5 mg/kg p.o. q24h until signs controlled.
- **Perianal fistula, sebaceous adenitis:** 5 mg/kg p.o. q24h. May be increased to q12h in non-responsive cases.
- **Immune-mediated disease:** 5 mg/kg p.o. q12h. A proportion of dogs may require higher doses and pharmacodynamic monitoring is therefore advised.

Cats:
- **Atopic dermatitis:** 7 mg/kg p.o. q24h until signs controlled.
- **Immune-mediated disease:** dosing strategies are not well defined but typically 3–5 mg/kg p.o. q12h or 5–7 mg/kg p.o. q24h.

References
Nuttall T, Reece D and Roberts E (2014) Life-long diseases need life-long treatment: long-term safety of ciclosporin in canine atopic dermatitis. *Veterinary Record* **174**, 3–12
Swann JW, Garden OA, Fellman CL *et al.* (2019) ACVIM consensus statement on the treatment of immune-mediated hemolytic anemia in dogs. *Journal of Veterinary Internal Medicine* **29**, 513–518

Cimetidine

(Zitac [d], Cimetidine*, Tagamet*) **POM-V, POM**

Formulations: Injectable: 100 mg/ml solution in 2 ml ampoule.
Oral: 100 mg, 200 mg tablets; 40 mg/ml syrup.

Action: Histamine (H2) receptor antagonist, reducing histamine-induced gastric acid secretion. Rapidly absorbed with high bioavailability; undergoes hepatic metabolism and renal excretion. Plasma half-life is about 2 hours. It is not an antiemetic. Has weak anti-androgenic effects.

Use:
- Management of idiopathic, uraemic or drug-related erosive gastritis, gastric and duodenal ulcers, oesophagitis, and hypersecretory conditions secondary to gastrinoma, mast cell neoplasia or short bowel syndrome. Efficacy against NSAID-induced ulcers is controversial.

Rebound gastric acid secretion may be seen on cessation of cimetidine, so therapy should be tapered. Concomitant treatment with sucralfate may be helpful. If used i.v., should be administered over 30 minutes to prevent cardiac arrhythmias and hypotension. Dosage should be reduced for animals with renal impairment. Less effective at reducing gastric acidity than more modern H2 blockers and proton pump inhibitors. Cimetidine has minimal prokinetic effects.

Safety and handling: Normal precautions should be observed.

Contraindications: No information available.

Adverse reactions: Rare, although hepatotoxicity and nephrotoxicity have been reported in humans. Adverse reactions are generally minor even at high doses, but thrombocytopenia has been reported in dogs. Transient and self-resolving slight swelling of mammary glands may be observed in bitches. In humans, cimetidine has also been associated with headache and decreased libido.

Drug interactions: Retards oxidative hepatic drug metabolism by binding to the microsomal cytochrome P450. May increase plasma levels of beta-blockers (e.g. propranolol), calcium-channel blockers (e.g. verapamil), diazepam, lidocaine, metronidazole, pethidine and theophylline. When used with other agents that cause leucopenia, may exacerbate the problem. Sucralfate may decrease bioavailability: although there is little evidence to suggest this is of clinical importance, it may be a wise precaution to administer sucralfate at least 2 hours before cimetidine. Stagger oral doses by 2 hours when used with other antacids, digoxin, itraconazole or maropitant.

DOSES
Dogs: 5 mg/kg p.o., i.v., i.m. q8h.
Cats: 2.5–5 mg/kg p.o., i.v., i.m. q12h.

References
Marks SL, Kook PH, Papich MG *et al.* (2018) ACVIM consensus statement: support for rational administration of gastrointestinal protectants to dogs and cats. *Journal of Veterinary Internal Medicine* **32**, 1823–1840

Cimicoxib
(Cimalgex [d]) **POM-V**

Formulations: Oral: 8 mg, 30 mg, 80 mg chewable tablets.

Action: Selectively inhibits COX-2 enzyme, thereby limiting the production of prostaglandins involved in inflammation.

Use:
- For the treatment of pain and inflammation associated with osteoarthritis and the management of perioperative pain due to orthopaedic or soft tissue surgery in dogs.

For perioperative use, one dose 2 hours before surgery, followed by 3–7 days of treatment, is indicated. All NSAIDs should be administered cautiously in the perioperative period. Although cimicoxib preferentially inhibits COX-2, it may still adversely affect renal perfusion during periods of hypotension. If hypotension during anaesthesia is anticipated, delay cimicoxib administration until the animal is fully recovered from anaesthesia and normotensive. Liver disease will prolong the metabolism of cimicoxib, leading to the potential for drug accumulation and overdose with repeated dosing. For the relief of pain and inflammation associated with osteoarthritis, an initial treatment period of 6 months is indicated; this can be extended depending on clinical need for analgesic treatment.

Safety and handling: Normal precautions should be observed.

Contraindications: Do not give to dogs <10 weeks. The safety of cimicoxib has not been determined in dogs <6 months; monitor dogs in this age group carefully for signs of NSAID-related adverse effects. Do not give to dehydrated, hypovolaemic or hypotensive animals, or those with GI disease or blood clotting problems. Administration to patients with concurrent renal or hepatic disease may carry additional risk; careful monitoring of patients is required if cimicoxib is administered to these patient groups. Do not give to pregnant or lactating bitches. Do not administer concurrently or within 24 hours of other NSAIDs. The optimal wash-out period between NSAID administration and glucocorticoid administration is unknown – allowing 3–5 days between the two classes of drugs is recommended.

Adverse reactions: GI signs are commonly reported but most cases are mild and recover without treatment. Stop therapy if signs persist beyond 1–2 days. Some animals develop signs with one NSAID and not another. A 3–5 day wash-out period should be allowed before starting therapy with another NSAID. Stop therapy immediately if GI bleeding is suspected. There is a small risk that NSAIDs may precipitate cardiac failure in humans and this risk in animals is unknown.

Drug interactions: No information available.

DOSES
Dogs: 2 mg/kg p.o. q24h administered with or without food.
Cats: Not authorized for cats.

Ciprofloxacin
(Ciloxan*) **POM**

Formulations: Ophthalmic: 0.3% solution in 5 ml bottle.

Action: Concentration-dependent inhibition of bacterial DNA gyrase.

Use:
- Broad-spectrum activity against wide range of Gram-negative and some Gram-positive aerobes; some activity against *Mycoplasma* and *Chlamydia* spp. Active against many ocular pathogens, including *Staphylococcus* spp. and *Pseudomonas aeruginosa*, although there is increasing resistance among staphylococci and streptococci.

Safety and handling: Normal precautions should be observed.

Contraindications: No information available.

Adverse reactions: May cause local irritation after application. In humans: local burning and itching, lid margin crusting, hyperaemia, taste disturbances, corneal staining, keratitis, lid oedema, lacrimation, photophobia, corneal infiltrates, nausea and visual disturbances.

Drug interactions: No information available.

DOSES
Classified as category B (Restrict) by the EMA.
See Appendix for guidelines on responsible antibiotic use.
Dogs, Cats: 1 drop to affected eye q6h. **Intensive therapy:** q30–120 min for short-term use (1–2 days).

Cisapride

CIL

(Cisapride) **POM**

Formulations: Oral: 2.5 mg, 5 mg tablets. Must be obtained from a compounding pharmacy. **VSP**

Action: GI prokinetic action by acting on 5-HT4 receptors on enteric cholinergic neurons, inducing depolarization and contraction of GI smooth muscle.

Use:

- Potentially useful in cases where there is reduced gastric motility and obstruction has been ruled out.
- May be part of the management of constipation and megacolon in cats that are mildly or moderately affected.
- Has been shown to increase lower oesophageal sphincter pressure in dogs so may be of benefit in canine patients for which this is desirable. Cisapride also decreased the frequency of gastro-oesophageal reflux in anesthetized dogs.

No evidence that cisapride is effective in the treatment of megaoesophagus in dogs; the canine oesophagus is primarily striated muscle with little smooth muscle to respond to cisapride.

Safety and handling: Due to the potential for side effects in humans, gloves should be worn when handling this drug and particular care taken to avoid accidental ingestion.

Contraindications: Do not use in cases of suspected gastrointestinal obstruction or perforation.

Adverse reactions: Vomiting, diarrhoea, abdominal pain. In human medicine, the drug was removed from the market because it was shown to cause QT prolongation and increase the risk of serious cardiac arrhythmias. This has not been reported in dogs or cats.

Drug interactions: Effects on motility could affect the absorption of other oral drugs so caution should be used when using drugs with a narrow therapeutic index. Metabolized by cytochrome P450 enzymes so use with caution if used with other drugs metabolized by these enzymes (e.g. ketoconazole, itraconazole, cimetidine, amiodarone, chloramphenicol). Drugs such as amiodarone, procainamide, quinidine, sotalol, and tricyclic antidepressants (e.g. amitriptyline) may increase the QT interval and this risk may be exacerbated by concurrent use of cisapride. Use with caution in animals with hepatic or renal dysfunction; may require reduced dosing due to decreased metabolism or clearance.

DOSES

Dogs: 0.1–0.5 mg/kg p.o. q8–12h; some recommend giving 30 minutes before feeding. Some sources state that gradually increasing doses up to 1 mg/kg p.o. q8h may be required (if tolerated).

Cats: Various doses have been suggested, including 2.5–5.0 mg/cat p.o. q8–12h and 0.5 mg/kg q8–12h. Dosages may be titrated upwards, if tolerated, to as high as 7.5 mg/cat p.o. q8h in large cats.

References

Burger DM, Wiestner T, Hubler M *et al.* (2006) Effect of anticholinergics (atropine, glycopyrrolate) and prokinetics (metoclopramide, cisapride) on gastric motility in Beagles and Labrador Retrievers. *Journal of Veterinary Medicine Series A* **53**, 97–107
Kempf J, Lewis F, Reusch CE *et al.* (2014) High-resolution manometric evaluation of the effects of cisapride and metoclopramide hydrochloride administered orally on lower esophageal sphincter pressure in awake dogs. *American Journal of Veterinary Research* **75**, 361–366

Cisatracurium

(Nimbex*) **POM**

Formulations: Injectable: 2 mg/ml, 10 mg/ml solutions.

Action: Inhibits actions of acetylcholine at neuromuscular junctions by binding competitively to nicotinic acetylcholine receptors on post-junctional membranes.

Use:
- Provision of neuromuscular blockade during anaesthesia.
- To improve surgical access through muscle relaxation, to facilitate positive pressure ventilation or for intraocular surgery.

Cisatracurium is one of the isomers that comprise atracurium; it is 3–5 times more potent than atracurium in dogs. This means that the plasma concentration of the epileptogenic by-product laudanosine is lower and there is less histamine release. Monitoring (using a nerve stimulator) and reversal of the neuromuscular blockade is recommended to ensure complete recovery before the end of anaesthesia. Hypothermia, acidosis and hypokalaemia will prolong the duration of action of neuromuscular blockade. Limited experimental and clinical studies suggest that cisatracurium has similar characteristics in cats to those described for dogs.

Safety and handling: Store in refrigerator.

Contraindications: Do not administer unless the animal is adequately anaesthetized and facilities to provide positive pressure ventilation are available.

Adverse reactions: Can precipitate the release of histamine after rapid i.v. administration, resulting in bronchospasm and hypotension. Diluting in normal saline and giving slowly i.v. minimizes these effects.

Drug interactions: Neuromuscular blockade is more prolonged when given in combination with volatile anaesthetics, aminoglycosides, clindamycin and lincomycin.

DOSES

Dogs: 0.05–0.1 mg/kg i.v. followed by additional doses of 0.03 mg/kg as required (based on monitoring of neuromuscular blockade).

Cats: A dose of 0.15 mg/kg i.v. followed by additional doses of 0.05 mg/kg as required (based on monitoring of neuromuscular blockade) produced a central eyeball position which was suitable for ophthalmic surgeries.

References

Adams WA, Senior JM, Jones RS *et al.* (2006) cis-Atracurium in dogs with and without porto-systemic shunts. *Veterinary Anaesthesia and Analgesia* **33**, 17–23

Van Wijnsberghe AS, Ida KK, Dmitrovic P, Tutunaru A and Sandersen C (2022) Neuro-muscular blockade effects of cisatracurium in 11 cats undergoing ophthalmological surgery anaesthetised with isoflurane. *Journal of Feline Medicine and Surgery* **24**, 402–406

Clarithromycin

(Klaricid*) **POM**

Formulations: Oral: 250 mg, 500 mg tablets; 125 mg/5 ml, 250 mg/5 ml suspensions; 250 mg granules sachet (to be dissolved in water). **Injectable:** 500 mg vial for reconstitution.

Action: Derived from erythromycin and with greater activity. Time-dependent macrolide antibacterial that binds to the 50S ribosome, inhibiting peptide bond and therefore protein formation.

Use:
- Active against Gram-positive cocci (some *Staphylococcus* spp. resistant), Gram-positive bacilli, some Gram-negative bacilli (e.g. *Pasteurella*) and some spirochaetes (e.g. *Helicobacter*). Some strains of *Actinomyces*, *Nocardia*, *Chlamydia* and *Rickettsia* also inhibited. Most strains of Enterobacteriaceae (*Pseudomonas*, *Escherichia coli*, *Klebsiella*) are resistant.
- Highly lipid-soluble and useful against intracellular pathogens.
- Particularly useful in management of respiratory tract infections, mild to moderate skin and soft tissue infections, and non-tuberculous mycobacterial infections. For the latter, use in combination with fluoroquinolones and rifampin.

Alternative to penicillin in penicillin-allergic humans as it has a similar, although not identical, antibacterial spectrum. Activity is enhanced in an alkaline pH; administer on an empty stomach. There is limited information regarding use in animals. Use with caution in animals with hepatic dysfunction. Reduce dose in animals with renal impairment.

Safety and handling: Normal precautions should be observed.

Contraindications: No information available.

Adverse reactions: In humans, similar adverse effects to those of erythromycin are seen, i.e. vomiting, cholestatic hepatitis, stomatitis and glossitis.

Drug interactions: May increase serum levels of several drugs, including methylprednisolone, theophylline, omeprazole and itraconazole. The absorption of digoxin may be enhanced.

DOSES

Classified as category C (Caution) by the EMA.

See Appendix for guidelines on responsible antibiotic use.

Dogs: 4–12 mg/kg i.v., p.o. q12h. Doses of 15–25 mg/kg p.o. total daily dose divided q8–12h are recommended in the treatment of leproid granuloma syndrome combined with rifampin 10–15 mg/kg p.o. q24h. These doses are empirical and are based on only a few reports.

Cats: 5–10 mg/kg i.v., p.o. q12h or 62.5 mg/cat p.o. These doses are empirical and are based on only a few reports. A variety of combination protocols have been used in the treatment of feline mycobacterial infections, e.g. combination of clarithromycin with a fluoroquinolone and either rifampin or clofazamine.

Clemastine (Meclastin)

(Tavegil*) **GSL**

`CIL`

Formulations: Oral: 1 mg tablets.

Action: Binds to H1 histamine receptors and prevents histamine from binding.

Use:
- Management of allergic disease.

Specific doses for cats have not been determined by pharmokinetic studies. In dogs, therapeutic levels are not usually achieved by oral administration. Use with caution in cases with urinary retention, angle-closure glaucoma and pyloroduodenal obstruction.

Safety and handling: Normal precautions should be observed.

Contraindications: No information available.

Adverse reactions: May cause sedation or hyperexcitability in high doses. May reduce seizure threshold.

Drug interactions: No information available.

DOSES
Dogs: 0.05–0.1 mg/kg p.o. q12h.
Cats: 0.1 mg/kg p.o. q12h.

Climbazole

(Vetruus CLX cleansing wipes) **general sale**

Formulations: Topical: chlorhexidine + Tris-EDTA + zinc gluconate + glycerine + climbazole + benzyl alcohol + propylene glycol wipes.

Action: Inhibits cytochrome P450-dependent synthesis of ergosterol in fungal cells, causing increased cell wall permeability and allowing leakage of cellular contents.

Use:
- Topical treatment of *Malassezia* skin infections. Additional systemic antifungal treatment may be required in generalized cases.

Safety and handling: Normal precautions should be observed.

Contraindications: None known.

Adverse reactions: None known.

Drug interactions: No information available.

DOSES
Dogs, Cats: May be applied daily–weekly.

References
Cavana P, Petit JY, Perrot S *et al.* (2015) Efficacy of a 2% climbazole shampoo for reducing *Malassezia* population sizes on the skin of naturally infected dogs. *Journal de Mycologie Medicale* **25**, 268–273

Clindamycin

(Antirobe [c,d], Clinacin [d], Clindacyl, Clindaseptin [c,d], Mycinor [d], Zodon [c,d]) **POM-V**

Formulations: Oral: 25 mg, 75 mg, 88 mg, 150 mg, 264 mg, 300 mg capsules and tablets; 25 mg/ml solution.

Action: Time-dependent lincosamide antibiotic that binds to the 50S ribosomal subunit, inhibiting peptide bond formation.

Use:
- Bone and joint infections associated with Gram-positive bacteria, pyoderma, toxoplasmosis and infections associated with the oral cavity.
- It is also recommended as part of the treatment for sepsis/bacteraemia and hospital-acquired pneumonia.
- Active against Gram-positive cocci (including penicillin-resistant staphylococci), many obligate anaerobes, mycoplasmas and protozoal infections (*Neospora caninum*, *Toxoplasma gondii*).

Attains high concentrations in bone and bile. Being a weak base, it becomes ion-trapped (and therefore concentrated) in fluids that are more acidic than plasma, such as prostatic fluid, milk and intracellular fluid. Clindamycin has complete cross-resistance with lincomycin and partial cross-resistance with erythromycin. Use with care in individuals with hepatic or renal impairment.

Safety and handling: Normal precautions should be observed.

Contraindications: No information available.

Adverse reactions: Colitis, vomiting and diarrhoea are reported. Although not a major problem in dogs and cats, discontinue drug if diarrhoea develops. In cats, may be associated with oesophagitis and oesophageal stricture; therefore, consider following solid dosage forms such as tablet administration with a small water or food bolus.

Drug interactions: May enhance the effect of non-depolarizing muscle relaxants (e.g. tubocurarine) and may antagonize the effects of neostigmine and pyridostigmine. Do not administer with macrolide, chloramphenicol or other lincosamide antimicrobials as these combinations are antagonistic.

DOSES

Classified as category C (Caution) by the EMA.
See Appendix for guidelines on responsible antibiotic use.
Dogs:
- 5.5 mg/kg p.o. q12h or 11 mg/kg p.o. q24h; in severe infection, can increase to 11 mg/kg q8–12h.
- **Toxoplasmosis/neosporosis:** 25 mg/kg p.o. daily in divided doses.

Cats:
- 5.5 mg/kg p.o. q12h or 11 mg/kg p.o. q24h.
- **Toxoplasmosis:** 25 mg/kg p.o. daily in divided doses; increased doses of 30–50 mg/kg p.o. daily have been recommended for CNS involvement.

References

Beatty JA, Swift N, Foster DJ *et al.* (2006) Suspected clindamycin-associated oesophageal injury in cats: five cases. *Journal of Feline Medicine and Surgery* **8**, 412–419
Hu HZ, Jeffery ND, Donnelly J *et al.* (2016) What is your neurologic diagnosis? *Journal of the American Veterinary Medical Association* **249**, 1007–1010

Clofazimine

(Clofazimine*) **POM**

Formulations: Oral: 100 mg capsules.

Action: Not entirely clear but appears to be antimycobacterial and has membrane disrupting properties.

Use:
- Mycobacterial infections, including feline leprosy.

Limited information available with most derived from human medicine. For feline mycobacterial infection, long-term treatment is required and combination therapy is utilized, e.g. with clarithromycin and doxycycline or fluoroquinolones. Monitor hepatic and renal function during treatment. Use with caution in hepatic and renal impairment.

Safety and handling: Normal precautions should be observed.

Contraindications: No information available.

Adverse reactions: In humans, the major adverse effects are nausea, diarrhoea, discoloration of skin, eyes and body fluids, and renal and hepatic impairment. Photosensitization can also occur and treated animals should be housed indoors.

Drug interactions: No information available.

DOSES

Classified as category A (Avoid) by the EMA.
See Appendix for guidelines on responsible antibiotic use.
Dogs, Cats: 4–8 mg/kg p.o. q24h. For the management of mycobacterial infections, the drug is used in combination therapy with other antimicrobials, including fluoroquinolones and clarithromycin, for several months. Refer to specialist texts.

Clomipramine

(Clomicalm [d]) **POM-V**

Formulations: Oral: 5 mg, 20 mg, 80 mg tablets.

Action: Both clomipramine and its primary metabolite desmethyl-clomipramine are active in blocking serotonin and noradrenaline reuptake in the brain, with resultant anxiolytic, antidepressant and anticompulsive effects.

Use:
- Authorized for use in association with a behaviour modification plan for the management of separation-related disorders in dogs.
- Also used in management of a wider range of anxiety-related disorders in dogs and cats, including compulsive behaviours, noise fears and urine spraying.
- Has been reported in the treatment of cataplexy in the dog, with resolution of signs after 3 months of treatment.

Care required before use in animals with a history of constipation, epilepsy, glaucoma, urinary retention or arrhythmias. Can be used alongside benzodiazepines.

Safety and handling: Normal precautions should be observed.

Contraindications: Patients sensitive to tricyclic or serotonin reuptake inhibitor antidepressants. Do not give with, or within 2 weeks of, monoamine oxidase inhibitors (e.g. selegiline). Not recommended for use in male breeding animals as testicular hypoplasia may occur.

Adverse reactions: May cause sporadic vomiting, changes in appetite or lethargy. Vomiting may be reduced by co-administration with a small quantity of food. May cause urinary retention in cats. The safety margin is quite low, with toxic side effects observed at 2–3 mg/kg, although the fatal dose is >10 times the recommended dose.

Drug interactions: May potentiate the effects of the antiarrhythmic drug quinidine, anticholinergic agents (e.g. atropine), other CNS active drugs (e.g. barbiturates, benzodiazepines, general anaesthetics, neuroleptics), sympathomimetics (e.g. adrenaline) and coumarin derivatives. Simultaneous administration with cimetidine may lead to increased plasma levels of clomipramine. Plasma levels of certain antiepileptic drugs, e.g. phenytoin and carbamazepine, may be increased by co-administration with clomipramine. Should not generally be used alongside other serotonergic agents given risk of serotonin syndrome, although use alongside trazodone may be considered in exceptional cases, so long as patient carefully monitored for signs of serotonin syndrome.

DOSES
Dogs: 1–2 mg/kg p.o. q12h.
Cats: 0.25–1 mg/kg p.o. q24h.

References
King JN, Simpson BS, Overall KL et al. (2000) Treatment of separation anxiety in dogs with clomipramine: results from a prospective, randomized, double-blind, placebo-controlled, parallel-group, multicenter clinical trial. Applied Animal Behaviour Science **67**, 255–275
Pfeiffer E, Guy N and Cribb A (1999) Clomipramine-induced urinary retention in a cat. The Canadian Veterinary Journal **40**, 265
Seksel K and Lindeman MJ (1998) Use of clomipramine in the treatment of anxiety-related and obsessive-compulsive disorders in cats. Australian Veterinary Journal **76**, 317–321

Clonazepam
(Klonopin*, Rivotril* and several others) **POM**

Formulations: Oral: 0.25 mg, 0.5 mg, 1.0 mg, 2 mg tablets; 0.5 mg/5 ml, 2 mg/5 ml solution.

Action: Long-acting benzodiazepine with anticonvulsant, muscle relaxant and anxiolytic properties. Enhances activity of gamma-aminobutyric acid (GABA) through binding at the benzodiazepine site of the $GABA_A$ receptor. Also affects glutamate decarboxylase activity.

Use:
- Management of muscular hypertonicity (episodic falling) in the Cavalier King Charles Spaniel.
- Anxiolytic for behaviour modification in both cats and dogs and for hyperaesthesia in cats.
- It has been used to treat epilepsy in cats but more suitable medications are available, including phenobarbital, imepitoin (although to date there have been no publications on its efficacy in cats), levetiracetam and diazepam.

Tolerance may develop following prolonged therapy, with reduction in clinical effect. Dogs may also show physical dependence. Care is required when withdrawing clonazepam after prolonged therapy and the dose should be tapered off.

Safety and handling: Normal precautions should be observed.

Contraindications: Avoid use in patients with marked CNS depression, respiratory depression, severe muscle weakness or hepatic impairment (may worsen hepatic encephalopathy). Also contraindicated in patients with acute narrow angle glaucoma.

Adverse reactions: Generally mild; sedation and respiratory suppression at higher doses are the most important. In cats, potential adverse effects include acute hepatic necrosis, sedation and ataxia.

Drug interactions: Drugs that result in hepatic enzyme induction, e.g. phenobarbital and phenytoin, may accelerate metabolism of clonazepam. Antifungal imidazoles may increase clonazepam levels.

DOSES

Dogs: 0.5 mg/kg p.o. q8–12h (suggested starting dose but there is a wide range of recommendations).

Cats: 0.5 mg/cat p.o. q12–24h (suggested starting dose but there is a wide range of recommendations).

References

Garosi LS, Platt SR and Shelton GD (2002) Hypertonicity in Cavalier King Charles Spaniels. *Journal of Veterinary Internal Medicine* **16**, 330

Moesta A (2014) Animal behavior case of the month. Spinning. *Journal of the American Veterinary Medical Association* **244**, 1149–1152

Clonidine

(Catapres*) **POM**

Formulations: Injectable: 150 µg (micrograms)/ml solution. **Oral:** 25 µg tablets.

Action: Stimulates the secretion of growth hormone releasing hormone (GHRH) from the hypothalamus.

Use:
- Diagnostic test used in patients suspected of pituitary dwarfism (hyposomatotropism) to assess the pituitary's ability to produce growth hormone (GH). Specialist texts should be consulted if attempting a clonidine stimulation test. Assessment of plasma insulin-like growth factor-1 (IGF-1) concentration in a single sample is a useful screening test for growth hormone disorders.
- Used in dogs to control panic-like responses and fear-based behavioural problems. Effect develops in about 30 minutes and lasts for 3–4 hours, so often needs to be used tactically (prn). Can be used over longer term but may take 1–2 weeks to see full response. Withdrawal must be done gradually to avoid hypertension.

Safety and handling: Normal precautions should be observed.

Contraindications: Use very cautiously in animals with renal or cardiovascular disease.

Adverse reactions: Transient sedation and bradycardia may develop.

Drug interactions: Care should be exercised when using with drugs that also lower blood pressure or heart rate. Should not be used concurrently with barbiturates, opiates or hypotensive agents (e.g. beta-blockers).

DOSES

Dogs:
- **Growth hormone stimulation:** 3–10 µg (micrograms)/kg i.v. once.
- **Behavioural modification:** 0.01–0.05 mg/kg as needed up to q12h (often with food).

Cats: No information available.

References
Ogata N and Dodman NH (2011) The use of clonidine in the treatment of fear-based behavior problems in dogs: an open trial. *Journal of Veterinary Behavior: Clinical Applications and Research* **6**, 130–137

Clopidogrel CIL
(Clopidogrel*, Plavix*) **POM**

Formulations: Oral: 18.75 mg, 75 mg tablets.

Action: Clopidogrel irreversibly binds to the ADP(2Y12) receptor on platelets, preventing both primary and secondary platelet aggregation in response to stimuli.

Use:
- Thromboprophylaxis in cats and dogs.

Commonly used to reduce the risk of thrombus formation in cats with advanced cardiac disease, thromboembolism in cats with a pre-existing thrombus, or recurrence of embolism in cats with a previous arterial thromboembolic event. Evidence suggests clopidogrel is superior compared with aspirin in delay of feline recurrent thromboembolic events secondary to cardiac disease. May be used in conjunction with aspirin (as the drugs act on different parts of the platelet activation cycle). May be substituted for aspirin if aspirin is not tolerated. Use with care in patients with renal or hepatic impairment.

Safety and handling: Normal precautions should be observed.

Contraindications: Bleeding disorders, GI ulceration.

Adverse reactions: Tablet formulations for humans are film-coated, which needs to be broken for appropriate dosing in cats. Many cats dislike the taste of the tablets when the film-coating is broken so it is recommended that the tablet be administered in a gelatin capsule to improve patient compliance. Taste of newer resized formulations anecdotally still not tolerated. In humans, skin reactions have been reported. Overdoses are expected to lead to bleeding disorders.

Drug interactions: High risk of bleeding complications if used with anticoagulants.

DOSES

Dogs: 1.1–4 mg/kg p.o. q24h. A single loading dose of 4–10 mg/kg p.o. may help achieve therapeutic concentrations more rapidly.

Cats: 18.75 mg/cat p.o. q24h. A single loading dose of 37.5 mg p.o. may help achieve therapeutic concentrations more rapidly.

References
Blais M-C, Bianco D, Goggs R *et al.* (2019) Consensus on the rational use of antithrombotics in veterinary critical care (CURATIVE): Domain 3—Defining antithrombotic protocols. *Journal of Veterinary Emergency and Critical Care* **29**, 60–74
Hogan DF, Fox PR, Jacob K *et al.* (2015) Secondary prevention of cardiogenic arterial thromboembolism in the cat: The double-blind, randomized, positive-controlled feline arterial thromboembolism; clopidogrel *versus* aspirin trial (FATCAT). *Journal of Veterinary Cardiology* **17(S1)**, 306–317

Clotrimazole

CIL

(Aurizon[d], Marbodex[d], Otomax[d], Otoxolan[d], Canesten*, Clotrimazole*, Lotriderm*) **POM-V, POM**

Formulations: Topical: 1% cream; 1% solution; 10 mg/ml suspension with dexamethasone and marbofloxacin (Aurizon, Marbodex, Otoxolan); 8.8 mg/ml suspension with gentamicin and betamethasone (Otomax). Many other products are available; some contain corticosteroids.

Action: Topical imidazole with an inhibitory action on the growth of pathogenic dermatophytes, *Aspergillus* and yeasts by inhibiting cytochrome P450-dependent ergosterol synthesis.

Use:
- Superficial fungal infections.
- Sinonasal infections including aspergillosis. Although evidence of additional benefit from clotrimazole administration is limited.

Safety and handling: Normal precautions should be observed.

Contraindications: No information available.

Adverse reactions: No information available.

Drug interactions: No information available.

DOSES

Dogs, Cats:
- Otic: instil 3–5 drops in ear q12h.
- Topical: apply to affected area and massage in gently q12h; if no improvement in 4 weeks, re-evaluate therapy or diagnosis.
- Nasal: instil 10 g (dogs up to 10 kg) or 20 g (dogs >10 kg) of 1% cream in each frontal sinus via trephine holes. Do not use this route (or seek specialist advice) if cribiform plate not intact.

Cloxacillin

(Opticlox[c,d], Orbenin[c,d]) **POM-V**

Formulations: Ophthalmic: Cloxacillin benzathine ester 16.7% suspension.

Action: Beta-lactamase-resistant penicillin which works in a time-dependent fashion. Binds to penicillin-binding proteins involved in cell wall synthesis, thereby decreasing bacterial cell wall strength and rigidity, and affecting cell division, growth and septum formation.

Use:
- Specifically indicated for ocular infections with beta-lactamase-producing *Staphylococcus*.
- Narrow-spectrum antimicrobial. Less active than penicillin G or V against *Streptococcus*.

Safety and handling: May cause a reaction in penicillin-sensitive individuals. Normal precautions should be observed.

Contraindications: No information available.

Adverse reactions: No information available.

Drug interactions: No information available.

DOSES

Classified as category D (Prudence) by the EMA.

See Appendix for guidelines on responsible antibiotic use.

Dogs, Cats: Apply 1/10 of a tube (0.3 g) q24h.

Co-amoxiclav (Amoxicillin/Clavulanate, Amoxycillin/Clavulanic acid)

(Clavaseptin c,d, Clavubactin c,d, Clavucill c,d, Clavudale c,d, Combimox, Kesium c,d, Nisinject d, Noroclav c,d, Synuclav c,d, Synulox c,d, Twinox, Augmentin*) **POM-V, POM**

Formulations: Injectable: 175 mg/ml suspension (140 mg amoxicillin, 35 mg clavulanate); 600 mg powder (500 mg amoxicillin, 100 mg clavulanate); 1.2 g powder (1 g amoxicillin, 200 mg clavulanate) for reconstitution (Augmentin). Oral: 40/10 mg, 50/12.5 mg, 200/50 mg, 250/62.5 mg, 400/100 mg, 500/125 mg tablets each containing amoxicillin and clavulanate in a ratio of 4:1. Palatable drops which when reconstituted with water provide 40 mg amoxicillin and 10 mg clavulanic acid per ml. Note variation in labelling of products. The preparation size may be labelled in relation to amoxicillin quantity only or the combined amoxicillin/clavulanic acid quantity.

Action: Amoxicillin binds to penicillin-binding proteins involved in bacterial cell wall synthesis, thereby decreasing cell wall strength and rigidity, affecting cell division, growth and septum formation. The addition of the beta-lactamase inhibitor clavulanate increases the antimicrobial spectrum against those organisms that produce beta-lactamase, such as *Staphylococcus* and *Escherichia coli*. Time-dependent action.

Use:
- Active against Gram-positive and Gram-negative aerobic organisms and many obligate anaerobes. Beta-lactamase-producing *Escherichia coli* and *Staphylococcus* are susceptible, but difficult Gram-negative organisms such as *Pseudomonas aeruginosa* and *Klebsiella* are often resistant.
- May be an appropriate choice for surgical prophylaxis (clean-contaminated and contaminated procedures), please refer to separate surgical prophylaxis guidelines and see 'adverse reactions' below.

Dose and dosing interval will be determined by infection site, severity and organism.

Safety and handling: Tablets are wrapped in foil moisture-resistant packaging; do not remove until ready to administer. Refrigerate oral suspension after reconstitution and discard after 10 days. The i.v. solution should be used immediately after reconstitution.

Contraindications: Avoid oral antibiotic agents in critically ill patients, as absorption from the GI tract may be unreliable; such patients may require i.v. formulation. Avoid use in animals which have displayed hypersensitivity reactions to other antimicrobials within the beta-lactam family (which includes cephalosporins).

Adverse reactions: Nausea, diarrhoea and skin rashes are the commonest adverse effects. There are reports of adverse reactions associated with the soluble intravenous preparations, particularly under general anaesthesia during use as surgical prophylaxis. This has included signs of allergic oedema, allergic pruritis, development of urticaria and hypotension. Some centres have opted to use alternative preparations such as the 2nd generation cephalosporin cefuroxime, and this may be associated with fewer adverse reactions.

Drug interactions: Do not mix in the same syringe as aminoglycosides. Synergism may occur between beta-lactam and aminoglycoside antimicrobials *in vivo*.

DOSES

Classified as category C (Caution) by the EMA.
See Appendix for guidelines on responsible antibiotic use.
Dogs, Cats:
- Parenteral:
  - 8.75–25 mg/kg (combined) i.v. q8h, i.m, s.c. q24h. Some susceptible infections require doses higher than the authorized dose or increased administration frequency; doses up to 25 mg/kg i.v. q8h are used to treat serious infections in humans.
  - **For surgical prophylaxis:** 22–25 mg/kg i.v. 30–60 min prior to surgery and then repeated q1.5–2h during surgery.
- Oral: 12.5–25 mg/kg (combined) p.o. q8–12h.

References
Gosling MJ and Martinez-Taboada F (2018) Adverse reactions to two intravenous antibiotics (Augmentin and Zinacef) used for surgical prophylaxis in dogs. *Veterinary Record* **182**, 80

Codeine `CIL`

(Pardale-V [d], Codeine*) **POM-V, POM**

Formulations: Oral: 3 mg/5 ml paediatric linctus; 3 mg/ml linctus; 5 mg/ml syrup; 15 mg, 30 mg, 60 mg tablets. Pardale-V is a veterinary formulation with 400 mg paracetamol + 9 mg codeine. However, to deliver the dose of codeine listed below would result in a very high dose of paracetamol and therefore Pardale-V tablets cannot be recommended as a source of codeine for general usage.

Action: Opioid analgesic.

Use:
- Cough suppression.
- Analgesia.
- Treatment of diarrhoea.

Safety and handling: Normal precautions should be observed.

Contraindications: Renal insufficiency, hypoadrenocorticism, increased intracranial pressure, hypothyroidism. Use with care in animals with severe respiratory compromise. Never administer Pardale-V to cats.

Adverse reactions: Sedation, ataxia, respiratory depression and constipation. May cause CNS stimulation in cats.

Drug interactions: No information available.

DOSES

Dogs:
- **Antitussive:** 1–2 mg/kg p.o. q6–12h. Do not use Pardale-V for codeine at this dose rate.
- **Analgesia:** 1–2 mg/kg p.o. q6–12h. Do not use Pardale-V for codeine at this dose rate.

Cats: Analgesia: 0.5–2 mg/kg p.o. q6–8h. Do not use formulation with paracetamol.

References
Kukanich B (2010) Pharmacokinetics of acetaminophen, codeine, and the codeine metabolites morphine and codeine-6-glucuronide in healthy Greyhound dogs. *Journal of Veterinary Pharmacology and Therapeutics* **33**, 15–21

Colchicine

CIL

(Colchicine*) **POM**

Formulations: Oral: 0.5 mg tablets.

Action: Colchicine inhibits collagen synthesis, may enhance collagenase activity and blocks the synthesis and secretion of serum amyloid A.

Use:
- Used in the prevention and management of Shar-Pei Autoinflammatory Disease (SPAID) or 'Shar-Pei fever', although very limited data exists to support its efficacy.

Only very limited and anecdotal evidence for its efficacy as an antifibrotic in dogs. No evidence for its efficacy as an antifibrotic in cats. No data to suggest it is beneficial in management of cirrhosis or chronic hepatitis. Due to the relatively high incidence of adverse reactions, this drug should be used with caution.

Safety and handling: Protect from light.

Contraindications: Pregnancy, severe renal impairment.

Adverse reactions: Adverse effects include vomiting, abdominal pain and diarrhoea. Rarely, renal damage, bone marrow suppression, myopathy and peripheral neuropathy may develop. Colchicine may increase serum ALP activity, decrease platelet counts and cause false-positive results when testing urine for RBCs and haemoglobin. Overdoses can be fatal.

Drug interactions: Possible increased risk of nephrotoxicity and myotoxicity when given with ciclosporin. NSAIDs, especially phenylbutazone, may increase the risks of thrombocytopenia, leucopenia or bone marrow depression when used concurrently with colchicine. Many anticancer chemotherapeutics may cause additive myelosuppressive effects when used with colchicine.

DOSES

Dogs: Initial dose: 0.01 mg/kg p.o. q24h and, if no adverse GI effects, increase in incremental amounts every 3−4 days to a maximum dose of 0.03 mg/kg p.o. q12h.
Cats: Not recommended.

Colestyramine (Cholestyramine)

(Questran*) **POM**

Formulations: Oral: 4 g powder sachet.

Action: Ion-exchange resin.

Use:
- In dogs for the reduction of serum cholesterol in idiopathic hypercholesterolaemia.
- Bile acid sequestration (may help alleviate diarrhoea in cases of fat malabsorption).
- May be used in digoxin overdose in dogs.

Safety and handling: Normal precautions should be observed.

Contraindications: No information available.

Adverse reactions: Constipation may develop. May cause taurine depletion in cats. May interfere with macronutrient and fat-soluble vitamin absorption.

Drug interactions: Colestyramine reduces the absorption of digoxin, anticoagulants, diuretics and thyroxine.

DOSES
Dogs:
- **Hyperlipidaemia:** 1–2 g/dog p.o. q12h.
- **Bile acid sequestration:** 1–2 g/dog p.o. q12h.

Cats: Anecdotally, 0.5 g/cat p.o q24h titrated upwards to effect.

Crisantaspase see **Asparaginase**

Cyclopentolate hydrochloride
(Minims cyclopentolate hydrochloride*) **POM**

Formulations: Ophthalmic: 0.5%, 1% solutions in single-use vials.

Action: Topical ocular parasympatholytic drug that induces pupillary dilation (mydriasis) and paralysis of the ciliary muscle (cycloplegia).

Use:
- Induce diagnostic mydriasis.
- Premedication for intraocular surgery.
- Treatment/prevention of synechia in uveitis.
- Cycloplegia to reduce ocular pain secondary to corneal and/or intraocular inflammation.

Safety and handling: Normal precautions should be observed.

Contraindications: Do not use in cases of glaucoma.

Adverse reactions: In cats, tear production can reduce for up to 36 hours and intraocular pressure can increase in normal individuals.

Drug interactions: No information available.

DOSES
Dogs: A single drop will cause pupillary dilation within 30 minutes that lasts for 72 hours, with maximum dilation at 12 hours.

Cats: A single drop will cause pupillary dilation within 20–40 minutes that lasts for 24–36 hours.

References
Costa D, Leiva M, Coyo N *et al.* (2016) Effect of topical 1% cyclopentolate hydrochloride on tear production, pupil size, and intraocular pressure in healthy Beagles. *Veterinary Ophthalmology* **19**, 449–453

Kovalcuka L and Nikolajenko M (2020) Changes in intraocular pressure, horizontal pupil diameter, and tear production during the use of topical 1% cyclopentolate in cats and rabbits. *Open Veterinary Journal* **10**, 59–67

A
B
C
D
E
F
G
H
I
J
K
L
M
N
O
P
Q
R
S
T
U
V
W
X
Y
Z

Cyclophosphamide

(Cyclophosphamide*, Endoxana*) **POM**

Formulations: Injectable: 100 mg, 200 mg, 500 mg, 1000 mg powder for reconstitution. **Oral:** 50 mg tablets. Available through specialist pharmacies as 2.5 mg, 5 mg, 7.5 mg, 10 mg, 12.5 mg, 15 mg and 20 mg capsules. **VSP**

Action: Metabolites crosslink DNA resulting in inhibition of DNA synthesis, RNA transcription and replication and function.

Use:

- Treatment of lymphoproliferative diseases and myeloproliferative disease.
- May have a role in management of certain sarcomas and carcinomas when included in metronomic chemotherapy protocols.

Use with caution in patients with renal failure; dose reduction may be required. Cyclophosphamide is no longer recommended as an immunosuppressant drug.

Safety and handling: Cytotoxic drug; see Appendix and specialist texts for further advice on chemotherapeutic agents.

Contraindications: No information available.

Adverse reactions: Myelosuppression, with the nadir usually occurring 5−14 days after the start of therapy; regular monitoring of WBCs recommended. A metabolite of cyclophosphamide (acrolein) may cause a sterile haemorrhagic cystitis. The cystitis may be persistent and may lead to bladder fibrosis and/or transitional cell carcinoma. This risk may be reduced by increasing water consumption and by giving furosemide to ensure adequate urine production. Other adverse effects include vomiting, diarrhoea, hepatotoxicity, nephrotoxicity, pulmonary infiltrates and fibrosis, and a reduction in hair growth rate.

Drug interactions: Increased risk of myelosuppression if thiazide diuretics given concomitantly. Absorption of orally administered digoxin may be decreased, may occur several days after dosing. Barbiturates increase cyclophosphamide toxicity due to increased rate of conversion to metabolites. Phenothiazines, ondansetron and chloramphenicol reduce cyclophosphamide efficacy. If administered with doxorubicin, there is an increased risk of cardiotoxicity. Insulin requirements are altered by cyclophosphamide.

DOSES

See Appendix for chemotherapy protocols and conversion of bodyweight to body surface area.

Dogs:

- **Lymphoid neoplasia:** 50 mg/m^2 p.o. q48h or 3−4 consecutive days/week; or 200−250 mg/m^2 p.o., i.v. q3wk as part of a multidrug chemotherapy protocol.
- **Metronomic chemotherapy:** 10−15 mg/m^2 p.o. q24−48h.
- **Multiple myeloma in patients refractory to melphalan:** 1 mg/kg p.o. q24h.
- **Macroglobulinaemia in patients refractory to chlorambucil:** 1 mg/kg p.o. q24h.

Cats: Lymphoid neoplasia: as for dogs, except 200−300 mg/m^2 in 'high dose' COP regimes.

References

Elmslie RE, Glowe P and Dow SW (2008) Metronomic therapy with cyclophosphamide and piroxicam effectively delays tumor recurrence in Dogs with Incompletely Resected Soft Tissue Sarcomas. *Journal of Veterinary Internal Medicine* **22**, 1373–1379

Teske E, van Straten G, van Noort R *et al.* (2002) Chemotherapy with cyclophosphamide, vincristine and prednisolone (COP) in cats with malignant lymphoma: new results with an old protocol. *Journal of Veterinary Internal Medicine* **16**, 179–186

Cyclosporin(e) see Ciclosporin

Cyproheptadine

(Periactin*) **POM**

CIL

Formulations: Oral: 4 mg tablets.

Action: Binds to and blocks the activation of H1 histamine and serotonin receptors.

Use:
- Management of allergic disease.
- Appetite stimulation.
- Also used in cats with aortic thromboembolism as serotonin, along with other mediators, is involved in collateral vasoconstriction. Maintenance of this collateral supply is important in recovery.

Use with caution in cases with urinary retention, angle-closure glaucoma and pyloroduodenal obstruction. Specific doses for dogs and cats have not been determined by pharmacokinetic studies and clinical effectiveness has not been established.

Safety and handling: Normal precautions should be observed.

Contraindications: No information available.

Adverse reactions: May cause mild sedation, polyphagia, weight gain. May reduce seizure threshold.

Drug interactions: No information available.

DOSES

Dogs, Cats: 0.1–0.5 mg/kg p.o. q8–12h.

Cytarabine (Cytosine arabinoside, Ara-C)

(Cytarabine*, Cytosar-U*) **POM**

Formulations: Injectable: 100 mg, 500 mg powders for reconstitution. 100 mg/ml, 100 mg/5 ml vials of solution for injection (larger bottles and stronger concentrations also available).

Action: The active nucleotide metabolite ara-CTP is incorporated into DNA and inhibits pyrimidine and DNA synthesis. Cytarabine is therefore S-phase-specific.

Use:
- Management of lymphoproliferative and myeloproliferative disorders. For dogs diagnosed with lymphoma with bone marrow or CNS involvement, addition of cytarabine into a VCAA combination protocol may improve survival time. Cytarabine is included in many rescue protocols for relapsed lymphoma.

- Cytarabine is widely used for the treatment of meningoencephalitis of unknown origin and other suspected immune-mediated neurological diseases that are unresponsive to steroids or have significant side effects from steroid treatment (e.g. steroid responsive meningitis). There is currently no general agreement on the best treatment protocol, but combination therapy of prednisolone and cytarabine is widely reported.

Safety and handling: Cytotoxic drug; see Appendix and specialist texts for further advice on chemotherapeutic agents. After reconstitution, store at room temperature and discard after 48 hours or if a slight haze develops.

Contraindications: Do not use if there is evidence of bone marrow suppression or substantial hepatic impairment.

Adverse reactions: Mainly GI (e.g. vomiting, diarrhoea, anorexia) and leucopenia (myelosuppression). As it is a myelosuppressant, careful haematological monitoring is required. Conjunctivitis, oral ulceration, neurotoxicity, hepatotoxicity and fever have also been seen. Calcinosis cutis has been reported at the site of injection in three dogs. There has been one case of possible drug induced pulmonary infiltrative disease.

Drug interactions: Oral absorption of digoxin is decreased. Activity of gentamicin may be antagonized. Simultaneous administration of methotrexate increases the effect of cytarabine.

DOSES

See Appendix for chemotherapy protocols and conversion of bodyweight to body surface area.

Dogs, Cats:

- **Lymphoproliferative neoplastic disease:** 100–150 mg/m^2 given i.v. or s.c. over 2–5 days (as part of a VCAA-based protocol); 100 mg/m^2 by CRI over 24–96 hours; 20 mg/m^2 intrathecally q1–5d. Or 200 mg/m^2 given i.v. (over 4 hours) or s.c. q2wk as part of the DMAC protocol. A dose of 300 mg/m^2 s.c. has been used as a rescue agent as part of a lomustine, methotrexate and cytarabine chemotherapy protocol in cats with relapsed lymphoma.
- **Meningoencephalitis of unknown origin:** various different regimes are described in the literature. CRI of cytarabine 200 mg/m^2 over 8 hours; CRI of cytarabine 100 mg/m^2 over 24 hours; 50 mg/m^2 s.c. q12h for 4 doses. Many regimes repeat the treatment over an increasing number of weeks (i.e. 3 week intervals, 4 week intervals, 5 week intervals) depending on disease remission. There is limited evidence to support a single dose over multiple treatments and it is probably case dependent as to clinical response and disease progression.

References

Marconato L, Bonfanti U, Stefanello D *et al.* (2008) Cytosine arabinoside in addition to VCAA-based protocols for the treatment of canine lymphoma with bone marrow involvement: does it make the difference? *Veterinary Comparative Oncology* **6**, 80–89

Zarfoss M, Schatzberg S, Venator K *et al.* (2006) Combined cytosine arabinoside and prednisone therapy for meningoencephalitis of unknown aetiology in 10 dogs. *Journal of Small Animal Practice* **47**, 588–595

Dacarbazine

(Carboxamide*, Dacarbazine*, DTIC*, Imidazole*) **POM**

Formulations: Injectable: 100 mg, 200 mg, 500 mg powders for reconstitution.

Action: Methylates nucleic acids and inhibits DNA, RNA and protein synthesis. Minimally immunosuppressive.

Use:
- Management of lymphoproliferative diseases (e.g. relapsed lymphoma), haemangiosarcoma, histiocytic sarcoma, melanoma and soft tissue sarcoma.

Use with caution in patients with renal or hepatic insufficiency. Can cause severe pain and extensive tissue damage with extravasation, and therefore must be administered via a preplaced i.v. catheter.

Safety and handling: Cytotoxic drug; see Appendix and specialist texts for further advice on chemotherapeutic agents.

Contraindications: Bone marrow suppression. Not recommended in cats, as it is unknown whether they can metabolize it adequately.

Adverse reactions: May be severe. Include myelosuppression and gastrointestinal adverse events, such as intense nausea and vomiting (consider premedication with an antiemetic). Considered a vesicant and can cause extravasation reactions.

Drug interactions: Phenobarbital and phenytoin increase the metabolic activation of dacarbazine. Do not use with other myelosuppressive drugs.

DOSES
See Appendix for chemotherapy protocols and conversion of bodyweight to body surface area.

Dogs: 200–250 mg/m^2 i.v. q24h on days 1–5. Repeat cycle q3–4wk. Or, dependent upon the chemotherapy protocol, 800–1000 mg/m^2 i.v. over a 4–8h period, may repeat q2–3wk provided the bone marrow has recovered.

Cats: Not recommended.

References
Griessmayr PC, Payne SE, Winter JE, Barber LG and Shofer FS (2009) Dacarbazine as single-agent therapy for relapsed lymphoma in dogs. *Journal of Veterinary Internal Medicine* **23**, 1227–1231

Dactinomycin (Actinomycin-D)

(Cosmegen*, Dactinomycin*, Lyovac*) **POM**

Formulations: Injectable: 0.5 mg powder for reconstitution.

Action: An antibiotic antineoplastic that inhibits DNA synthesis and function. Inhibition of RNA and protein synthesis may also contribute to cytotoxic effects.

Use:
- Has been used in rescue protocols for canine lymphoma and also in some sarcomas and carcinomas.

Use with caution with pre-existing bone marrow depression, hepatic dysfunction or infection. The drug is vesicant and will cause tissue

A
B
C
D
E
F
G
H
I
J
K
L
M
N
O
P
Q
R
S
T
U
V
W
X
Y
Z

damage if extravasated, and therefore must be administered via a preplaced catheter.

Safety and handling: Potent cytotoxic drug that should only be prepared and administered by trained personnel. See Appendix and specialist texts for further advice on chemotherapeutic agents.

Contraindications: The P-glycoprotein pump actively transports dactinomycin, hence use with caution in breeds susceptible to the *ABCB1* mutation (e.g. collies, Australian Shepherds).

Adverse reactions: Myelosuppression is the main dose-limiting toxicity. GI and hepatic toxicity may also occur. Can increase the risk of urate stone formation in susceptible breeds. Risk of anaphylaxis; consider premedication with antihistamine prior to injection.

Drug interactions: May add to cardiotoxicity if used concurrently or sequentially with doxorubicin.

DOSES
See Appendix for chemotherapy protocols and conversion of bodyweight to body surface area.

Dogs: 0.5–0.75 mg/m^2 slow i.v. (over 20 min) q1–3wk.

Cats: No information available.

References
Alvarez FJ, Kisseberth WC, Gallant SL and Couto CG (2006) Dexamethasone, melphalan, actinomycin D, cytosine arabinoside (DMAC) protocol for dogs with relapsed lymphoma. *Journal of Veterinary Internal Medicine* **20**, 1178–1183
Siedlecki CT, Kass PH, Jakubiak MJ *et al.* (2006) Evaluation of an actinomycin-D-containing combination chemotherapy protocol with extended maintenance therapy for canine lymphoma. *Canadian Veterinary Journal* **47**, 52–59

Dantrolene
(Dantrium*) **POM**   `CIL`

Formulations: Oral: 25 mg, 100 mg capsules. Injectable: Vials of 20 mg dantrolene powder + 3 g mannitol + sodium hydroxide for reconstitution.

Action: Uncouples the excitation contraction process by preventing the release of calcium ions from the sarcoplasmic reticulum in striated muscle. As vascular smooth muscle and cardiac muscle are not primarily dependent on calcium release for contraction they are not usually affected.

Use:
- Management of muscle spasms (e.g. urethral muscle spasm, tetanus).
- Prevention (oral) or treatment (i.v.) of malignant hyperthermia.

Each vial should be reconstituted with 60 ml of water. Before administration, the solution must be clear and without visible particles.

Safety and handling: Normal precautions should be observed. Protect from light and use each re-constituted vial within 6 hours.

Contraindications: No information available.

Adverse reactions: Injectable preparation has pH 9.5 and is highly irritant when extravasated. Ideally administer via a large vein or inject into a fast-running infusion to reduce the likelihood of thrombophlebitis. Diuresis follows i.v. administration, reflecting its formulation with mannitol. Chronic use is associated with hepatitis and pleural effusion; monitor liver function during therapy. Generalized muscle weakness, including the respiratory muscles, has been reported after overdose; initiate symptomatic supportive therapy and monitor the patient carefully, particularly with respect to efficacy of respiration.

Drug interactions: Do not combine with calcium-channel blockers.

DOSES

Dogs, Cats:
- **Malignant hyperthermia:** 2–5 mg/kg i.v.
- **Other indications:** 0.5–2 mg/kg p.o. q12h.

References
Haraschak JL, Langston VC, Wang R *et al.* (2014) Pharmacokinetic evaluation of oral dantrolene in the dog. *Journal of Veterinary Pharmacology and Therapeutics* **37**, 286–294

Darbepoetin
(Aranesp*) **POM**

`CIL`

Formulations: Injectable: 25–500 µg (micrograms) pre-filled syringes for injection (total dose).

Action: Stimulates division and differentiation of RBCs. Darbepoetin is a derivative of human erythropoietin that has been chemically modified to prolong its half-life. It may be less prone to produce anti-erythropoietin antibodies than other recombinant human erythropoietin.

Use:
- Treatment of anaemia associated with chronic renal failure and FeLV-associated anaemia.

Monitoring and/or supplementation of iron may be necessary, especially if the response to treatment is poor. It is also used to treat anaemic human patients with cancer and rheumatoid arthritis.

Safety and handling: Normal precautions should be observed.

Contraindications: Conditions where high serum concentrations of erythropoietin already exist (e.g. haemolytic anaemia, anaemia due to blood loss), where anaemia is due to iron deficiency or where uncontrolled systemic hypertension is present.

Adverse reactions: Local and systemic allergic reactions may rarely develop (skin rash at the injection site, pyrexia, arthralgia and mucocutaneous ulcers). The production of cross-reacting anti-EPO antibodies can cause pure red cell aplasia. Hypertension and seizures have also been reported.

Drug interactions: No information available.

DOSES

Dogs, Cats: For stimulating erythropoiesis (induction dose): 0.25–1 µg (micrograms)/kg s.c. weekly until PCV is normal, then increasing dose interval for maintenance. Some authors recommend starting at the 1 µg/kg dose for improved efficacy. Dosing interval >21 days failed to maintain a response to treatment in one study (dogs).

References
Chalhoub S, Langston CE and Farrelly J (2012) The use of darbepoetin to stimulate erythropoiesis in anemia of chronic kidney disease in cats: 25 cases. *Journal of Veterinary Internal Medicine* **26**, 363–369

Polzin DJ (2013) Evidence-based step-wise approach to managing chronic kidney disease in dogs and cats. *Journal of Veterinary Emergency and Critical Care* **23**, 205–215

Deferoxamine (Desferrioxamine)

(Desferal*) **POM**

Formulations: Injectable: 500 mg vial for reconstitution.

Action: Deferoxamine chelates iron, and the complex is excreted in the urine.

Use: To remove iron from the body following poisoning.

Safety and handling: Normal precautions should be observed.

Contraindications: Avoid in severe renal disease.

Adverse reactions: i.m. administration is painful. Anaphylactic reactions and hypotension may develop if administered rapidly i.v.

Drug interactions: No information available.

DOSES

Dogs, Cats: 40 mg/kg i.m. q4–8h or 15 mg/kg/h slow i.v. infusion.

References

Haldane SL and Davis RM (2009) Acute toxicity in five dogs after ingestion of a commercial snail and slug bait containing iron EDTA. *Australian Veterinary Journal* **87**, 284–286

Delmadinone

(Tardak) **POM-V**

Formulations: Injectable: 10 mg/ml suspension.

Action: Progestogens suppress follicle-stimulating hormone and luteinizing hormone production.

Use:
- Used in the treatment of hypersexuality (male dog and cat).
- Treatment of prostatic hypertrophy.
- Management of peri-anal gland adenomas.
- Treatment of hormonally driven canine aggression.

Dogs that show a reduced level of aggression when treated with delmadinone will not automatically show the same behavioural response to surgical castration because the drug also has a central calming effect. In situations of fear- or anxiety-related aggressive behaviour, the surgical approach can exacerbate the behaviour.

Safety and handling: Normal precautions should be observed.

Contraindications: Avoid in patients with severe renal or hepatic impairment or diabetes mellitus.

Adverse reactions: Possible adverse effects include a transient reduction in fertility and libido, polyuria and polydipsia, an increased appetite and hair colour change at the site of injection.

Drug interactions: Cortisol response to ACTH stimulation is significantly suppressed after just one dose of delmadinone.

DOSES

Dogs: Benign prostatic hypertrophy: 1.5–2 mg/kg (dogs <10 kg); 1–1.5 mg/kg (10–20 kg); 1 mg/kg (>20 kg) i.m., s.c. repeated after 8 days if no response. Animals that respond to treatment may need further treatment after 3–4 weeks.

Cats: Hypersexuality: 1.5 mg/kg i.m., s.c. repeated after 8 days if no response. Animals that respond to treatment may need further treatment after 3–4 weeks.

References
Albouy M, Sanquer A, Maynard L and Eun HM (2008) Efficacies of osaterone and delmadinone in the treatment of benign prostatic hyperplasia in dogs. *Veterinary Record* **163**, 179–183

Deltamethrin
(Canishield [d], Scalibor Protectorband [d]) **NFA-VPS**

Formulations: Topical: 4% deltamethrin collar: 0.76 g (for small and medium dogs), 1 g (for large dogs).

Action: Acts as a sodium 'open channel blocker' resulting in muscular convulsions and death in arthropods. It also repels ticks and insects.

Use:
- Control of tick infestation (*Ixodes ricinus*, *Rhipicephalus sanguineus*).
- Prevention of feeding by phlebotomine sandflies and mosquitoes (*Culex pipiens pipiens*) on dogs for up to 6 months.
- Persistent flea (*Ctenocephalides felis*) killing activity for 16 weeks (Canishield).

Collar exerts full effect after 1 week.

Safety and handling: Wash hands after fitting the collar. Avoid letting children, in particular those under 2-years of age, touch the collar, play with it or put it into their mouth. Highly toxic to aquatic animals (remove collar before letting dog swim in rivers) and bees, also toxic to birds.

Contraindications: Do not use on dogs <7 weeks old. Avoid use on dogs with skin lesions. Do not use on cats.

Adverse reactions: Rarely, dermatitis around the neck, GI and neuro-muscular disturbances can occur. Diazepam should be administered in the event of accidental ingestion.

Drug interactions: No information available.

DOSES
See Appendix for guidelines on responsible parasiticide use.
Dogs: One collar q5–6months.
Cats: Do not use.

ʟ-Deprenyl see **Selegiline**
Desferrioxamine see **Deferoxamine**

Deslorelin
(Suprelorin [c,d]) **POM-V**

Formulations: Implant containing 4.7 mg (6 months) or 9.4 mg (12 months) of active product.

Action: Gonadotropin-releasing hormone superagonist. Receptors are stimulated in the first 2 weeks after application, but then die down through overstimulation, thereby decreasing release of luteinizing hormone and follicle-stimulating hormone. This leads to cessation of testosterone and sperm production.

Use:
- Temporary chemical castration.

Infertility (no spermatogenesis and reduced libido) is achieved from 6 weeks for up to 6 or 12 months. Treated dogs should still be kept away from bitches in oestrus for 6 weeks following initial treatment (separation unnecessary following subsequent implantations provided the product is administered every 6 or 12 months). Rarely, matings may occur during the treatment period but will not result in pregnancy. Dogs <10 kg may not recover their testosterone concentrations for 18 months. Deslorelin stabilizes the bladder wall and can improve incontinence either with or without concurrent sphincter-enhancing treatment. In tom cats, deslorelin implants cause chemical castration for 2–4 years. The product should be implanted subcutaneously in the loose skin on the back between the lower neck and the lumbar area. Avoid injection of the implant into fat, as release of the active substance might be impaired in areas of low vascularization. The biocompatible implant does not require removal; however, should it be necessary to end treatment, implants can be removed under local anaesthesia.

Safety and handling: People who are or may become pregnant should not handle this drug.

Contraindications: Use in bitches causes induction of oestrus within a few days, followed by a long anoestrus period.

Adverse reactions: Moderate swelling at the implant site may be observed for 14 days. A significant decrease in testicle size will be seen during treatment.

Drug interactions: No information available.

DOSES
Dogs: 1 implant per male dog, repeat after 6 (4.7 mg) or 12 (9.4 mg) months (depending on size of implant).
Cats: 1 implant (4.7 mg) per male cat.

References
Fontaine C (2015) Long-term contraception in a small implant: A review of suprelorin (deslorelin) studies in cats. *Journal of Feline Medicine and Surgery* **17**, 766–771

Desmopressin
(DDAVP*, Desmospray*, Desmotabs*) **POM**

Formulations: Intranasal: 100 μg (micrograms)/ml solution; 10 μg metered spray. **Injectable:** 4 μg/ml solution. **Oral:** 100 μg, 200 μg tablets.

Action: Binds to and stimulates arginine vasopressin receptors in the collecting ducts of the kidney. Desmopressin, a vasopressin analogue, has a longer duration of action than vasopressin and, unlike vasopressin, has no vasoconstrictor activity. Also increases von Willebrand factor, factor VIII and plasminogen concentrations.

Use:
- Diagnosis and treatment of central diabetes insipidus.

- To boost plasma levels of factor VIII and von Willebrand factor in patients with mild to moderate haemophilia A or von Willebrand's disease. Severe forms of these diseases are not successfully treated with desmopressin.

Further advice on the use of this drug as a therapeutic trial (or a modified water deprivation test) should be obtained from *BSAVA Manual of Canine and Feline Endocrinology*. Assess adrenocortical function before performing the test. Desmopressin will decrease urine output for any condition that is even partially mediated via arginine vasopressin. Response to desmopressin does not confirm diabetes insipidus.

Safety and handling: Normal precautions should be observed.

Contraindications: Do not use in patients with hyponatraemia, renal disease, dehydration or hypercalcaemia.

Adverse reactions: No information available.

Drug interactions: No information available.

DOSES

Dogs:
- **Diabetes insipidus treatment:** 1–4 µg (micrograms)/dog i.v., i.m.; 5–20 µg or 0.05–0.2 ml/dog intranasally or on to the conjunctiva q8–24h; 5 µg/kg p.o. q8–24h (maximum dose 400 µg q8h). The dose and frequency of dosing can be increased or decreased according to response.
- **Coagulopathies:** 1–4 µg/kg i.v. once, diluted in 20 ml saline and administered over 10 min.
- **Diabetes insipidus diagnosis (modified water deprivation test):** 1–4 µg/dog i.v. once. This test is now very rarely used. A therapeutic trial of desmopressin may be more approrpiate once other differentials have been excluded.

Cats: 5 µg (micrograms)/cat or 0.05 ml (1–2 drops) intranasally or on to the conjunctiva q8–24h; 5 µg/cat p.o. q8–24h. The dose and frequency of dosing can be increased or decreased according to response.

References
Shiel RE (2012) Disorders of vasopressin production. In: *BSAVA Manual of Canine and Feline Endocrinology 4th edn*, ed. CT Mooney and ME Peterson, pp. 15–27. BSAVA Publications, Gloucester

Desoxycortone pivalate
(Desoxycorticosterone pivalate)
(Zycortal [d]) **POM-V**

Formulations: Injectable: 25 mg/ml prolonged-release suspension.

Action: Mineralocorticoid.

Use:
- Long-acting replacement therapy for mineralocorticoid deficiency in dogs and cats with primary hypoadrenocorticism.

It is important that hypoadrenocorticism has been definitively diagnosed before starting treatment. Any dog presenting with severe hypovolaemia, dehydration, pre-renal azotaemia and inadequate tissue perfusion (i.e. an 'Addisonian crisis') must be rehydrated with intravenous fluid therapy before starting mineralocorticoid treatment. Use lower doses in dogs with congestive heart disease, severe renal disease, primary hepatic failure or oedema.

Safety and handling: Normal precautions should be observed. The vials are stable for several months once opened. Before use, shake gently to resuspend the product and continue to move the loaded syringe before injection to prevent precipitation.

Contraindications: None.

Adverse reactions: Rarely, pain is seen on initial injection but repeated injections are not painful in the same animal. Overdoses may cause polyuria and hypokalaemia. Vomiting, anorexia, polyuria/polydipsia, muzzle swelling and anaphylaxis have been reported.

Drug interactions: Avoid concurrent use of aldosterone antagonists (spironolactone) and other drugs that may reduce potassium (e.g. furosemide, thiazides).

DOSES
Dogs: Initial dose: 1.5–2.2 mg/kg s.c. Many dogs given the authorized dose of 2.2 mg/kg require lower subsequent doses. For this reason, many authorities start at the lower dose of 1.5 mg/kg s.c., particularly in larger dogs. The dose must be titrated to effect for each individual according to response to therapy and monitoring of electrolyte levels. The final dose can be between 1.0 and 2.7 mg/kg.

Cats: Initial dose: 2.2 mg/kg. Experience is limited but higher doses seem to be needed.

References
Carr AP (2016) How best to treat Addison's disease in dogs? *Veterinary Record* **179**, 96–97
Farr H, Mason BL and Longhofer SL (2020) Randomised clinical non-inferiority trial comparing two formulations of desoxycortone pivalate for the treatment of canine primary hypoadrenocorticism. *Veterinary Record* **187**, e12

Dexamethasone   `CIL`

(Aurizon [d], Dexadreson [c,d], Dexafast [c,d], Dexafort [c,d], Dexa-ject [c,d], Duphacort Q [c,d], Rapidexon [c,d], Voren, Dexamethasone*, Maxidex*, Maxitrol*) **POM-V, POM**

Formulations: Ophthalmic: 0.1% solution (Maxidex, Maxitrol). Maxitrol also contains polymyxin B and neomycin. **Injectable:** 2 mg/ml solution; 1 mg/ml, 3 mg/ml suspensions; 4 mg/ml (1.32 mg/ml sodium phosphate + 2.67 mg/ml phenylpropionate salts) (Voren); 2.5 mg/ml dexamethasone + 7.5 mg/ml prednisolone suspension. **Topical:** 0.9 mg/ml suspension with clotrimazole and marbofloxacin (Aurizon). **Oral:** 0.5 mg tablets. 1 mg of dexamethasone is equivalent to 1.1 mg of dexamethasone acetate, 1.3 mg of dexamethasone isonicotinate or dexamethasone sodium phosphate, or 1.4 mg of dexamethasone trioxa-undecanoate.

Action: Alters the transcription of DNA, leading to alterations in cellular metabolism which cause reduction in inflammatory response.

Use:
- Anti-inflammatory (lower doses) and immunosuppressive (higher doses) action.
- Assessment of adrenal function in suspected hypercortisolism. Consult specialist texts and laboratories for advice on the performance and interpretation of dexamethasone suppression tests.

- Emergency treatment of hypoadrenocorticism.
- To prevent and treat anaphylaxis associated with transfusion or chemotherapeutic agents.

Anti-inflammatory potency is 7.5 times greater than prednisolone. On a dose basis 0.15 mg dexamethasone is equivalent to 1 mg prednisolone. Dexamethasone has a long duration of action and low mineralocorticoid activity and is particularly suitable for short-term high-dose therapy in conditions where water retention would be a disadvantage. Unsuitable for long-term daily or alternate-day use. Animals receiving chronic therapy should be tapered off steroids when discontinuing the drug. The use of long-acting steroids in most cases of shock and spinal injury is of no benefit and may be detrimental.

Safety and handling: Normal precautions should be observed.

Contraindications: Do not use in pregnant animals. Systemic corticosteroids are generally contraindicated in patients with renal disease and diabetes mellitus. Impaired wound healing and delayed recovery from infections may be seen. Topical corticosteroids are contraindicated in ulcerative keratitis.

Adverse reactions: A single dose of dexamethasone or dexamethasone sodium phosphate suppresses adrenal gland function for up to 32 hours. Prolonged use of glucocorticoids suppresses the hypothalamic–pituitary–adrenal axis, causing adrenal atrophy, increased liver enzyme activities, cutaneous atrophy, weight loss, polyuria/polydipsia, vomiting and diarrhoea. GI ulceration may develop. Hyperglycaemia and decreased serum T4 values may be seen in patients receiving dexamethasone.

Drug interactions: There is an increased risk of GI ulceration if used concurrently with NSAIDs. The risk of developing hypokalaemia is increased if corticosteroids are administered concomitantly with amphotericin B or potassium-depleting diuretics (furosemide, thiazides). Dexamethasone antagonizes the effect of insulin. The metabolism of corticosteroids may be enhanced by phenytoin or phenobarbital and decreased by antifungals such as itraconazole.

DOSES
See Appendix for immunosuppression protocols.
Dogs:
- **Ophthalmic:** Apply small amount of ointment to affected eye(s) q6–24h or 1 drop of solution in affected eye(s) q6–12h.
- **Otic:** 10 drops in ear q24h for 7–14 days (authorized dose; many authorities use less).
- **Hypoadrenocorticism:** 0.2 mg/kg i.v. Repeat daily until able to use oral medication.
- **Inflammation:** 0.05–0.2 mg/kg i.m., s.c., p.o. q24h for 3–5 days maximum.
- **Prevention and treatment of anaphylaxis:** 0.5 mg/kg i.v. once.
- **Immunosuppression:** 0.3–0.5 mg/kg i.m., s.c., p.o. q24h for up to 5 days.
- **Assessment of adrenal function (low-dose dexamethasone suppression test):** 0.01–0.015 mg/kg i.v. once.

Cats:
- **Ophthalmic, cerebral oedema, inflammation, anaphylaxis, immunosuppression:** doses as for dogs.
- **Assessment of adrenal function (dexamethasone suppression test):** 0.1–0.15 mg/kg i.v. once.

A
B
C
D
E
F
G
H
I
J
K
L
M
N
O
P
Q
R
S
T
U
V
W
X
Y
Z

Dexmedetomidine

(Dexdomitor [c,d], Sedadex [c,d], Sileo [d]) **POM-V**

Formulations: Injectable: 0.5 mg/ml. **Oral:** 0.1 mg/ml gel.

Action: Agonist at peripheral and central alpha-2 adrenoreceptors producing dose-dependent sedation, muscle relaxation and analgesia.

Use:

- To provide sedation and premedication when used alone or in combination with opioid analgesics.
- Dexmedetomidine combined with ketamine is used to provide a short duration (20–30 min) of surgical anaesthesia in cats.
- Dexmedetomidine is also being increasingly used in very low doses to manage emergence excitation in dogs and cats during recovery from anaesthesia and for the provision of analgesia when administered by CRI.
- Oromucosal gel authorized in dogs for the alleviation of acute noise anxiety, but may also be used to reduce the stress of travel and veterinary visits.

Dexmedetomidine is the pure dextroenantiomer of medetomidine. As the levomedetomidine enantiomer is largely inactive, dexmedetomidine is twice as potent as the racemic mixture (medetomidine). Administration of dexmedetomidine reduces the biological load presented to the animal, resulting in quicker metabolism of concurrently administered anaesthetic drugs and a potentially faster recovery from anaesthesia. Dexmedetomidine is a potent drug that causes marked changes in the cardiovascular system, including an initial peripheral vasoconstriction that results in an increase in blood pressure and a compensatory bradycardia. Vasoconstriction wanes after 20–30 minutes, while blood pressure returns to normal values. Heart rate remains low due to the central sympatholytic effect of alpha-2 agonists. These cardiovascular changes result in a fall in cardiac output; in healthy animals central organ perfusion is well maintained at the expense of redistribution of blood flow away from the peripheral tissues. Respiratory system function is well maintained; respiration rate may fall but is accompanied by an increased depth of respiration. Oxygen supplementation is advisable in all animals that have received dexmedetomidine for sedation. The duration of analgesia from a 5 µg (micrograms)/kg dose of dexmedetomidine is approximately 1 hour. Combining dexmedetomidine with an opioid provides improved analgesia and sedation. Lower doses of dexmedetomidine should be used in combination with other drugs. Reversal of dexmedetomidine sedation or premedication with atipamezole at the end of the procedure shortens the recovery period, which is advantageous. Analgesia should be provided with other classes of drugs before atipamezole.

Safety and handling: Normal precautions should be observed with the injectable form. Gloves should be worn when handling the gel formulation.

Contraindications: Do not use in animals with cardiovascular or other systemic disease. Use of dexmedetomidine in geriatric patients is not advisable. It should not be used in pregnant animals, nor in animals likely to require or receiving sympathomimetic amines. Due to effects on blood glucose, use with caution in diabetic animals.

Adverse reactions: Causes diuresis by suppressing arginine vasopressin secretion, a transient increase in blood glucose by decreasing endogenous insulin secretion, mydriasis and decreased intraocular pressure. Vomiting after i.m. administration is common, so dexmedetomidine should be avoided when vomiting is contraindicated (e.g. foreign body, raised intraocular pressure). Vomiting is a recognized occassional side effect of the oromucosal gel. Spontaneous arousal from deep sedation following stimulation can occur with all alpha-2 agonists; aggressive animals sedated with dexmedetomidine must still be managed with caution.

Drug interactions: No information available.

DOSES
When used for sedation is generally given as part of a combination. See Appendix for sedation protocols in cats and dogs.

Dogs: Control of noise anxiety: 125 µg (micrograms)/m² applied to the oral mucosa 30–60 minutes before the onset of the noise stimulus, or after the first signs. Dosing can be repeated after 2 hours up to a maximum of 5 occasions.

Dogs, Cats:
- **Premedication:** 2–10 µg (micrograms)/kg i.v., i.m, s.c. in combination with an opioid (use lower end of dose range i.v.).
- **Emergence excitation:** 1 µg/kg i.v. can be given to manage emergence excitation during recovery from anaesthesia, although administration around the time of extubation will prolong the recovery period from anaesthesia and treated animals should be monitored carefully.
- **Perioperative analgesia and rousable sedation:** 1–2 µg/kg/h CRI is indicated, although the efficacy of analgesia will be improved in most animals if dexmedetomidine is used as an adjunct to opioid analgesia.

The authorized dose range of dexmedetomidine for dogs and cats is very broad. High doses (>10 µg/kg) are associated with greater physiological disturbances than doses of 1–10 µg/kg. Using dexmedetomidine in combination with opioids in the lower dose range can provide good sedation and analgesia with minimal side effects.

References
Granholm M, Mckusick BC, Westerholm FC and Aspegrén JC (2007) Evaluation of the clinical efficacy and safety of intramuscular and intravenous doses of dexmedetomidine and medetomidine in dogs and their reversal with atipamezole. *Veterinary Record* **160**, 891–897
Korpivaara M, Laapas K, Huhtinen M, Schöning B and Overall K (2017) Dexmedetomidine oromucosal gel for noise-associated acute anxiety and fear in dogs—a randomised, double-blind, placebo-controlled clinical study. *Veterinary Record* **180**, 356

Dexrazoxane
(Cardioxane*, Zinecard*) **POM**

Formulations: Intravenous: 500 mg vials which, when reconstituted, produce a 20 mg/ml solution for infusion.

Action: Prevents the formation of anthracycline-iron complex free radicals thought to be the cause of anthracycline induced cardiotoxicity and extravasation reactions.

Use: Used to manage complications associated with the use of anthracycline chemotherapeutics.

Safety and handling: Wear gloves when handling.

Contraindications: Unknown.

Adverse reactions: Myelosuppression is documented in humans; it may also decrease the clinical efficacy of anthracycline anti-neoplastic agents.

Drug interactions: Unknown.

DOSES
Dogs:
- Extravasation injury: terminate doxorubicin infusion and administer 1000 mg/m^2 i.v. into a separate infusion (ideally within 6 hours). Repeat on day 2 (1000 mg/m^2 i.v.) and day 3 (500 mg/m^2 i.v.). Lower doses (250–500 mg/m^2 i.v.) have also been shown to be effective.
- Prevention of doxorubicin cardiotoxicity: 10 times the administered dose of doxorubicin i.v. over 5–10 minutes, 10 minutes prior to doxorubicin.

Cats: Unknown.

References
FitzPatrick WM, Dervisis NG and Kitchell BE (2010) Safety of concurrent administration of dexrazoxane and doxorubicin in the canine cancer patient. *Veterinary and Comparative Oncology* **8**, 273–282
Venable RO, Saba CF, Endicott MM and Northrup NC (2012) Dexrazoxane treatment of doxorubicin extravasation injury in four dogs. *Journal of the American Veterinary Medical Association* **240**, 304–307

Dextrose see Glucose

Diazepam   CIL
(Diazedor ^{c,d}, Ziapam ^{c,d}, Diazemuls*, Diazepam*, Diazepam Rectubes*, Stesolid Rectal Tubes*) **POM-V, POM**

Formulations: Injectable: 5 mg/ml solution or emulsion; 2 mg/5 ml solution. Oral: 2 mg, 5 mg, 10 mg tablets. Rectal: 2 mg/ml (1.25 ml, 2.5 ml tubes), 4 mg/ml (2.5 ml tube) solutions.

Action: Enhances activity of the major inhibitory central nervous system neurotransmitter, gamma-aminobutyric acid (GABA), through binding to the benzodiazepine site of the GABA$_A$ receptor.

Use:
- Anticonvulsant: diazepam is the drug of choice for the short-term emergency control of severe epileptic seizures and status epilepticus in dogs and cats.
- Anxiolytic: used in behavioural medicine for anxiety- and fear-related disorders in dogs and cats, especially where there are signs of panic.
- Skeletal muscle relaxant (e.g. urethral muscle spasm and tetanus).
- Used in cats as an appetite stimulant and, due to the longer half-life in cats, can be used as mainenance therapy for epilepsy.

The anti-seizure effect in the dog is only maintained for around 20 minutes and should always be used as part of a balanced emergency seizure protocol; not effective as maintenance anti-seizure medication in the dog due to its short half-life. Diazepam is indicated in dogs with marked spinal pain due to muscle spasm, in combination with conventional analgesics. It may also be used in combination with ketamine to offset muscle hypertonicity associated with ketamine, and with opioids and/or acepromazine for pre-anaesthetic medication in critically ill animals. Provides very poor sedation or even excitation when used alone in healthy animals. Its amnesic properties mean it can be used during or immediately following an aversive experience to minimize the impact of such exposure. Best if used approximately 30 minutes before a fear-inducing event. Higher range doses are required for amnesic activity. Although it has been used for the management of urine spraying in cats, a high relapse rate upon withdrawal should be expected. Diazepam has a high lipid solubility, which facilitates its oral absorption and rapid central effects. Liver disease will prolong duration of action. In the short term, repeated doses of diazepam or a CRI will lead to drug accumulation and prolonged recovery in both species but particularly in cats, in which it may also cause liver injury. Flumazenil (a benzodiazepine antagonist) will reverse the effects of diazepam. The development of dependence to benzodiazepines may occur after regular use, even with therapy of only a few weeks, and the dose should be gradually reduced in these cases if the benzodiazepine is being withdrawn. Chronic dosing leads to a shortened half-life due to activation of the hepatic microsomal enzyme system and tolerance to the drug may develop in dogs.

Safety and handling: Substantial adsorption of diazepam may occur on to some plastics and this may cause a problem when administering diazepam by continuous i.v. infusion. The use of diazepam in PVC infusion bags should be avoided; giving sets should be kept as short as possible and should not contain a cellulose propionate volume-control chamber. If diazepam is given by continuous i.v. infusion, compatible materials include glass, polyolefin, polypropylene and polyethylene.

Contraindications: Benzodiazepines should be avoided in patients with CNS depression, respiratory depression, severe muscle weakness or hepatic impairment (as may worsen hepatic encephalopathy). They are also contraindicated in the long-term treatment of canine and feline behavioural disorders due to the risks of disinhibition and interference with memory and learning.

Adverse reactions: Sedation, muscle weakness and ataxia are common. Rapid i.v. injection or oral overdose may cause marked paradoxical excitation (including aggression) and elicit signs of pain in normal dogs; i.v. injections should be made slowly (over at least 1 min for each 5 mg). Intramuscular injection is painful and results in erratic drug absorption. Rectal administration is effective for emergency control of seizures if i.v. access is not possible, but the time to onset is delayed to 5–10 min. The duration of action may be prolonged after repeated doses in rapid succession, in older animals, those with liver dysfunction and those receiving beta-1 antagonists. Fulminant hepatic necrosis in cats has been associated with repeated oral administration. The propylene glycol formulation of injectable diazepam can cause thrombophlebitis, therefore the emulsion formulation is preferred for i.v. injection.

Drug interactions: Do not dilute or mix with other agents. Due to extensive metabolism by the hepatic microsomal enzyme system, interactions with other drugs metabolized in this way are common. Cimetidine and omeprazole inhibit metabolism of diazepam and may prolong clearance. Concurrent use of phenobarbital may lead to a decrease in the half-life of diazepam. An enhanced sedative effect may be seen if antihistamines or opioid analgesics are administered with diazepam, and diazepam will reduce the dose requirement of other anaesthetic agents. The effects of digoxin may be increased when given with diazepam. Diazepam may be used in combination with tricyclic antidepressant therapy for the management of more severe behavioural responses.

DOSES
When used for sedation is generally given as part of a combination. See Appendix for sedation protocols in cats and dogs.

Dogs:
- Anxiolytic: 0.5–2.0 mg/kg p.o. prn.
- Sedation and premedication: 0.2–0.5 mg/kg i.v., i.m.
- Skeletal muscle relaxation: 2–10 mg/dog p.o. q8–12h.
- Emergency management of seizures, including status epilepticus: bolus dose of 0.5–1 mg/kg i.v., or intrarectally if venous access is not available. Time to onset of clinical effect is 2–3 min for i.v. use; therefore, repeat every 10 min if no clinical effect, up to 3 times. Additional doses may be administered if appropriate supportive care facilities are available (for support of respiration).
- CRI for control of status epilepticus or cluster seizures: initial rate 0.5–2 mg/kg/h, titrated to effect.

Cats:
- Anxiolytic: 0.2–0.4 mg/kg p.o. q8h.
- Appetite stimulant: 0.1–0.2 mg/kg i.v. once.
- Behavioural modification of urine spraying and muscle relaxation: 1.25–5 mg/cat p.o. q8h. The dose should be gradually increased to achieve the desired effect without concurrent sedation.
- Emergency management of seizures, including status epilepticus: bolus dose of 0.5–1 mg/kg i.v., or intrarectally if venous access is not available. Time to onset of clinical effect is 2–3 min for i.v. use; therefore, repeat every 10 min if there is no clinical effect, up to maximum of 3 times.
- CRI for the control of status epilepticus or cluster seizures: initial rate of 0.5 mg/kg/h. Care should be taken to avoid overdosing; discontinue if cats demonstrate excessive sedation. Consider monitoring liver parameters.
- Maintenance for epilepsy: 0.5–2 mg/kg q8–12h. However, oral diazepam has been associated with an idiosyncratic fatal hepatotoxicosis and therefore other safer anti-convulsants should be considered first.

References
Ferreira JP, Dzikit TB, Zeiler GE *et al.* (2015) Anaesthetic induction and recovery characteristics of a diazepam–ketamine combination compared with propofol in dogs. *Journal of the South African Veterinary Association* **86**, 1258

Patterson EN (2014) Status epilepticus and cluster seizures. *Veterinary Clinics of North America: Small Animal Practice* **44**, 1103–1112

Diazoxide
CIL

(Eudemine*) **POM**

Formulations: Injectable: 15 mg/ml solution (special order).
Oral: 50 mg tablets.

Action: A diuretic that causes vasodilation and inhibits insulin secretion by blocking calcium mobilization.

Use:
- Used to manage hypoglycaemia caused by hyperinsulinism in dogs.
- In humans, it is also used in the short-term management of acute hypertension.

Safety and handling: Normal precautions should be observed.

Contraindications: No information available.

Adverse reactions: The commonest adverse effects are anorexia, vomiting and diarrhoea (potentially alleviated by adminstering with food). Hypotension, tachycardia, bone marrow suppression, pancreatitis, cataracts and electrolyte and fluid retention may occur. Drug efficacy may diminish over a period of months.

Drug interactions: Phenothiazines and thiazide diuretics may increase the hyperglycaemic activity of diazoxide, while alpha-adrenergic blocking agents (e.g. phenoxybenzamine) may antagonize the effects of diazoxide.

DOSES
Dogs:
- **Hypoglycaemia:** 5 mg/kg p.o. q12h initially, increasing gradually to 30 mg/kg p.o. q12h.

Cats: No information available.

References
Cook S, McKenna M, Glanemann B, Sandhu R and Scudder C (2020) Suspected congenital hyperinsulinism in a Shiba Inu dog. *Journal of Veterinary Internal Medicine* **34**, 2086–2090

Dichlorophen

(Various authorized proprietary products) **AVM-GSL**

Formulations: Oral: 250 mg, 500 mg, 750 mg tablets.

Action: Cestocide which acts by interfering with oxidative phosphorylation.

Use: Control of tapeworm infections in dogs and cats >6 months old. Effective against *Taenia* and *Dipylidium* but not *Echinococcus*. Affected worms are dislodged and disintegrate during their passage along the alimentary tract so they are not easily recognizable when passed 6–8 hours after dosing. Administer tablets whole or crushed in food.

Safety and handling: Normal precautions should be observed.

Contraindications: Do not administer to animals <1.25 kg or <6 months.

Adverse reactions: Vomiting may be seen. Rarely, salivation, hyperaesthesia and loss of coordination.

Drug interactions: No information available.

DOSES
See Appendix for guidelines on responsible parasiticide use.

Dogs, Cats: 250 mg total dose (animals <2.5 kg), 500 mg/2.5 kg (larger animals) p.o. Give maximum 6 tablets at one time, and give the rest 3 hours later if there is no vomiting. The tablets are best administered immediately before the main feed of the day and may be given whole or crushed and given in food. Animals should be treated every 4–6 months. Do not repeat the treatment if vomiting occurs shortly after dosing. Do not repeat the treatment in <10 days.

Diclofenac

(Voltarol Ophtha*, Voltarol Ophtha Multidose*) **POM**

Formulations: Ophthalmic: 0.1% solution in 5 ml bottle and in single-use vial.

Action: COX inhibitor that produces local anti-inflammatory effects.

Use:

- Used in cataract surgery to prevent intraoperative miosis and reflex (axonal) miosis caused by ulcerative keratitis.
- Used to control pain and inflammation associated with corneal surgery and in ulcerative keratitis when topical corticosteroid use is contraindicated.

Safety and handling: Normal precautions should be observed.

Contraindications: No information available.

Adverse reactions: As with other topical NSAIDs, diclofenac may cause local irritation. Topical NSAIDs should be used with caution in ulcerative keratitis as they can delay epithelial healing. Topical NSAIDs, and most specifically diclofenac, have been associated with an increased risk of corneal 'melting' (keratomalacia) in humans, although this has not been reported in the veterinary literature. Topical NSAIDs have the potential to increase intraocular pressure and should be used with caution in dogs and cats with glaucoma Regular monitoring is advised.

Drug interactions: Ophthalmic NSAIDs may be used safely with other ophthalmic pharmaceuticals, although concurrent use of drugs which adversely affect the corneal epithelium (e.g. gentamicin) may lead to increased corneal penetration of the NSAID. The concurrent use of topical NSAIDs with topical corticosteroids has been identified as a risk factor in humans for precipitating corneal problems.

DOSES

Dogs, Cats: 1 drop q30min for 2 hours prior to cataract surgery (there is a wide variation in protocols for cataract surgery).

References

Lanuza R, Rankin AJ, KuKanich B and Meekins JM (2015) Evaluation of systemic absorption and renal effects of topical ophthalmic flurbiprofen and diclofenac in healthy cats. *Veterinary Ophthalmology* **19(S1)**, 24–29

Digoxin

(Digoxin*, Lanoxin*, Lanoxin PG*) **POM** `CIL`

Formulations: Oral: 62.5 µg (micrograms), 125 µg, 250 µg tablets; 50 µg/ml elixir. Injectable: 250 µg/ml.

Action: Acts as an antiarrhythmic. Digoxin slows the ventricular response rate (heart rate) in atrial fibrillation by having a vagomimetic effect, predominantly acting at the AV node, therefore slowing AV nodal conduction. May also be used in other supraventricular tachyarrhythmias. Has a secondary mild positive inotropic effect. Inhibits Na^+/K^+ ATPase, leading to an increase in intracellular sodium. Sodium is exchanged for calcium, resulting in an increase in intracellular calcium and hence positive inotropic effect. The combination of a slower heart rate and increased force of contraction increases cardiac output in patients with supraventricular tachyarrhythmias. Digoxin improves baroreceptor reflexes that are impaired in heart failure.

Use:
- Management of supraventricular tachyarrhythmias.
- It is primarily used to control the ventricular rate in cases of heart failure with concurrent atrial fibrillation. Effective to decrease the ventricular rate in dogs with atrial fibrillation either as monotherapy or in combination with diltiazem. Digoxin/diltiazem combination therapy results in more effective rate control than monotherapy.

Serum levels should be checked after 7–10 days, with a sample taken at 6–8 hours after a dose. The bioavailability of digoxin varies between the different formulations (tablets ~60%, elixir ~75%, i.v. ~100%). If toxic effects are seen or the drug is ineffective, serum levels of digoxin should be assessed; the ideal therapeutic level is a trough serum concentration in the region of 0.6–1.2 ng (nanograms)/ml. The dose provided below achieves a therapeutic serum digoxin concentration (1.0–2.0 ng/ml) while minimizing adverse effects in dogs. Decreased doses or an increase in dosing intervals may be required in geriatric patients, obese animals or those with significant renal dysfunction. The intravenous formulation is rarely indicated and, if used, should be administered very slowly and with extreme care.

Safety and handling: Normal precautions should be observed.

Contraindications: Frequent ventricular arrhythmias or atrioventricular block. Considered to be contraindicated in cases of feline hypertrophic cardiomyopathy. Do not use if hypokalaemia present.

Adverse reactions: Cats are more sensitive than dogs to the toxic effects of digoxin. Hypokalaemia predisposes to toxicity in all species. Signs of toxicity include anorexia, vomiting, diarrhoea, depression or trigger arrhythmias (e.g. AV block, bigeminy, paroxysmal ventricular or atrial tachycardias with block, and multiform ventricular premature contractions). Lidocaine and phenytoin may be used to control digoxin-associated arrhythmias. Intravenous administration may cause vasoconstriction.

Drug interactions: Antacids, chemotherapy agents (e.g. cyclophosphamide, cytarabine, doxorubicin, vincristine), cimetidine and metoclopramide may decrease digoxin absorption from the GI tract. The following may increase the serum level, decrease the elimination rate or enhance the toxic effects of digoxin: amiodarone, antimuscarinics, diazepam, erythromycin, loop and thiazide diuretics (hypokalaemia), oxytetracycline, quinidine and verapamil. Spironolactone may enhance or decrease the toxic effects of digoxin.

DOSES
Dogs: Tablets: 2.5–3.5 µg (micrograms)/kg p.o. q12h based on lean bodyweight (decrease dose by 10% for elixir). Maximum dose 0.25 mg/dog p.o. q12h. Start at lower end of dose range and titrate upwards carefully based on clinical response and serum therapeutic levels. **Only use i.v. if essentially indicated:** 2.2–4.4 µg/kg i.v. q12h.

Cats: Tablets: 10 µg (micrograms)/kg p.o. q24–48h, equating to ¼ of a 125 µg tablet/cat q24–48h. Start at lower dose range and titrate upwards. **Only use i.v. if essentially indicated:** 1–1.6 µg/kg i.v. q12h.

References
Gelzer ARM, Kraus MS, Rishniw M *et al.* (2009) Combination therapy with digoxin and diltiazem controls ventricular rate in chronic atrial fibrillation in dogs better than digoxin or diltiazem monotherapy: A Randomized Crossover Study in 18 Dogs. *Journal of Veterinary Internal Medicine* **23**, 499–508

Diltiazem

CIL

(Hypercard^c, Adizem*, Angitil*, Dilcardia*, Diltiazem*, Dilzem*, Slozem*, Tildiem*, Viazem*, Zemret*) **POM-V, POM**

Formulations: Oral: 10 mg (Hypercard), 60 mg modified-release (-MR) tablets. Long-acting (-SR) preparations authorized for humans, such as Dilcardia SR (60 mg, 90 mg, 120 mg capsules), are available but their pharmacokinetics have been little studied in animals to date. **Injectable:** 10 mg/ml (check concentration prior to use as strength may vary).

Action: Non-dihydropyridine calcium channel blocker. It inhibits inward movement of calcium ions through slow (L-type) calcium channels in myocardial cells, cardiac conduction tissue and vascular smooth muscle. Diltiazem is less potent than the dihydropyridine calcium channel blockers (e.g. amlodipine) at causing vasodilation of coronary and peripheral vessels. Diltiazem causes a reduction in myocardial contractility (negative inotrope, although less marked than verapamil), depressed electrical activity (retarded atrioventricular conduction) and decreased vascular resistance (vasodilation of cardiac vessels and peripheral arteries and arterioles).

Use:
- Primarily used to control supraventricular tachyarrhythmias in dogs and cats.
- Authorized for use in cats with hypertrophic cardiomyopathy although beta-adrenergic blockers are more commonly used.
- Effective to decrease the ventricular rate in dogs with atrial fibrillation either as monotherapy or in combination with digoxin.

Digoxin/diltiazem combination therapy results in more effective rate control than monotherapy. Diltiazem is preferred to verapamil by many because it has effective antiarrhythmic properties with minimal negative inotropy. Diltiazem is less effective than amlodipine in the management of hypertension. Reduce the dose in patients with hepatic or renal impairment.

Safety and handling: Normal precautions should be observed.

Contraindications: Diltiazem is contraindicated in patients with second or third degree AV block, marked hypotension or sick sinus syndrome, and should be used cautiously in patients with systolic dysfunction or acute or decompensated CHF.

Adverse reactions: Bradycardia in dogs and vomiting in cats are the commonest adverse effects. Lethargy can be seen in both species.

Drug interactions: If diltiazem is administered concurrently with beta-adrenergic blockers (e.g. propranolol), there may be additive negative inotropic and chronotropic effects. The co-administration of diltiazem and beta-blockers is not recommended. The activity of diltiazem may be adversely affected by calcium salts or vitamin D. There are conflicting data regarding the effect of diltiazem on serum digoxin levels and monitoring of these levels is recommended if the drugs are used concurrently. Cimetidine inhibits the metabolism of diltiazem, thereby increasing plasma concentrations. Diltiazem enhances the effect of theophylline, which may lead to toxicity. It may affect quinidine and ciclosporin concentrations. May displace highly protein-bound agents from plasma proteins. May increase intracellular vincristine levels by inhibiting outflow of the drug from the cell.

DOSES

Dogs: 0.05–0.25 mg/kg i.v. over 1–2 min; 0.5–2.0 mg/kg p.o. q8h for modified-release products; up to 3.0 mg/kg p.o. q12h for sustained-/extended-release preparations (little evidence established with -SR products). Lower doses are preferred in the presence of heart failure. Long-acting preparations have been used at a dose of 10 mg/kg p.o. q24h but there is little experience with such formulations in animals. In refractory supraventricular tachyarrhythmias, doses up to 4 mg/kg p.o. q8h have been reported.

Cats: 0.05–0.25 mg/kg i.v. over 1–2 min; 0.5–2.5 mg/kg p.o. q8h; one 10 mg tablet for cats of 3–6.25 kg p.o. q8h.

References

Gelzer ARM, Kraus MS, Rishniw M *et al.* (2009) Combination therapy with digoxin and diltiazem controls ventricular rate in chronic atrial fibrillation in dogs better than digoxin or diltiazem monotherapy: A Randomized Crossover Study in 18 Dogs. *Journal of Veterinary Internal Medicine* **23**, 499–508

Johnson LM, Atkins CE, Keene BW and Bai SA (1996) Pharmacokinetic and pharmacodynamic properties of conventional and CD-formulated diltiazem in cats. *Journal of Veterinary Internal Medicine* **10**, 316–320

Dimercaprol (British anti-lewisite)

(Dimercaprol*) **POM**

Formulations: Injectable: 50 mg/ml solution in peanut oil.

Action: Chelates heavy metals.

Use:
- Treatment of acute toxicity caused by arsenic, gold, bismuth and mercury.
- Used as an adjunct (with edetate calcium disodium) in acute lead poisoning.

Safety and handling: Normal precautions should be observed.

Contraindications: Severe hepatic failure.

Adverse reactions: Intramuscular injections are painful. Dimercaprol-metal complexes are nephrotoxic. This is particularly so with iron, selenium or cadmium; do not use for these metals. Alkalinization of urine during therapy may have protective effects for the kidney. Avoid in chronic lead or mercury poisoning (as can mobilize metal uptake from other tissues to the brain).

Drug interactions: Iron salts should not be administered during therapy.

DOSES

Dogs, Cats: Heavy metal toxicity: 2.5–5 mg/kg i.m. q4h for 2 days, then progressively increase dosing interval to q12h until recovery. (Note: the 5 mg/kg dose should only be used on the first day when severe acute intoxication occurs.) Aggressive supportive therapy should be maintained throughout the treatment period.

References

Bahri EL (2003) Dimercaprol. *Compendium on Continuing Education for the Practising Veterinarian – North American Edition* **25**, 698–700

Dimethylsulfoxide (DMSO)

(Rimso-50*) **POM**

Formulations: Injectable: 50%, 90% liquid; medical grade only available as a 50% solution, other formulations are available as an industrial solvent. **Topical:** 70%, 90% gel; 70% cream.

Action: The mechanism of action is not well understood. Antioxidant activity has been demonstrated in certain biological settings and is thought to account for the anti-inflammatory activity.

Use:

- Treatment of extravasation of cytotoxic vesicant (e.g. doxorubicin).
- Intravesical adminstration for haemorrhagic cystitis induced by cyclophosphamide.
- Although efficacy is unproven it has been used in the treatment of renal amyloidosis.
- Anecdotal evidence for use in the resolution of canine calcinosis cutis.

DMSO is very rapidly absorbed through the skin following administration by all routes and is distributed throughout the body. Metabolites of DMSO are excreted in the urine and faeces. DMSO is also excreted through the lungs and skin, producing a characteristic sulphuric odour. Humans given DMSO experience a garlic-like taste sensation after administration.

Safety and handling: Should be kept in a tightly closed container because it is very hygroscopic. Gloves should be worn during topical application and the product should be handled with care.

Contraindications: Unknown.

Adverse reactions: Changes in refractive index and lens opacities have been seen in dogs given high doses of DMSO chronically; these are slowly reversible upon discontinuation of the drug. Other adverse effects include local irritation and erythema caused by local histamine release. Administration of i.v. of solutions with concentrations >20% may cause haemolysis and diuresis. In the treatment of calcinosis cutis, rapid resorption of calcium could result in calcification of renal tissue; monitoring serum calcium is recommended.

Drug interactions: DMSO should not be mixed with other potentially toxic ingredients when applied to the skin because of profound enhancement of systemic absorption. The use of dexrazoxane and DMSO in combination should possibly be discouraged (as DMSO may decrease the activity of dexrazoxane).

DOSES

Dogs:

- **Calcinosis cutis:** apply 90% solution to half the affected area every other day.
- **Renal amyloidosis:** 80 mg/kg s.c. 3 times/week; 125–300 mg/kg p.o. q24h.
- **Topical:** apply 90% solution to affected areas q8–12h. Total daily dose should not exceed 20 ml. Do not apply for longer than 14 days.

Note that data to support these dose recommendations are limited.

Cats: No information available.

References

Tolon JMC, Jimenez JJE, Irizar IG and Trasobares PC (2018) Resolution of iatrogenic calcinosis cutis in a dog through topical application of DMSO. *Veterinary Record Case Reports* **6**, 1–2

Venable RO, Saba CF, Endicott MM and Northrup NC (2012) Dexrazoxane treatment of doxorubicin extravasation injury in four dogs. *Journal of the American Veterinary Medical Association* **240**, 304–307

Dinotefuran

(Vectra 3D [d], Vectra Felis [c]) **POM-V**

Formulations: Topical spot-on: 6.4 mg dinotefuran + 0.6 mg pyriproxyfen + 46.6 mg permethrin per kg available in 5 sizes (Vectra 3D); 42.3 mg dinotefuran + 4.23 mg pyriproxyfen per kg available in one size (Vectra Felis).

Action: Flea adulticide. Nicotinic acetylcholine receptor agonist. Synergist activity with permethrin observed *in vitro*.

Use:
- For the treatment and prevention of fleas (dogs/cats) and ticks (dogs).
- The permethrin-containing product has repellent activity against sandflies, mosquitoes and stable flies.

Remains effective after animal is immersed in water (swimming/bathing).

Safety and handling: Do not smoke, eat or drink when handling product.

Contraindications: Not for animals <7 weeks, dogs <1.5 kg or cats <0.6 kg. Not for use in pregnancy or lactation.

Adverse reactions: In rare cases, behavioural disorder signs such as hyperactivity, vocalization or anxiety, lethargy or anorexia, and vomiting and diarrhoea, and neurological signs such as muscle tremor have been reported. Vectra Felis: erythema, scaling, alopecia at site of application. Transient neurological signs.

Drug interactions: No information available.

DOSES

See Appendix for guidelines on responsible parasiticide use.

Dogs, Cats: One spot-on monthly.

References

Halos L, Fourie JJ, Fankhauser B and Beugnet F (2016) Knock-down and speed of kill of a combination of fipronil and permethrin for the prevention of *Ctenocephalides felis* flea infestation in dogs. *Parasites and Vectors* **9**, 57

Dinoprost tromethamine (Prostaglandin F2)

(Enzaprost, Lutalyse) **POM-V**

Formulations: Injectable: 5 mg/ml solution.

Action: Stimulates uterine contraction, causes cervical relaxation.

Use: Stimulation of uterine contractions in the treatment of open pyometra, although aglepristone is the first treatment of choice as it is much better tolerated.

Safety and handling: People who are or may become pregnant and asthmatics should not handle this drug.

Contraindications: Do not use for the treatment of closed pyometra as there is a risk of uterine rupture.

Adverse reactions: Hypersalivation, panting, tachycardia, vomiting, urination, defecation, transient hyperthermia, locomotor incoordination and mild CNS signs have been reported. Such effects usually diminish within 30 minutes of drug administration. There is no adverse effect on future fertility.

Drug interactions: No information available.

DOSES

Dogs: Open pyometra: 0.1–0.25 mg/kg s.c. q12h until the uterus is empty; usually 3–5 days treatment required.

Cats: 0.1 or 0.25 mg/kg s.c. q12–24h.

Dioctyl sodium sulfosuccinate see Docusate sodium

Diphenhydramine

(Nytol*) **P**

Formulations: Oral: 25 mg tablets; 2 mg/ml solution. Other products are available of various concentrations and most contain other active ingredients.

Action: The antihistaminergic (H1) effects are used to reduce pruritus and prevent motion sickness. It is also a mild anxiolytic and sedative.

Use: To control mild pruritus in cats and dogs, and prevent motion sickness in dogs.

Safety and handling: Normal precautions should be observed.

Contraindications: Urine retention, glaucoma and hyperthyroidism.

Adverse reactions: Paradoxical excitement and apparent nervousness may be seen in dogs and cats.

Drug interactions: An increased sedative effect may occur if used with benzodiazepines or other anxiolytics/hypnotics. Avoid the concomitant use of other sedative agents. Diphenhydramine may enhance the effect of adrenaline and partially counteract anticoagulant effects of heparin.

DOSES

Dogs:
- **Antiemesis:** 2–4 mg/kg p.o. q6–8h.
- **Suppression of pruritus:** 1–2 mg/kg p.o. q8–12h.

Cats: 2–4 mg/kg p.o. q6–8h; 1 mg/kg i.v., i.m. q8h.

Diphenoxylate (Co-phenotrope) CIL
(Lofenoxal*, Lomotil* (with atropine)) **POM**

Formulations: Oral: 2.5 mg diphenoxylate + 0.025 mg atropine tablets.

Action: Opioid that increases intestinal segmental smooth muscle tone, decreases the propulsive activity of smooth muscle, and decreases electrolyte and water secretion into the intestinal lumen. Atropine is added in a sub-therapeutic dose to discourage abuse by diphenoxylate overdose.

Use:
- Management of acute diarrhoea and irritable bowel syndrome in dogs. Concurrent correction of water and electrolyte imbalance is indicated while investigations into the cause of the diarrhoea are undertaken.
- Treatment of chronic cough due to its antitussive properties.

Safety and handling: Normal precautions should be observed.

Contraindications: Do not use in animals with liver disease, intestinal obstruction, neoplastic or toxic bowel disease.

Adverse reactions: Sedation, constipation and ileus. Little is known about the safety and efficacy of diphenoxylate in cats; adverse behavioural effects (excitement) may occur.

Drug interactions: Diphenoxylate may potentiate the sedative effects of barbiturates and other tranquillizers.

DOSES
Dogs:
- **Antidiarrhoeal:** 0.05–0.1 mg/kg diphenoxylate p.o. q6–8h.
- **Antitussive:** 0.2–0.4 mg/kg diphenoxylate p.o. q8–12h. Monitor for constipation and use stool softeners if required.

Cats: No information available.

Dobutamine
(Dobutamine*, Dobutrex*, Posiject*) **POM**

Formulations: Injectable: 12.5 mg/ml, 50 mg/ml solutions (**NB:** check vial strength prior to administration).

Action: Dobutamine is a direct-acting synthetic catecholamine and derivative of isoprenaline with direct beta-1 adrenergic agonist effects and mild beta-2 and alpha-1 adrenergic effects at standard doses. Positive inotropy results primarily from stimulation of the beta-1 adrenoreceptors of the heart, while producing less marked chronotropic, arrhythmogenic and vasodilatory effects. Dobutamine does not cause the release of endogenous noradrenaline.

Use:
- Short-term inotropic support of patients with heart failure due to systolic dysfunction (e.g. dilated cardiomyopathy), septic and cardiogenic shock.
- It is used to support myocardial function during anaesthesia in animals that are hypotensive when reduced myocardial contractility is suspected as the primary cause.

Dobutamine is a potent and short-acting drug, therefore, it should be given in low doses by CRI; accurate dosing is important. The dose of dobutamine should be adjusted according to clinical effect, therefore, monitoring of arterial blood pressure during administration is advisable. Ideally, blood pressure should be measured directly via an arterial catheter during dobutamine infusion for greater accuracy. All sympathomimetic drugs have proarrhythmic properties, therefore ECG should be monitored during infusion. The dose should be titrated upwards until improvement in blood pressure, perfusion or clinical status is seen, or adverse effects (usually tachyarrhythmias) develop. The beneficial effects of dobutamine diminish over 48 hours due to down regulation of beta receptors.

Safety and handling: Dilute to a 25 µg (micrograms)/ml solution in dextrose or normal saline and store solution in the fridge when not in use. Degradation of dobutamine solution causes a pink discoloration. The reconstituted solution is stable for at least 24 hours, after which time discoloured solutions should be discarded.

Contraindications: Avoid in patients with a cardiac outflow obstruction (e.g. aortic stenosis).

Adverse reactions: Dobutamine is short-acting, therefore, adverse reactions such as tachycardia, proarrhythmia and hypertension can usually be managed by stopping the drug infusion. Hypokalaemia can develop with prolonged use; this can predispose to tachyarrhythmias. Complex ventricular arrhythmias may also be treated with lidocaine. Use cautiously in cases of atrial fibrillation as may increase ventricular rate. Prior and concurrent treatment with digoxin is recommended. Nausea, vomiting and seizures are also possible (particularly in cats).

Drug interactions: Diabetic patients treated with dobutamine may experience increased insulin requirements. Increased systemic vascular resistance may develop if dobutamine is administered with beta-blocking drugs such as propranolol, doxapram or monoamine oxidase inhibitors (e.g. selegiline). Concomitant use with halothane may result in an increased incidence of arrhythmias.

DOSES

Dogs: 2.5–5 µg (micrograms)/kg/min i.v. CRI. Start at the bottom end of the dose range and increase slowly until the desired effect is achieved. Higher end dose ranges up to 20 µg/kg/min i.v. CRI have been reported. Adverse effects (tachycardia, arrhythmia) are more commonly seen at doses >10 µg/kg/min. Administer with an i.v. infusion pump or other i.v. flow controlling device.

Cats: 1–5 µg (micrograms)/kg/min i.v. CRI. Start at the bottom end of the dose range and increase slowly until the desired effect is achieved. Adverse effects are more commonly seen at doses >2.5 µg/kg/min. Administer with an i.v. infusion pump or other i.v. flow controlling device. Doses over 5 µg/kg/min i.v. CRI are reported; may cause seizures.

References
Boller M, Boller EM, Oodegard S and Otto CM (2012) Small animal cardiopulmonary resuscitation requires a continuum of care: proposal for a chain of survival for veterinary patients. *Journal of the American Veterinary Medicine Association* **240**, 26–28

Docusate sodium (Dioctyl sodium sulfosuccinate, DSS)

(Co-danthrusate*, Dioctyl*, Docusol*, DulcoEase*, Norgalax*, Waxsol*) **P, GSL**

Formulations: Oral: 100 mg capsules (Dioctyl); 2.5 mg/ml (Docusol Paediatric Solution), 10 mg/ml (Docusol), 50 mg dantron + 60 mg docusate/5 ml (Co-danthrusate) liquids. **Rectal:** 120 mg enema (Norgalax). **Topical:** 0.5% (Waxsol), 5% (Molcer) docusate in water-miscible base. Docusate is also a component of many other mixed topical preparations.

Action: Anionic surfactant acting as emulsifying, wetting and dispersing agent.

Use: Constipation and ceruminous otitis.

Safety and handling: Normal precautions should be observed.

Contraindications: Intestinal obstruction.

Adverse reactions: Avoid the concurrent use of docusate and mineral oil.

Drug interactions: No information available.

DOSES
Dogs:
- **Constipation:** 50–100 mg p.o. q12–24h; 10–15 ml of 5% solution mixed with 100 ml of water instilled per rectum prn.
- **Otitis:** a few drops in the affected ear q8–12h or 5–15 min prior to flushing.

Cats:
- **Constipation:** 50 mg p.o. q12–24h; 2 ml of a 5% solution mixed with 50 ml of water instilled per rectum prn.
- **Otitis:** dose as for dogs.

Dog appeasing pheromone (DAP)

(Adaptil) **general sale**

Formulations: Plug-in diffuser, topical environmental spray, collar. NOT to be confused with Adaptil tablets which are a nutraceutical.

Action: The mixture is based on derivatives of the dermal secretions produced by the bitch after whelping, which reassure puppies in their immediate environment and so help to keep them within the safety of the den. The signal causes an emotional bias in the perception of the environment which does not require learning. A similar signal appears to form part of the social signal regulating maintenance of stable social groups of adult dogs. Associated limbic activity is believed to help antagonize the effect of certain perceived potential threats in the environment, but does not cause sedation or reduce the startle response.

Use:
- Helps control signs of stress associated with separation, noise sensitivity, travel, introduction to a new home, visits to a novel environment (e.g. veterinary clinic) and other anxiogenic circumstances (e.g. kennels).

The diffuser should be placed in the room most frequently occupied by the dog or where the inappropriate behaviour most frequently occurs.

For behavioural problems involving attachment-related issues with the owner, a treatment period of 3 months is recommended. The spray can be used inside and outside the home environment. It can be used in cars, hospitalization cages, kennels, indoor pens or refuge areas, and applied directly on to bedding. The collar formulation is particularly useful to help control reactions which occur outside the home. If multiple dogs are affected by a problem, each dog should wear a collar and/or possibly a diffuser considered for problems based around the home. Do not spray directly on to animals or near an animal's face. The collar formulation should not be used for animals with a known reactivity to collars. Avoid contact with water when the collar is in use as this may wash out the active ingredients.

Safety and handling: Normal precautions should be observed.

Contraindications: No information available.

Adverse reactions: No information available.

Drug interactions: None known, although anecdotally an apparently synergistic action with benzodiazepines has been reported in some instances. Can be used safely alongside psychopharmacy.

APPLICATION

Dogs: The diffuser is active over an area of approximately 50–70 m^2, although this may be reduced in the presence of air-conditioning. If the total target area exceeds this, a second diffuser should be used; a collar may be preferable in the case of an air-conditioned environment. One vial will last for approximately 4 weeks of continuous use. It should not be repeatedly switched on and off. Follow manufacturer's instructions for each formulation. In the house, spray can complement the use of the diffuser device where a more local application is needed. Spray 8–10 pumps on to the required surface 15 minutes before the effect is required, and before the dog is introduced into the environment, to allow the alcohol carrier to evaporate. The effect should last for 1–2 hours, although each animal will respond individually. The application can be renewed after 1–2 hours or when the effects appear to be reducing.

Cats: Not generally applicable, but the diffuser may be used to reduce tension between cats in dogs in multispecies households. By relaxing the dog, problems related to stress in the cat may be reduced.

References

Estellés MG and Mills DS (2006) Signs of travel-related problems in dogs and their response to treatment with dog appeasing pheromone. *Veterinary Record* **159**, 143–148

Landsberg GM, Beck A, Lopez A *et al.* (2015) Dog-appeasing pheromone collars reduce sound-induced fear and anxiety in beagle dogs: a placebo-controlled study. *Veterinary Record* **177**, 260

Mills DS, Ramos D, Estelles MG and Hargrave C (2006) A triple blind placebo-controlled investigation into the assessment of the effect of Dog Appeasing Pheromone (DAP) on anxiety related behaviour of problem dogs in the veterinary clinic. *Applied Animal Behaviour Science* **98**, 114–126

Sheppard G and Mills DS (2003) Evaluation of dog-appeasing pheromone as a potential treatment for dogs fearful of fireworks. *Veterinary Record* **152**, 432–436

Domperidone

(Domperidone*, Motilium*) **POM**

Formulations: Oral: 10 mg tablets; 1 mg/ml suspension.

Action: Antiemetic with a similar mechanism of action to metoclopramide, but with fewer adverse CNS effects as it cannot penetrate the blood–brain barrier. It is gastrokinetic in humans but may not be prokinetic in dogs. It has also been shown to enhance the innate cell-mediated immune response.

Use:
- Treatment of vomiting; however, maropitant is authorized for veterinary use and there is more clinical experience with metoclopramide and ondansetron.
- A strategic domperidone-based treatment programme has shown some efficacy in reducing the risk of developing clinical canine leishmaniosis in a high-prevalence area.

Safety and handling: Normal precautions should be observed.

Contraindications: Intestinal obstruction or perforation, severe hepatic impairment. Contraindicated in humans with known existing prolongation of cardiac conduction intervals, significant electrolyte disturbances or underlying cardiac disease, but no information available for dogs and cats. Use with caution in dog breeds (e.g. collies) that may have *ABCB1* mutations.

Adverse reactions: There is little information on the use of this drug in veterinary medicine, but it may cause gastroparesis in dogs. May increase plasma prolactin, leading to galactorrhea. Domperidone is banned for human use in the USA because it has been associated with prolongation of the QT interval and has been linked to increased risk of cardiac arrhythmias or sudden cardiac death in humans. Dose-dependent adverse behavioural effects (excitement, aggression) and motor impairment have been seen in cats.

Drug interactions: Do not use concurrently with Class 1A or Class III antiarrhythmics (e.g. amiodarone, quinidine, sotalol), erythromycin or cisapride.

DOSES

Dogs:
- **Vomiting:** 2–5 mg/dog q8h.
- **Preventive strategy for leishmaniosis in a high-prevalence area:** 0.5 mg/kg q24h for 30 consecutive days, repeated every 4 months.

Cats: Vomiting: 2–5 mg/cat q8h.

References

Fernandez M, Tabar MD, Arcas A *et al.* (2018) Comparison of efficacy and safety of preventive measures used against canine leishmaniasis in southern European countries: longitudinal retrospective study in 1647 client-owned dogs (2012–2016). *Veterinary Parasitology* **263**, 10–17

Sabaté D, Llinás J, Homedes J *et al.* (2014) A single-centre, open-label, controlled, randomized clinical trial to assess the preventive efficacy of a domperidone-based treatment programme against clinical canine leishmaniasis in a high prevalence area. *Preventive Veterinary Medicine* **115**, 56–63

Dopamine

(Dopamine*) **POM**

Formulations: Injectable: 200 mg in 5 ml vial (40 mg/ml solution), 800 mg in a 5 ml vial (160 mg/ml solution). **NB:** check vial strength prior to administration.

Action: Dopamine is an endogenous catecholamine and precursor of noradrenaline, with direct and indirect (via release of noradrenaline) agonist effects on dopaminergic and beta-1 and alpha-1 adrenergic receptors.

Use:

- Treatment of shock following correction of fluid deficiencies.
- Treatment of acute heart failure.
- Support of blood pressure during anaesthesia.

Dobutamine is preferred for support of systolic function in patients with heart failure. Dopamine is a potent and short-acting drug, therefore it should be given in low doses by CRI and accurate dosing is important. Dopamine should be diluted in normal saline to an appropriate concentration. At low doses (<10 μg (micrograms)/kg/min), dopamine acts on dopaminergic and beta-1 adrenergic receptors, causing some vasodilation, increased force of contraction and heart rate, and resulting in an increase in cardiac output and organ perfusion; systemic vascular resistance remains largely unchanged. At higher doses (>10 μg/kg/min), dopaminergic effects are overridden by alpha effects, resulting in an increase in systemic vascular resistance and reduced peripheral blood flow. Dopamine has been shown to vasodilate mesenteric blood vessels via DA1 receptors. There may be an improvement in urine output but this may be entirely due to inhibition of proximal tubule sodium ion reabsorption and an improved cardiac output and blood pressure rather than directly improving renal blood flow. The dose of dopamine should be adjusted according to clinical effect, therefore, monitoring of arterial blood pressure during administration is advisable and should ideally be performed via an arterial catheter. All sympathomimetic drugs have pro-arrhythmic properties; ECG monitoring is advised.

Safety and handling: Solution should be discarded if it becomes discoloured.

Contraindications: Discontinue or reduce the dose of dopamine should cardiac arrhythmias arise.

Adverse reactions: Nausea, vomiting, tachyarrhythmias and changes in blood pressure are the most common adverse effects. Hypotension may develop with low doses and hypertension may occur with high doses. Sudden increases in blood pressure may cause severe bradycardia. All dopamine-induced arrhythmias are most effectively treated by stopping the infusion. Extravasation of dopamine causes necrosis and sloughing of surrounding tissue due to ischaemia. Should extravasation occur, infiltrate the site with a solution of 5–10 mg phentolamine in 10–15 ml of normal saline using a syringe with a fine needle.

Drug interactions: Risk of severe hypertension when monoamine oxidase inhibitors, doxapram and oxytocin are used with dopamine. Halothane may increase myocardial sensitivity to catecholamines. The effects of beta-blockers and dopamine are antagonistic.

DOSES

Dogs: 2–10 µg (micrograms)/kg/min i.v. CRI; titrate to effect. Ensure adequate volume replacement prior to use.

Cats: 1–5 µg (micrograms)/kg/min i.v. CRI; titrate to effect. Ensure adequate volume replacement prior to use.

NB: in dogs and cats, a CRI of 1–10 µg/kg/min i.v. will have predominantly beta-1 effects, whereas a CRI of 10–15 µg/kg/min i.v. will have beta-1 and alpha-1 effects. Monitor closely for adverse effects during administration.

Dorzolamide

CIL

(CoSopt*, Dorzolamide*, Dorzolamide with Timolol*, Trusopt*) **POM**

Formulations: Ophthalmic drops: 20 mg/ml (2%) (Trusopt), 2% dorzolamide + 0.5% timolol (CoSopt); 5 ml bottle, single-use vials (CoSopt, Trusopt).

Action: Reduces intraocular pressure (IOP) by reducing the rate of aqueous humour production by inhibiting the formation of bicarbonate ions within the ciliary body epithelium.

Use: In the control of all types of glaucoma in dogs and cats, either alone or in combination with other topicals. Dorzolamide/timolol combination may be more effective in dogs than either drug alone; in cats, maximal IOP lowering efficiency occurs with dorzolamide alone. It may be less tolerated than brinzolamide because of its pH of 5.6.

Safety and handling: Normal precautions should be observed.

Contraindications: Severe hepatic or renal impairment. Timolol causes miosis and is therefore not the drug of choice in uveitis or anterior lens luxation.

Adverse reactions: Local irritation, blepharitis, keratitis, salivation, inappetence. Dorzolamide may cause more local irritation than brinzolamide. Timolol can cause bradycardia and hypotension. Rarely, dorzolamide has been reported to cause hypokalaemia in cats, and metabolic acidosis in dogs, as a result of systemic absorption.

Drug interactions: No information available.

DOSES

Dogs, Cats: 1 drop per eye q8–12h.

References

Beckwith-Cohen B, Bentley E, Gasper DJ *et al.* (2015) Keratitis in six dogs after topical treatment with carbonic anhydrase inhibitors for glaucoma. *Journal of American Veterinary Medical Association* **247**, 1419–1426

Thiessen CE, Tofflemire KL, Makielski KM *et al.* (2016) Hypokalemia and suspected renal tubular acidosis associated with topical carbonic anhydrase inhibitor therapy in a cat. *Journal of Veterinary Emergency and Critical Care* **26**, 870–874

Doxepin
(Sinepin*, Sinequan*, Zonalon*) **POM**

Formulations: Oral: 25 mg, 50 mg capsules.

Action: Doxepin blocks noradrenaline and serotonin reuptake in the brain, resulting in antidepressive activity, while the H1 and H2 blockage result in antipruritic effects. Its metabolite, desmethyldoxepin, is also psychoactive.

Use:
- Management of pruritus and psychogenic dermatoses where there is a component of anxiety, including canine acral lick dermatitis and compulsive disorders.

There are no good published trial data as to its efficacy in this context at the suggested doses; other agents, e.g. amitriptyline or clomipramine (which is an authorized preparation in dogs), are preferable.

Safety and handling: Normal precautions should be observed.

Contraindications: Hypersensitivity to tricyclic antidepressants, glaucoma, history of seizure or urinary retention and severe liver disease.

Adverse reactions: Sedation, dry mouth, diarrhoea, vomiting, excitability, arrhythmias, hypotension, syncope, increased appetite, weight gain and, less commonly, seizures and bone marrow disorders have been reported in humans.

Drug interactions: Should not be used with monoamine oxidase inhibitors or drugs which are metabolized by cytochrome P450 2D6, e.g. chlorphenamine and cimetidine. Should not generally be used alongside other serotonergic agents given risk of serotonin syndrome, although use alongside trazodone may be considered in exceptional cases; monitor carefully for signs of serotonin syndrome.

DOSES
Dogs: 3–5 mg/kg p.o. q8–12h, maximum dose 150 mg q12h.
Cats: 0.5–1.0 mg/kg p.o. q12–24h.

Doxorubicin (Adriamycin)
(Doxorubicin*) **POM**

Formulations: Injectable: 10 mg, 50 mg powders for reconstitution; 10 mg (2 mg/ml) solution.

Action: Inhibits DNA synthesis and function in a variety of ways. The drug likely acts throughout the cell cycle.

Use:
- Used in the managment of several malignancies, including lymphoma, soft tissue sarcoma, osteosarcoma and haemangiosarcoma.
- May have a role in the management of carcinomas in the dog and soft tissue sarcomas in the cat.

May be used alone or in combination with other antineoplastic therapies. Premedication with i.v. chlorphenamine or dexamethasone is recommended. Doxorubicin is highly irritant and must be administered via a preplaced i.v. catheter. The reconstituted drug should be administered over a minimum period of 10 minutes into the side port of a freely running i.v. infusion of 0.9% NaCl. Do not use heparin flush. Use with care in breeds predisposed to cardiomyopathy. May need to reduce dose in patients with liver disease. Use with caution in patients previously treated with radiation as can cause radiation recall. See specialist texts for protocols and further advice.

Safety and handling: Potent cytotoxic drug that should only be prepared and administered by trained personnel. See Appendix and specialist texts for further advice on chemotherapeutic agents. After reconstitution, the drug is stable for at least 48 hours at 4°C. A 1.5% loss of potency may occur after 1 month at 4°C but there is no loss of potency when frozen at −20°C. Filtering through a 0.22 µm (micrometre) filter will ensure adequate sterility of the thawed solution. Store unopened vials under refrigeration.

Contraindications: Do not use in patients with existing cardiac disease. Do not use in cats with renal disease/dysfunction.

Adverse reactions: Allergic reactions have been reported; acute anaphylactic reactions should be treated with adrenaline, steroids and fluids. Doxorubicin causes a dose-dependent cumulative cardiotoxicity in dogs (leading to cardiomyopathy and CHF). The risk of cardio-toxicity is greatly increased when the cumulative dose is >240 mg/m^2. It may also cause tachycardia and arrhythmias on administration; monitor with clinical exam/auscultation, ECG and/or echocardiography. Anorexia, vomiting, severe leucopenia, thrombocytopenia, haemorrhagic gastroenteritis and nephrotoxicity (in cats if dosages >100 mg/m^2) are the major adverse effects. A CBC and platelet count should be monitored whenever therapy is given. If neutrophil count drops below 2.5×10^9/l or platelet count drops below 50×10^9/l, treatment should be suspended. Once counts have stabilized, doxorubicin can be restarted at the same dose or reduced as required. If haematological toxicity occurs again, or if GI toxicity is recurrent, the dose should be reduced by 10–25%. Extravasation injuries secondary to perivascular administration may be serious, with severe tissue ulceration and necrosis possible. Dexrazoxane can be used to treat extravasation if it occurs. Ice compresses may also be beneficial (applied for 15 min q6h). Dogs with the *ABCB1* mutation may be at higher risk of toxicity.

Drug interactions: Do not mix doxorubicin with other drugs. Barbiturates increase plasma clearance of doxorubicin. Concurrent administration with cyclophosphamide increases the risk of nephrotoxicity in cats. The agent causes a reduction in serum digoxin levels. Doxorubicin is incompatible with heparin; concurrent use will lead to precipitate formation. Do not use with spinosad: increased risk of toxicity. Glucosamine may reduce the effectiveness of doxorubicin.

DOSES
See Appendix for chemotherapy protocols and conversion of bodyweight to body surface area.

Dogs: All uses: 30 mg/m^2 i.v. q3wk. In dogs weighing <15 kg a dose of 1 mg/kg should be used. Maximum total dose not to exceed 240 mg/m^2.

Cats: All uses: 1 mg/kg or 20–25 mg/m^2 i.v. q3–5wk. Maximum total dose not to exceed 240 mg/m^2.

References
Lori JC, Stein TJ and Thamm DH (2010) Doxorubicin and cyclophosphamide for the treatment of canine lymphoma: a randomized, placebo-controlled study. *Veterinary and Comparative Oncology* **8**, 188–195

Doxycycline

(Doxybactin [c,d], Ronaxan [c,d]) **POM-V**

Formulations: Oral: 20 mg, 50 mg, 100 mg, 200 mg, 400 mg tablets. A paste is available on a named patient basis. **VSP**

Action: Time-dependent antimicrobial agent inhibiting protein synthesis at the initiation step by interacting with the 30S ribosomal subunit.

Use:
- Antibacterial (including spirochaetes such as *Helicobacter* and *Campylobacter*), antirickettsial, antimycoplasmal (e.g. *Mycoplasma haemofelis*) and antichlamydial activity.
- It is the drug of choice to treat feline chlamydiosis; treatment may be required for 3–4 weeks in cats.
- It is also an adjunctive treatment for canine heartworm disease as it eliminates the symbiont *Wolbachia*.

It is not affected by, and does not affect, renal function as it is excreted in faeces, and is therefore recommended when tetracyclines are indicated in animals with renal impairment. Being extremely lipid-soluble, it penetrates well into prostatic fluid and bronchial secretions. Administer with food.

Safety and handling: Normal precautions should be observed.

Contraindications: Do not administer to pregnant animals. Do not administer if there is evidence of oesophagitis or dysphagia.

Adverse reactions: Nausea, vomiting and diarrhoea. Oesophagitis and oesophageal ulceration may develop; administer with food or a water bolus to reduce this risk. Administration during tooth development may lead to discoloration of the teeth, although the risk is less than with other tetracyclines. Doxycycline hyclate (the salt used in the authorized form of doxycycline in the UK) produces an acidic solution, while doxycycline monohydrate is much less acidic. Doxycycline monohydrate has been associated with reduced development of oesophageal ulceration in humans.

Drug interactions: Absorption of doxycycline is reduced by antacids, calcium, magnesium and iron salts, although the effect is less marked than that seen with water-soluble tetracyclines. Phenobarbital and phenytoin may increase its metabolism, thus decreasing plasma levels.

DOSES

Classified as category D (Prudence) by the EMA.
See Appendix for guidelines on responsible antibiotic use.
Dogs, Cats: 10 mg/kg p.o. q24h with food.
- For heartworm treatment: 10 mg/kg p.o. q12h with food for 4 weeks.

References
American Heartworm Society (2020) *Highlights of the Current Canine Guidelines for the Prevention, Diagnosis, and Management of Heartworm* (Dirofilaria immitis) *Infection in Dogs.* American Heartworm Society, Holly Springs, NC
Schulz BS, Zauscher S, Ammer H *et al.* (2013) Side effects suspected to be related to doxycycline use in cats. *Veterinary Record* **172**, 184

Edetate calcium disodium (CaEDTA)

(Ledclair*) **POM**

Formulations: Injectable: 200 mg/ml solution.

Action: Heavy metal chelating agent.

Use:
* Treatment of lead and zinc poisoning.

Dilute strong solution to a concentration of 10 mg/ml in 5% dextrose before use. Blood lead levels may be confusing; monitor clinical signs during therapy. Measure blood lead levels 2–3 weeks after completion of treatment in order to determine whether a second course is required or if the animal is still being exposed to lead. Ensure there is no heavy metal in the GI tract before administering (e.g. use laxatives). Use in zinc toxicity controversial – removal from GI tract alone usually sufficient and avoids chelator side effects.

Safety and handling: Normal precautions should be observed.

Contraindications: Use with caution in patients with impaired renal function.

Adverse reactions: Reversible nephrotoxicity is usually preceded by other clinical signs of toxicity (e.g. depression, vomiting, diarrhoea). Dogs showing GI effects may benefit from zinc supplementation (when treating lead toxicity). Injections are painful.

Drug interactions: No information available.

DOSES

Dogs, Cats: 25 mg/kg s.c. q6h for 2–5 days. The total daily dose should not exceed 2 g. Dogs that respond slowly or have an initial (pretreatment) blood lead level of >4.5 µmol (micromoles)/l may need another 5-day course of treatment after a rest period of 5 days.

Eltrombopag

(Revolate*) **POM**

Formulations: Oral: 25 mg, 50 mg tablets.

Action: Thrombopoietin receptor agonists stimulate haematopoietic stem cells and other progenitor cells in the bone marrow of megakaryocyte lineage to differentiate and proliferate.

Use:
* Treatment of pancytopenia.

Reported to have been used in a dog with idiopathic aplastic pancytopenia and in a dog with acquired pancytopenia secondary to lomustine overdose (concurrently treated with granulocyte-macrophage colony-stimulating factor). Typically used alongside immunosuppressives for the treatment of aplastic pancytopenia, chronic immune (idiopathic) thrombocytopenia purpura, thrombocytopenia associated with chronic hepatis C infection and acquired severe aplastic anaemia in humans, its use in dogs is less well defined.

Safety and handling: Normal precautions should be observed.

Contraindications: In humans, to be avoided during pregnancy and to be used with caution in patients with hepatic or kidney impairment.

Adverse reactions: In humans, a wide range of adverse reactions have been reported including abdominal pain, vomiting, diarrhoea, constipation, inappetence, nausea, depression, anxiety, lethargy, cough, dyspnoea, dry eye, dry mouth, pyrexia, skin lesions, pruritus muscle spasms, musculoskeletal pain, jaundice and hepatic encephalopathy.

Drug interactions: In humans, it is advised that each dose is taken 4 hours before or after any foods containing calcium or medicines containing aluminium, calcium, iron, magnesium, zinc or selenium, as these may interfere with absorption.

DOSES
Dogs: No dose has been established in dogs or cats. For the treatment of pancytopenia, doses ranging from 0.9 to 1.25 mg/kg p.o. q24h have been reported in dogs. Proposed treatment duration ranges from 10 days to 2 months.

Cats: No information available.

References
Aspinall S, Desmas I and Bazelle J (2021) Use of eltrombopag and granulocyte colony-stimulating factor in treatment of lomustine overdose in a dog. *Vet Record Case Reports* **9**, e174

Kelly D, Lamb V and Juvet F (2020) Eltrombopag treatment of a dog with idiopathic aplastic pancytopenia. *Journal of Veterinary Internal Medicine* **34**, 890–892

Emodepside
(Dronspot[c], Felpreva[c], Procox[d], Profender[c]) **POM-V**

Formulations: Topical: 21.4 mg/ml emodepside with praziquantel solution in spot-on pipettes for cats (Profender/Dronspot: 3 sizes); emodepside with praziquantel and tigolaner (Felpreva). Oral: 0.9 mg/ml solution or tablets with toltrazuril (Procox).

Action: Stimulates pre-synaptic secretin receptors resulting in paralysis and death of the parasite.

Use:
- Treatment of roundworms (adult and immature) and tapeworms (adult) in cats including *Toxocara cati*, *Toxascaris leonina*, *Ancylostoma tubaeforme*, *Aelurostrongylus abstrusus*, *Dipylidium caninum*, *Taenia taeniaeformis*, *Echinococcus multilocularis*.
- Treatment of queens during late pregnancy to prevent lactogenic transmission to the offspring of *Toxocara cati* (L3 larvae).
- Product with tigolaner; treatment of fleas, *Otodectes cynotis*, *Notoedres cati*.
- Do not shampoo until substance has dried.

Safety and handling: People who are or may become pregnant should not handle this drug. Harmful to aquatic organisms.

Contraindications: Do not use in cats <8 weeks or <0.5 kg. Do not use Felpreva in cats <10 weeks or <1 kg.

Adverse reactions: Ingestion may result in salivation or vomiting.

Drug interactions: Emodepside is a substrate for P-glycoprotein. Co-treatment with other drugs that are P-glycoprotein substrates/inhibitors (these include ciclosporin, ivermectin, ranitidine and many steroids and opiates) could cause problems but there are no reports of this.

DOSES

See Appendix for guidelines on responsible parasiticide use.

Dogs: No information available – **see Toltrazuril for Procox dose**.

Cats: Endoparasites: minimum dose 0.14 ml/kg (3 mg/kg) applied topically once per treatment cycle. For the lungworm *Aelurostrongylus abstrusus*, two treatments administered 2 weeks apart are effective.

Enalapril
(Enacard) **POM-V**

Formulations: Oral: 1 mg, 2.5 mg, 5 mg, 10 mg, 20 mg tablets.

Action: ACE inhibitor. It inhibits conversion of angiotensin I to angiotensin II and inhibits the breakdown of bradykinin. Overall effect is a reduction in preload and afterload via venodilation and arteriodilation, decreased salt and water retention via reduced aldosterone production and inhibition of the angiotensin-aldosterone-mediated cardiac and vascular remodelling. Efferent arteriolar dilation in the kidney can reduce intraglomerular pressure and therefore glomerular filtration. This may decrease proteinuria.

Use:
- Indicated for treatment of congestive heart failure caused by mitral regurgitation or dilated cardiomyopathy in dogs. Can be used in combination with other drugs to treat heart failure (e.g. pimobendan, spironolactone, digoxin).
- Can also be used for heart failure in cats.
- Management of proteinuria associated with chronic renal insufficiency, glomerular disorders and protein-losing nephropathies.
- May reduce blood pressure in hypertension.

ACE inhibitors are more likely to cause or exacerbate prerenal azotaemia in hypotensive animals and those with poor renal perfusion (e.g. acute, oliguric renal failure). Use cautiously if hypotension, hyponatraemia or outflow tract obstruction are present. Regular monitoring of blood pressure, serum creatinine, urea and electrolytes is strongly recommended with ACE inhibitor treatment. The use of ACE inhibitors in cats with cardiac disease stems from extrapolation from theoretical benefits and studies showing a benefit in other species with heart failure and different cardiac diseases (mainly dogs and humans).

Safety and handling: Normal precautions should be observed.

Contraindications: Do not use in cases of cardiac output failure or hypotension.

Adverse reactions: Potential adverse effects include hypotension, hyperkalaemia and azotaemia. Monitor blood pressure, serum creatinine and electrolytes when used in cases of heart failure. Dosage should be reduced if there are signs of hypotension (weakness, disorientation). Anorexia, vomiting and diarrhoea are rare. No adverse effects were seen in normal dogs given 15 mg/kg/day for up to 1 year. Not recommended for breeding, pregnant or lactating bitches, as safety has not been established.

Drug interactions: Concomitant treatment with potassium-sparing diuretics (e.g. spironolactone) or potassium supplements could result in hyperkalaemia. However, in practice, spironolactone and ACE inhibitors appear safe to use concurrently. There may be an increased risk of nephrotoxicity and decreased clinical efficacy when used with NSAIDs. There is a risk of hypotension with concomitant administration of diuretics, vasodilators (e.g. anaesthetic agents, antihypertensive agents) or negative inotropes (e.g. beta-blockers).

DOSES

Dogs:
- **Cardiac disease:** 0.5 mg/kg p.o. q24h increasing to 0.5 mg/kg p.o. q12h after 2 weeks in the absence of a clinical response.
- **Protein-losing nephropathy:** 0.25–1 mg/kg p.o. q12–24h.
- **Hypertension:** 0.5 mg/kg p.o. q12h. Can be titrated upwards slowly to effect. Doses up to 3 mg/kg have been used.

Cats: Cardiac disease, protein-losing nephropathy: 0.25–0.5 mg/kg p.o. q12–24h.

Enilconazole

(Imaverol [d]) **POM-VPS**

Formulations: Topical: 100 mg/ml (10%) liquid.

Action: Inhibition of cytochrome P450-dependent synthesis of ergosterol in fungal cells, causing increased cell wall permeability and allowing leakage of cellular contents.

Use:
- Fungal infections of the skin.
- Topical treatment of sinonasal aspergillosis.

Safety and handling: Normal precautions should be observed.

Contraindications: No information available.

Adverse reactions: Hepatotoxic if swallowed. Avoid contact with eyes. Hypersalivation, GI signs and muscle signs reported in cats.

Drug interactions: No information available.

DOSES

Dogs:
- **Dermatological indications:** dilute 1 volume enilconazole in 50 volumes of water to produce a 2 mg/ml (0.2%) solution. Apply every 3 days for 3–4 applications.
- **Nasal aspergillosis:** 10 mg/kg instilled once via endoscopically-placed sinus catheter (maintain *in situ* for 15 minutes). Dilute the solution of enilconazole (100 mg/ml) 10:90 with water. Make up a fresh solution as required.

Cats: Dermatological indications: doses as for dogs.

References
Moriello KA (2004) Treatment of dermatophytosis in dogs and cats: review of published studies. *Veterinary Dermatology* **15**, 99–107
Vangrinsven E, Girod M, Goossens D *et al.* (2018) Comparison of two minimally invasive enilconazole perendoscopic infusion protocols for the treatment of canine sinonasal aspergillosis. *The Journal of Small Animal Practice* **59**, 777–782

Enrofloxacin

(Baytril [c,d], Enrocare [c,d], Enrotron [c,d], Enrox, Enroxil [d], Fenoflox [c,d], Floxabactin [c,d], Powerflox, Quinoflox, Xeden [c,d], Zobuxa) **POM-V**

Formulations: Injectable: 25 mg/ml, 50 mg/ml. Oral: 15 mg, 50 mg, 100 mg, 150 mg, 200 mg, 250 mg tablets; 25 mg/ml solution.

Action: Enrofloxacin is a concentration-dependent antimicrobial which inhibits bacterial DNA gyrase. Pulse dosing regimens may be effective, particularly against Gram-negative bacteria.

Use:

- Use should be based on antimicrobial susceptibility testing, wherever possible and where lower tier antimicrobials would not be effective.
- Active against *Mycoplasma* and many Gram-positive and Gram-negative organisms, including *Pasteurella*, *Staphylococcus*, *Pseudomonas aeruginosa*, *Klebsiella*, *Escherichia coli*, *Mycobacterium*, *Proteus* and *Salmonella*. Relatively ineffective against obligate anaerobes.

Fluoroquinolones are highly lipophilic drugs that attain high concentrations within cells in many tissues and are particularly effective in the management of soft tissue, urogenital (including prostatic) and skin infections. Can be used in combination protocols for mycobacterial infections, although newer fluoroquinolones may be more effective. Administration by i.v. route is not authorized but has been used in cases of severe sepsis. If this route is used, dilute to 10 times the volume in 0.9% sodium chloride and administer slowly as the carrier contains potassium (ideally 35–45 minutes).

Safety and handling: Normal precautions should be observed.

Contraindications: Fluoroquinolones are relatively contraindicated in growing dogs, as cartilage abnormalities have been reported in young dogs (but not cats). Enrofloxacin is not authorized in cats <8 weeks of age; dogs <1 year of age; large-breed dogs <18 months of age.

Adverse reactions: In cats, irreversible retinal blindness has occurred at dosing rates higher than those currently recommended, although at least one case reported in the literature was being dosed at 5 mg/kg q24h. Retinal damage has not been reported with other fluoro-quinolones. Enrofloxacin should be used with caution in epileptic animals until further information is available, as in humans it can potentiate adverse CNS effects when administered concurrently with NSAIDs.

Drug interactions: Absorbents and antacids containing cations (Mg^{2+}, Al^{3+}) may bind fluoroquinolones, preventing their absorption from the GI tract. Their absorption may also be inhibited by sucralfate and zinc salts; separate dosing by at least 2 hours. Fluoroquinolones increase plasma theophylline concentrations. Cimetidine may reduce the clearance of fluoroquinolones and so should be used with caution with these drugs. Some fluoroquinolones may decrease the metabolism and increase nephrotoxicity of ciclosporin and tacrolimus in humans and therefore concurrent use in animals is best avoided until more research has been performed. May increase the action of orally administered anticoagulants.

DOSES

See Appendix for guidelines on responsible antibiotic use.

Dogs: 5 mg/kg p.o., s.c. q24h. Higher doses (10 mg/kg q24h) should be considered for certain sites, including the prostate gland. Even higher doses may be necessary for certain isolates of *Pseudomonas aeruginosa*. Contact the manufacturer to discuss individual cases.

Cats: 5 mg/kg s.c. q24h; 2.5 mg/kg p.o. q12h or 5 mg/kg p.o. q24h. Use with caution due to risk of retinal damage and consider alternative fluoroquinolones.

References

Cummings KJ, Aprea VA and Altier C (2015) Antimicrobial resistance trends among canine *Escherichia coli* isolates obtained from clinical samples in the northeastern USA, 2004–2011. *Canadian Veterinary Journal* **56**, 393–398

Federico S, Carrano R, Capone D *et al.* (2006) Pharmacokinetic interaction between levofloxacin and ciclosporin or tacrolimus in kidney transplant recipients: ciclosporin, tacrolimus and levofloxacin in renal transplantation. *Clinical Pharmacokinetics* **45**, 169–75

Ford MM, Dubielzig RR, Giuliano EA *et al.* (2007) Ocular and systemic manifestations after oral administration of a high dose of enrofloxacin in cats. *American Journal of Veterinary Research* **68**, 190–202

Ephedrine

(Enurace[d], Ephedrine hydrochloride*) **POM-V, POM**

Formulations: Oral: 10 mg, 15 mg, 30 mg, 50 mg tablets. **Injectable:** 3 mg/ml, 30 mg/ml solutions. **Nasal:** 0.5% and 1% drops.

Action: Non-catecholamine sympathomimetic. Stimulates alpha- and beta-adrenergic receptors directly, and indirectly through endogenous release of noradrenaline. Also causes contraction of internal urethral sphincter muscles and relaxation of bladder muscles. Compared with more powerful sympathomimetics, e.g. oxymetazoline and xylometazoline, there is less of a rebound effect.

Use:
- Treatment of hypotension during anaesthesia. As well as constricting peripheral vessels, it has a positive inotropic effect and accelerates heart rate, thereby assisting in bradycardia. Effects tend to wane after 2 or 3 doses, due to exhaustion of endogenous noradrenaline stores.
- Also used orally in the treatment of urinary incontinence. Can be used in conjunction with phenylpropanolamine. Polyuria should be excluded before treatment is given for urinary incontinence, as many conditions that cause polyuria would be exacerbated by ephedrine.
- Proposed for treatment of nasal congestion (and may be of some benefit in influenza in cats).

Use with caution in dogs and cats with cardiovascular disease, partial urethral obstruction, hypertension, diabetes mellitus, hypercortisolism, hyperthyroidism or other metabolic disorders.

Safety and handling: People who are or may become pregnant should not handle this drug.

Contraindications: Do not use in pregnant or lactating animals or those with glaucoma.

Adverse reactions: Even at recommended therapeutic doses, may cause more generalized sympathetic stimulation (panting, mydriasis, CNS stimulation) and cardiovascular effects (tachycardia, atrial fibrillation and vasoconstriction). May also cause reduction of the motility and tone of the intestinal wall.

Drug interactions: Synergistic with other sympathomimetics. Volatile anaesthetics will enhance the sensitivity of the myocardium to the effects of ephedrine. Concomitant use with cardiac glycosides (digoxin) and tricyclic antidepressants (amitriptyline) can cause arrhythmias. Will enhance effects of theophylline and may cause hypertension when given with monoamine oxidase inhibitors (e.g. selegeline).

DOSES
Dogs:
- **Hypotension:** 0.05–0.2 mg/kg i.v., repeat as necessary; duration of effect is short (5–15 min). Effects tend to wane after 2 or 3 doses.
- **Urinary incontinence:** 1 mg/kg p.o. q12h. Dose should be adjusted according to effect up to a maximum dose of 2.5 mg/kg p.o. q12h.
- **Nasal congestion:** No dose determined. Suggest start at 1 drop of 0.5% solution intranasally q12h. If giving orally, suggest 0.5 mg/kg p.o. q12h.

Cats:
- **Hypotension:** 0.05–0.1 mg/kg i.v., repeat as necessary; duration of effect is short (5–15 min). Effects tend to wane after 2 or 3 doses.
- **Nasal congestion:** 1 drop of 0.5% solution intranasally q12h. Oral formulations not convenient for administration to most cats.

Epinephrine see Adrenaline

Epirubicin (4'-Epi-doxorubicin)
(Epirubicin*, Pharmorubicin*) **POM**

Formulations: Injectable: 10 mg, 20 mg, 50 mg powder for reconstitution; 2 mg/ml solution.

Action: Cytotoxic anthracycline glycoside antibiotic that has demonstrated efficacy against several human neoplasms. Epirubicin is a semisynthetic stereoisomer of doxorubicin. Intracellularly, its metabolism results in production of cytotoxic free radicals. It also binds irreversibly to DNA, thereby preventing replication, and can alter cell membrane functions.

Use:
- Treatment of lymphoma (similar efficacy to doxorubicin) and also as an adjunct in the management of splenic haemangiosarcoma, canine histiocytic sarcoma and sporadically in other sarcomas and carcinomas.
- Epirubicin has been used in cats with feline injection site sarcomas.

It may be used alone or in combination with other antineoplastic therapies. The drug must be given i.v. Premedication with i.v. chlorphenamine or dexamethasone is recommended. As extravasation of the drug is likely to result in severe tissue necrosis, an indwelling intravenous catheter taped in place is essential. The reconstituted drug should be administered over a minimum period of 10 minutes into the side port of a freely running i.v. infusion of 0.9% NaCl. Reported to be less cardiotoxic than doxorubicin, epirubicin should still be used with caution in patients with or predisposed to cardiac disease.

Safety and handling: Potent cytotoxic drug that should only be prepared and administered by trained personnel. See Appendix and specialist texts for further advice on chemotherapeutic agents. After reconstitution, the drug is stable for 24 hours at room temperature. Store under refrigeration for up to 28 days. Protection from light is not necessary.

Contraindications: No information available.

Adverse reactions: Acute anaphylactic reactions should be treated with adrenaline, steroids and fluids. Epirubicin may cause a dose-dependent cumulative cardiotoxicity in dogs (leading to cardiomyopathy and congestive heart failure) but possibly at a lower incidence than doxorubicin does. This rarely develops in dogs given a total dose of <240 mg/m^2. It may also cause tachycardia and arrhythmias on administration. Dogs with pre-existing cardiac disease should be routinely monitored with physical examination/auscultation, ECGs and/or echocardiograms. Anorexia, vomiting, pancreatitis, severe leucopenia, thrombocytopenia, haemorrhagic gastroenteritis and nephrotoxicity are major adverse effects. CBC and platelet count should be monitored whenever therapy is given. If the neutrophil count drops below 2.5×10^9 or the platelet count drops below 50×10^9, treatment should be suspended. Once the counts have stabilized, epirubicin may then be restarted at the same dose or lower if desired. If haematological toxicity occurs again, or if GI toxicity is recurrent, the dose should be reduced by 10–25%. Dogs with the *ABCB1* mutation may be at higher risk of toxicity.

Drug interactions: Epirubicin is incompatible with heparin: a precipitate will form. Increased risk of myelosuppression when used in combination with cyclophosphamide. In humans, cimetidine increased the area under the dose curve of epirubicin by 50%; it should not be used concurrently.

DOSES
See Appendix for chemotherapy protocols and conversion of bodyweight to body surface area.
Dogs (all uses): 30 mg/m^2 i.v. q3wk; maximum total dose not to exceed 240 mg/m^2. In dogs weighing <10 kg, a dose of 1 mg/kg should be used.
Cats: 25 mg/m^2 or 1 mg/kg i.v. q3wk.

References
Bray J and Polton G (2016) Neoadjuvant and adjuvant chemotherapy combined with anatomical resection of feline injection-site sarcoma: results in 21 cats. *Veterinary and Comparative Oncology* **14**, 147–160
Elliott JW, Cripps P, Marrington AM *et al.* (2013) Epirubicin as part of a multi-agent chemotherapy protocol for canine lymphoma. *Veterinary and Comparative Oncology* **11**, 185–198

Epoetin alfa, epoetin beta see Erythropoietin

Eprinomectin

(Broadline [c], Nexgard Combo [c]) **POM-V**

Formulations: Topical: 4 mg/ml eprinomectin with fipronil, S-methoprene and praziquantel spot-on solution in 2 pipette sizes (Broadline); 4 mg/ml eprinomectin with esafoxolaner and praziquantel spot-on solution in 2 pipette sizes (Nexgard Combo).

Action: Interacts with GABA- and glutamate-gated channels, leading to flaccid paralysis of parasites.

Use:

Broadline:

- Treatment and prevention of fleas and ticks, and treatment of nematodes, including feline lungworm and vesical worms (*Capillaria plica*), in cats.
- Prevention of heartworm disease (*Dirofilaria immitis* larvae) for 1 month.
- The praziquantel component confers tapeworm control. The fipronil component treats notoedric mange (*Notoedres cati*) and aids in the control of *Neotrombicula autumnalis*, and *Cheyletiella* spp. The S-methoprene component confers ovicidal and larvicidal activity against fleas.

Nexgard Combo:

- Fleas, ticks, heartworm prevention, feline lungworm and *Capillaria*, as above.
- Treatment of infestations by ear mites (*Otodectes cynotis*).
- Treatment of notoedric mange (caused by *Notoedres cati*).
- Treatment of infections with tapeworms (*Dipylidium caninum, Taenia taeniaeformis, Echinococcus multilocularis, Joyeuxiella pasqualei* and *Joyeuxiella fuhrmanni*).
- Treatment of infections with gastrointestinal nematodes (L3, L4 larvae and adults of *Toxocara cati*, L4 larvae and adults of *Ancylostoma tubaeforme* and *Ancylostoma ceylanicum*, and adult forms of *Toxascaris leonina* and *Ancylostoma braziliense*).

Safety and handling: Normal precautions should be observed when administering. Likely to be toxic to aquatic organisms. Take care with disposal.

Contraindications: Cats <0.6 kg or <7 weeks (Broadline), <0.8 kg or <8 weeks (Nexgard Combo). Not intended for use in dogs.

Adverse reactions: Mild clumping of the hair is often seen after application.

Drug interactions: May have interactions with other P-glycoprotein substrates such as ciclosporin, itraconazole, loperamide and many steroids and opiates but none reported.

DOSES

See Appendix for guidelines on responsible parasiticide use.

Dogs: No information available.

Cats: 1 pipette per cat according to bodyweight. Repeat monthly.

References

Kvaternick V, Kellermann M, Knaus M *et al.* (2014) Pharmacokinetics and metabolism of eprinomectin in cats when administered in a novel topical combination of fipronil, (S)-methoprene, eprinomectin and praziquantel. *Veterinary Parasitology* **202**, 2–9

Erythromycin

(Erythrocin, Erythroped*) **POM-V, POM**

Formulations: Oral: 250 mg, 500 mg tablets/capsules; 250 mg/5 ml suspension.

Action: Time-dependent macrolide antibacterial that binds to the 50S ribosome (close to binding site for chloramphenicol), inhibiting peptide bond formation.

Use: Not commonly used in dogs and cats.
- Has a similar antibacterial spectrum to penicillins. It is active against Gram-positive cocci (some *Staphylococcus* species are resistant), Gram-positive bacilli and some Gram-negative bacilli (*Pasteurella*). Some strains of *Actinomyces*, *Nocardia*, *Chlamydophila* and *Rickettsia* are also inhibited by erythromycin. Most of the Enterobacteriaceae (*Pseudomonas*, *Escherichia coli*, *Klebsiella*) are resistant.
- It may be considered to treat canine enteric *Campylobacter*, although isolation rates are similar between healthy dogs and those with diarrhoea so treatment is rarely indicated.
- Erythromycin acts as a GI prokinetic by stimulating motilin receptors.

Being a lipophilic weak base, it is concentrated in fluids that are more acidic than plasma, including milk, prostatic fluid and intracellular fluid. Resistance to erythromycin can be quite high, particularly in staphylococcal organisms. Different esters of erythromycin are available. It is likely that the kinetics will differ and possible that the toxicity will differ depending on the ester used. Activity is enhanced in an alkaline pH. As the base is acid labile, it should be administered on an empty stomach.

Safety and handling: Normal precautions should be observed.

Contraindications: In humans, the erythromycin estolate salt has been implicated in causing cholestatic hepatitis. Although not demonstrated in veterinary medicine, this salt should be avoided in animals with hepatic dysfunction.

Adverse reactions: The commonest adverse effect is GI upset (vomiting and diarrhoea are common). Care should be taken in cases of hepatic or renal impairment.

Drug interactions: Erythromycin may enhance the absorption of digoxin from the GI tract and increase serum levels of ciclosporin, cisapride, methylprednisolone, theophylline and terfenadine. The interactions with terfenadine and cisapride proved particularly significant in human medicine, leading to fatal or near-fatal arrhythmias in some patients receiving both drugs. Erythromycin should not be used in combination with other macrolide, lincosamide or chloramphenicol antimicrobials as antagonism may occur.

DOSES

Classified as category C (Caution) by the EMA.
See Appendix for guidelines on responsible antibiotic use.
Dogs, Cats:
- Antibiosis: 10 mg/kg p.o. q8h.
- GI prokinetic: 0.5–1 mg/kg p.o. q8h.

References

Husnik R, Gaschen FP, Fletcher JM and Gaschen L (2020) Ultrasonographic assessment of the effect of metoclopramide, erythromycin, and exenatide on solid-phase gastric emptying in healthy cats. *Journal of Veterinary Internal Medicine* **34**, 1440–1446

Marks SL, Rankin SC, Byrne BA and Weese JS (2011) Enteropathogenic bacteria in dogs and cats: diagnosis, epidemiology, treatment, and control. *Journal of Veterinary Internal Medicine* **25**, 1195–1208

Rutherford S, Gaschen F, Husnik R, Fletcher J and Gaschen L (2022) Ultrasonographic evaluation of the effects of azithromycin on antral motility and gastric emptying in healthy cats. *Journal of Veterinary Internal Medicine* **36**, 508–514

Erythropoietin (Epoetin alfa, Epoetin beta) CIL
(Eprex*, Neorecormon*) **POM**

Formulations: Injectable: Various concentrations available as pre-filled syringes: ranging from 1667 IU/ml to 50,000 IU/ml solutions (Neorecormon); or 2000 IU/ml, 4000 IU/ml, 10,000 IU/ml, 40,000 IU/ml solutions (Eprex). Eprex is epoetin alfa. Neorecormon is epoetin beta.

Action: Stimulates division and differentiation of RBCs.

Use:
- Recombinant human erythropoietin (r-HuEPO) is predominantly used to treat anaemia associated with chronic renal failure and cats with FeLV-associated anaemia.

Monitoring and/or supplementation of iron may be necessary, especially if response to treatment is poor. Darbepoetin may be a better choice in many cases. Also used to treat anaemic human patients with cancer and rheumatoid arthritis.

Safety and handling: Normal precautions should be observed.

Contraindications: Conditions where high serum concentrations of erythropoietin already exist (e.g. haemolytic anaemia, anaemia due to blood loss), where anaemia is due to iron deficiency or where uncontrolled systemic hypertension is present.

Adverse reactions: Local and systemic allergic reactions may rarely develop (skin rash at the injection site, pyrexia, arthralgia and muco-cutaneous ulcers). The production of cross-reacting antibodies to r-HuEPO occurs in 20%–70% of treated dogs and cats 4 weeks or more after treatment. These antibodies reduce the efficacy of the drug and can cause pure red cell aplasia. The drug should be discontinued if this develops.

Drug interactions: No information available.

DOSES

Dogs, Cats: For stimulating erythropoiesis (induction dose): 100 IU/kg i.v., s.c. epoetin alfa/beta 3 times/week until packed cell volume (PCV) is at lower end of target range, then gradually reduce frequency of dosing to maintain this PCV (typical maintenance dose is 50–100 IU/kg once or twice a week). Dose changes should only be made at 3-weekly intervals.

References

Polzin DJ (2013) Evidence-based step-wise approach to managing chronic kidney disease in dogs and cats. *Journal of Veterinary Emergency and Critical Care* **23**, 205–215

Randolph JE, Scarlett J, Stokol T *et al.* (2004) Clinical efficacy and safety of recombinant canine erythropoietin in dogs with anemia of chronic renal failure and dogs with recombinant human erythropoietin-induced red cell aplasia. *Journal of Veterinary Internal Medicine* **18**, 81–91

Esafoxolaner

(Nexgard Combo [c]) **POM-V**

Formulations: Topical: 12 mg/ml esafoxolaner with eprinomectin and praziquantel spot-on solution in 2 pipette sizes.

Action: Esafoxolaner is the (*S*)-enantiomer of afoxolaner and belongs to the isoxazoline class, which is active against arthropods. Esafoxolaner acts as an antagonist at ligand-gated chloride channels, in particular those gated by the neurotransmitter gamma-aminobutyric acid (GABA).

Use:
- Treatment of fleas and ticks, *Notoedres cati* and *Otodectes cynotis*.

Combnation with eprinomectin and praziquantel confers action against gastrointestinal nematodes and tapeworms and lungworms.

Safety and handling: Normal precautions should be observed.

Contraindications: Do not use in cats <0.8 kg or <8 weeks.

Adverse reactions: Transient hypersalivation, diarrhoea, transient skin reactions at the application site (alopecia, pruritus), anorexia, lethargy and emesis.

Drug interactions: No information available.

DOSES
See Appendix for guidelines on responsible parasiticide use.
Dogs: No information available.
Cats: 1 pipette per cat according to bodyweight. Repeat monthly.

References
Beugnet F (2021) NexGard® Combo (esafoxolaner, eprinomectin, praziquantel), a new endectoparasiticide spot-on formulation for cats. *Parasite* **28**, E1

Esmolol

(Brevibloc*) **POM**

Formulations: Injectable: 10 mg/ml solution.

Action: An ultra-short-acting beta blocker. Relatively cardioselective and blocks beta-1 adrenergic receptors in the heart. Has a negative inotropic and chronotropic action which can lead to a decreased myocardial oxygen demand. Blood pressure is reduced. Has an antiarrhythmic effect through its blockade of adrenergic stimulation of the heart.

Use:
- Therapy of, or as an assessment of the efficacy of beta-adrenergic blockers in the treatment of, supraventricular tachycardias (including atrial fibrillation, atrial flutter and atrial tachycardia).

Its effect is brief, persisting only 10–20 minutes after i.v. infusion. Other antiarrhythmic therapy must be used for chronic or maintenance therapy.

Safety and handling: Normal precautions should be observed.

Contraindications: Patients with bradyarrhythmias, acute or decompensated congestive heart failure. Relatively contraindicated in animals with medically controlled congestive heart failure as it is poorly tolerated. Do not administer concurrently with alpha-adrenergic agonists.

Adverse reactions: Most frequently seen in geriatric patients with chronic heart disease or in patients with acute or decompensated heart failure. Include bradycardia, AV block, myocardial depression, heart failure, syncope, hypotension, hypoglycaemia, bronchospasm and diarrhoea. Depression and lethargy are occasionally seen and are a result of esmolol's high lipid solubility and penetration into the CNS. Esmolol may reduce the glomerular filtration rate and therefore exacerbate any pre-existing renal impairment.

Drug interactions: The hypotensive effect of esmolol is enhanced by many agents that depress myocardial activity including anaesthetics, phenothiazines, antihypertensives, diuretics and diazepam. There is an increased risk of bradycardia, severe hypotension, heart failure and AV block if esmolol is used concurrently with calcium channel blockers. Concurrent digoxin administration potentiates bradycardia. Esmolol may increase serum digoxin levels by up to 20%. Morphine may increase esmolol serum concentration by up to 50%. Esmolol may enhance the effects of muscle relaxants. The bronchodilatory effects of theophylline may be blocked by esmolol.

DOSES
Dogs, Cats: 0.05–0.5 mg/kg i.v. bolus over 5 min; 25–200 µg (micrograms)/kg/min CRI.

Estriol (Oestriol)
(Incurin⁽ᵈ⁾) **POM-V**

Formulations: Oral: 1 mg tablets.

Action: Synthetic, short-acting oestrogen with a high affinity for oestrogen receptors in the lower urogenital tract. It increases muscle tone, improving urodynamic function.

Use:
* Management of urethral sphincter mechanism incompetence that develops in spayed bitches.

Safety and handling: Normal precautions should be observed. Pregnant or breastfeeding people should handle with caution.

Contraindications: Do not use in intact bitches. Do not use if polyuria/polydipsia present. Manufacturer states that this drug should not be used in animals <1 year old.

Adverse reactions: Oestrogenic effects are seen in 5–9% of bitches receiving 2 mg q24h. Low risk of bone marrow suppression (consider monitoring CBC for long-term use).

Drug interactions: Concurrent administration with phenylpropanolamine may potentiate efficacy.

DOSES
Dogs: Starting dose: 1 mg/dog p.o. q24h. If treatment is successful reduce the dose to 0.5 mg/dog p.o. q24h. If treatment is unsuccessful increase to 2 mg/dog p.o. q24h. Alternate-day dosing can be considered once a response has been seen. The minimum effective dose is 0.5 mg/dog p.o. q24–48h. The maximum dose is 2 mg/dog p.o. q24h.
Cats: Do not use.

References
Hamaide AJ, Grand J-G, Farnir F *et al.* (2006) Urodynamic and morphologic changes in the lower portion of the urogenital tract after administration of estriol alone and in combination with phenylpropanolamine in sexually intact and spayed female dogs. *American Journal of Veterinary Research* **67**, 901–908

Ethanol

(Alcohol*) **POM**

Formulations: Injectable: medical grade alcohol is a 95% solution. To prepare a solution for i.v. use, dilute to 20% in sterile water and administer through a 22 µm (micrometre) filter. Other commercially available forms of alcohol are less safe as they usually contain other substances that make i.v. administration hazardous (vodka is likely to be the least dangerous).

Action: Competitive inhibition of alcohol dehydrogenase.

Use:
- Prevents metabolization of ethylene glycol (antifreeze) or methanol to toxic metabolites.
- To cleanse and degrease skin.

When treating ethylene glycol toxicity, adjust dose to maintain blood ethanol levels above 35 mg/dl in dogs (which as a guide is about half the legal limit to drive in humans). Monitor fluid and electrolyte balance during ethanol therapy. Unlikely to be effective if administered >8 hours after toxin ingestion or acute renal failure has already developed. Fomepizole, if available, is safer and more effective than ethanol.

Safety and handling: Normal precautions should be observed.

Contraindications: No information available.

Adverse reactions: Ethanol will cause diuresis and may cause additive depression that will mask CNS signs of ethylene glycol toxicity. Adverse events occur frequently with intravenous ethanol infusions. Oral administration commonly associated with gastric irritation, vomiting.

Drug interactions: Avoid concurrent fomepizole administration (increases risk of alcohol toxicity).

DOSES

Dogs: 5.5 ml/kg of 20% ethanol solution given i.v. q4h for 5 treatments, then i.v. q6h for 4 additional treatments. Alternatively, give an i.v. loading dose of 1.3 ml/kg of 30% solution then begin a CRI of 0.42 ml/kg/h for 48 hours. For clinically mild cases (minimal CNS signs), particularly if using vodka, oral administration is also possible but adverse effects are common with this route.

Cats: 5 ml/kg of 20% ethanol solution i.v. q6h for 5 treatments, then q8h for 4 additional treatments.

References
Connally HE, Thrall MA and Hamar DW (2010) Safety and efficacy of high-dose fomepizole compared with ethanol as therapy for ethylene glycol intoxication in cats. *Journal of Veterinary Emergency and Critical Care* **20**, 191–206

Famciclovir

CIL

(Famciclovir*, Famvir*) **POM**

Formulations: Oral: 125 mg, 250 mg, 500 mg tablets; 100 mg/ml paste.

Action: Inhibits viral replication (viral DNA polymerase); depends on viral thymidine kinase for phosphorylation.

Use:
- Management of feline herpesvirus (FHV-1) infections.

Famciclovir is a prodrug for penciclovir, which is closely related to aciclovir. Famciclovir is virostatic and is unable to eradicate latent viral infection. Dose recommendations have varied because of complex and non-linear pharmacokinetics in cats.

Safety and handling: Normal precautions should be observed.

Contraindications: No information available.

Adverse reactions: GI signs are the most common side effects. Monitor haematology, biochemistry and urinalysis in cats with known concurrent disease and those expected to receive the drug for long periods. Reduce dose frequency in cats with renal insufficiency (as in humans).

Drug interactions: No information available.

DOSES

Dogs: No information available.

Cats: 90 mg/kg q12h.

References
Thomasy SM and Maggs DJ (2016) A review of antiviral drugs and other compounds with activity against feline herpesvirus type 1. *Veterinary Ophthalmology* **19(S1)**, 119–130

Famotidine

CIL

(Famotidine*) **POM**

Formulations: Oral: 20 mg, 40 mg tablets.

Action: Histamine (H2) receptor antagonist blocking histamine-induced gastric acid secretion. Many times more potent than cimetidine, but has poorer oral bioavailability (37%). Famotidine is not antiemetic.

Use:
- Management of gastric and duodenal ulcers, idiopathic, uraemic or drug-related erosive gastritis, oesophagitis, and hypersecretory conditions secondary to gastrinoma, mast cell neoplasia or short bowel syndrome.

Currently, cimetidine is the only anti-ulcer drug with a veterinary market authorization. Famotidine has little effect on GI motility in humans. In healthy dogs, famotidine did increase intragastric pH, but to a lesser degree than omeprazole and not to a degree that would suggest therapeutic efficacy when assessed by criteria used for humans with acid-related disease. Famotidine was less effective than omeprazole in preventing exertion-induced gastritis in racing sled dogs. When given every day, effect on gastric pH diminished with time in studies in dogs and cats. Combination therapy with pantoprazole was not superior to pantoprazole alone. Famotidine was not helpful in reducing GI adverse effects in dogs receiving piroxicam for cancer.

Safety and handling: Normal precautions should be observed.

Contraindications: No information available.

Adverse reactions: Good safety profile. In humans, famotidine has fewer side effects than cimetidine.

Drug interactions: Famotidine is devoid of many of the interactions of the H2 related antagonist cimetidine.

DOSES
Dogs, Cats: All uses: 0.5–1.0 mg/kg p.o. q12–24h.

References
Bersenas AM, Mathews KA, Allen DG et al. (2005) Effects of ranitidine, famotidine, pantoprazole, and omeprazole on intragastric pH in dogs. *American Journal of Veterinary Research* **66**, 425–431

Tolbert K, Bissett S, King A et al. (2011) Efficacy of oral famotidine and 2 omeprazole formulations for the control of intragastric pH in dogs. *Journal of Veterinary Internal Medicine* **25**, 47–54

Febantel see **Pyrantel**

Feline facial fraction F3 (Feline facial pheromone F3)

(Feliway Classic, Feliway Optimum, Zenifel, ZenSylk, various others (difficult to verify formulation)) **general sale**

Formulations: Plug-in diffuser, topical environmental spray. Feliway spray also contains Valerian extract and Zenifel has historically contained Nepeta (catnip) extract. Some supposed pheromone products for calming cats may not contain F3. Feliway Optimum is an engineered variant, which claims superior efficacy to Feliway Classic and additional Cat Appeasing Pheromone effects.

Action: A synthetic analogue of the F3 fraction of the 'feline facial pheromones' that are used in facial marking of the physical environment by cats. F3 stimulates receptors in the vomeronasal organ, resulting in limbic activity that has a calming effect in the presence of particular classes of stimuli, especially those associated with threats to physical resources, such as unfamiliar cats and novel odours.

Use:
- Management of indoor urine marking, inappropriate scratching and changes to the animal's physical environment at home or outside (e.g. during transport, within the cattery or the veterinary clinic).
- Management of situational anxiety-related disorders.
- It can aid handling for anaesthesia induction and during other medical examinations when the spray may be applied to the consultation or preparation table.

The diffuser should be placed in the room most frequently occupied by the cat and/or where the inappropriate behaviour most frequently occurs. The pump spray should not mark or stain but it is sensible to patch-test fabrics and polished surfaces before using extensively. For best results, allow the spray to come to room temperature before it is applied and adopt appropriate cleaning regimes for indoor marking. Rinse well after using an enzymatic cleaner and allow areas to dry after cleaning before applying the F3 spray; residual enzymatic action may break down the active ingredient. The diffuser is active over an area of approximately 50–70 m². If the total target area exceeds this or air conditioning is in use, a second diffuser should be used, or the spray form used as well. Do not repeatedly switch the diffuser on and off; it is designed to be left on at all times.

Safety and handling: Humans with known sensitivity to the ingredients should avoid using the product in their homes.

Contraindications: No information available.

Adverse reactions: No information available.

Drug interactions: None.

DOSES

Dogs: Not applicable.

Cats: Pump spray: F3 is applied to the environment in locations where the inappropriate behaviour is occurring and in locations that are of behavioural significance. Familiarization signal for cats in potentially stressful situations, or in new environments: apply spray 30 minutes before the cat has access to the area. Existing urine marking: apply one dose (one depression of the nozzle) daily from about 10 cm from the soiled site at a height of about 20 cm from the floor. In multicat households, the spray should be applied 2–3 times/day on previously marked sites and once a day on other locations which are of behavioural significance. When using to prevent urine marking, spray once per day in locations of behavioural significance.

References

Mills DS and Mills CB (2001) Evaluation of a novel method for delivering a synthetic analogue of feline facial pheromone to control urine spraying by cats. *Veterinary Record* **149**, 197–199

Pereira JS, Fragoso S, Beck A *et al.* (2016) Improving the feline veterinary consultation: the usefulness of Feliway spray in reducing cats' stress. *Journal of Feline Medicine and Surgery* **18**, 959–964

Fenbendazole

(Granofen [c,d], Panacur [c,d], Various authorized proprietary products) **AVM-GSL, NFA-VPS**

Formulations: Oral: 222 mg/g (22%), 440 mg/g (44%) granules; 25 mg/ml (2.5%), 100 mg/ml (10%) oral suspension; 187.5 mg/g (18.75%) oral paste.

Action: Inhibits fumarate reductase system of parasites, thereby blocking the citric acid cycle, and reduces glucose absorption by parasites.

Use: Treatment of ascarids (including larval stages), hookworms, whipworms, tapeworms (*Taenia*), *Giardia* spp., *Oslerus osleri*, *Aelurostrongylus abstrusus*, *Angiostrongylus vasorum*, *Capillaria aerophila*, *Ollulanus tricuspis*, *Physaloptera rara* and *Paragonimus kellicotti* infections. Has 60–70% efficacy against *Dipylidium caninum*. Unlike some other benzimidazoles, fenbendazole is safe to use in pregnant animals.

Safety and handling: Normal precautions should be observed.

Contraindications: No information available.

Adverse reactions: Bone marrow hypoplasia has been reported in a dog.

Drug interactions: No information available.

DOSES
See Appendix for guidelines on responsible parasiticide use.
Dogs:
- GI nematodes and cestodes:
  - Puppies <6 months: 50 mg/kg p.o. q24h for 3 days. For puppies >2 kg, an extra 2 ml is required daily for each additional kg bodyweight. Treat at 2 weeks, 5 weeks and again before leaving the breeder's premises. Treatment may also be required at 8 and 12 weeks
  - Adult dogs: 100 mg/kg p.o. as a single dose. Routine treatment of adult dogs with minimal exposure to infection is advisable 2–4 times per year. More frequent treatment at 6- and 8-weekly intervals is advisable for dogs in kennels
  - Pregnant bitches: 25 mg/kg p.o. q24h from day 40 of pregnancy continuously to 2 days post-whelping (approximately 25 days).
- *Angiostrongylus vasorum:* 50 mg/kg p.o. q24h for 21 days, although the dose and duration of treatment has yet to be defined.
- *Oslerus (Filaroides) osleri:* 50 mg/kg p.o. q24h for 7 days, although a repeat course of treatment may be required in some cases.
- Giardiasis: 50 mg/kg p.o. q24h for 3 days.

Cats:
- GI nematodes and cestodes
  - Kittens <6 months: 50 mg/kg p.o. q24h for 3 consecutive days. Treat at 2 weeks, 5 weeks and again before leaving the breeder's premises
  - Adult cats: 100 mg/kg p.o. as a single dose. Routine treatment of adult cats with minimal exposure to infection is advisable 2–4 times per year
  - Pregnant queens: single treatment of 100 mg/kg.
- *Aelurostrongylus abstrusus:* 50 mg/kg p.o. q24h for 3 days.
- Giardiasis: 50 mg/kg p.o. q24h for 3–5 days with treatment repeated after 2 weeks if clinical signs reoccur.

References
Willesen JL, Kristensen AT, Jensen AL *et al.* (2007) Efficacy and safety of imidacloprid/moxidectin spot-on solution and fenbendazole in the treatment of dogs naturally infected with *Angiostrongylus vasorum*. *Veterinary Parasitology* **147**, 258–264

Fentanyl

(Fentadon[d], Durogesic*, Fentanyl*, Fentora*, Sublimaze*) **POM-V CD SCHEDULE 2, POM CD SCHEDULE 2**

Formulations: Oral: 100 μg (microgram), 200 μg, 400 μg, 600 μg, 800 μg tablets. **Injectable:** 50 μg/ml solution. **Transdermal:** 12.5 μg/h, 25 μg/h, 50 μg/h, 75 μg/h, 100 μg/h patches.

Action: Synthetic pure mu receptor agonist.

Use:
- Very potent opioid analgesic (50 times more potent than morphine) used to provide profound intraoperative analgesia in dogs and cats.
- Can also be used at low dose rates for postoperative analgesia.
- Transdermal fentanyl patches can be used to provide analgesia for up to 72 hours after surgery or for the management of chronic pain.

Use of potent opioids during anaesthesia contributes to a balanced anaesthesia technique, therefore the dose of other concurrently administered anaesthetic agents should be reduced. Fentanyl has a rapid onset of action after i.v. administration and short duration of action (10–20 min depending on dose). After prolonged administration (>4 hours) or high doses, its duration of action is significantly prolonged as tissues become saturated. It can be used intraoperatively to provide analgesia by intermittent bolus doses or by CRI. Postoperatively, fentanyl can be given by CRI to provide analgesia, doses at the low end of the dose range should be used and respiratory function monitored. Its clearance is similar to morphine while its elimination half-life is longer, reflecting its higher lipid solubility and volume of distribution. Following transdermal patch application, it takes approximately 7 hours in cats and 24 hours in dogs to attain adequate plasma concentrations to provide analgesia. Alternative forms of analgesia must be provided during this period, or patches must be placed before surgery. Systemic plasma concentrations of fentanyl can be very variable after transdermal absorption from patches and some animals may not develop adequate plasma concentrations to achieve analgesia. Therefore, it is preferable to use transdermal fentanyl as an adjunctive analgesic in combination with other drugs. Direct application of heat sources to transdermal fentanyl patches (e.g. during anaesthesia) will significantly increase the uptake of fentanyl and may result in higher than expected plasma concentrations. Oral administration of fentanyl tablets is unlikely to provide adequate analgesia due to a high first pass metabolism in cats and dogs.

Safety and handling: If animals are sent home with transdermal fentanyl patches, the owners must be warned about the dangers of patch ingestion by humans or other animals.

Contraindications: No information available.

Adverse reactions: Intraoperative administration is likely to cause respiratory depression; therefore, respiration should be monitored using capnometry and facilities must be available to provide positive pressure ventilation. Rapid i.v. injection can cause severe bradycardia, even asystole; the drug should be given slowly. A reduction in heart rate is likely whenever fentanyl is given. Atropine can be administered to counter bradycardia if necessary. Apart from the effects on heart rate, fentanyl has limited other effects on cardiovascular function when used at clinical dose rates.

Drug interactions: Fentanyl can be used to reduce the dose requirement for other anaesthetic drugs in patients with cardiovascular instability or systemic disease.

DOSES

Dogs:
- **Intraoperative analgesia:** 5 µg (micrograms)/kg i.v. q20min; 2.5–10 µg/kg/h by CRI during anaesthesia, reduced to 1–5 µg/kg/h during the postoperative period. CRI should be preceded by a loading dose given slowly i.v. (2.5–10 µg/kg).
- **Transdermal patch:** 4 µg/kg/h (e.g. 100 µg/h patch for a 25 kg dog).

Cats:
- **Intraoperative analgesia:** 5 µg (micrograms)/kg bolus, repeated injections may be required q20min. During anaesthesia: CRI as for dogs.
- **Transdermal patch:** 25 µg/h patch for cats 3–5 kg; in smaller cats and kittens the 12.5 µg/h patch can be applied.

References
Ambros B, Alcorn J, Duke-Novakovski T et al. (2014) Pharmacokinetics and pharmacodynamics of a constant rate infusion of fentanyl (5 µg/kg/h) in awake cats. *American Journal of Veterinary Research* **75**, 716–721

Filgrastim (Granulocyte colony stimulating factor, G-CSF)

(Neupogen*) **POM**

Formulations: Injectable: 30 million IU (300 µg (micrograms))/ml solution.

Action: Filgrastim is recombinant human granulocyte colony stimulating factor (rhG-CSF). Activates proliferation and differentiation of granulocyte progenitor cells, and enhances granulopoiesis.

Use:
- Management of febrile patients, particularly those receiving cytotoxic drugs with neutrophil counts <1×10^9/l.
- As an adjunct in the treatment of neutropenia due to infections (e.g. canine ehrlichiosis, parvovirus, FeLV or FIV), bone marrow neoplasia or cyclic haemopoiesis in dogs.

There are few reports on the use of G-CSF in dogs or cats. In humans it is indicated in the management of neutropenia, especially in patients receiving high-dose chemotherapy. Neutrophil counts rise within 24 hours. Following discontinuation of therapy, neutrophil counts drop to normal after 5 days.

Safety and handling: Normal precautions should be observed.

Contraindications: Dogs or cats that have developed antibodies to G-CSF (with resultant neutropenia) should not receive it in the future.

Adverse reactions: Normal dogs produce neutralizing antibodies to rhG-CSF. This limits repeated use and may result in neutropenia. This does not appear to be the case in canine chemotherapy patients. A variety of adverse effects have been reported in humans, including musculoskeletal pain, transient hypotension, dysuria, allergic reactions, proteinuria, haematuria, splenomegaly and increased liver enzymes. Reported adverse effects are bone pain at high doses and irritation at the injection site.

Drug interactions: Steroids and lithium may potentiate the release of neutrophils during G-CSF therapy. Concurrent administration with chemotherapy may increase incidence of adverse effects. G-CSF should be given at least 24 hours after the last dose of chemotherapy, as the stimulatory effects of G-CSF on haemopoietic precursors renders them more susceptible to the effects of chemotherapy.

DOSES

Dogs, Cats: 100,000–500,000 IU (1–5 micrograms)/kg s.c. q24h for 3–5 days.

References
Mishu L, Callahan G, Allebban Z et al. (1992) Effects of recombinant canine granulocyte colony-stimulating factor on white blood cell production in clinically normal and neutropenic dogs. *Journal of the American Veterinary Medical Association* **200**, 1957–1964

Finasteride

(Proscar*) **POM**

Formulations: Oral: 5 mg tablets.

Action: Competitively inhibits dihydrotestosterone (DHT) production within the prostate. DHT is the main hormonal stimulus for the development of benign prostatic hypertrophy.

Use: Treatment of benign prostatic hypertrophy as an alternative to castration. Extended treatment course (<8 weeks) may be required for full efficacy. Not authorized for veterinary use and therefore should only be used when delmadinone or osaterone are not appropriate.

Safety and handling: People who are or may become pregnant should not handle this drug.

Contraindications: Do not use in sexually developing dogs.

Adverse reactions: Secreted into semen and causes fetal anomalies.

Drug interactions: No information available.

DOSES

Dogs: 5 mg/dog p.o. q24h.

Cats: Not used.

References

Angrimani DSR, Brito MM, Rui BR, Nichi M and Vannucchi CI (2020) Reproductive and endocrinological effects of Benign Prostatic Hyperplasia and finasteride therapy in dogs. *Scientific Reports* **10**, 14834

Fipronil

(Broadline[c], Effipro[c,d], Frontline[c,d], Frontect and many others) **AVM-GSL, NFA-VPS, POM-V**

Formulations: Topical: 10% w/v fipronil spot-on pipettes in a wide range of sizes (Frontline and many others); some formulations combined with other drugs including *S*-methoprene (Frontline Combo/Plus), pyriproxyfen (Effipro Duo), permethrin (Frontect), eprinomectin, *S*-methoprene and praziquantel (Broadline). Also 0.25% w/v fipronil spray in alcohol base (Effipro and Frontline sprays) in a range of sizes.

Action: Fipronil interacts with ligand-gated (GABA) chloride channels, blocking pre- and post-synaptic transfer of chloride ions, resulting in death of parasites on contact.

Use:

- Exhibits an insecticidal and acaricidal activity against fleas (*Ctenocephalides* spp.), ticks (*Rhipicephalus* spp., *Dermacentor* spp., *Ixodes* spp.) and feline and canine lice (*Felicola subrostratus*, *Trichodectes canis*).
- May aid in the control of *Neotrombicula autumnalis*, *Sarcoptes* spp. and *Cheyletiella* spp.
- Kills and repels sandflies (*Phlebotomus perniciosus*) and mosquitoes (*Aedes albopictus*) for 3 weeks (+ permethrin).
- Repels (anti-feeding activity) and kills stable flies (*Stomoxys calcitrans*) for 5 weeks (+ permethrin).

Effective against flea infestation for approximately 2 months and against tick infestations for up to 1 month. See relevant monographs for additional information on efficacy of other compounds included in specific formulations. Bathing between 48 hours before and 24 hours after application is not recommended. Can be used in pregnant and lactating females. When treating flea infestations, treatment of the environment is also recommended.

Safety and handling: Normal precautions should be observed. Spray contains alcohol, use away from naked flames.

Contraindications: Fipronil spot-on: do not use in dogs <2 kg, cats <1 kg, or dogs or cats <8 weeks of age. Fipronil spray may be used in puppies and kittens from 2 days old. Fipronil may be harmful to aquatic organisms. Do not use fipronil, *S*-methoprene, eprinomectin and praziquantel combination (Broadline) in dogs.

Adverse reactions: Local pruritus or alopecia may occur at the site of application.

Drug interactions: No information available

DOSES
See Appendix for guidelines on responsible parasiticide use.
Dogs:
- **Flea infestations:** spray 3–6 ml/kg (6–12 pumps/kg 100 ml application, 2–4 pumps/kg 250 ml or 500 ml application) or apply 1 pipette per dog according to bodyweight. Treatment should be repeated not more frequently than every 4 weeks.
- *Neotrombicula autumnalis*, *Sarcoptes* spp. and *Cheyletiella* spp. **infestations:** spray should be used every 1–2 weeks.

Cats: Spray 3–6 ml/kg (6–12 pumps/kg 100 ml application) or apply 1 pipette per cat. Treatment should be repeated monthly.

References
Curtis CF (2004) Current trends in the treatment of *Sarcoptes*, *Cheyletiella* and *Otodectes* mite infestations in dogs and cats. *Veterinary Dermatology* **15**, 108–114

Firocoxib
(Previcox [d]) **POM-V**

Formulations: Oral: 57 mg, 227 mg tablets.

Action: NSAID that selectively inhibits the COX-2 enzyme, thereby limiting the production of prostaglandins involved in inflammation. Also has analgesic and antipyretic effects.

Use:
- Relief of pain and inflammation associated with osteoarthritis and with soft tissue, orthopaedic and dental surgery in dogs.

When used for perioperative pain, it is recommended to give the first dose 2 hours before surgery. Studies investigating the safety of firocoxib in dogs were only carried out for 90 days; animals receiving firocoxib for more prolonged periods should be monitored carefully for NSAID-induced side effects. Administration of firocoxib to animals with renal disease must be carefully evaluated. Firocoxib may have a synergistic role with platinum-based chemotherapeutic agents in the treatment of transitional cell carcinomas of the urinary bladder and may have some antitumour effects on its own.

Safety and handling: Normal precautions should be observed.

Contraindications: All NSAIDs should be administered cautiously in the perioperative period as they may adversely affect renal perfusion during periods of hypotension. If hypotension during anaesthesia is anticipated, delay firocoxib administration until the animal is fully recovered and normotensive. Do not give to dehydrated, hypovolaemic or hypotensive patients or those with GI disease or blood clotting problems. Do not give to pregnant or lactating bitches, animals <10 weeks old or <3 kg. Do not use in cats.

Adverse reactions: GI signs may occur in all animals after NSAID administration. Stop therapy if this persists beyond 1–2 days. Some animals develop signs with one NSAID and not another. A 3–5 day wash-out period should be allowed before starting another NSAID after cessation of therapy. Stop therapy immediately if GI bleeding is suspected. There is a small risk that NSAIDs may precipitate cardiac failure in humans and this risk in animals is unknown. Liver disease will prolong the metabolism of firocoxib, leading to the potential for drug overdose with repeated dosing.

Drug interactions: Do not administer concurrently or within 24 hours of other NSAIDs. The optimal wash-out period between NSAID administration and glucocorticoid administration is unknown – allowing 3–5 days between the two classes of drugs is recommended. Do not administer with other potentially nephrotoxic agents, e.g. aminoglycosides.

DOSES
Dogs: 5 mg/kg p.o. q24h, with or without food.
Cats: Do not use.

References
Ryan WG, Moldave K and Carithers D (2006) Clinical effectiveness and safety of a new NSAID, Firocoxib: a 1000 dog study. *Veterinary Therapeutics* **7**, 119–126
Steagall PV, Mantovani FB, Ferreira TH *et al.* (2007) Evaluation of the adverse effects of oral firocoxib in healthy dogs. *Journal of Veterinary Pharmacology and Therapeutics* **30**, 218–223

Florfenicol
(Neptra [d], Osurnia [d]) **POM-V**

Formulations: Topical: 1.2 g ear gel containing 10 mg florfenicol + 10 mg terbinafine + 1 mg betamethasone acetate (Osurnia); 1 ml ear drop solution containing 16.7 mg florfenicol + 16.7 mg terbenafine + 2.2 mg Mometasone furoate (Neptra).

Action: Florfenicol inhibits bacterial protein synthesis and is a broad-spectrum time-dependent antimicrobial. Its activity includes Gram-negative and Gram-positive bacteria including *Staphylococcus pseudintermedius*.

Use:
- Although authorized for systemic use in some food animals, florfenicol is currently only authorized for use in the treatment of otitis externa in the dog.

It is recommended to clean and dry the external ear canal before the first administration of the product and repeat application after 7 days (Osurnia). It is recommended not to repeat ear cleaning until 21 days after the second administration of the product. Neptra has a longer duration of action of up to 28 days.

Safety and handling: Store in the refrigerator (Osurnia).

Contraindications: Otic preparation: do not use in pregnant or breeding animals, in dogs with generalized demodicosis or if the tympanic membrane is not intact. Not for use in dogs <2 months or <1.4 kg (Osurnia), or <3 months or <4 kg (Neptra).

Adverse reactions: Rare incidence of transient deafness mainly in older dogs. Keratoconjunctivitis sicca, corneal ulcers, local irritant reactions and hypersensitivity responses (angio-oedema, urticaria, shock) are reported rarely.

Drug interactions: None reported when used by otic route.

DOSES
Classified as category C (Caution) by the EMA.
See Appendix for guidelines on responsible antibiotic use.
Dogs:
- Osurnia: 1.2 g (10 mg florfenicol) administered into affected ear and repeated once after 7 days.
- Neptra: 1 ml (16.7 mg florfenicol) administered into affected ear.

Cats: Not authorized.

References
King SB, Doucette KP, Seewald W and Forster SL (2018) A randomized, controlled, single-blinded, multicenter evaluation of the efficacy and safety of a once weekly two dose otic gel containing florfenicol, terbinafine and betamethasone administered for the treatment of canine otitis externa. *BMC Veterinary Research* **14**, 307

Fluconazole

CIL

(Diflucan*, Fluconazole*) **POM**

Formulations: Oral: 50 mg, 150 mg, 200 mg capsules; 40 mg/ml suspension. Injectable: 2 mg/ml solution.

Action: Inhibition of the synthesis of ergosterol in fungal cell membranes, causing increased cell wall permeability and allowing leakage of cellular contents.

Use:
- Effective against *Blastomyces*, *Candida*, *Cryptococcus*, *Coccidioides*, *Histoplasma* and *Microsporum canis* infections and variably effective against *Aspergillus* and *Penicillium* infections.

It attains therapeutic concentrations in the CNS and respiratory tract. It is excreted by the kidney, producing high concentrations in urine. Reduce dose in animals with renal impairment and liver disease. This drug should be used until clinical signs have resolved and the organism is no longer present – this may take up to 2 months in some cases.

Safety and handling: Normal precautions should be observed.

Contraindications: Do not use in pregnant/lactating animals.

Adverse reactions: Adverse effects may include nausea and diarrhoea. May be hepatotoxic.

Drug interactions: Fluconazole (due to inhibition of cytochrome P450-dependent liver enzymes) may increase plasma theophylline concentrations. In humans, fluconazole has led to terfenadine toxicity when the two drugs were administered together. Fluconazole increases ciclosporin blood levels.

DOSES

Dogs:
- **Fungal infections:** 2.5–10 mg/kg p.o. q12h. Individual dose adjustment may be necessary, guided by adverse effects or lack of efficacy.
- **Urinary candidiasis:** 5–10 mg/kg q24h.

Cats:
- **Ocular/CNS cryptococcosis:** 50–100 mg/cat i.v., p.o. q24h.
- **Systemic infections:** give double the calculated dose on day 1. Doses up to 100 mg/cat q12h are sometimes used for systemic/CNS *Cryptococcus* infection.
- **Dermatophytosis, nasal cryptococcosis:** 5 mg/kg p.o. q24h. For dermatophytosis, administer for 3 periods of 7 days, with 7 days without treatment in between.
- **Urinary candidiasis:** 5–10 mg/kg q24h.

References
KuKanich K, KuKanich B, Lin Z et al. (2020) Clinical pharmacokinetics and outcomes of oral fluconazole therapy in dogs and cats with naturally occurring fungal disease. *Journal of Veterinary Pharmacology and Therapeutics* **43**, 547–556
Pennisi MG, Hartmann K, Lloret A et al. (2013) Cryptococcosis in cats: ABCD guidelines on prevention and management. *Journal of Feline Medicine and Surgery* **15**, 611–618

Flucytosine

(Ancotil*) **POM**

Formulations: Injectable: 10 mg/ml solution. Flucytosine tablets are available from special order manufacturers or specialist importing companies. **VSP**

Action: Fungal cells convert flucytosine (5-FC) into 5-fluorouracil (5-FU), which inhibits DNA and RNA synthesis in the cell. Mammalian cells are spared.

Use:
- Treatment of cryptococcosis (often in conjunction with amphotericin B or itraconazole) particularly if involving meninges.
- Treatment of systemic and urinary yeast infections (e.g. candidiasis).

Little used in veterinary medicine compared with other antifungals. Use flucytosine with caution in patients with hepatic or renal impairment; reduce the dose and monitor haematological, renal and hepatic parameters. Resistance can develop quickly when used as a sole agent. Penetrates well into cerebrospinal fluid.

Safety and handling: Normal precautions should be observed.

Contraindications: No information available.

Adverse reactions: Drug eruptions, including toxic epidermal necrolysis. Vomiting and diarrhoea may develop as well as myelosuppression, renal and hepatic toxicity; alleviate by dosing over 15 minutes. Flucytosine may be teratogenic.

Drug interactions: Synergy with amphotericin B has been demonstrated, although there is an increased risk of nephrotoxicity.

DOSES

Dogs: 25–35 mg/kg i.v. q8h or 50–65 mg/kg p.o. q8h.
Cats: 25–50 mg/kg i.v. q6h or 50–65 mg/kg p.o. q8h.

References
Pennisi MG, Hartmann K, Lloret A et al. (2013) Cryptococcosis in cats: ABCD guidelines on prevention and management. *Journal of Feline Medicine and Surgery* **15**, 611–618

Fludrocortisone

CIL

(Fludrocortisone acetate*) **POM**

Formulations: Oral: 0.1 mg tablets. Also available on a named patient basis in 0.25 mg and 0.5 mg sizes.

Action: Aldosterone analogue that increases potassium excretion and sodium retention but which also has some glucocorticoid properties.

Use:
- Treatment of adrenocortical insufficiency (Addison's disease) when authorized product (desoxycortone pivalate) is not suitable in an individual patient.

Fludrocortisone is about 125 times more potent as a mineralocorticoid than hydrocortisone but it is also about 12 times more potent as a glucocorticoid (and therefore about 3 times more potent than prednisolone). Monitor absolute sodium and potassium concentrations (not just the ratio) 4–6 hours post pill. Some dogs only require q24h dosing but in such cases the sodium and potassium concentrations should also be checked pre pill. Supplemental doses of prednisolone may be required at times of metabolic or physical stress.

Safety and handling: Normal precautions should be observed. Some formulations require refrigeration.

Contraindications: No information available.

Adverse reactions: Hypertension, oedema (including cerebral oedema) and hypokalaemia with overdosages. Long-term overdose may result in clinical signs of hypercortisolism.

Drug interactions: Hypokalaemia may develop if fludrocortisone is administered concomitantly with amphotericin B or potassium-depleting diuretics (furosemide, thiazides).

DOSES

Dogs: Hypoadrenocorticism: start at 0.01 mg/kg p.o. q12h. Check serum electrolytes at 5–7 days and adjust dose as needed to maintain serum sodium and potassium within normal ranges. Most patients when stable require <0.05 mg/kg p.o. q12h.

Cats: Hypoadrenocorticism: dose as for dogs (very few reports).

References

Roberts E, Boden LA and Ramsey IK (2016) Factors that affect stabilisation times of canine spontaneous hypoadrenocorticism. *Veterinary Record* **179**, 98

Flumazenil

(Romazicon*) **POM**

Formulations: Injectable: 0.1 mg/ml solution available as 5 ml and 10 ml vials.

Action: Flumazenil binds to and rapidly displaces benzodiazepines from the benzodiazepine receptor, thereby reversing their sedative and anxiolytic effects within 1–2 minutes. The duration of action of flumazenil is short (1 hour); dosing may need to be repeated.

Use: To reverse the sedative and respiratory depressant effects of benzodiazepines such as midazolam and diazepam.

Safety and handling: Normal precautions should be observed.

Contraindications: Flumazenil is contraindicated in human patients with suspected tricyclic antidepressant overdose as it can cause seizures.

Adverse reactions: The use of flumazenil has been associated with seizures in humans receiving long-term benzodiazepine administration for sedation. Be prepared to manage seizures should they occur.

Drug interactions: Can cause seizures in human patients with suspected tricyclic antidepressant overdose.

DOSES
Dogs, Cats: 0.01–0.1 mg/kg i.v., can be repeated if marked respiratory depression reoccurs. It takes 6–10 minutes for flumazenil to reach peak effects after i.v. administration. Start at the low end of the dose range.

Flumethrin see Imidacloprid

Fluoxetine `CIL`
(Reconcile [d], Prozac*) **POM-V, POM**

Formulations: Oral: 8 mg, 16 mg, 32 mg, 64 mg tablets (Reconcile); 20 mg tablets and liquid forms are also available.

Action: Fluoxetine and its primary metabolite norfluoxetine block serotonin reuptake in the brain, resulting in antidepressive activity and a raising in motor activity thresholds. It also has minor noradrenaline reuptake inhibition properties, but is considered a selective serotonin reuptake inhibitor (SSRI).

Use:
- Authorized for the management of canine separation anxiety in association with a behaviour modification plan.
- Used for the management of a wide range of anxiety-related conditions, including compulsive disorders and some forms of aggression in dogs.
- Fluoxetine has been used in the cat to control urine spraying and other anxiety-related behaviour problems, such as psychogenic alopecia and certain forms of aggression.
- Use in aggression should be with a specifically constructed behaviour modification plan and with caution.

Safety and handling: Normal precautions should be observed.

Contraindications: Known sensitivity to fluoxetine or other SSRIs, history of seizures.

Adverse reactions: Common reactions include lethargy, decreased appetite and vomiting, which may result in minor weight loss. Trembling, restlessness and other GI disturbances may also occur and must be distinguished from a paradoxical increase in anxiety which has been reported in some cases. Owners should be warned of a potential increase in aggression in response to medication.

Drug interactions: Fluoxetine should not be used within 2 weeks of treatment with a monoamine oxidase inhibitor (MAOI) (e.g. selegiline) and an MAOI should not be used within 6 weeks of treatment with fluoxetine. Fluoxetine, like other SSRIs, antagonizes the effects of anticonvulsants and so is not recommended for use with epileptic patients or in association with other agents which lower seizure threshold, e.g. phenothiazines. Caution is warranted if fluoxetine is used concomitantly with aspirin or other anticoagulants since the risk of increased bleeding in the case of tissue trauma may be increased. Should not generally be used alongside other serotonergic agents given risk of serotonin syndrome, although use alongside trazodone may be considered in exceptional cases, so long as patient carefully monitored for signs of serotonin syndrome.

DOSES
Dogs: 1–2 mg/kg p.o. q24h.
Cats: 0.5–1.0 mg/kg p.o. q24h.

References
Simpson B S, Landsberg GM, Reisner IR et al. (2007) Effects of reconcile (fluoxetine) chewable tablets plus behavior management for canine separation anxiety. Veterinary Therapeutics **8**, 18–31

Fluralaner
(Bravecto[d], Bravecto plus spot-on[c], Bravecto spot-on[c,d])
POM-V

Formulations: Oral: 5 sizes of chewable tablets for dogs, delivering 25–56 mg fluralaner/kg (Bravecto). **Topical:** 280 mg/ml solution, 3 sizes for cats, 5 sizes for dogs (Bravecto spot-on); 280 mg/ml fluralaner + 14 mg/ml moxidectin, 3 sizes for cats (Bravecto plus spot-on).

Action: Fluralaner acts at ligand-gated chloride channels, in particular those gated by the neurotransmitter GABA, thereby blocking pre- and post-synaptic transfer of chloride ions across cell membranes.

Use:
- Treatment of fleas and ticks in dogs and cats.
- Treatment of ear mite (Otodectes cynotis) in cats.
- Treatment of Demodex canis.
- Treatment of Sarcoptes scabiei in dogs.
- Reduction of the risk of infection with Babesia canis.

Onset of action: fleas within 8 hours and ticks within 12 hours (Ixodes ricinus). Immediate and persistent tick killing activity for 12 weeks for Ixodes ricinus, Dermacentor reticulatus and D. variabilis, 8 weeks for Rhipicephalus sanguineus. Parasites need to start feeding on the host to become exposed to fluralaner; therefore the risk of the transmission of parasite-borne diseases cannot be excluded. Can be used in breeding, pregnant and lactating dogs.

Safety and handling: Normal precautions should be observed.

Contraindications: Do not use in dogs <8 weeks or <2 kg, or cats <11 weeks or <1.2 kg. Use with caution in dogs with pre-existing epilepsy. The product should not be administered at intervals shorter than 8 weeks.

Adverse reactions: Oral: mild GI signs may occur; convulsions and lethargy have been reported very rarely. Spot-on: erythema and alopecia at application site. Cats: apathy, tremors, anorexia, vomiting and hypersalivation.

Drug interactions: Fluralaner is highly bound to plasma proteins and might compete with other highly bound active substances such as NSAIDs and the coumarin derivative warfarin.

DOSES
See Appendix for guidelines on responsible parasiticide use.

Dogs: 25–56 mg/kg p.o. q3months or 1 pipette per dog according to bodyweight q3months.

Cats: 1 pipette per cat according to bodyweight q3months.

References
Crosaz O, Chapelle E, Cochet-Faivre N *et al.* (2016) Open field study on the efficacy of oral fluralaner for long-term control of flea allergy dermatitis in client-owned dogs in Ile-de-France region. *Parasites and Vectors* **9**, 174

Taenzler J, de Vos C, Roepke RK *et al.* (2017) Efficacy of fluralaner against *Otodectes cynotis* infestations in dogs and cats. *Parasites and Vectors* **10**, 30

Flurbiprofen
(Ocufen*) **POM**

Formulations: Ophthalmic: 0.03% solution in single-use vials.

Action: Inhibits prostaglandin synthesis, producing an anti-inflammatory and analgesic action. Prostaglandins also play a role in the miosis produced during intraocular surgery by constricting the iris sphincter independently of cholinergic mechanisms.

Use:
- Before cataract surgery.
- It is also useful for anterior uveitis and ulcerative keratitis when topical corticosteroids are contraindicated.

Topical NSAIDs have the potential to increase intraocular pressure and should be used with caution in dogs and cats with glaucoma.

Safety and handling: Normal precautions should be observed.

Contraindications: No information available.

Adverse reactions: As with other topical NSAIDs, flurbiprofen may cause local irritation. Topical NSAIDs can be used in ulcerative keratitis but with caution as they can delay epithelial healing. Topical NSAIDs have been associated with an increased risk of corneal 'melting' (keratomalacia) in humans, although this has not been reported in the veterinary literature. Regular monitoring is advised.

Drug interactions: Ophthalmic NSAIDs may be used safely with other ophthalmic pharmaceuticals, although concurrent use of drugs which adversely affect the corneal epithelium (e.g. gentamicin) may lead to increased corneal penetration of the NSAID. The concurrent use of topical NSAIDs with topical corticosteroids has been identified as a risk factor in humans for precipitating corneal problems.

DOSES
Dogs, Cats: 1 drop per eye q6–12h depending on severity of inflammation. **Preoperatively:** 1 drop q30min for 4 doses (pre-surgery protocols vary widely).

References
Lanuza R, Rankin AJ, KuKanich B *et al.* (2015) Evaluation of systemic absorption and renal effects of topical ophthalmic flurbiprofen and diclofenac in healthy cats. *Veterinary Ophthalmology* **19(S1)**, 24–29

Fluticasone

(Flixotide*) **POM**

CIL

Formulations: Inhalational: 50 µg (microgram), 125 µg, 250 µg metered inhalations (Evohaler).

Action: Binds to specific nuclear receptors and affects gene transcription such that many aspects of inflammation are suppressed.

Use:
- Used as an inhaled corticosteroid in the management of inflammatory airway disease in dogs and cats.

Administer via commercially available chambers and masks specifically designed for veterinary use. Not useful for acute bronchospasm.

Safety and handling: Normal precautions should be observed.

Contraindications: No information available.

Adverse reactions: Inhaled steroids are known to suppress the hypothalamic–pituitary–adrenal axis, although they are considered generally safer than systemic steroids. Chronic use occasionally associated with local opportunistic infection, e.g. demodicosis.

Drug interactions: No information available.

DOSES

Dogs: Chronic inflammatory tracheobronchial disease: 125–500 µg (micrograms)/dog q12–24h.

Cats: Feline lower airway disease: 50–250 µg (micrograms)/cat q12–24h.

References

Cohn LA, DeClue AE, Cohen RL *et al.* (2010) Effects of fluticasone propionate dosage in an experimental model of feline asthma. *Journal of Feline Medicine and Surgery* **12**, 91–96
Kirschvink N, Leemans J, Delvaux F *et al.* (2006) Inhaled fluticasone reduces bronchial responsiveness and airway inflammation in cats with mild chronic bronchitis. *Journal of Feline Medicine and Surgery* **8**, 45–54

Fomepizole (4-Methylpyrazole)

(Antizol*) **POM**

Formulations: Injectable: 1.5 g/1.5 ml vial; dilute 1:19 (i.e. 1.5 ml vial added to 28.5 ml of 0.9% saline, giving a 50 mg/ml solution). Discard after 72 hours. Available from special order manufacturers or specialist importing companies.

Action: Competitive inhibition of alcohol dehydrogenase.

Use: Treatment of ethylene glycol (antifreeze) toxicity. Available for import on a named-patient basis.

Safety and handling: Normal precautions should be observed.

Contraindications: No information available.

Adverse reactions: No information available.

Drug interactions: Increases risk of ethanol toxicity if co-administered.

DOSES

Dogs: 20 mg/kg i.v. over 30 min initially, then 15 mg/kg i.v. slowly over 15–30 min 12 h and 24 h later, then 5 mg/kg i.v. q12h until ethylene glycol concentration is negligible or the dog has recovered. Most effective if started within 8 hours of intoxication.

Cats: 125 mg/kg slow i.v. then 31.25 mg/kg i.v. q12h for 3 additional doses. Efficacy has been shown if treated within 3 hours of ingestion.

References

Tart KM and Powell LL (2011) 4-Methylpyrazole as a treatment in naturally occurring ethylene glycol intoxication in cats. *Journal of Veterinary Emergency and Critical Care* **21**, 268–272

Framycetin

(Canaural [c,d]) **POM-V**

Formulations: Topical: 5 mg/g suspension (Canaural also contains fusidic acid, nystatin and prednisolone).

Action: Aminoglycosides inhibit bacterial protein synthesis and require an oxygen-rich environment to be effective, thus they are ineffective in low-oxygen sites (abscesses, exudates), making all obligate anaerobic bacteria resistant. Their mechanism of killing is concentration-dependent, leading to a marked post-antibiotic effect, allowing pulse-dosing regimens which may limit toxicity.

Use:
- Treatment of ear infections. Framycetin is particularly effective against Gram-negative bacteria, although the combination preparation Canaural has a broad spectrum of activity.

Safety and handling: Normal precautions should be observed.

Contraindications: Do not use in animals with a perforated tympanum. Do not use in conjunction with other products known to be ototoxic.

Adverse reactions: Aminoglycosides are potentially ototoxic, and alaxia, deafness and nystagmus may be observed in animals where drops have been administered with a perforated tympanum. Local irritation.

Drug interactions: No information available.

DOSES

Classified as category C (Caution) by the EMA.
See Appendix for guidelines on responsible antibiotic use.

Dogs, Cats: 5–10 drops per ear q12h. In small animals, 2–5 drops may be a more feasible volume to instill.

Frunevetmab

(Solensia [c]) **POM-V**

Formulations: Injectable: 1 ml vials containing 7 mg frunevetmab.

Action: Frunevetmab is a feline monoclonal antibody that targets nerve growth factor (NGF). The inhibition of NGF-mediated cell signalling has been demonstrated to provide relief from pain associated with osteoarthritis.

Use:
- Indicated for the alleviation of pain associated with osteoarthritis in cats.

Continuation of treatment should be based on the individual response of each animal. If a positive response is not observed, consider alternative treatments.

Safety and handling: Store in the fridge between 2 and 8°C. Protect from light. Avoid excessive shaking or foaming of the solution. Due to the role of NGF in ensuring normal fetal nervous system development, people who are or may become pregnant, or who are breastfeeding should not handle this drug. In the case of accidental self-injection, seek medical advice immediately and show the package leaflet or label to the physician.

Contraindications: Do not use in cats <12 months or <2.5 kg. Do not use in animals intended for breeding or in pregnant or lactating animals. The safety of frunevetmab has not been established in cats with International Renal Interest Society stage 3 or 4 kidney disease. Use of the product in such cases should be based on a benefit-risk assessment.

Adverse reactions: Mild reactions at the injection site, such as pruritus, dermatitis and alopecia, occurred commonly in studies.

Drug interactions: There are no safety data on the concurrent long term use of NSAIDs with frunevetmab in cats. In clinical trials in humans, rapidly progressive osteoarthritis has been reported in patients receiving antiNGF monoclonal antibody therapy and NSAIDs for more than 90 days. Cats have no reported equivalent of human rapidly progressive osteoarthritis. If vaccines are to be administered at the same time as treatment with frunevetmab, different sites should be used.

DOSES
Dogs: Do not use.

Cats: 1–2.8 mg/kg s.c. once a month. Administer one vial to cats between 2.5 and 7 kg, administer 2 vials to cats >7 kg.

References
Enomoto M, Mantyh PW, Murrell J, Innes JF and Lascelles BDX (2019) Anti-nerve growth factor monoclonal antibodies for control of pain in cats and dogs. *Veterinary Record* **184**, 23

Gruen ME, Myers JAE, Tena JS *et al.* (2021) Frunevetmab, a felinized anti-nerve growth factor monoclonal antibody, for the treatment of pain from osteoarthritis in cats. *Journal of Veterinary Internal Medicine* **35**, 2752–2762

Furosemide (Frusemide) `CIL`

(Dimazon [c,d], Frusecare, Frusedale [c,d], Libeo [d], Frusol*)
POM-V, POM

Formulations: Injectable: 50 mg/ml solution. Oral: 10 mg, 20 mg, 40 mg tablets; 20 mg/5 ml, 40 mg/5 ml, 50 mg/5 ml sugar-free solutions.

Action: Loop diuretic, inhibiting the $Na^+/K^+/Cl^-$ cotransporter in the thick ascending limb of the loop of Henle. The net effect is a loss of sodium, potassium, chloride and water in the urine. It also increases excretion of calcium, magnesium and hydrogen as well as renal blood flow and glomerular filtration rate. Transient venodilation may occur following i.v. administration and, in some species, bronchodilation may occur; the exact mechanism for both is unclear.

Use:

- Management of acute and chronic CHF. The use of diuretic monotherapy for the chronic management of heart failure due to mild regurgitation or dilated cardiomyopathy in dogs is not recommended, as patients receiving concomitant therapy with pimobendan and ACE inhibitors (and spironolactone in dogs with mitral regurgitation) have a better clinical outcome.
- Treatment of hypercalcaemia.
- Promotion of diuresis in acute renal failure (questionable efficacy).

Use with caution in patients with severe electrolyte depletion, hepatic failure and diabetes mellitus. Evidence for efficacy in non-cardiogenic pulmonary oedema is lacking.

Safety and handling: Normal precautions should be observed.

Contraindications: Dehydration and anuria. Do not use in pericardial effusion where cardiac tamponade is confirmed. Can be used after effusion drainage to assist in management of right-sided heart failure symptoms if necessary.

Adverse reactions: Hypokalaemia, hypochloraemia, hypocalcaemia, hypomagnesaemia and hyponatraemia; dehydration, polyuria/polydipsia and prerenal azotaemia occur readily. A marked reduction in cardiac output can occur in animals with severe pulmonary disease, low-output heart failure, hypertrophic cardiomyopathy, pericardial or myocardial disorders, cardiac tamponade and severe hypertension. Other adverse effects include ototoxicity (especially in cats), GI disturbances, leucopenia, anaemia, weakness and restlessness.

Drug interactions: Nephrotoxicity/ototoxicity associated with aminoglycosides may be potentiated when furosemide is also used. Furosemide may induce hypokalaemia, thereby increasing the risk of digoxin toxicity. Increased risk of hypokalaemia if given with acetazolamide, corticosteroids, thiazides and theophylline. Concurrent administration of NSAIDs with furosemide may decrease efficacy and may predispose to nephrotoxicity, particularly in patients with poor renal perfusion. Furosemide may inhibit the muscle relaxation qualities of tubocurarine but increase the effects of suxamethonium.

DOSES

Dogs, Cats:

- **Acute, life-threatening CHF:** 1–2 mg/kg i.v., i.m. q0.5–4h prn, based on improvement in respiratory rate and effort. Once clinical signs improve, increase dosing interval to q4–12h, monitor urea, creatinine and electrolytes, and start oral therapy once tolerated. Use lower end of dose range for cats and monitor response. Ensure no pleural effusion present.
- **Chronic CHF:** 1–5 mg/kg p.o. q6–12h. Typical maintenance doses for mild to moderate CHF are 1–2 mg/kg p.o. q8–24h (dogs) and 1–2 mg/kg p.o. q12–48h (cats). The goal is to use the lowest dose of furosemide that effectively controls clinical signs. Doses in excess of 12 mg/kg/day are unlikely to be beneficial and warrant the addition of a different class of diuretic (e.g. thiazide) or transfer to alternative diuretic (e.g. torasemide) to control refractory failure. In patients with ascites, use of s.c. instead of p.o. furosemide can have a marked clinical benefit due to improved bioavailability.

- **Hypercalcaemia:** hydrate before therapy. Give 2–4 mg/kg i.v., s.c., p.o. q8–24h. Maintain hydration status and electrolyte balance with normal saline and added KCl. Furosemide generally reduces serum calcium levels by 0.5–1.5 mmol/l.
- **Acute renal failure/oliguria:** Replace fluid deficit and subsequently closely monitor fluid input and output. Give furosemide at 2 mg/kg i.v. If no diuresis within 1 hour, repeat dose at 2–4 mg/kg i.v. (and again if no response at 2 hours). Alternatively, bolus dose with 1–2 mg/kg i.v. followed by CRI at 0.1–2 mg/kg/h.

References

Ames MK, Atkins CE, Lantis AC et al. (2013) Effect of furosemide and high-dosage pimobendan administration on the renin-angiotensin-aldosterone system in dogs. *American Journal of Veterinary Research* **74**, 2–8

Peddle GD, Singletary GE, Reynolds CA et al. (2012) Effect of torsemide and furosemide on clinical, laboratory, radiographic and quality of life variables in dogs with heart failure secondary to mitral valve disease. *Journal of Veterinary Cardiology* **14**, 253–259

Fusidic acid

(Betafuse[d], Canaural[c,d], Isaderm[d], Isathal[c,d], Trigoderm[d])
POM-V

Formulations: Topical: 5 mg/g fusidate suspension (Canaural also contains framycetin, nystatin and prednisolone); 0.5% fusidic acid + 0.1% betamethasone gel (Betafuse, Isaderm, Trigoderm); 1% fusidic acid viscous solution (Isathal).

Action: Inhibits bacterial protein synthesis.

Use:
- Active against Gram-positive bacteria, particularly *Staphylococcus pseudintermedius*.
- Used topically in the management of staphylococcal infections of the conjunctiva, skin or ear.

Fusidic acid is able to penetrate skin and penetrate the cornea, gaining access to the anterior chamber of the eye. The carbomer gel vehicle in the ocular preparation may also be efficacious as a surface lubricant.

Safety and handling: Avoid contamination of the container on application.

Contraindications: Do not use preparations containing corticosteroids in pregnant animals.

Adverse reactions: No information available.

Drug interactions: No information available.

DOSES

Classified as category D (Prudence) by the EMA.
See Appendix for guidelines on responsible antibiotic use.
Dogs:
- Otic: 5–10 drops per affected ear q12h. In small animals, 2–5 drops may be a more feasible volume to instill.
- Ophthalmic: 1 drop per eye q12h.
- Skin: apply to affected area q12h for 5 days.

Cats: Otic, Ophthalmic: doses as for dogs.

References

Clark SM, Loeffler A and Bond R (2015) Susceptibility *in vitro* of canine methicillin-resistant and -susceptible staphylococcal isolates to fusidic acid, chlorhexidine and miconazole: opportunities for topical therapy of canine superficial pyoderma. *Journal of Antimicrobial Chemotherapy* **70**, 2048–2052

Loeffler A, Baines SJ, Toleman MS *et al.* (2008) In vitro activity of fusidic acid and mupirocin against coagulase-positive staphylococci from pets. *Journal of Antimicrobial Chemotherapy* **62**, 1301–130

A
B
C
D
E
F
G
H
I
J
K
L
M
N
O
P
Q
R
S
T
U
V
W
X
Y
Z

Gabapentin (Gabapentinum) [CIL]

(Gabapentin*, Neurontin*) **POM CD SCHEDULE 3**

Formulations: Oral: 100 mg, 300 mg, 400 mg capsules; 600 mg, 800 mg film-coated tablets; 50 mg/ml solution.

Action: The precise mechanism of action of gabapentin is unknown but it appears to bind to a specific modulating protein of the voltage-gated calcium channels, resulting in a decreased release of excitatory neurotransmitters. Gabapentin is structurally related to GABA and does increase levels of GABA in the CNS but does not appear to alter GABA binding, uptake or release. The mode of action of the analgesic effect may be due to down-regulation of excitatory neurotransmitters in the dorsal horn of the spinal cord or its inhibitory effect on dorsal horn N-methyl-D-aspartate receptors.

Use:
- Adjunctive therapy in the treatment of seizures refractory to treatment with conventional therapy, although the supporting evidence in dogs is weak.
- Treatment of chronic pain states, such as neuropathic pain and possibly postoperative pain.
- Studies have shown it to be effective in improving quality of life in dogs with syringomyelia and effective in reducing the amount of opioid required postoperatively.
- A double-blind, placebo-controlled crossover trial showed the effectiveness of a single dose for storm phobia.

After multiple dosing, peak plasma concentrations of gabapentin are usually achieved within 2 hours of a dose, and steady state achieved within 1–2 days. It is partially metabolized by the liver before renal excretion and has an elimination half-life of 3–4 hours. Abrupt discontinuation of the drug has precipitated seizures in humans; therefore, tapered withdrawal is recommended. Monitoring of serum levels does not appear useful in dogs or humans. Use with caution in patients with renal impairment, behavioural abnormalities or severe hepatic disease.

Safety and handling: Normal precautions should be observed.

Contraindications: Avoid oral solutions containing xylitol which may be toxic to dogs at higher doses.

Adverse reactions: The most commonly reported adverse effect in dogs is mild sedation and ataxia. False-positive readings have been reported with some urinary protein tests in human patients taking gabapentin. Hepatic toxicity has been reported as a rare side effect in human patients.

Drug interactions: The absorption of gabapentin from the GI tract is reduced by antacids containing aluminium with magnesium; it is recommended that gabapentin is taken at least 2 hours after the administration of such antacids. Cimetidine has been reported to reduce the renal clearance of gabapentin but the product information does not consider this to be of clinical importance.

DOSES

Dogs: 10–20 mg/kg p.o. q6–8h (starting dose; incremental dose increases are recommended).
- **For storm phobia:** single dose of 25–30 mg/kg given 90 minutes before a storm.

Cats: 5–10 mg/kg p.o. q8–12h (starting dose; incremental dose increases are recommended).

References

Bleuer-Elsner S, Medam T and Masson S (2021) Effects of a single oral dose of gabapentin on storm phobia in dogs: A double-blind, placebo-controlled crossover trial. *Veterinary Record* **189**, e453

KuKanich B (2013) Outpatient oral analgesics in dogs and cats beyond nonsteroidal antiinflammatory drugs: an evidence-based approach. *Veterinary Clinics of North America: Small Animal Practice* **43**, 1109–1125

Muñana KR (2013) Management of refractory epilepsy. *Top Companion Animal Medicine* **28**, 67–71

Ganciclovir
(Virgan*) **POM**

Formulations: Topical: 0.15% eye gel in 5 g tube.

Action: Inhibits viral replication (viral DNA polymerase); depends on viral thymidine kinase for phosphorylation.

Use:
* Management of ocular feline herpesvirus-1 (FHV-1) infections.

In vitro studies show that ganciclovir is at least 10 times more effective against FHV-1 than aciclovir. Anecdotal reports of its topical use are promising, but neither the safety nor the pharmacokinetics has been reported in cats. Cannot eradicate latent viral infection. In refractory and severe cases of FHV-1 ulceration, combined therapy including topical or systemic antiviral medication can be used

Safety and handling: Normal precautions should be observed.

Contraindications: No information available.

Adverse reactions: Ocular irritation may occur and the frequency of application should be reduced if this develops. Treatment should not be continued for >3 weeks.

Drug interactions: No information available.

DOSES
Dogs: No information available.
Cats: Apply small amount to affected eye q4–6h (maximum 3 weeks).

References

Thomasy SM and Maggs DJ (2016) A review of antiviral drugs and other compounds with activity against feline herpesvirus type 1. *Veterinary Ophthalmology* **19(S1)**, 119–130

Gelatine (Oxypolygelatine, Polygeline)
(Gelofusine*, Haemaccel*) **POM**

Formulations: Injectable: 4% solution of succinylated gelatine in 0.7% sodium chloride (Gelofusine); 35 g/dl degraded urea-linked gelatine with NaCl, KCl and $CaCl_2$ (Haemaccel).

Action: Promotes retention of fluid within the vascular system through the exertion of oncotic pressure.

Use:
* The expansion and maintenance of blood volume in various forms of shock including hypovolaemic and haemorrhagic shock.

The main difference between gelatine-based solutions and other synthetic colloids is that they have lower molecular weights (and hence are excreted rapidly) and appear to have few antigenic or anticoagulative effects. The plasma half-life of most gelatines is approximately 8 hours (oxypolygelatine 2–4 hours), so the duration of plasma expansion is much shorter than with hydroxyethyl starch. There appears to be little effect on coagulation or blood loss following gelatine administration. Use with caution in animals with congestive heart failure or renal insufficiency as will increase risk of circulatory overload.

Safety and handling: Normal precautions should be observed.

Contraindications: No information available.

Adverse reactions: Anaphylactoid reactions to gelatine solutions are rare; it is uncertain whether these reactions represent a specific immune response. In human medicine, there are concerns over the safety of these solutions when used in patients with kidney disease.

Drug interactions: No information available.

DOSES

Dogs, Cats: 10–20 ml/kg i.v. bolus. In normal circumstances do not exceed replacement of >25% of circulating blood volume with gelatines in a 24-hour period.

References
Glowaski MM, Moon-Passat PF, Erb HN *et al.* (2003) Effects of oxypolygelatin and dextran 70 on hemostatic variables in dogs. *Veterinary Anaesthesia and Analgesia* **30**, 202–210

Gemcitabine
(Gemzar*) **POM**

Formulations: Injectable: Lyophilized powder for reconstitution before use. 200 mg (in 10 ml vials) and 1 g (in 50 ml vials).

Action: Metabolites of the drug inhibit the enzyme ribonucleotide reductase and compete with endogenous nucleotides for incorporation into DNA strands, thereby inhibiting DNA synthesis. Acts primarily in S phase.

Use:
- Used in dogs with bladder urothelial carcinoma, lymphoma and various carcinomas.
- Described for use in cats with exocrine pancreatic carcinoma.
- May also be useful as a radiosensitizer for some tumours.

Limited clinical use at present. In humans, gemcitabine has been used in cases of pancreatic carcinoma, small cell lung carcinoma, lymphoma, bladder and other soft tissue carcinomas. Seek specialist advice before using this drug.

Safety and handling: Potent cytotoxic drug that should only be prepared and administered by trained personnel. See Appendix and specialist texts for further advice on chemotherapeutic agents.

Contraindications: Contraindicated in patients with known hypersensitivity to gemcitabine. Do not use in patients with pre-existing bone marrow suppression. Should be used with caution in patients with reduced hepatic or renal function.

Adverse reactions: May cause myelosuppression and gastrointestinal adverse events. Retinal haemorrhage may also occur. Death due to treatment-related complications has been described.

Drug interactions: Not reported at present.

DOSES

See Appendix for chemotherapy protocols and conversion of bodyweight to body surface area.

Dogs: High dose: 800–900 mg/m^2 i.v. over 30–60 minutes every 7–14 days for 4 doses. **Low dose:** 25–50 mg/m^2 i.v. over 30–60 minutes once or twice a week as per protocols. Some studies report doses of 2 mg/kg i.v. over 20–30 minutes (in 0.9% NaCl) combined with carboplatin no more than every 7 days.

Cats: Low dose: 20–25 mg/m^2 or 2 mg/kg as a 20 minute i.v. infusion every 7 days.

References

Dominguez PA, Dervisis NG, Cadile CD *et al.* (2009) Combined gemcitabine and carboplatin therapy for carcinomas in dogs. *Journal of Veterinary Internal Medicine* **23**, 130–137

Marconato L, Finotello R, Bonfanti U *et al.* (2015) An open-label phase 1 dose-escalation clinical trial of a single intravenous administration of gemcitabine in dogs with advanced solid tumors. *Journal of Veterinary Internal Medicine* **29**, 620–625

Gentamicin

(Clinagel Vet, Easotic [d], Genta, Otomax [d], Tiacil [c,d], Genticin*) **POM-V, POM**

Formulations: Injectable: 40 mg/ml solution (human preparation), 100 mg/ml solution (Genta). **Ophthalmic:** 0.3% w/w gel; 0.5% w/v drops. **Otic:** 1505 IU/ml gentamicin with miconazole and hydrocortisone (Easotic), 2640 IU/ml gentamicin with clotrimazole and betamethasone (Otomax).

Action: Aminoglycosides irreversibly bind to the 30S ribosome subunit, inhibiting bacterial protein synthesis. They require an oxygen-rich environment to be effective, thus they are ineffective in low-oxygen sites (abscesses, exudates), making all obligate anaerobic bacteria resistant. Their mechanism of killing is concentration-dependent, leading to a marked post-antibiotic effect, allowing pulse-dosing regimens which may limit toxicity.

Use:
- Active against Gram-negative bacteria, but some staphylococcal and streptococcal (*Streptococcus faecalis*) species are also susceptible.
- When used for empiric therapy of serious infections, gentamicin is usually given in conjunction with a penicillin and/or metronidazole to provide broad-spectrum cover.

All obligate anaerobic bacteria and many haemolytic streptococci are resistant. Use in domestic animals is limited by nephrotoxicity and, more rarely, ototoxicity and neuromuscular blockade. Cats are more sensitive to toxic effects. Microbial resistance is a concern, although many bacteria resistant to gentamicin may be susceptible to amikacin. Aminoglycosides are more active in an alkaline environment. Geriatric animals or those with reduced renal function should only be given this drug systemically when absolutely necessary, although dosing q24h should reduce the likelihood of nephrotoxicity. Sepsis, dehydration, hypokalaemia, prolonged treatment and fever all increase the risk of nephrotoxicity. Therapeutic drug monitoring should be considered if possible and is highly recommended if nephrotoxicity risk factors are present. Peak level (30–60 minutes post i.v. dose) should be >20 µg (micrograms)/ml and trough level should be <1 µg/ml.

Safety and handling: Normal precautions should be observed.

Contraindications: Do not use the otic preparation if the tympanum is perforated. Do not use in conjunction with other drugs considered to be nephrotoxic. For systemic use, do not exceed 7 days treatment duration.

Adverse reactions: Gentamicin delays epithelial healing of corneal ulcers and may cause local irritation. Nephrotoxicity and ototoxicity (auditory and vestibular) are potential side effects. Cellular casts in urine sediment are an early sign of impending nephrotoxicity; however, urine must be examined immediately to detect their presence, and their absence is not a guarantee of safety. Serum creatinine levels rise later and fatal acute renal failure may be inevitable when they do. Gentamicin should not be used during pregnancy.

Drug interactions: Avoid concurrent use of other nephrotoxic, ototoxic or neurotoxic agents (e.g. amphotericin B, furosemide). Increase monitoring and adjust dosages when these drugs must be used together. Aminoglycosides may be chemically inactivated by beta-lactam antibiotics (e.g. penicillins, cephalosporins) or heparin *in vitro* (avoid mixing in the same syringe). The effect of non-depolarizing muscle relaxants (e.g. atracurium, pancuronium, vecuronium) may be enhanced by aminoglycosides. Synergism may occur when aminoglycosides are used with beta-lactam antimicrobials.

DOSES

Classified as category C (Caution) by the EMA.

See Appendix for guidelines on responsible antibiotic use.

Dogs:
- Otic: 4–8 drops (depending on weight of the animal) in affected ear or apply ointment to affected area q12h. Easotic preparation: apply 1 ml to each ear q24h using a metered or single dose delivery system.
- Ophthalmic: 1 drop per eye q6–8h. 1 cm gel per eye q8–12h.
- Systemic: 5–10 mg/kg slowly i.v. (over 30 min), i.m., s.c. q24h.

Cats:
- Ophthalmic: Dose as for dogs.
- Systemic: 5–8 mg/kg slowly i.v. (over 30 min), i.m., s.c. q24h.

Glipizide

CIL

(Glipizide*, Minodiab*) **POM**

Formulations: Oral: 2.5 mg, 5 mg tablets.

Action: Increases insulin secretion (if functional reserve of beta-cells), thereby reducing blood glucose.

Use:
- Management of type II diabetes mellitus in cats whose owners are unwilling or unable to give insulin.

Glipizide use may accelerate beta-cell loss. May be effective alone or administered with insulin to reduce insulin requirements. It is ineffective when there is an absolute insulin deficiency, or when insulin resistance or ketosis is present. An effect on blood glucose may not be seen for 4–8 weeks. Administer with food. Preferred to metformin and glibenclamide, as better researched.

Safety and handling: Normal precautions should be observed.

Contraindications: Do not use if ketosis present. Do not use if there is evidence of reduced hepatic or renal function.

Adverse reactions: Glipizide may cause GI disturbances (e.g. vomiting) and sensitivity reactions (e.g. jaundice, rashes, fever). May cause hypoglycaemia.

Drug interactions: The effects of glipizide may be enhanced by ACE inhibitors, NSAIDs, chloramphenicol, potentiated sulphonamides and fluoroquinolones.

DOSES

Dogs: Do not use.

Cats: 2.5–5 mg p.o. q12h. Start at the lower end of the dose range, increasing the dose as required if no adverse effects are reported after 2 weeks.

References

Feldman EC, Nelson RW and Feldman MS (1997) Intensive 50-week evaluation of glipizide administration in 50 cats with previously untreated diabetes mellitus. *Journal of the American Veterinary Medical Association* **210**, 772–777

Glucagon

(Glucagen*) **POM**

Formulations: Injectable: 1 mg vial for reconstitution.

Action: Binds to specific receptor and counteracts most of the effects of insulin.

Use:
- Treatment of insulin overdose. Use only when feeding and glucose administration has failed to maintain a response. Duration of activity is unknown in dogs but likely to be 1–2 hours. Blood glucose levels should be monitored hourly.

Safety and handling: Store at room temperature until reconstituted and then use immediately.

Contraindications: Normoglycaemia.

Adverse reactions: Vomiting is the main adverse reaction reported in humans. Anaphylaxis may occur but is rare. Experience with dogs is too limited to provide clear guidance.

Drug interactions: No information available.

DOSES

Dogs, Cats: 50 ng (nanograms)/kg i.v., i.m. once followed by infusion of 10–15 ng/kg/min i.v., i.m.; may increase up to 40 ng/kg/min i.v., i.m. depending on blood glucose measurements.

References

Datte K, Guillaumin J, Barrett S *et al.* (2016) Retrospective evaluation of the use of glucagon infusion as adjunctive therapy for hypoglycemia in dogs: 9 cases (2005–2014). *Journal of Veterinary Emergency and Critical Care (San Antonio)* **26**, 775–781

Glucose (Dextrose)

(Aqupharm [c,d], Vetivex [c,d], 50% Glucose for injection*)
POM-V, POM-VPS, POM

Formulations: Injectable: 0.9% w/v sodium chloride + 5.5% w/v glucose monohydrate (Aqupharm No. 3 and Vetivex 3); 0.18% w/v sodium chloride + 4.4% w/v glucose monohydrate (Aqupharm No. 18 and Vetivex 6); other electrolyte solutions with glucose for i.v. use: glucose 40% and 50% w/v.

Action: Source of energy for cellular metabolism. Osmotic agent.

Use:
- Dilute glucose solutions are used for fluid replacement (primarily where intracellular and interstitial losses have occurred).
- Concentrated glucose solutions are used parenterally as an energy source or in the treatment of hypoglycaemia.

Patients requiring parenteral nutritional support will require mixtures comprising combinations of amino acids, glucose solutions and fat. Solutions containing >5% glucose are hypertonic and irritant if administered other than i.v. 50% solutions contain 1.7 kcal/ml (8.4 kJ/ml) glucose and are extremely hypertonic (2525 mOsm/l). Use with caution in patients with insulin resistance and diabetes mellitus.

Safety and handling: Multi-use vials of 5% glucose or higher rapidly support bacterial growth and strict aseptic technique is required; single patient use is advised.

Contraindications: No information available.

Adverse reactions: 10–50% solutions are irritant and hyperosmolar; administer through a jugular catheter or dilute appropriately. Glucose infusions may produce severe hypophosphataemia in some patients with prolonged starvation. If glucose loading produces signs of hyperglycaemia, insulin may be added to correct it. See comments under Amino acid solutions for use in parenteral nutrition solutions.

Drug interactions: No information available.

DOSES

Dogs:
- **Fluid therapy:** fluid requirements depend upon the degree of dehydration and ongoing losses. **See Parenteral fluids table in Appendix.**
- **Parenteral nutrition:** the amount required will be governed by the animal's physiological status, the parenteral nutrition admixture and its ability to tolerate high blood glucose levels. Generally, glucose is used to supply 40–60% of the energy requirement. Seek specialist advice before giving parenteral nutrition. **See Amino acid solutions**.
- **Hypoglycaemia:** 1–5 ml 50% dextrose i.v. slowly over 10 min. (**NB:** 1 ml/kg/h of 50% glucose is needed to meet minimum needs for maintenance.)

Cats: Doses as for dogs for fluid therapy and hypoglycaemia. Specific advice regarding nutrient admixtures and the use of concentrated glucose solutions for provision of energy in cats requiring nutritional support should be sought.

Glyceryl trinitrate (Nitroglycerin(e))

(Deponit*, Glyceryl trinitrate*, Glytrin*, Minitran*, Nitrocine*, Nitronal*, Percutol*, Transderm-Nitro*) **POM**

Formulations: Topical: 2% ointment to be applied to skin (Percutol) equating to dose of up to 800 µg (micrograms)/kg/h per inch; 5 mg/24h, 10 mg/24h, 15 mg/24h transdermal patches (Deponit, Minitran, Nitro-Dur, Transderm-Nitro). **Oral:** 300 µg, 500 µg sublingual tablets (Glyceryl trinitrate). **Injectable:** 1 mg/ml solutions (Nitrocine, Nitronal).

Action: Systemic vasodilator. Although a potent coronary vasodilator, its major benefit in small animals follows from a reduction in venous return as a consequence of venodilation. A decrease in venous return reduces left ventricular filling pressures.

Use:
- Short-term management of cardiogenic oedema (particularly acute pulmonary oedema) in animals with congestive heart failure.

It is normally only used for 1–2 days. Its efficacy is debatable. Rotate application sites; suggested sites include the thorax, groin and inside the ears. Rub ointment well into the skin.

Safety and handling: Owners should be cautioned to avoid contact with areas where the ointment has been applied and to wear non-permeable gloves when applying.

Contraindications: Hypotension, hypovolaemia, cerebral haemorrhage, head trauma.

Adverse reactions: Hypotension (reduce dose), tachycardia and a rash at the site of application. Tachyphylaxis can occur. Headaches are common in humans and may be an adverse effect in animals.

Drug interactions: Concurrent use of ACE inhibitors, anaesthetics, beta-blockers, calcium-channel blockers, corticosteroids and diuretics may enhance the hypotensive effect. NSAIDs may antagonize its hypotensive effects.

DOSES

Dogs: 6–50 mm (¼–2 inch) Percutol applied topically to the skin q6–8h; extrapolate dose to transdermal patches when Percutol not available. Closely monitor clinical signs and blood pressure. Where it is used chronically for the management of heart failure (e.g. nocturnal dyspnoea), use q24h to avoid tolerance.
- **Anecdotal use of patches has been reported:** dogs <5 kg: 1 x 5 mg/24h patch q24h; small/medium dogs: 1 x 10 mg/24h patch q24h; large/giant dogs: 2 x 10 mg/24h patch q24h.

Cats: 3–6 mm (¼ inch) topically to the skin q6–8h; extrapolate dose to transdermal patches when Percutol not available. Closely monitor clinical signs and blood pressure.
- **Anecdotal use of patches:** cats 1 x 5 mg/24h patch q24h.

References

Ferasin L, Sturgess CP, Cannon MJ *et al.* (2003) Feline idiopathic cardiomyopathy: a retrospective study of 106 cats (1994–2001). *Journal of Feline Medicine and Surgery* **5**, 151–159

Glycopyrronium (Glycopyrrolate)
(Robinul*) **POM**

Formulations: Injectable: 200 µg (micrograms)/ml solution.

Action: Blocks the action of acetylcholine at muscarinic receptors at the terminal ends of the parasympathetic nervous system, reversing parasympathetic effects. Its quaternary structure prevents it from crossing the blood–brain barrier and so it is devoid of central effects.

Use:
- Potent antisialagogue agent and has been used preoperatively to decrease oral and bronchial secretions.
- It is also used to inhibit vagal efferent activity and manage bradycardias caused by the administration of potent opioid drugs.
- Glycopyrronium is used with long-acting anticholinesterase drugs (e.g. neostigmine, pyridostigmine) during antagonism of neuromuscular block.

Glycopyrronium is longer acting than atropine. Routine administration of glycopyrronium prior to anaesthesia as part of premedication is no longer recommended. It causes a reduction in oral and bronchial secretions by decreasing the water content, therefore, secretions become more sticky. Administration of potent opioids in the perioperative period can promote bradyarrhythmias but it is better to monitor heart rate and give glycopyrronium to manage a low heart rate if necessary. Administration of very low doses of glycopyrronium i.v. can cause exacerbation of bradyarrhythmias due to a vagal stimulatory effect; giving another dose i.v. will usually cause an increase in heart rate. Glycopyrronium is devoid of central effects and therefore does not cause mydriasis

Safety and handling: Normal precautions should be observed.

Contraindications: No information available.

Adverse reactions: Tachycardias following overdose of glycopyrronium are usually transient and do not require management. Ventricular arrhythmias may be treated with lidocaine if severe. The incidence of adverse effects is lower than that seen with atropine.

Drug interactions: When mixed with alkaline drugs (e.g. barbiturates), a precipitate may form. Antimuscarinics may enhance the actions of sympathomimetics and thiazide diuretics. The following may enhance the activity of glycopyrronium: antihistamines, quinidine, pethidine, benzodiazepines and phenothiazines. Combining glycopyrronium and alpha-2 adrenergic agonists is not recommended.

DOSES
Dogs, Cats:
- **Management of vagally mediated bradyarrhythmias:** 2–10 µg (micrograms)/kg i.v., i.m.
- **Neuromuscular blockade antagonism:** glycopyrronium (10 µg/kg i.v. once) with neostigmine (50 µg/kg i.v. once).

References
Jang M, Son WG and Lee I (2015) Fentanyl-induced asystole in two dogs. *Journal of Small Animal Practice* **56**, 411–413

Sinclair MD, O'Grady MR, Kerr CL and McDonnell WN (2003) The echocardiographic effects of romifidine in dogs with and without prior or concurrent administration of glycopyrrolate. *Veterinary Anaesthesia and Analgesia* **30**, 211–219

Grapiprant

(Galliprant [d]) **POM-V**

Formulations: Oral: 20 mg, 60 mg, 100 mg tablets.

Action: Grapiprant is a piprant NSAID. It is a specific EP4 receptor antagonist; this receptor normally binds PGE2 to produce pain and inflammation associated with osteoarthritis.

Use:
- Management of mild to moderate pain caused by osteoarthritis in dogs >9 months of age.

Safety and handling: Wash hands after handling the product.

Contraindications: Mild decreases in serum albumin and total protein, most often within the reference range, have been observed in dogs treated with grapiprant but were not associated with any clinically significant observations or events. Use with caution in dogs suffering from pre-existing liver, cardiovascular or renal dysfunction or from GI disease. The EP4 receptor is involved in ulcer healing in the GI tract and is abundant in cardiac tissue, the clinical significance of this is unknown. The safety of the veterinary medicinal product has not been established in dogs <9 months of age and in dogs weighing <3.6 kg. It is not authorized for use in cats.

Adverse reactions: In clinical studies, the following mild and generally transient adverse reactions were observed: vomiting, soft-formed faeces, diarrhoea and inappetence. In very rare cases, haematemesis or haemorrhagic diarrhoea was reported following clinical use post authorization in the USA.

Drug interactions: The concurrent use of grapiprant with other anti-inflammatory agents such as NSAIDs and steroids has not been studied and should be avoided.

DOSES

Dogs: 2 mg/kg once daily. Administer on an empty stomach (one hour before the next meal).

Cats: Not authorized for use in cats.

References

Kirkby Shaw K, Rausch-Derra LC and Rhodes L (2015) Grapiprant: an EP4 prostaglandin receptor antagonist and novel therapy for pain and inflammation. *Veterinary Medicine and Science* **2**, 3–9

Rausch-Derra L, Huebner M, Wofford J and Rhodes L (2016) A prospective, randomized, masked, placebo-controlled multisite clinical study of grapiprant, an EP4 prostaglandin receptor antagonist (PRA), in dogs with osteoarthritis. *Journal of Veterinary Internal Medicine* **30**, 756–763

GS-441524   CIL

Formulations: Oral: 50 mg palatable breakable tablets. **VSP**

Action: Nucleoside analogue that terminates the RNA chain of the viral RNA-dependent RNA polymerase. It acts as an alternative substrate for viral RNA synthesis, resulting in RNA chain termination during viral RNA transcription.

Use:
- Used in cases of confirmed or strongly suspected feline infectious peritonitis.

Safety and handling: Normal precautions should be observed. Store at room temperature.

Contraindications: Use with care in animals with significant renal or hepatic disease.

Adverse reactions: Raised renal parameters (e.g. symmetric dimethyl-arginine) have been reported as have raised liver enzyme activities (e.g. alanine aminotransferase). Effusions, especially pleural effusion, can worsen for 1–2 days. Neurological signs may appear or worsen during the first few days of treatment. There may be a transient increase in serum globulins but this should resolve before 6 weeks of treatment.

Drug interactions: There are no known drug interactions.

DOSES

Dogs: Not applicable.

Cats: Minimum doses:
- **Effusive (wet) FIP without ocular or neurological signs:** 10–12 mg/kg p.o. q24h.
- **Dry FIP with ocular signs:** 15 mg/kg p.o. q24h.
- **Dry FIP with neurological signs:** 10 mg/kg p.o. q12h. Some protocols also involve remdesivir.
- Recommended total treatment duration of 84 days.

References
Taylor S and Barker E (2021) FIP: *Hope on the horizon for cats with FIP.* Vet Times, last reviewed February 2022

Heparin (low molecular weight) (Dalteparin, Enoxaparin)

(Clexane (enoxaparin)*, Fragmin (dalteparin)*) **POM**

Formulations: Injectable: 2500 IU/ml, 100,000 IU/ml ampoules (Dalteparin); 25,000 IU/ml multidose vial plus various pre-filled syringes at concentrations of 12,500 IU/ml and 25,000 IU/ml (Dalteparin); pre-filled syringes of 100 mg/ml (Enoxaparin). 100 mg Enoxaparin is equivalent to 10,000 IU of anti-Factor Xa activity.

Action: Low molecular weight heparin (LMWH) is an anticoagulant that inhibits Factor Xa and thrombin. When compared with unfractionated heparin (UFH), LMWH has reduced anti-IIa activity relative to anti-Xa activity (ratio of anti-Xa to anti-IIa is 2–4:1 compared with UFH 1:1). Thus, at therapeutic doses LMWH has minimal effect on activated partial thromboplastin time (aPTT). Therapeutic monitoring of LMWH is by anti-Xa activity (but this may not be practical or necessary given its more reliable and consistent pharmacokinetics).

Use:
- Treatment of thromboembolic complications and hypercoagulable syndromes (e.g. pulmonary thromboembolism, immune-mediated haemolytic anaemia (IMHA)).
- LMWH is also used in the treatment of myocardial infarction, atrial fibrillation, deep vein thrombosis and pulmonary thromboembolism in humans.
- Its use in disseminated intravascular coagulation (DIC) is controversial as no beneficial effect has been shown in controlled clinical trials in humans. LMWH is no longer used to try to prevent DIC.

Heparins are only effective if sufficient AT III is present. Heparin therapy is only one aspect of the management of DIC: addressing the precipitating cause, administration of fluids, fresh whole blood, aspirin and diligent monitoring of coagulation tests (aPTT, PT), fibrin degradation products and fibrinogen are all important factors. The doses of heparin are controversial, with some texts recommending lower or higher doses, the use of CRI, or preincubation with plasma. The aim of therapy is to achieve anti-Factor Xa activity of 0.35–0.7 IU/ml (although in many cases this may not be practical to measure). This therapeutic target is extrapolated from humans but no data are available to determine if this decreases risk for thromboembolic complications in dogs or cats. Cats appear to require higher dosages of LMWH to achieve proposed therapeutic targets. LMWH has better pharmacokinetic properties than UFH and its actions are more predictable in humans. It is considerably more expensive than UFH.

Safety and handling: Normal precautions should be observed.

Contraindications: Bleeding disorders or severe renal dysfunction.

Adverse reactions: If an overdosage occurs, protamine can be used as an antidote. Heparin should not be administered i.m. as it may result in haematoma formation. Its use in DIC may worsen haemorrhage, especially if the patient is thrombocytopenic. Heparin-induced thrombocytopenia syndrome is a serious concern in human patients but has not been reported in dogs or cats.

Drug interactions: Use with caution with other drugs that can cause changes in coagulation status (e.g. aspirin, NSAIDs). Heparin may antagonize ACTH, corticosteroids or insulin. Heparin may increase plasma levels of diazepam. The actions of heparin may be partially counteracted by antihistamines, digoxin and tetracyclines. Do not mix other drugs in the same syringe as heparin.

DOSES

Dogs:
- 100–175 IU/kg s.c. q8h (Dalteparin).
- 0.8 mg/kg s.c. q6h (Enoxaparin).
- Anticoagulation: 80–150 IU/kg s.c. q4–8h.

Cats:
- 75 IU/kg s.c. q6h (Dalteparin).
- 0.75–1 mg/kg s.c. q6–12h (Enoxaparin).
- Anticoagulation: 80–150 IU/kg s.c. q4–8h.

References

Blais MC, Bianco D, Goggs R *et al.* (2019) Consensus on the Rational Use of Antithrombics in Veterinary Critical Care (CURATIVE): Domain 3 – Defining antithrombotic protocols. *Journal of Veterinary Emergency and Critical Care* **29**, 60 – 74

Sharp CR, deLaforcade AM, Koenigshof AM *et al.* (2019) Consensus on the Rational Use of Antithrombics in Veterinary Critical Care (CURATIVE): Domain 4 – Refining and monitoring antithrombotic therapies. *Journal of Veterinary Emergency and Critical Care* **29**, 75 – 87

Heparin (unfractionated) (UFH)
(Heparin*, Hepsal*) **POM**

Formulations: Injectable: 1,000–25,000 IU/ml solutions; 10 IU/ml, 100 IU/ml in saline.

Action: Heparin is an anticoagulant that exerts its effects primarily by enhancing the binding of antithrombin III (AT III) to factors IIa, IXa, Xa, XIa and XIIa; it is only effective if adequate AT III is present. The AT III/clotting factor complex is subsequently removed by the liver. Heparin inactivates thrombin and blocks the conversion of fibrinogen to fibrin. The inhibition of Factor XII activation prevents the formation of stable fibrin clots. Heparin does not significantly change the concentrations of clotting factors, nor does it lyse pre-existing clots.

Use:
- Management of hypercoagulable conditions with associated increased risk of thromboembolic events (e.g. immune-mediated haemolytic anaemic, cardiomyopathy in cats, protein-losing nephropathy).

Therapy must be carefully monitored as the activity of UFH is somewhat less predictable than low molecular weight heparin (LMWH), ideally via Anti-Xa activity (which may not be practical).

Safety and handling: Normal precautions should be observed.

Contraindications: Major bleeding disorders, increased risk of haemorrhage, thrombocytopenia.

Adverse reactions: If an overdosage occurs, protamine can be used as an antidote. Heparin should not be administered i.m. as it may result in haematoma formation. Its use in disseminated intravascular coagulation may worsen haemorrhage, especially if the patient is thrombocytopenic. Heparin-induced thrombocytopenia syndrome is a serious concern in human patients but has not been reported in dogs or cats.

Drug interactions: Use with caution with other drugs that can cause changes in coagulation status (e.g. aspirin, NSAIDs). Heparin may antagonize ACTH, corticosteroids and insulin. Heparin may increase plasma levels of diazepam. The actions of heparin may be partially counteracted by antihistamines, digoxin and tetracyclines. Do not mix other drugs in the same syringe as heparin.

DOSES

Dogs: Anticoagulation: 150–300 IU/kg s.c. q6h; adjust dosage so that the aPTT is 1.5–2.0 times normal or anti-Factor Xa activity is between 0.35 and 0.7 IU/ml (see LMWH for more information); 100 IU/kg bolus i.v. then 480–900 IU/kg q24h (20–37.5 IU/kg/h) by CRI.
Cats: Anticoagulation: 250–300 IU/kg s.c. q8h.

References

Blais MC, Bianco D, Goggs R *et al.* (2019) Consensus on the Rational Use of Antithrombics in Veterinary Critical Care (CURATIVE): Domain 3–Defining antithrombotic protocols. *Journal of Veterinary Emergency and Critical Care* **29**, 60–74

Diquelou A, Barbaste C, Gabaig AM *et al.* (2005) Pharmacokinetics and pharmaco-dynamics of a therapeutic dose of unfractionated heparin (200 U/kg) administered subcutaneously or intravenously to dogs. *Veterinary Clinical Pathology* **34**, 237–242

Helmond SE, Polzin DJ, Armstrong PJ *et al.* (2010) Treatment of immune-mediated hemolytic anemia with individually adjusted heparin dosing in dogs. *Journal of Veterinary Internal Medicine* **24**, 597–605

Human chorionic gonadotrophin see Chorionic gonadotrophin

Hyaluronate

(An-HyPro, ClinaDry, Remend Corneal Lubricant, Remend Corneal Repair Gel, Hyabak*, Hylo-Forte*, Hylo-Tear*, Vismed Multi*) **P**

Formulations: Ophthalmic: 0.1%, 0.15%, 0.2%, 0.4% solution in 10 ml bottle; 0.4% and 0.75% Hyasent-S (modified, cross-linked hyaluronic acid) in Remend products.

Action: Viscoelastic fluid with mucomimetic properties; increases corneal epithelial migration. Sodium hyaluronate is also available in different formulations as a viscoelastic for intraocular surgery.

Use:
• Used as a tear replacement.
• Management of quantitative (keratoconjunctivitis sicca) and qualitative tear film disorders.

It has longer corneal contact time than the aqueous tear substitutes.

Safety and handling: Normal precautions should be observed.

Contraindications: No information available.

Adverse reactions: It is tolerated well and ocular irritation is unusual.

Drug interactions: No information available.

DOSES

Dogs, Cats: 1 drop per eye q4–6h, although it can be used hourly if required.

Hydralazine

(Hydralazine*) **POM**

Formulations: Oral: 25 mg, 50 mg tablets.

Action: Hydralazine acts chiefly on arteriolar smooth muscle causing vasodilation; it is able to decrease systemic vascular resistance to about 50% of the baseline value. The effects of hydralazine are to reduce afterload and increase heart rate, stroke volume and cardiac output.

Use:
- Afterload reducer as adjunctive therapy of congestive heart failure in dogs secondary to severe or refractory mitral value insufficiency.
- It can be used to treat systemic hypertension (not typically as a first-line drug).

Hospitalization with frequent monitoring of blood pressure is advised during its use. As hydralazine may cause sodium and water retention, concomitant use of diuretic therapy is often necessary. Give with food if possible.

Safety and handling: Normal precautions should be observed.

Contraindications: Hypovolaemia, hypotension, renal impairment or cerebral bleeding.

Adverse reactions: Reflex tachycardia, severe hypotension (monitor and adjust doses as necessary), anorexia and vomiting (the latter two effects are commonly seen in cats).

Drug interactions: The hypotensive effects of hydralazine may be enhanced by ACE inhibitors (e.g. enalapril, benazepril), anaesthetics, beta-blockers (e.g. propranolol), calcium-channel blockers (e.g. diltiazem, verapamil), corticosteroids, diuretics and NSAIDs. Sympathomimetics (e.g. phenylpropanolamine) may cause tachycardia. The pressor response to adrenaline may be reduced

DOSES

Dogs: 0.5–3 mg/kg p.o. q8–12h. Start at low dose (0.5–1 mg/kg q12h), monitor blood pressure regularly and increase to 2–3 mg/kg q12h if necessary.

Cats: 2.5–10 mg/cat p.o. q12h. Start at low dose and titrate upwards cautiously as above if necessary.

References

Häggström J, Hansson K, Karlberg BE *et al.* (1996) Effects of long-term treatment with enalapril or hydralazine on the renin-angiotensin-aldosterone system and fluid balance in dogs with naturally acquired mitral valve regurgitation. *American Journal of Veterinary Research* **57**, 1645–1652

Hydrochlorothiazide `CIL`

(Co-amilozide*, Moduret*, Moduretic*) **POM**

Formulations: Oral: 25 mg hydrochlorothiazide + 2.5 mg amiloride, 50 mg hydrochlorothiazide + 5 mg amiloride tablets.

Action: Thiazide diuretic that inhibits reabsorption of sodium and chloride in the distal convoluted tubule by blocking the sodium/chloride symporter, resulting in sodium, chloride and water loss in the urine. It also causes excretion of potassium, magnesium and bicarbonate. It is formulated with a potassium-sparing diuretic (amiloride). Part of the diuretics used in 'sequential nephron blockade'.

Use:
- Additional therapy for CHF when the clinical signs have become refractory to furosemide/torasemide. However, loop-diuretic therapy should still be continued when using hydrochlorthiazide to gain the beneficial effect of sequential nephron blockade.
- It may also be used in the prevention of calcium oxalate urolithiasis.
- Thiazides have antihypertensive effects, although the exact mechanism is unclear.

Safety and handling: Normal precautions should be observed.

Contraindications: Renal impairment, as it tends to reduce glomerular filtration rate. Electrolyte disturbances. Hydrochlorothiazide is a potent diuretic which can lead to loss of Na, K and Cl.

Adverse reactions: Hyperglycaemia, hypokalaemia, hyponatraemia, hypochloraemia and volume contraction. It enhances the effects of the renin–angiotensin–aldosterone system in heart failure.

Drug interactions: Increased possibility of hypokalaemia developing if thiazides are used concomitantly with corticosteroids or loop diuretics (furosemide). Thiazide-induced hypokalaemia may increase the risk of digoxin toxicity. Thus, concomitant use of potassium-sparing diuretics (e.g. spironolactone) or potassium supplementation may be necessary during prolonged administration. The concurrent administration of vitamin D or calcium salts with thiazides may exacerbate hypercalcaemia.

DOSES
Dogs: 0.5–4 mg/kg p.o. q12–24h. Start at low dose and titrate upwards every 5–10 days, to effect. Monitor urea, creatinine, electrolytes and blood pressure before increasing dose.
Cats: 1–2 mg/kg p.o. q12–24h. Start at low dose and titrate upwards cautiously as above.

References
Atkins CE and Häggström J (2012) Pharmacologic management of myxomatous mitral valve disease in dogs. *Journal of Veterinary Cardiology* **14**, 165–184

Hydrocortisone
(Efcortesol*, Solu-cortef*) **POM**

Formulations: Topical: 0.5%, 1% creams; 1% solution; cutaneous spray (Cortavance). **Injectable:** 25 mg/ml solution; 100 mg, 500 mg powders for reconstitution (Solu-cortef). **Oral:** 10 mg, 20 mg tablets.

Action: Alters the transcription of DNA, leading to alterations in cellular metabolism. It has both glucocorticoid and mineralocorticoid activity.

Use:
- Topical anti-inflammatory for treatment of inflammatory and pruritic dermatoses in dogs (e.g. atopic dermatitis).
- Early management of acute hypoadrenocorticism.
- Treatment of critical illness-related corticosteroid insufficiency (CIRCI) has been described in dogs and cats with fluid-loaded, vasopressor-resistant septic shock, but a dose has not been established.

Hydrocortisone has only a quarter of the glucocorticoid potency of prednisolone and one thirtieth that of dexamethasone. On a dose basis,

4 mg hydrocortisone is equivalent to 1 mg prednisolone. Animals receiving chronic therapy should be tapered off steroids when discontinuing the drug (even following topical administration). The use of steroids in most cases of shock or spinal cord injury is of no benefit and may be detrimental.

Safety and handling: Wear gloves when applying topically as the cream is absorbed through skin.

Contraindications: Do not use in pregnant animals. Systemic corticosteroids are generally contraindicated in patients with renal disease and diabetes mellitus.

Adverse reactions: Excessively rapid correction of hyponatraemia in cases of acute hypoadrenocorticism may cause brain damage and so, in severely hyponatraemic animals, initial doses should be reduced by 50% or postponed until the rate of correction using saline has been established. Delay starting treatment until post-stimulation cortisol collected as hydrocortisone will interfere with the assay. Catabolic effects of glucocorticoids lead to weight loss and cutaneous atrophy. Iatrogenic hypercortisolism may develop (PU/PD, elevated liver enzymes). Vomiting and diarrhoea, or GI ulceration may develop. Glucocorticoids may increase urine glucose levels and decrease serum T3 and T4 values. Prolonged use of glucocorticoids suppresses the hypothalamic–pituitary–adrenal axis and causes adrenal atrophy. Impaired wound healing and delayed recovery from infections may be seen.

Drug interactions: Increased risk of GI ulceration if used concurrently with NSAIDs. Glucocorticoids antagonize the effect of insulin. Antiepileptic drugs (phenobarbital) may accelerate the metabolism of corticosteroids and antifungals (e.g. itraconazole) may decrease it. There is an increased risk of hypokalaemia when corticosteroids are used with acetazolamide, amphotericin and potassium-depleting diuretics (furosemide, thiazides).

DOSES

Dogs:
- **Topically:** apply spray or a thin layer of cream to affected area q6–12h.
- **Hypoadrenocorticism:** 0.5 mg/kg/h i.v. by CRI in acute Addisonian crisis and 0.125 mg/kg p.o. q12h for maintenance.
- **Anti-inflammatory:** 0.5 mg/kg p.o. q12h.

Cats: Topical use as for dogs. Its use in feline hypoadrenocorticism has not been documented.

References

Creedon JMB (2014) Controversies surrounding critical illness-related corticosteroid insufficiency in animals. *Journal of Veterinary Emergency and Critical Care* **25**, 107–112

Gunn E, Shiel RE and Mooney CT (2016) Hydrocortisone in the management of acute hypoadrenocorticism in dogs: a retrospective series of 30 cases. *Journal of Small Animal Practice* **57**, 227–233

Summers AM, Culler C, Yaxley PE and Guillaumin J (2021) Retrospective evaluation of the use of hydrocortisone for treatment of suspected critical illness-related corticosteroid insufficiency (CIRCI) in dogs with septic shock (2010–2017): 47 cases. *Journal of Veterinary Emergency and Critical Care* **31**, 371–379

Hydrocortisone aceponate

(Cortavance ^d, Easotic ^d, Hydrocortisone aceponate Ecuphar ^d) **POM-V**

Formulations: Topical: 76 ml spray (0.584 mg/ml) (Cortavance); suspension for ears: 1.11 mg/ml hydrocortisone aceponate + 15.1 mg/ml miconazole + 1505 IU/ml gentamicin (Easotic).

Action: Hydrocortisone aceponate is a pro-drug that is biotransformed in the epidermis to its active form, hydrocortisone 17-propionate.

Use:
- Treatment of inflammatory and pruritic dermatoses including acute otitis externa and acute exacerbations of recurrent otitis externa associated with bacteria and *Malassezia*.

Minimizes systemic side effects (such as increases in liver enzyme activities, depression of cortisol response to ACTH stimulation). Microbial infections should be treated appropriately prior to use. Patients should be monitored appropriately during long-term use. Use with caution in dogs <7 months old as glucocorticoids are known to slow growth. Total body surface treated should not exceed a surface corresponding to a treatment of two flanks from the spine to the mammary chains including the shoulders and the thighs.

Safety and handling: Normal precautions should be observed.

Contraindications: Do not use on ulcerated skin (Cortavance). Do not use if the ear drum is perforated (Easotic).

Adverse reactions: Protracted use of any topical glucocorticoid can result in epidermal atrophy. The otic preparation may result in aural erythema and rarely transient hearing loss in geriatric dogs.

Drug interactions: No information available.

DOSES

Dogs: Cortavance: 2 pumps of spray per 10 cm × 10 cm square of skin for 7 days. This delivers 1.52 µg (micrograms) of hydrocortisone aceponate per cm^2. **Easotic:** 1 pump (1 ml) per ear q24h for 5 days.
Cats: Dose not established.

References
Bonneau S, Skowronski V and Maynard L (2006) Efficacy of a 0.0584% hydrocortisone aceponate spray in the treatment of pruritic inflammatory skin disease in dogs. *Veterinary Dermatology* **17**, 354–355

Hydroxycarbamide (Hydroxyurea) `CIL`

(Hydrea*) **POM**

Formulations: Oral: 100 mg and 1 g tablets; 300 mg and 500 mg capsules.

Action: Inhibits ribonucleotide reductase, which converts ribonucleotides to deoxyribonucleotides (important precursors for DNA synthesis and repair). It acts primarily in the S-phase, but may also arrest cells at the G1-S border.

Use:
- Treatment of polycythaemia vera, chronic myeloid leukaemia (CML) and chronic granulocytic leukaemia.

- Treatment of mast cell tumours and part of adjunctive treatment of canine meningiomas.

Once in remission, reduce dosage frequency as required. Perform haematology initially weekly for 1 month, then every 2 weeks for 1 month, then monthly if tolerated. Haematology must be monitored weekly at the start of drug therapy in cats, as they are at greater risk of myelosuppression compared with dogs. Use with caution in patients with renal dysfunction; dose reduction may be required.

Safety and handling: Cytotoxic drug; see Appendix and specialist texts for further advice on chemotherapeutic agents.

Contraindications: Patients with bone marrow suppression. Use with caution in patients with a history of urate stones, renal disease/dysfunction and those that have received previous chemotherapy and/or radiotherapy.

Adverse reactions: Myelosuppression, GI signs (nausea, vomiting, diarrhoea, anorexia), dysuria and skin reactions (stomatitis, sloughing of nails, alopecia). Myelosuppression is dose-limiting; monitor haematological parameters at regular intervals. In cats given very high doses (>500 mg), methaemoglobinaemia is reported. Normal doses are associated with increased diastolic blood pressure and heart rate but decreased systolic blood pressure, QT and PR intervals, maximum left ventricular systolic and end-diastolic pressures.

Drug interactions: No information available but advisable not to use with other myelosuppressive agents.

DOSES
See Appendix for chemotherapy protocols and conversion of bodyweight to body surface area.
Dogs:
- CML: 50 mg/kg p.o. q24h for 1–2 weeks then q48h.
- Polycythaemia vera or CML: 50–80 mg/kg p.o. q3d or 1 g/m^2 p.o. q24h until haematology is normal.
- Mast cell tumours: 60 mg/kg p.o. q24h for 14 days; then 30 mg/kg p.o. q24h.
- Meningioma: 20 mg/kg p.o. q24h or 50 mg/kg p.o. 3 times a week.

Cats: 10 mg/kg q12–24h until remission; then taper to lowest effective frequency by monitoring haematocrit; or 25 mg/kg p.o. 3 times a week.
- Meningioma: 20 mg/kg p.o. q24h.

References
Evans LM and Caylor KB (1995) Polycythemia vera in a cat and management with hydroxyurea. *Journal of the American Animal Hospital Association* **31**, 434–438
Rassnick KM, Al-Sarraf R, Bailey DB *et al.* (2010) Phase II open-label study of single-agent hydroxyurea for treatment of mast cell tumours in dogs. *Veterinary and Comparative Oncology* **8**, 103–111

Hydroxyurea see Hydroxycarbamide

Hydroxyzine `CIL`
(Atarax*, Ucerax*) **POM**

Formulations: Oral: 10 mg, 25 mg tablets; 2 mg/ml syrup.

Action: Binds to H1 histamine receptors, preventing histamine from binding. Hydroxyzine is metabolized to cetirizine.

Use:
- Management of allergic disease in dogs and cats, although specific doses have not been determined by pharmacokinetic studies.

Use with caution in cases with urinary retention, angle closure glaucoma and pyloroduodenal obstruction. Has been reported to result in QT interval prolongation in humans.

Safety and handling: Normal precautions should be observed.

Contraindications: No information available.

Adverse reactions: May cause mild sedation. May reduce seizure threshold.

Drug interactions: No information available.

DOSES
Dogs, Cats: 2.0–2.2 mg/kg q8–12h.

References
Bizikova P, Papich MG and Olivry T (2008) Hydroxyzine and cetirizine pharmacokinetics and pharmacodynamics after oral and intravenous administration of hydroxyzine to healthy dogs. *Veterinary Dermatology* **19**, 348–357

Hyoscine see Butylscopolamine

Hypromellose
(Hypromellose*, Isopto Plain*) **P**

Formulations: Ophthalmic: 0.3%, 0.5% solutions in 10 ml dropper bottle; 0.32% (single-use vial). Large variety of other formulations also available.

Action: Cellulose based, aqueous tear substitute to replace aqueous component of trilaminar tear film (lacrimomimetic).

Use:
- Lubrication of dry eyes.
- In cases of keratoconjunctivitis sicca, it will improve ocular surface lubrication, tear retention and patient comfort while lacrostimulation therapy (e.g. topical ciclosporin) is initiated.
- It may also be used as a vehicle base for compounding ophthalmic drugs.

Compliance may be poor if used more frequently than q4h: consider using a longer acting tear replacement.

Safety and handling: Normal precautions should be observed.

Contraindications: No information available.

Adverse reactions: No information available.

Drug interactions: No information available.

DOSES
Dogs, Cats: 1 drop per eye q8h (or more frequently if needed).

References
Grahn GH and Storey ES (2004) Lacrimostimulants and lacrimomimetics. *Veterinary Clinics of North America: Small Animal Practice* **34**, 739–753

Imepitoin

(Pexion^d) **POM-V**

Formulations: Oral: 100 mg, 400 mg tablets.

Action: Imepitoin inhibits seizures via potentiation of the $GABA_A$ receptor-mediated inhibitory effects on the neurons. Imepitoin also has a weak calcium-channel blocking effect, which may contribute to its anticonvulsive properties.

Use:

- Imepitoin and phenobarbital are the initial medications of choice for the management of epileptic seizures due to idiopathic epilepsy in dogs. The choice of initial medication is guided by patient requirements: imepitoin has a more rapid onset of action than phenobarbital (a steady state does not need to be achieved), does not require the determination of serum concentrations and has a less severe adverse effect profile; however, phenobarbital is less expensive and more efficacious. Imepitoin is well tolerated in healthy cats at similar doses to dogs but its efficacy to control seizures is yet to be proven in cats.
- Imepitoin is authorized for the reduction of anxiety and fear associated with noise phobia in dogs. It may also be used in combination with a behaviour modification plan for the treatment of anxiety in dogs in relation to both social stimuli (e.g. crowds, strangers) and non-social stimuli (e.g. noises, novel items, new environments), once any role of pain has been controlled. Should be used with caution in dogs displaying aggressive behaviour and associated risks should be managed. It may be used alongside serotonergic agents to enhance anxiolysis.

Safety and handling: Normal precautions should be observed.

Contraindications: Severely impaired liver, kidney and heart function.

Adverse reactions: The most frequent adverse effect reported is sedation, particularly in dogs receiving higher doses or concurrent phenobarbital therapy. A cutaneous adverse reaction has been reported. Other adverse effects are generally mild and transient and include polyphagia, hyperactivity, polyuria, polydipsia, somnolence, hypersaliva-tion, emesis, ataxia, apathy, diarrhoea, prolapsed nictitating membrane, decreased sight and a paradoxical increase in sensitivity to sound.

Drug interactions: Imepitoin has been used in combination with phenobarbital in a small number of cases and no harmful clinical interactions were reported.

DOSES

See Appendix for guidelines on responsible parasiticide use.

Dogs: 10–30 mg/kg p.o. q12h. Doses towards the higher end of the range appear to be more effective. For the control of acute anxiety, an initial dose of 30 mg/kg p.o. q12h is recommended; in more chronic cases, the dose may be titrated up from an initial dose of 10 mg/kg p.o. q12h or down to 5 mg/kg p.o. q12h as necessary, dependent on initial response.

Cats: Imepitoin is well tolerated in healthy cats at similar doses to dogs (10–30 mg/kg p.o. q12h) but its efficacy to control seizures or anxiety remains unproven.

References

Engel O, Müller HW, Klee R, Francke B and Mills DS (2019) Effectiveness of imepitoin for the control of anxiety and fear associated with noise phobia in dogs. *Journal of Veterinary Internal Medicine* **33**, 2675–2684

Gallucci A, Gagliardo T, Menchetti M *et al.* (2015) Efficacy of imepitoin as first choice drug in treatment of 53 naïve dogs affected by idiopathic epilepsy. In: Proceedings of the 28th Symposium ESVN-ECVN. *Journal of Veterinary Internal Medicine* **30**, 446

Rundfeldt C, Tipold A and Löscher W (2015) Efficacy, safety, and tolerability of imepitoin in dogs with newly diagnosed epilepsy in a randomized controlled clinical study with long-term follow up. *BMC Veterinary Research* **11**, 228

Imidacloprid

(Advantage [c,d], Advantix [d], Advocate [c,d], Moxiclear [c,d], Prinovoxc [c,d], Seresto [c,d], several other products) **POM-V, NFA-VPS**

Formulations: Topical: 100 mg/ml imidacloprid either as sole agent or with moxidectin or permethrin (e.g. Advantix, Advocate, Moxiclear, Prinovox) in spot-on pipettes of various sizes. Also used in collars impregnated with 1.25 g imidacloprid + 4.5 g flumethrin (Seresto). Numerous GSL and non-authorized formulations.

Action: Binds to post-synaptic nicotinic receptors resulting in paralysis and death of fleas and their larvae.

Use:
- Treatment and prevention of flea infestations in dogs and cats.

For the treatment of flea infestations, the additional use of an approved insect growth regulator is recommended and the product should be applied every 4 weeks to all in-contact cats and dogs. May be used in nursing bitches and queens. The combined product with flumethrin or moxidectin has additional preventative and treatment indications.

Safety and handling: Many combinations contain products that are dangerous to aquatic organism and birds. Treated dogs should not swim in surface water for 48 hours and collars should be removed before swimming.

Contraindications: Do not use in unweaned puppies and kittens <8 weeks. The flumethrin-impregnated collar is not recommended in pregnancy and lactation and should not be used in kittens <10 weeks or puppies <7 weeks. Do not use the permethrin-containing product on cats. Moxidectin/imadocloprid not for kittens <9 weeks or <1 kg, or puppies <7 weeks.

Adverse reactions: Transient pruritus and erythema may occur at the site of application. Diazepam should be administered in the event of accidental ingestion of the combined product with flumethrin. Spot-on products taste bitter, may cause salivation if ingested. Transient lethargy, agitation and inappetence may occur.

Drug interactions: No information available.

DOSES

See Appendix for guidelines on responsible parasiticide use.

Dogs: Fleas and ticks: 10 mg/kg topically every month. In dogs >40 kg, an appropriate combination of pipettes should be applied. Collars should be replaced every 8 months.

Cats: Fleas: 10–20 mg/kg topically every month. Collars should be replaced every 8 months.

References
Horak IG, Fourie JJ and Stanneck D (2012) Efficacy of slow-release collar formulations of imidacloprid/flumethrin and deltamethrin and of spot-on formulations of fipronil/(s)-methoprene, dinotefuran/pyriproxyfen/permethrin and (s)-methoprene/amitraz/fipronil against *Rhipicephalus sanguineus* and *Ctenocephalides felis felis* on dogs. *Parasites and Vectors* **5**, 79

Imidapril
(Prilium) **POM-V**

Formulations: Oral: 75 mg, 150 mg powders for reconstitution.

Action: ACE inhibitor. It inhibits conversion of angiotensin I to angiotensin II and inhibits the breakdown of bradykinin. Overall effect is a reduction in preload and afterload via venodilation and arteriodilation, decreased salt and water retention via reduced aldosterone production and inhibition of the angiotensin-aldosterone-mediated cardiac and vascular remodelling. Efferent arteriolar dilation in the kidney can reduce intraglomerular pressure and therefore glomerular filtration. This may decrease proteinuria.

Use:
- Treatment of CHF caused by mitral regurgitation or dilated cardiomyopathy in dogs. No data available on cats. Often used in conjunction with diuretics when heart failure is present as most effective when used in these cases. Can be used in combination with other drugs to treat heart failure (e.g. pimobendan, spironolactone, digoxin).
- Management of proteinuria associated with chronic renal insufficiency, glomerular disorders and protein-losing nephropathies.
- May reduce blood pressure in hypertension.

ACE inhibitors are more likely to cause or exacerbate prerenal azotaemia in hypotensive animals and those with poor renal perfusion (e.g. acute, oliguric renal failure). Use cautiously if hypotension, hyponatraemia or outflow tract obstruction are present. Regular monitoring of blood pressure, serum creatinine, urea and electrolytes is strongly recommended with ACE inhibitor treatment. The use of ACE inhibitors in cats with cardiac disease stems from extrapolation from theoretical benefits and studies showing a benefit in other species with heart failure and different cardiac diseases (mainly dogs and humans).

Safety and handling: Normal precautions should be observed.

Contraindications: Do not use in animals with acute renal failure, congenital heart disease, haemodynamically relevant stenoses (e.g. aortic stenosis), obstructive hypertrophic cardiomyopathy or hypovolaemia.

Adverse reactions: Potential adverse effects include hypotension, hyperkalaemia and azotaemia. Monitor blood pressure, serum creatinine and electrolytes when used in cases of heart failure. Dosage should be reduced if there are signs of hypotension (weakness, disorientation). Anorexia, vomiting and diarrhoea are rare. Doses of up to 5 mg/kg/day have been well tolerated in healthy dogs. Not recommended for breeding, pregnant or lactating bitches, as safety has not been established. The safety of imidapril has not been established in dogs <4 kg.

Drug interactions: Concomitant use of potassium-sparing diuretics (e.g. spironolactone) or potassium supplements could result in hyperkalaemia. However, in practice, spironolactone and ACE inhibitors appear safe to use concurrently. There may be an increased risk of nephrotoxicity and decreased clinical efficacy when used with NSAIDs. There is a risk of hypotension with concomitant administration of diuretics, vasodilators (e.g. anaesthetic agents, antihypertensive agents) or negative inotropes (e.g. beta-blockers).

DOSES
Dogs: 0.25 mg/kg p.o. q24h (for dogs weighing >4 kg).
Cats: 0.5 mg/kg p.o. q24h (anecdotal dose; no data available).

References
Amberger C, Chetboul V, Bomassi E *et al.* (2004) Comparison of the effects of imidapril and enalapril in a prospective, multicentric, randomized trial in dogs with naturally acquired heart failure. *Journal of Veterinary Cardiology* **6**, 9–16
Besche B, Chetboul V, Lachaud Lefay MP *et al.* (2007) Clinical evaluation of imidapril in congestive heart failure in dogs: results of the EFFIC study. *Journal of Small Animal Practice* **48**, 265–270

Imidocarb dipropionate
(Imizol) **POM-V**

Formulations: Injectable: 85 mg/ml imidocarb solution containing 121.15 mg/ml imidocarb dipropionate (active agent). Authorized for use in cattle.

Action: Interferes with parasite nucleic acid metabolism.

Use:
* Treatment of *Babesia canis* infection in dogs.

The safety and effectiveness of imidocarb have not been fully determined in puppies or in breeding, lactating or pregnant animals. Reduce dose with renal, hepatic or pulmonary compromise. Clinical/parasitological cure is often not achieved with smaller *Babesia* species, although one prospective study showed an imidocarb-containing multidrug protocol to have reasonable efficacy against *B. gibsoni*.

Safety and handling: Normal precautions should be observed.

Contraindications: Do not administer i.v.

Adverse reactions: Cholinergic signs (e.g. salivation, vomiting and occasionally diarrhoea, panting, restlessness) may develop after dosing. These may be alleviated by atropine. Mild injection site inflammation lasting one to several days and which may ulcerate has been reported. Anaphylactoid reactions have been reported in cattle but not in dogs.

Drug interactions: Avoid concurrent use of anticholinesterases.

DOSES
See Appendix for guidelines on responsible parasiticide use.
Dogs: 6.6 mg/kg imidocarb dipropionate i.m., s.c. once, repeated in 2–3 weeks. Dose should be calculated based on Imizol containing 121.15 mg/ml imidocarb dipropionate. Premedication with atropine (0.05 mg/kg) to minimize side effects could be considered.
Cats: 2.5 mg/kg imidocarb dipropionate i.m. once can improve clinical signs in cats infected with large babesial species. Dose should be

calculated based on Imizol containing 121.15 mg/ml imidocarb dipropionate. Alternative agents are preferable for smaller species (e.g. *Babesia felis*), however parasitological cure is rare and controlled therapeutic trials are lacking.

References
Baneth G (2018) Antiprotozoal treatment of canine babesiosis. *Veterinary Parasitology* **254**, 58–63
Lin EC, Chueh LL, Lin CN *et al.* (2012) The therapeutic efficacy of two antibabesial strategies against *Babesia gibsoni. Veterinary Parasitology* **186**, 159–164

Imipramine

(Tofranil, Imipramine*) **POM**

`CIL`

Formulations: Oral: 10 mg, 25 mg tablets.

Action: Imipramine blocks noradrenaline and serotonin reuptake in the brain, resulting in antidepressive activity.

Use:
- It has been suggested that it may be particularly useful for the control of panic disorders, but quality evidence is lacking. Suggested uses include the management of panic-related, generalized and separation anxieties, especially when these conditions are associated with urine elimination.
- It might also be used to aid control of narcolepsy, supersubmissive urination and excitatory urination, and may assist learning in anxious subjects.

Veterinary authorized products, e.g. clomipramine or imepitoin, may be preferable for initial use, although not authorized for all of these indications. It is suggested that imipramine is less sedating than amitriptyline. Use with caution in young animals.

Safety and handling: Normal precautions should be observed.

Contraindications: Glaucoma, history of seizures or urinary retention, severe liver disease, hypersensitivity to tricyclic antidepressants.

Adverse reactions: Sedation, dry mouth, diarrhoea, vomiting, excitability, arrhythmias, hypotension, syncope and increased appetite are reported in humans.

Drug interactions: Should not be used with monoamine oxidase inhibitors or drugs that are metabolized by cytochrome P450 2D6 (e.g. chlorphenamine, cimetidine). Should not generally be used alongside other serotonergic agents given risk of serotonin syndrome, although use alongside trazodone may be considered in exceptional cases, so long as patient carefully monitored for signs of serotonin syndrome.

DOSES
Dogs: 1–2 mg/kg p.o. q12h or 2–4 mg/kg p.o. q24h.
Cats: 0.5–1 mg/kg p.o. q12–24h.

Immunoglobulins

(Flebogamma*, Gammagard*, Kiovig*) **POM**

Formulations: Injectable: 2.5 g, 5 g, 10 g vials for reconstitution.

Action: Has both immediate and long-term effects; however, the exact modes of action are unclear. Binding to Fc receptors and providing anti-idiotype antibodies may explain the immediate effects. The longer term effects on immune system autoregulation may be associated with a reaction with a number of membrane receptors on T cells, B cells and monocytes, which are pertinent to autoreactivity and induction of tolerance to self.

Use:
- Treatment of some severe immune-mediated diseases in dogs.
- Efficacy has been demonstrated in immune-mediated thrombocytopenia (comparable to that achieved with vincristine) and in acute canine polyradiculoneuritis. However, use in immune-mediated haemolytic anaemia remains controversial.

Its use has not been systematically investigated for other immune-mediated diseases. Use should therefore be reserved for exceptional cases where other treatments have failed.

Safety and handling: Vials may be stored at room temperature but once reconstituted must be used immediately.

Contraindications: Avoid in patients with increased plasma protein levels.

Adverse reactions: Anaphylactic reactions are a risk but have not been recorded in dogs.

Drug interactions: None known but use with care in patients receiving drugs with strong protein-binding action and vaccines.

DOSES
See Appendix for immunosuppression protocols.

Dogs: 0.5–1.0 g/kg i.v. over 6–8 hours. Higher doses of up to 2.2 g/kg are used in some studies.

Cats: No information available.

References
Balog K, Huang AA, Sum SO et al. (2013) A prospective randomized clinical trial of vincristine versus human intravenous immunoglobulin for acute adjunctive management of presumptive primary immune-mediated thrombocytopenia in dogs. *Journal of Veterinary Internal Medicine* **27**, 536–541

Spurlock NK and Prittie JE (2011) A review of current indications, adverse effects, and administration recommendations for intravenous immunoglobulin. *Journal of Veterinary Emergency and Critical Care* **21**, 471–483

Indoxacarb

(Activyl [c,d], Activyl Tick Plus [d]) **POM-V, NFA-VPS**

Formulations: Topical: spot-on solution for dogs and cats containing 195 mg/ml in pipettes of various sizes (Activyl); spot-on solution for dogs and cats containing 150 mg/ml indoxacarb and permethrin (Activyl Tick Plus).

Action: Acts on voltage-dependent sodium channels in susceptible insects.

Use:
- Treatment of flea infestations (*Ctenocephalides felis*).

Developing stages of fleas in the immediate environment are killed on contact. As indoxacarb is a pro-drug bioactivated by insect enzymes and the active component has a much higher affinity for insect sodium channels, it is very specific for insect cells. Developing stages of fleas in the immediate environment of the treated pet are killed on contact. Formulations with permethrin also provide prevention of tick infestations (*Ixodes ricinus* and *Rhipicephalus sanguineus*). If ticks are present on the dog at the time of application, they may not be killed within 48 hours.

Safety and handling: Normal precautions should be observed. May be harmful to aquatic organisms.

Contraindications: Do not use on dogs and cats <8 weeks, dogs <1.5 kg (<1.2 kg for Activyl Tick Plus) or cats <0.6 kg. **Do not use permethrin product on cats.**

Adverse reactions: Transient pruritus at the site of application can occur, and rarely GI signs.

Drug interactions: No information available.

DOSES
See Appendix for guidelines on responsible parasiticide use.
Dogs: 15 mg/kg (equivalent to 0.077 ml/kg Activyl or 0.1 ml/kg Activyl Tick Plus). Apply monthly.
Cats: 25 mg/kg (equivalent to 0.128 ml/kg Activyl). Apply monthly. The combined formulation is not authorized for cats.

References
Dryden MW, Payne PA, Smith V *et al* (2013) Evaluation of indoxacarb and fipronil (s)-methoprene topical spot-on formulations to control flea populations in naturally infested dogs and cats in private residences in Tampa FL, USA. *Parasites and Vectors* **28**, 6

Fisara P, Sargent RM, Shipstone M *et al.* (2014) An open, self-controlled study on the efficacy of topical indoxacarb for eliminating fleas and clinical signs of flea-allergy dermatitis in client-owned dogs in Queensland, Australia. *Journal of Veterinary Dermatology* **25**, 195–198

Insulin

(Caninsulin[c,d], Prozinc [c,d], Actrapid*, Humulin*, Hypurin*, Insulatard*, Lantus*) **POM-V, POM**

Formulations: Injectable: 40 IU/ml, 100 IU/ml suspensions (for s.c. injection); 100 IU/ml solution (for s.c., i.v. or i.m. injection). There are many preparations (including soluble) authorized for use in humans; however, veterinary authorized preparations (lente and PZI), when available, are preferential for both legal and clinical reasons. Both PZI and the lente formulation are authorized for cats and dogs. An injection pen and cartridges are available for the lente formulation.

Action: Binds to specific receptors on the cell surface that stimulate the formation of glycogen from glucose, lipid from free fatty acids, protein from amino acids and many other metabolic effects.

Use:
- Treatment of diabetes mellitus.
- Adjunctive therapy in the management of hyperkalaemia associated with urinary tract obstruction.

There are various formulations of insulins from various species. Neutral (soluble) insulin is the normal crystalline form. Lente insulins rely on a combination of different concentrations of zinc to produce a range of sizes of zinc-insulin crystals to provide different durations of activity and should be shaken vigorously prior to administration. Protamine zinc uses zinc and protamine (a protein) to provide an extended duration of action. Glargine insulin (Lantus) is a pH sensitive, long-acting formulation that precipitates at the site of injection. Further advice on the use of insulin should be obtained from an authoritative source such as the *BSAVA Manual of Canine and Feline Endocrinology*. Hyperkalaemia associated with hypoadrenocorticism is often associated with hypoglycaemia and insulin should be avoided in those cases.

Type	Route	Onset	Peak effect in dog (hours)	Peak effect in cat (hours)	Duration of action in dog (hours)	Duration of action in cat (hours)
Soluble (neutral)	i.v.	Immediate	0.5–2	0.5–2	1–4	1–4
	i.m.	10–30 min	1–4	1–4	3–8	3–8
	s.c.	10–30 min	1–5	1–5	4–8	4–8
Isophane (NPH)	s.c.	0.5–3 h	2–10	2–8	6–24	4–12
Lente (mixed IZS)	s.c.	30–60 min	2–10	2–8	8–24	6–14
Ultralente (crystalline IZS)	s.c.	2–8 h	4–16	4–16	8–28	8–24
PZI	s.c.	1–4 h	4–14	3–12	6–28	6–24
Glargine	s.c.	1–4 h	6–10	3–12	18–28	12–24

IZS = insulin zinc suspension; NPH = neutral protamine Hagedorn; PZI = protamine zinc insulin. Note that all times are approximate averages and insulin doses need to be adjusted for individual patients.

Trade name	Species of insulin	Types available
Caninsulin	Porcine	Lente
Lantus*	Human	Glargine
Humulin*	Human	Neutral, Isophane
Hypurin*	Bovine	Neutral, Isophane, Lente, PZI
	Porcine	Neutral, Isophane
Insulatard*	Human or porcine	Isophane
Prozinc	Human	PZI

Safety and handling: Normal precautions should be observed. Insulin should be stored in a refrigerator (preferably not in the door); however, formulations using insulin pens have been shown to be stable at room temperature. Ensure use of appropriate syringes for the concentration of insulin.

Contraindications: Hypoglycaemia.

Adverse reactions: Overdosage results in hypoglycaemia and hypokalaemia.

Drug interactions: Corticosteroids, ciclosporin, thiazide diuretics and thyroid hormones may antagonize the hypoglycaemic effects of insulin. Anabolic steroids, beta-adrenergic blockers (e.g. propranolol), phenylbutazone, salicylates and tetracycline may increase insulin's effect. Administer with caution and monitor patients closely if digoxin is given concurrently. Beta-adrenergic agonists, such as terbutaline, may prevent or lessen insulin-induced hypoglycaemia in humans. This effect has not been investigated in dogs or cats.

DOSES

Dogs:
- **Diabetes mellitus:** initially 0.25–0.5 IU/kg (dogs >25 kg) or 0.5–1 IU/kg (dogs <25 kg) of lente insulin s.c. q12h. Adjust dose and frequency of administration by monitoring clinical effect (consider RVC Pet Diabetes App). Blood glucose curves may help when control is suboptimal.
- **Diabetic ketoacidosis:** 0.2 IU/kg soluble insulin i.m. initially followed by 0.1 IU/kg i.m. q1h. Alternatively, i.v. infusions may be given at 0.025–0.06 IU/kg/h of soluble insulin. Run approximately 50 ml of i.v. solution through tubing as insulin adheres to plastic; change insulin/saline solution q6h.
- **Hyperkalaemic myocardial toxicity (not in hypoadrenocorticism):** give a bolus of 0.5 IU/kg of soluble insulin i.v. followed by 2–3 g of dextrose/unit of insulin. Half the dextrose should be given as a bolus and the remainder administered i.v. over 4–6 hours.

Cats:
- **Diabetes mellitus:** initially 0.25 IU/kg of lente insulin s.c. q12h or 0.2–0.4 IU/kg of PZI insulin s.c. q12h. Adjust dose and frequency of administration by monitoring clinical effect. Urine results, blood glucose curves and/or fructosamine levels can assist surveillance.
- **Diabetic ketoacidosis:** doses as for dogs.
- **Hyperkalaemic myocardial toxicity:** doses as for dogs.

References
Gilor C and Fleeman LM (2022) One hundred years of insulin: Is it time for smart? *Journal of Small Animal Practice* **63**, 645–660
Gomez MejiasY (2021) Insulin choice in feline diabetes mellitus. *Veterinary Evidence* **6(3)**
Mooney CT and Peterson ME (2012) *BSAVA Manual of Canine and Feline Endocrinology, 4th edn.* BSAVA Publications, Gloucester

Interferon omega

(Virbagen omega [c,d]) **POM-V**

Formulations: 10 million units/vial powder with solvent for reconstitution.

Action: Interferons are cytokines that have many effects on immunity and immune cell function.

Use:
- Shown to reduce mortality and clinical signs of the enteric form of parvovirus infection in dogs.
- Treatment of early-stage FeLV infection, albeit with limited success, as shown by a reduction in mortality.
- Limited reports of use in feline infectious peritonitis, acute feline calicivirus infection and feline chronic gingivostomatitis.

The effect of treatment on cats with an FeLV-associated tumour is not known. No reduction in mortality is seen if the drug is used to treat

FIV-infected cats. In refractory and severe cases of feline herpesvirus-1 infection, combined therapy including oral or topical antiviral medication and topical interferon can be used. Has also been used topically in the management of herpetic keratitis in cats, however, is of questionable efficacy.

Safety and handling: In case of accidental self-injection, seek medical advice immediately and take the package insert or the label.

Contraindications: No information available.

Adverse reactions: Transient fatigue, hyperthermia, vomiting and mild diarrhoea may be observed (i.v. administration to cats increases the risk of these reactions). In addition, a slight decrease in WBCs, platelets and RBCs, and increases in the concentration of liver enzyme activities may be observed. Side effects such as the induction of immune-mediated diseases have been reported with long-term administration in humans. Ocular irritation has been seen in cats.

Drug interactions: Vaccines should not be administered concurrently until the animal has clinically recovered. The use of supplementary supportive treatments such as antibiotics and NSAIDs improves prognosis, and no interactions have been observed with these.

DOSES
Dogs: Parvovirus: 2.5 million units/kg i.v. q24h for 3 days.
Cats:
- **Parenteral:** 1–2.5 million units/kg i.v., s.c. q24–48h for up to 5 doses; then reduced, according to clinical effect, to twice weekly and then once weekly. Specific protocols within this dose range have been published for FeLV, FIP, FCV and chronic gingivostomatitis; consult the manufacturer for further advice.
- **Ophthalmic:** For ophthalmic use, reconstitute a 10 million unit vial with 1 ml of the solvent supplied and make up to 4 ml with sterile saline; decant into 0.2 ml aliquots and keep in freezer. To use, take a 0.2 ml aliquot of the diluted solution and add to 0.8 ml hypromellose. 1 drop of a diluted solution per eye up to q6h for 10 days, then 1 drop q8–12h for a further 3 weeks.

References
de Mari K, Maynard L, Eun HM *et al.* (2003) Treatment of canine parvoviral enteritis with interferon-omega in a placebo-controlled field trial. *Veterinary Record* **152**, 105–108
Thomasy SM and Maggs DJ (2016) A review of antiviral drugs and other compounds with activity against feline herpesvirus type 1. *Veterinary Ophthalmology* **19(S1)**, 119–130

Iron salts (Ferrous fumarate, Ferrous gluconate, Ferrous sulphate, Iron dextran)
(Gleptosil, CosmoFer*, Diafer*, Monofer*, Venofer*)
POM-VPS, POM, GSL

Formulations: Injectable: 50 mg/ml iron dextran (CosmoFer), 50 mg/ml iron(III) isomaltoside (Monofer), 100 mg/ml iron(III) isomaltoside (Monofer), 200 mg/ml iron dextran (Gleptosil and several other formulations authorized for pigs), 20 mg/ml iron sucrose (Venofer). Oral: 200 mg $FeSO_4$ tablets (ferrous sulphate), ferrous gluconate and other formulations in variable tablet and liquid preparations; ferrous fumarate preparations also typically contain folic acid. Although ferrous and ferric iron formulations are available, ferrous forms have superior absorption and are recommended.

Action: Essential for oxygen-binding in haemoglobin, electron transport chain and oxidative phosphorylation, and other oxidative reactions in metabolism.

Use:

- Treatment of iron-deficiency anaemia and conditions where RBC synthesis is high and iron stores are depleted. Iron supplementation is also used in chronic kidney disease.

The oral route should be used if possible. Iron absorption is complex and dependent in part on physiological demand, diet composition, current iron stores and dose. Valid reasons for administering iron parenterally are failure of oral therapy due to severe GI adverse effects, continuing severe blood loss, iron malabsorption or a non-compliant patient. Modified-release preparations should be avoided as they are ineffective; iron is absorbed in the duodenum and the release of iron from modified-release preparations occurs lower down the GI tract. Absorption is enhanced if administered 1 hour before or several hours after feeding. Reduce dosage if GI side effects occur.

Safety and handling: Normal precautions should be observed.

Contraindications: Severe infection or inflammation, intolerance to the oral preparation, any anaemia other than iron-deficiency anaemia, presence of GI ulcers. Also contraindicated in patients with hepatic, renal (particularly pyelonephritis) or cardiac disease or untreated urinary tract infections.

Adverse reactions: Parenteral iron may cause arrhythmias, anaphylaxis, shunting of iron to reticuloendothelial stores and iron overload. Pain often seen when injecting. Oral iron may cause nausea, vomiting, constipation and diarrhoea. The faeces of animals treated with oral iron may be dark in appearance. High doses may be teratogenic and embryotoxic (injectable iron dextran).

Drug interactions: Chloramphenicol can delay the response to iron dextran and its concurrent use should be avoided. Oral preparations bind to tetracyclines and penicillamine, causing a decrease in efficacy. Antacids, milk and eggs significantly decrease the bioavailability of oral iron.

DOSES

Dogs:

- Iron deficiency anaemia:
  - 1–2 mg/kg elemental iron p.o. q8–12h.
  - 5 mg/kg ferrous sulphate p.o. q8–12h.
- **Iron supplementation in chronic kidney disease:** 100–300 mg/dog ferrous sulphate p.o. q24h; provides 33–99 mg elemental iron.

Cats:

- 1–2 mg/kg elemental iron p.o. 8–12h.
- 5 mg/kg ferrous sulphate p.o. q8–12h.
- 50–100 mg/cat ferrous sulphate p.o. q24h; provides 16.5–49.5 mg elemental iron.

Isoflurane

(Isoba [c,d], Isocare [c,d], Isofane [c,d], IsoFlo [c,d], Isoflurane Vet [c,d], Iso-vet [c,d], Vetflurane [c,d]) **POM-V**

Formulations: Inhalational: 250 ml bottle of liquid isoflurane.

Action: The mechanism of action of volatile anaesthetic agents is not fully understood.

Use:
• Induction and maintenance of anaesthesia.

Isoflurane is potent and highly volatile so should only be delivered from a suitable calibrated vaporizer. It is less soluble in blood than halothane but more soluble than sevoflurane, therefore, induction and recovery from anaesthesia are quicker than halothane but slower than sevoflurane. The concentration of isoflurane required to maintain anaesthesia depends on the other drugs used in the anaesthesia protocol; the concentration should be adjusted according to clinical assessment of anaesthetic depth. Minimum alveolar concentration approximately 1.2–1.7% in most species. Isoflurane has a pungent smell and induction to anaesthesia using chambers or masks may be less well tolerated in small dogs and cats compared with halothane and sevoflurane.

Safety and handling: Measures should be adopted to prevent contamination of the environment with isoflurane during anaesthesia and when handling the agent.

Contraindications: No information available.

Adverse reactions: Isoflurane causes dose-dependent hypotension through vasodilation, particularly in skeletal muscle. This adverse effect does not wane with time. Isoflurane is a more potent respiratory depressant than halothane and respiratory depression is dose-dependent. Isoflurane does not sensitize the myocardium to catecholamines to the extent that halothane does, but can generate arrhythmias in certain conditions. Isoflurane is not metabolized by the liver (0.2%) and has less effect on liver blood flow compared with halothane.

Drug interactions: Sedatives, opioid agonists and N_2O reduce the concentration of isoflurane required to achieve surgical anaesthesia. The duration of action of non-depolarizing neuromuscular blocking agents is longer with isoflurane compared with halothane.

DOSES

Dogs: The expired concentration required to maintain surgical anaesthesia in 50% of dogs is approximately 1.2% (minimum alveolar concentration). Administration of other anaesthetic agents and opioid analgesics reduces the dose requirement of isoflurane; the dose should be adjusted according to individual requirement. 3–5% isoflurane concentration is required to induce anaesthesia in unpremedicated patients.

Cats: The expired concentration required to maintain surgical anaesthesia in 50% of cats is approximately 1.6% (minimum alveolar concentration).

References

Duke T, Caulkett NA and Tataryn JM (2006) The effect of nitrous oxide on halothane, isoflurane and sevoflurane requirements in ventilated dogs undergoing ovariohysterectomy. *Veterinary Anaesthesia and Analgesia* **33**, 343–350

March PA and Muir WW III (2003) Minimum alveolar concentration measures of central nervous system activation in cats anaesthetized with isoflurane. *American Journal of Veterinary Research* **64**, 1528–1533

Ispaghula (Psyllium)

(Fybogel*, Ispagel*) **GSL**

Formulations: Oral: granules, powder.

Action: Bulk-forming agent that increases faecal mass and stimulates peristalsis. Moderately fermentable in the colon and the resultant volatile fatty acids exert an osmotic laxative effect.

Use:
- Management of impacted anal sacs, diarrhoea and constipation, and the control of stool consistency after surgery.
- May be used as part of the management of canine idiopathic large bowel diarrhoea/irritable bowel syndrome.

Available preparations are for humans and often fruit-flavoured and may be effervescent when mixed with water. They can be added to food for animals.

Safety and handling: Normal precautions should be observed.

Contraindications: Bowel obstruction.

Adverse reactions: Constipation or, if excess is given, diarrhoea and bloating may occur.

Drug interactions: No information available.

DOSES

Dogs: All uses: 1–2 teaspoonfuls with meals (anecdotal).

Cats: All uses: ½–1 teaspoonful with meals (anecdotal).

References

Alves JC, Santos A, Jorge P and Pitães A (2021) The use of soluble fibre for the management of chronic idiopathic large-bowel diarrhoea in police working dogs. *BMC Veterinary Research* **17**, 100

Leib MS (2000) Treatment of chronic idiopathic large-bowel diarrhoea in dogs with a highly digestible diet and soluble fiber: a retrospective review of 37 cases. *Journal of Veterinary Internal Medicine* **14**, 27–32

Itraconazole

CIL

(Itracovet[c], Itrafungol[c], Sporanox*) **POM-V, POM**

Formulations: Oral: 100 mg capsules, 10 mg/ml oral solution.

Action: Triazole antifungal agent that inhibits the cytochrome systems involved in the synthesis of ergosterol in fungal cell membranes, causing increased cell wall permeability and allowing leakage of cellular contents.

Use:
- Treatment of aspergillosis, candidiasis, blastomycosis, coccidioidomycosis, cryptococcosis, sporotrichosis, histoplasmosis, dermatophytosis and *Malassezia*.
- Itraconazole is authorized in the form of an oral solution for the treatment of *Microsporum canis* dermatophytosis in cats and has been used successfully to treat ringworm in Persian cats without the need for clipping.

It is widely distributed in the body, although low concentrations are found in tissues with low protein contents, e.g. CSF, ocular fluid and saliva.

Safety and handling: Normal precautions should be observed.

Contraindications: Pregnancy. Avoid use if liver disease is present.

Adverse reactions: Vomiting, diarrhoea, anorexia, salivation, depression and apathy, abdominal pain, hepatic toxicosis, ulcerative dermatitis, limb oedema and occasional serious cutaneous drug eruptions have been reported. Reasonable to assume dose-related suppression of adrenal function (similar to that described for ketoconazole).

Drug interactions: In humans, antifungal imidazoles and triazoles inhibit the metabolism of antihistamines (particularly terfenadine), oral hypoglycaemics, antiepileptics, cisapride, ciclosporin and glucocorticoids. Although not as well studied in veterinary species, itraconazole is known to increase the bioavailability of ciclosporin in cats. Antacids, omeprazole, H2 antagonists and adsorbents may reduce the absorption of itraconazole. Plasma concentrations of digoxin, benzodiazepines, glucocorticoids and vincristine may be increased by itraconazole. Datasheet advises against concurrent administration with cefovecin or tolfenamic acid in cats. Itraconazole extends the activity of methylprednisolone.

DOSES

Dogs, Cats: General use: 5 mg/kg p.o. q24h. 4–20 weeks of treatment may be needed, dependent upon culture results. Pulse dosing (7 days on, 7 days off repeated x3) has been described for dermatophytosis in cats.

References

Frymus T, Gruffydd-Jones T, Pennisi MG *et al.* (2013) Dermatophytosis in cats: ABCD guidelines on prevention and management. *Journal of Feline Medicine and Surgery* **15**, 598–604

Kaolin CIL

(Kaogel VP, Pro-Kolin) **AVM-GSL, general sale**

Formulations: Oral: Aqueous suspension containing 0.99 g Kaolin Light per 5 ml (Kaogel VP). Combination products with pre-/probiotics, pectin, magnesium trisilicate, aluminium hydroxide and phosphate, bismuth salts, calcium carbonate or tincture of morphine are also available.

Action: Adsorbent antidiarrhoeal agent with possible antisecretory effect.

Use: Treatment of diarrhoea of nonspecific origin in cats and dogs. Although stool consistency may improve, studies do not show that fluid balance is corrected or that the duration of morbidity is shortened.

Safety and handling: Normal precautions should be observed.

Contraindications: Intestinal obstruction or perforation.

Adverse reactions: No information available.

Drug interactions: May decrease the absorption of lincomycin, trimethoprim and sulphonamides.

DOSES

Dogs, Cats: 0.5–1.0 ml/kg p.o. as a total daily dose. May be given as a divided dose 3–4 times daily.

Ketamine

(Anaestamine [c,d], Anesketin [c,d], Ketamindor [c,d], Ketaset [c,d], Ketavet [c,d], Narketan-10 [c,d], Vetalar-V [c,d]) **POM-V CD SCHEDULE 2**

Formulations: Injectable: 100 mg/ml solution.

Action: Antagonizes the excitatory neurotransmitter glutamate at N-methyl-D-aspartate (NMDA) receptors in the CNS. It interacts with opioid receptors in a complex fashion, antagonizing mu receptors, while showing agonist actions at delta and kappa receptors. It does not interact with GABA receptors.

Use:
- Provision of chemical restraint or dissociative anaesthesia.
- Ketamine may also provide profound visceral and somatic analgesia and inhibits central sensitization through NMDA receptor blockade.
- Used to provide perioperative analgesia as an adjunctive agent, although optimal doses to provide analgesia have not been elucidated.

Dissociative anaesthesia is associated with mild stimulation of cardiac output and blood pressure, modest respiratory depression and the preservation of cranial nerve reflexes. The eyes remain open during anaesthesia and should be protected using a bland ophthalmic ointment. Used alone at doses adequate to provide general anaesthesia, ketamine causes skeletal muscle hypertonicity and movement may occur that is unrelated to surgical stimulation. These effects are normally controlled by the co-administration of alpha-2 adrenergic agonists and/or benzodiazepines. When ketamine is combined with alpha-2 agonists (such as medetomidine or dexmedetomidine), reversal of the alpha-2 agonist should be delayed until 30 minutes after ketamine administration.

Safety and handling: Normal precautions should be observed.

Contraindications: Not recommended for animals whose eyes are at risk of perforation or who have raised intraocular pressure. The evidence that ketamine increases intracranial pressure is weak.

Adverse reactions: Cardiovascular depression, rather than stimulation, and arrhythmias may arise in animals with a high sympathetic nervous system tone (e.g. animals in shock or severe cardiovascular disease). Tachycardias can also arise after administration of high i.v. doses. Respiratory depression may be marked in some animals. Ketamine may result in 'spacey', abnormal behaviour for 1–2 hours during recovery. Prolonged administration of ketamine by infusion may result in drug accumulation and prolonged recovery.

Drug interactions: No information available.

DOSES
When used for sedation is generally given as part of a combination. See Appendix for sedation protocols in cats and dogs.
Dogs:
- **Perioperative analgesia:** intraoperatively: 10 μg (micrograms)/kg/min; postoperatively: 2–5 μg/kg/min; both preceded by a 250–500 μg/kg loading dose. There is some evidence to suggest that a 10 μg/kg/min dose may be too low to provide adequate analgesia continuously, although other evidence-based dose recommendations are lacking.
- **Induction of anaesthesia (combined with diazepam or midazolam) as part of a volatile anaesthetic technique:** 2 mg/kg i.v.
- **Induction of general anaesthesia combined with medetomidine or dexmedetomidine to provide a total injectable combination:** ketamine (5–7 mg/kg i.m.) combined with medetomidine (40 μg/kg i.m.) or dexmedetomidine (20 μg/kg i.m.).

Cats:
- **General anaesthesia:** combinations of ketamine (5–7.5 mg/kg i.m.) combined with medetomidine (80 μg (micrograms)/kg i.m.) or dexmedetomidine (40 μg/kg i.m.) will provide 20–30 min general anaesthesia. Reduce the doses of both drugs when given i.v.
- **Perioperative analgesia:** doses as for dogs.

References
Pascoe PJ, Ilkiw JE, Craig C et al. (2007) The effects of ketamine on the minimum alveolar concentration of isoflurane in cats. *Veterinary Anaesthesia and Analgesia* **34**, 31–39
Wagner AE, Walton JA, Hellyer PW et al. (2002) Use of low doses of ketamine administered by constant rate infusion as an adjunct for postoperative analgesia in dogs. *Journal of the American Veterinary Medical Association* **221**, 72–75

Ketoconazole
(Fungiconazol [d]) **POM-V**

Formulations: Oral: 200 mg, 400 mg tablets.

Action: Broad-spectrum imidazole that inhibits the cytochrome systems involved in the synthesis of ergosterol in fungal cell membranes, causing increased cell wall permeability and allowing leakage of cellular contents. It also inhibits the synthesis of cortisol in mammalian adrenal glands.

Use:
- Authorized for the treatment of *Microsporum canis*, *Microsporum gypseum* and *Trichophyton mentagrophytes*.
- May also be useful in the treatment of aspergillosis, candidiasis, blastomycosis, coccidioidomycosis, cryptococcosis, sporotrichosis and *Malassezia* dermatitis.
- May be effective in medical management of hypercortisolism where trilostane and mitotane are not available or tolerated but is generally less effective than either.
- In combination with ciclosporin to reduce the dose of ciclosporin required. Concomitant use of ketoconazole is likely to increase blood levels of ciclosporin.
- Can be used with amphotericin B in systemic fungal disease and in such cases the dose of amphotericin is reduced. See specialist texts for details.

Safety and handling: Normal precautions should be observed.

Contraindications: Do not use in animals with hepatic insufficiency.

Adverse reactions: Hepatotoxicity (not recognized in the dog unless high doses are used but routine monitoring of liver function tests is recommended), anorexia, vomiting and alterations in coat colour. Thrombocytopenia and adrenal insufficiency at high doses. Ketoconazole possibly has teratogenic effects. Has been associated with cataract development in dogs.

Drug interactions: Ketoconazole inhibits cytochrome P450 and may decrease elimination of drugs metabolized by this system. The absorption of ketoconazole may be impaired by drugs that increase the pH of gastric contents, e.g. antacids, antimuscarinics, proton-pump inhibitors and H2 blockers; stagger dosing of these drugs around ketoconazole dose. Ketoconazole extends the activity of methylprednisolone. In humans, antifungal imidazoles and triazoles inhibit the metabolism of antihistamines, oral hypoglycaemics and antiepileptics.

DOSES
Dogs:
- **Antifungal therapy:** 5–10 mg/kg p.o. after meals, once daily. Several months of treatment may be required depending on the organism and site of infection. Doses up to 40 mg/kg/day are recommended to treat CNS or nasal infections (often in conjunction with amphotericin B); ketoconazole does not attain therapeutic levels in the CNS at 'normal' doses.
- **Hypercortisolism:** 5 mg/kg p.o. q12h for 7 days, increasing to 10 mg/kg p.o. q12h for 14 days if no adverse effects seen. Perform an ACTH stimulation test after 14 days and if there is inadequate suppression gradually increase the dose to 15–30 mg/kg p.o. q12h.

Cats: Not recommended.

References
Kazuaki S and Minoru S (2015) Possible drug–drug interaction in dogs and cats resulted from alteration in drug metabolism. A mini review. *Journal of Advanced Research* **6**, 383–392

Ketoprofen

(Ketofen [c,d]) **POM-V**

Formulations: Injectable: 1% solution. **Oral:** 5 mg, 20 mg tablets.

Action: COX-1 inhibition reduces the production of prostaglandins, while lipoxygenase enzyme inhibition has a potent effect on the vascular and cellular phases of inflammation. It has antipyretic, analgesic and anti-inflammatory effects.

Use:
- Relief of acute pain from musculoskeletal disorders and other painful disorders in the dog and cat.
- Management of chronic pain from osteoarthritis in the dog.

Ketoprofen is not COX-2 selective and is not authorized for preoperative administration to cats and dogs. Do not administer perioperatively until the animal is fully recovered from anaesthesia and normotensive. Liver disease will prolong the metabolism of ketoprofen, leading to the potential for drug accumulation and overdose with repeated dosing. Accurate dosing of ketoprofen in cats is essential. Administration of ketoprofen to animals with renal disease must be carefully evaluated.

Safety and handling: Normal precautions should be observed.

Contraindications: Do not give to dehydrated, hypovolaemic or hypotensive patients or those with GI disease or blood clotting problems. Do not give to pregnant animals or animals <6 weeks of age.

Adverse reactions: GI signs may occur in all animals after NSAID administration. Stop therapy if this persists beyond 1–2 days. Some animals develop signs with one NSAID and not another. A 3–5 day wash-out period should be allowed before starting another NSAID after cessation of therapy. Stop therapy immediately if GI bleeding is suspected. There is a small risk that NSAIDs may precipitate cardiac failure in humans and this risk in animals is unknown.

Drug interactions: Do not administer concurrently or within 24 hours of other NSAIDs and glucocorticoids. Do not administer with other potentially nephrotoxic agents, e.g. aminoglycosides.

DOSES

Dogs: 2 mg/kg s.c., i.m., i.v. q24h, may be repeated for up to 3 consecutive days; 0.25 mg/kg p.o. q24h for up to 30 days in total; or 1 mg/kg p.o. q24h for up to 5 days. Oral dosing for 4 days may follow a single injection of ketoprofen on day one.

Cats: 2 mg/kg s.c. q24h, may be repeated for up to 3 consecutive days; 1 mg/kg p.o. q24h for up to 5 days. Oral dosing for 4 days may follow a single injection of ketoprofen on day one.

References

Narito T, Sato R, Tomizawa N *et al.* (2006) Safety of reduced dosage ketoprofen for long term oral administration in dogs. *American Journal of Veterinary Research* **67**, 1115–1120

Tobias KM, Harvey RC and Byarlay JM (2006) A comparison of four methods of analgesia in cats following ovariohysterectomy. *Veterinary Anaesthesia and Analgesia* **33**, 381–389

Ketorolac

(Acular*) **POM**

Formulations: Ophthalmic: 0.5% drops in 5 ml bottle.

Action: COX inhibitor that reduces the production of prostaglandins and therefore reduces inflammation.

Use: Treatment of anterior uveitis and ulcerative keratitis when topical corticosteroids are contraindicated. Topical NSAIDs have the potential to increase intraocular pressure and should be used with caution in dogs predisposed to glaucoma.

Safety and handling: Normal precautions should be observed.

Contraindications: No information available.

Adverse reactions: As with other topical NSAIDs, ketorolac may cause local irritation. Topical NSAIDs can be used in ulcerative keratitis but with caution as they can delay epithelial healing. Topical NSAIDs have been associated with an increased risk of corneal 'melting' (keratomalacia) in humans, although this has not been reported in the veterinary literature. Regular monitoring is advised.

Drug interactions: Ophthalmic NSAIDs may be used safely with other ophthalmic pharmaceuticals, although concurrent use of drugs which adversely affect the corneal epithelium (e.g. gentamicin) may lead to increased corneal penetration of the NSAID. The concurrent use of topical NSAIDs with topical corticosteroids has been identified as a risk factor in humans for precipitating corneal problems.

DOSES

Dogs, Cats: 1 drop per eye q6−24h depending on severity of inflammation.

Lactulose

CIL

(Duphalac*, Lactugal*, Lactulose*, Laevolac*) **P**

Formulations: Oral: 3.1–3.7 g/5 ml (or 10 g/15 ml) lactulose in a syrup base. Lactugal is equivalent to 62.0–74.0% w/v of lactulose.

Action: A non-absorbable sugar that is metabolized by colonic bacteria leading to the formation of low molecular weight organic acids (lactic, formic and acetic). These acids increase osmotic pressure, causing a laxative effect, and acidify colonic contents trapping ammonia as ammonium ions (which are then expelled with the faeces). Also increases the population of lactobacilli and bifidobacteria in the colon.

Use:
- Used to reduce blood ammonia in hepatic encephalopathy.
- Treatment of constipation.

Reduce the dose if diarrhoea develops. Cats and some dogs do not like the taste of lactulose. An alternative is lactitol (β-galactosidosorbitol) as a powder to add to food (500 mg/kg/day in 3 or 4 doses, adjusted to produce 2 or 3 soft stools per day), although its efficacy in the management of hepatic encephalopathy has not been extensively evaluated.

Safety and handling: Normal precautions should be observed.

Contraindications: Do not administer orally to severely encephalopathic animals at risk of inhalation. Do not use in animals with GI obstruction or those at risk of perforation. Use with caution in diabetic patients.

Adverse reactions: Excessive doses cause flatulence, diarrhoea, cramping and dehydration.

Drug interactions: Synergy may occur when lactulose is used with other laxatives. Oral antacids may reduce the colonic acidification efficacy of lactulose. Lactulose syrup contains some free lactose and galactose, and so may alter insulin requirements in diabetic patients. With increasing dose, the pH of the colon decreases, and therefore drugs which are released in the colon pH-dependently (e.g. 5-aminosalicylic acid) can be inactivated.

DOSES

Dogs:
- **Constipation and chronic hepatic encephalopathy:** 0.5–1.0 ml/kg p.o. q8–12h. Monitor and adjust therapy to produce 2 or 3 soft stools per day.
- **Acute hepatic encephalopathy:** 20 ml/kg of a solution comprising 3 parts lactulose and 7 parts warm water per rectum as a 20–30 minute retention enema. Repeat every 4–6 hours.

Cats:
- **Constipation and chronic hepatic encephalopathy:** 0.5–5 ml p.o. q8–12h. Monitor and adjust therapy to produce 2 or 3 soft stools per day.
- **Acute hepatic encephalopathy:** 1–10 ml/kg of a solution comprising 3 parts lactulose to 7 parts warm water per rectum as a 20–30 minute retention enema. Repeat every 4–6 hours.

References

Gow AG (2017) Hepatic encephalopathy. *Veterinary Clinics of North America: Small Animal Practice* **47**, 585–599

Lidbury JA, Cook AK and Steiner JM (2016) Hepatic encephalopathy in dogs and cats. *Journal of Veterinary Emergency and Critical Care* **26**, 471–487

Lamivudine (3TC) CIL

(Epivir*, Zeffix*, several generic preparations) **POM**

Formulations: Oral: 10 mg/ml solution; 100 mg tablets.

Action: A nucleoside reverse transcriptase inhibitor that inhibits viral replication.

Use:
- Treatment of cats with feline immunodeficiency virus.

In cats not showing clinical signs, it may delay the onset of the clinical phase. In cats showing clinical signs, it may improve recovery in combination with other therapies. Lamivudine (3TC) when combined with zidovudine seems to be more effective at reducing viral load and increasing CD4/CD8 ratios over a 1 year period than zidovudine on its own. These studies used small numbers of cats. Haematological monitoring is recommended.

Safety and handling: Normal precautions should be observed.

Contraindications: Anaemia.

Adverse reactions: Unknown, but cytopenias can be predicted.

Drug interactions: Unknown.

DOSES
Dogs: Not applicable.
Cats: 25 mg/kg p.o. q12h.

References
Gómez NV, Fontanals A, Castillo V *et al.* (2012) Evaluation of different antiretroviral drug protocols on naturally infected feline immunodeficiency virus (FIV) cats in the late phase of the asymptomatic stage of infection. *Viruses* **4**, 924–939

Lanthanum carbonate (Lantharenol)

(Fosrenol*) **POM, general sale**

Formulations: Oral: 500 mg, 750 mg, 1 g chewable tablets (lanthanum carbonate).

Action: Binds ingested phosphate in the gut; resultant insoluble complexes are not absorbed.

Use:
- Reduction of serum phosphate in azotaemia.

Hyperphosphataemia is implicated in the progression of chronic renal failure. Phosphate-binding agents are usually only used if low phosphate diets are unsuccessful. Monitor serum phosphate levels at 4–6 week intervals and adjust dosage accordingly if trying to achieve target serum concentrations. When using lanthanum, water should be available at all times. Dose adjustments should be based on serum phosphate levels.

Safety and handling: Normal precautions should be observed.

Contraindications: It is not advisable to introduce the drug for the first time during an acute crisis: always stabilize the patient before making any dietary alterations to enhance acceptance.

Adverse reactions: None known.

Drug interactions: Should be given at least 1 hour before or 3 hours after other medications.

DOSES

Dogs: Chronic kidney disease: 100 mg/kg/day p.o. divided between meals.

Cats: Chronic kidney disease: 400–800 mg/cat/day with a recommended starting dose of 400 mg/day. The dose should be divided according to the feeding schedule (it is important to give some with every meal).

References

Polzin DJ (2013) Evidence-based stepwise approach to managing chronic kidney disease in dogs and cats. *Journal of Veterinary Emergency and Critical Care* **23**, 205–215

Latanoprost `CIL`

(Latanoprost*, Xalatan*) **POM**

Formulations: Ophthalmic: 50 µg (micrograms)/ml (0.005%) solution in 2.5 ml bottle (Xalatan) or 0.2 ml preservative-free vials (Monopost).

Action: Agonist for receptors specific for prostaglandin F. It reduces intraocular pressure by increasing outflow.

Use:
- Management of primary canine glaucoma including emergency management of acute primary glaucoma. Often used in conjunction with other topical antiglaucoma drugs such as carbonic anhydrase inhibitors.
- Management of lens subluxation and posterior luxation despite being contraindicated in anterior lens luxation.

Latanoprost has comparable activity to travoprost. Efficacy in the cat is variable; it has been shown to reduce intraocular pressure acutely in cats with primary glaucoma but suitability and efficacy for long-term use is unknown.

Safety and handling: Check requirements for storage at room temperature or refrigeration.

Contraindications: Uveitis and anterior lens luxation. Avoid in pregnant animals.

Adverse reactions: Miosis in dogs and cats; blood-aqueous barrier disruption; conjunctival hyperaemia and mild irritation may develop. Increased iridal pigmentation has been noted in humans but not in dogs.

Drug interactions: Do not use in conjunction with thiomersal-containing preparations.

DOSES

Dogs: 1 drop per eye once daily (evening), or q8–12h.

Cats: Detailed information not available.

References

McDonald JE, Kiland JA, Kaufman PL *et al.* (2016) Effect of topical latanoprost 0.005% on intraocular pressure and pupil diameter in normal and glaucomatous cats. *Veterinary Ophthalmology* **19(S1)**, 13–23

Leflunomide

(Arava*) **POM**

Formulations: Oral: 10 mg, 15 mg, 20 mg, 100 mg tablets.

Action: Inhibits T and B lymphocyte proliferation, suppresses immunoglobulin production, and interferes with leucocyte adhesion and diapedesis, usually through inhibition of tyrosine kinases. Also inhibits dihydro-orotate dehydrogenase, an enzyme involved in the de novo pathway of pyrimidine synthesis.

Use:
- Treatment of systemic histiocytosis.
- Used in canine immune-mediated diseases.

Clinical veterinary experience of this drug is limited.

Safety and handling: Disposable gloves should be worn to handle or administer tablets. Staff and clients should be warned that excreta (including saliva) may contain traces of the parent drug or its metabolites, and should be handled with due care. Do not split or crush the tablets.

Contraindications: Bone marrow suppression, pre-existing infections, liver dysfunction.

Adverse reactions: Anorexia, lethargy, myelosuppression and haematemesis. In humans, leflunomide can cause severe hepatotoxicity, myelosuppression and interstitial lung disease.

Drug interactions: In humans, live virus vaccines, tolbutamide, rifampin and isoniazid should not be given concomitantly.

DOSES
See Appendix for immunosuppression protocols.
Dogs: 2 mg/kg p.o. q24h initially. Doses up to 4 mg/kg p.o. q24h are also described.
Cats: Rheumatoid arthritis (in combination with methotrexate): 10 mg (total dose) p.o. q24h, after significant improvement, reduce to 10 mg p.o. twice weekly.

References
Mehl ML, Tell L, Kyles AE *et al.* (2012) Pharmacokinetics and pharmacodynamics of A77 1726 and leflunomide in domestic cats. *Journal of Veterinary Pharmacology and Therapeutics* **35**, 139–146
Sato M, Veir JK, Legare M and Lappin MR (2017) A retrospective study on the safety and efficacy of leflunomide in dogs. *Journal of Veterinary Internal Medicine* **31**, 1502–1507

Lenograstim (rhG-CSF)

(Granocyte*) **POM**

Formulations: Injectable: 33.6 million IU (263 µg (microgram)) vial for reconstitution.

Action: Recombinant human granulocyte-colony stimulating factor (rhG-CSF). Activates proliferation and differentiation of granulocyte progenitor cells, enhances granulopoiesis.

Use:
- Management of febrile patients with neutrophil counts <1 x 10^9/l.

There are few reports on the use of G-CSF in dogs and cats; filgrastim is more commonly used.

Safety and handling: Normal precautions should be observed.

Contraindications: No information available.

Adverse reactions: Normal dogs produce neutralizing antibodies to rhG-CSF. This limits repeated use and may result in neutropenia. This does not appear to be the case in canine chemotherapy patients. A variety of adverse effects have been reported in humans, including musculoskeletal pain, transient hypotension, dysuria, allergic reactions, proteinuria, haematuria and increased liver enzymes. Reported adverse effects in dogs are bone pain at high doses and irritation at the injection site.

Drug interactions: In humans, steroids and lithium may potentiate the release of neutrophils during G-CSF therapy. Concurrent administration with chemotherapy may increase incidence of adverse effects. G-CSF should be given at least 24 hours after the last dose of chemotherapy as the stimulatory effects of G-CSF on haemopoietic precursors renders them more susceptible to the effects of chemotherapy.

DOSES
See Appendix for conversion of bodyweight to body surface area.
Dogs: 19.2 million IU/m^2 i.v. (over 30 min), s.c. q24h for 3–5 days.
Cats: No information available.

Levetiracetam (*S*-Etiracetam) `CIL`
(Desitrend*, Keppra*, Levetiracetum*) **POM**

Formulations: Oral: 250 mg, 500 mg, 750 mg and 1 g tablets; 100 mg/ml oral solution; 250 mg, 500 mg, 1 g granule sachets. Injectable: 500 mg/5 ml vials.

Action: The mechanism of anticonvulsant action is unknown but it has been shown to bind to the pre-synaptic vesicle protein SV2A within the brain, modulating the release of neurotransmitters, which may protect against seizures.

Use:
- Adjunctive maintenance therapy in dogs and cats presenting with epileptic seizures refractory to conventional therapy. Good tolerability reported in patients with structural epilepsy.
- May be more effective than phenobarbital at treating myoclonic seizures in cats.
- As a primary therapy where phenobarbital is contraindicated; however, efficacy is significantly worse than phenobarbital in newly diagnosed epileptic dogs.
- Used at a higher dose, in addition to conventional maintenance therapy, as pulse therapy for cluster seizures. CRI can be used for emergency control of status epilepticus.

Levetiracetam is rapidly absorbed from the GI tract with peak plasma concentrations reached in <2 hours of oral dosing. Steady state is rapidly achieved within 2 days. Plasma protein binding is minimal. The plasma half-life is around 3–4 hours in dogs. It will also reach target serum concentrations if administered rectally. Withdrawal of levetiracetam therapy or transition to or from another type of antiepileptic therapy should be done gradually. Use with caution and in reduced doses in patients with renal impairment; in humans, renal elimination of levetiracetam correlates with creatinine clearance.

Safety and handling: Normal precautions should be observed.

Contraindications: Severe renal disease.

Adverse reactions: The most commonly reported adverse effects include sedation and ataxia in dogs and reduced appetite. Behavioural changes have also been associated with its use. Hypersalivation and lethargy may occur in cats.

Drug interactions: Minimal, although there is some evidence to suggest that phenobarbital increases levetiracetam clearance, reducing the half-life and peak levels.

DOSES

Dogs, Cats:

- Maintenance therapy (as adjunct or sole anticonvulsant): 20–30 mg/kg p.o. q8–12h.
- Pulse therapy for severe cluster seizures (in addition to maintenance therapy): 30 mg/kg p.o. q6–8h for the duration of the cluster (usually 2–3 days) and then incrementally reduced and stopped until the start of the next cluster. Incremental increases in dose if required.
- **Status epilepticus:** a maximum of 60 mg/kg i.v. bolus q8h (response may be seen at lower doses and suggested starting dose is 30 mg/kg) or CRI of 8 mg/kg/h, incrementally increased to effect if required.
- The parenteral preparation can be given at 40 mg/kg per rectum, if oral or i.v. administration is not possible.

References

Hardy BT, Patterson EE, Cloyd JM et al. (2012) Double-masked, placebo-controlled study of intravenous levetiracetam for the treatment of status epilepticus and acute repetitive seizures in dogs. *Journal of Veterinary Internal Medicine* **26**, 334–340

Muñana KR (2013) Management of refractory epilepsy. *Topics in Companion Animal Medicine* **28**, 67–71

Levothyroxine see L-Thyroxine

Lidocaine (Lignocaine)

(EMLA, Intubeaze[c], Lignol[c,d], Locaine, Locovetic, Lidoderm*) **POM-V**

Formulations: Injectable: 1%, 2% solutions (some contain adrenaline). Topical: 2% solution (Intubeaze), 4% solution (Xylocaine); 2.5% cream with prilocaine (EMLA); 5% transdermal patches (Lidoderm).

Action: Local anaesthetic action is dependent on reversible blockade of the sodium channel, preventing propagation of an action potential. Sensory nerve fibres are blocked before motor nerve fibres, allowing a selective sensory blockade at low doses. Lidocaine also has class 1b antiarrhythmic actions, decreasing the rate of ventricular firing, action potential duration and absolute refractory period, and increasing relative refractory period. Lidocaine has a rapid onset of action and intermediate duration of action. Addition of adrenaline to lidocaine increases the duration of action by reducing the rate of systemic absorption.

Use:

- Provision of local or regional analgesia using perineural, infiltration,

local i.v. or epidural techniques. It is generally recommended that adrenaline-free solutions be used for epidural administration.
- Intratesticular lidocaine has been shown to reduce haemodynamic responses to castration in dogs and cats and is recommended to provide intraoperative analgesia during castration and reduce the requirement for inhalational anaesthesia.
- Also used to provide systemic analgesia when given i.v. by CRI.
- First-line therapy for rapid or haemodynamically significant ventricular arrhythmias.
- May also be effective for some supraventricular arrhythmias, such as bypass-mediated supraventricular tachycardia, and for cardioversion of acute-onset or vagally-mediated atrial fibrillation.
- Widely used topically to desensitize mucous membranes (such as the larynx prior to intubation).
- EMLA cream is used to anaesthetize the skin before vascular cannulation.

EMLA cream must be placed on the skin for approximately 45–60 minutes to ensure adequate anaesthesia; covering the skin with an occlusive dressing promotes absorption. EMLA is very useful to facilitate venous catheter placement in dogs and cats. The pharmacokinetics of transdermal lidocaine patches have been evaluated in dogs and cats; bioavailability of transdermal lidocaine is low in cats and dogs compared with humans. The analgesic efficacy and clinical usefulness of transdermal lidocaine has not yet been evaluated in either species. Infusions of lidocaine reduce the inhaled concentrations of anaesthetic required to produce anaesthesia and prevent central sensitization to surgical noxious stimuli. Systemic lidocaine is best used in combination with other analgesic drugs to achieve balanced analgesia. Lidocaine will accumulate after prolonged administration, leading to a delayed recovery. Cats are very sensitive to the toxic effects of local anaesthetics, therefore, it is important that doses are calculated and administered accurately.

Safety and handling: Normal precautions should be observed.

Contraindications: Do not give to cats by CRI during the perioperative period due to the negative haemodynamic effects. Do not give lidocaine solutions containing adrenaline i.v. Do not use solutions containing adrenaline for complete ring block of an extremity because of the danger of ischaemic necrosis.

Adverse reactions: Depression, seizures, muscle fasciculations, vomiting, bradycardia and hypotension. If reactions are severe, decrease or discontinue administration. Seizures may be controlled with i.v. diazepam. Monitor the ECG carefully during therapy. Cats tend to be more sensitive to the CNS effects. The propellant used in unauthorized aerosol preparations (e.g. Xylocaine spray) is alleged to have caused laryngeal oedema in cats and should not be used to desensitize the larynx prior to intubation.

Drug interactions: Cimetidine and propranolol may prolong serum lidocaine clearance if administered concurrently. Other antiarrhythmics may cause increased myocardial depression.

DOSES
Note: 1 mg/kg is 0.05 ml/kg of a 2% solution.
Dogs:
- **Local anaesthesia:** apply to the affected area with a small gauge

needle to an appropriate volume. Total dose that should be injected is 4 mg/kg.
- **Topical:** apply thick layer of cream to the skin and cover with a bandage for 45–60 min prior to venepuncture.
- **Analgesia by CRI:** 1 mg/kg loading dose (given slowly over 10–15 min) followed by 20–100 µg (micrograms)/kg/min. Adjust according to pain assessment and be aware of the likelihood of accumulation allowing an empirical reduction in dose rate over time.
- **Ventricular arrhythmias:** 2–8 mg/kg i.v. in 2 mg/kg boluses followed by CRI of 0.025–0.1 mg/kg/min.

Cats:
- **Local anaesthesia:** doses as for dogs.
- **Ventricular arrhythmias:** 0.25–2.0 mg/kg i.v. slowly in 0.25–0.5 mg/kg boluses followed by CRI of 0.01–0.04 mg/kg/min.
- Avoid systemic lidocaine for analgesia in cats due to the risk of drug accumulation, toxicity and negative haemodynamic effects.

References

Huuskonen V, Hughs JM, Estaca Banon E and West E (2013) Intratesticular lidocaine reduces the response to surgical castration in dogs. *Veterinary Anaesthesia and Analgesia* **40**, 74–82

Modal ER, Erikson T, Kirpensteijn J *et al.* (2013) Intratesticular and subcutaneous lidocaine alters the intraoperative haemodynamic responses and heart rate variability in male cats undergoing castration. *Veterinary Anaesthesia and Analgesia* **40**, 63–73

Lignocaine see Lidocaine

Lincomycin

(Lincocin, Lincoject [c,d]) **POM-V**

Formulations: Injectable: 100 mg/ml solution. **Oral:** powder for solution.

Action: Binds to 50S ribosomal subunit, inhibiting bacterial protein synthesis with a time-dependent mechanism. Being a weak base, it is ion-trapped in fluid that is more acidic than plasma and therefore concentrates in prostatic fluid, milk and intracellular fluid.

Use:
- Active against Gram-positive cocci (including penicillin-resistant staphylococci) and many obligate anaerobes.
- The lincosamides (lincomycin and clindamycin) are particularly indicated for staphylococcal bone and joint infections.

Clindamycin is more active than lincomycin, particularly against obligate anaerobes, and is better absorbed from the gut. Administer slowly if using i.v. route.

Safety and handling: Normal precautions should be observed.

Contraindications: Rapid i.v. administration should be avoided since this can result in collapse due to cardiac depression and peripheral neuromuscular blockade.

Adverse reactions: Human patients may develop colitis. Patients developing diarrhoea (particularly if it is haemorrhagic) while taking the medication should be monitored carefully. Exercise caution in patients with liver disease.

Drug interactions: The action of neuromuscular blocking agents may be enhanced if given with lincomycin. The absorption of lincomycin may be reduced by kaolin. Lincosamide antimicrobials should not be used in combination with chloramphenicols or macrolides as these combinations are antagonistic.

DOSES

Classified as category C (Caution) by the EMA.
See Appendix for guidelines on responsible antibiotic use.
Dogs, Cats:
- **Parenteral:** 22 mg/kg i.m. q24h; 11 mg/kg i.m. q12h or 11–22 mg/kg slow i.v. q12–24h.
- **Oral:** 22 mg/kg p.o. q12h or 15 mg/kg p.o. q8h.

Liothyronine (T3, L-Tri-iodothyronine)
POM

Formulations: Oral: 20 µg (microgram) tablets.

Action: Increases T3 concentrations.

Use:
- Diagnosis of feline hyperthyroidism (T3 suppression test).
- Suggested in the treatment of canine hypothyroidism where levothyroxine has been unsuccessful; however, evidence is scant.

Safety and handling: Normal precautions should be observed.

Contraindications: No information available.

Adverse reactions: Signs of overdosage include tachycardia, excitability, nervousness and excessive panting.

Drug interactions: The actions of catecholamines and sympatho-mimetics are enhanced by thyroxine. Diabetic patients receiving thyroid hormones may have altered insulin requirements; monitor carefully during the initiation of therapy. Oestrogens may increase thyroid requirements by increasing thyroxine-binding globulin. The therapeutic effect of digoxin may be reduced by thyroid hormones. In addition, many drugs may affect thyroid function tests and therefore monitoring of therapy.

DOSES
Dogs: Hypothyroidism: 2–6 µg (micrograms)/kg p.o. q8–12h.
Cats: T3 suppression test: administer 20 µg (micrograms)/cat p.o. q8h for 7 doses.

Lipid infusions
(ClinOleic*, Intralipid*, Ivelip*, Lipidem*, Lipofundin*, Omegaven*) **POM**

Formulations: Injectable: 10% solution contains soya oil emulsion, glycerol, purified egg phospholipids and phosphate (15 mmol/l) for i.v. use only. Contains 2 kcal/ml (8.4 kJ/ml), 268 mOsm/l. Other human products are available and vary in composition and concentration.

Action: Support intermediary metabolism, reverse negative energy balance, provide some essential fatty acids and sequester lipid-soluble sustances in plasma compartment.

Use:
- Used parenterally in animals receiving nutritional support, to provide fat for energy production and essential fatty acids for cellular metabolism and support of the immune system.
- Can also be used to bind lipid-soluble toxins, e.g. following unintentional intravenous administration of bupivacaine or topical avermectins.

Lipid emulsions are isosmolar with plasma and can be infused into a peripheral vein to provide parenteral nutrition. Due to the complex requirements of providing i.v. nutrition, including careful patient monitoring and the need for strict aseptic practice, in all cases product literature and specialist advice should be consulted. Use with caution in patients with known insulin resistance or at risk of developing pancreatitis. **See also Amino acid solutions and Glucose.**

Safety and handling: Do not use if separation of the emulsion occurs.

Contraindications: Insulin resistance (e.g. diabetes mellitus) and hyperlipidaemia.

Adverse reactions: Reactions include occasional febrile episodes mainly seen with 20% emulsions 20% and 30% lipid products have a higher rate of complications including vasculitis, thrombosis, fever and other metabolic complications and are not recommended. Rare anaphylactic responses are reported in humans. Early reports of hepatic failure, pancreatitis, cardiac arrest and thrombocytopenia detailed in human literature appear to have been complications of prolonged treatment.

Drug interactions: Consult specific product data sheet(s). Lines for i.v. parenteral feeding (lipid, glucose, amino acids or nutrient admixtures) should be dedicated for that use alone and should not be used for administration of other medications. Interference with biochemical measurements, such as those for blood gases and calcium, may occur if samples are taken before fat has been cleared. Daily checks are necessary to ensure complete clearance from the plasma in conditions where fat metabolism may be disturbed. Additives may only be mixed with fat emulsions where compatibility is known. **See Amino acid solutions for additional information.**

DOSES

Dogs:
- **Parenteral nutrition:** the amount required will be governed by the patient's physiological status and whether partial or total parenteral nutrition is provided. Generally, lipid infusions are used to supply 30% (partial peripheral) to 40–60% of energy requirements.
- **Treatment of lipid-soluble toxicosis:** administer 1.5–5 ml/kg i.v. of 20% lipid solution as bolus, followed by 0.25–0.50 ml/kg/min i.v. for 30–60 min. Boluses of 1.5 ml/kg can be repeated. Infusions of 0.5 ml/kg/min can be administered for a maximum of 24 hours.

Cats:
- **Parenteral nutrition:** the amount required will be governed by the patient's physiological status and its tolerance of lipids. Generally, peripheral parenteral nutrition is provided by amino acids in cats and lipids are used as an energy source in a nutrient admixture for

infusion through central venous access (total parenteral nutrition) to supply 40–60% of energy requirements.
- **Treatment of lipid-soluble toxicosis:** doses as for dogs.

References
Fernandez AL, Lee JA, Rahilly L et al. (2011) The use of intravenous lipid emulsion as an antidote in veterinary toxicology. *Journal of Veterinary Emergency and Critical Care* **21**, 309–320

Kang JH and Yang MP (2008) Effect of a short-term infusion with soybean oil-based lipid emulsion on phagocytic responses of canine peripheral blood polymorphonuclear neutrophilic leukocytes. *Journal of Veterinary Internal Medicine* **22**, 1166–1173

Liquid paraffin see Paraffin

Lithium carbonate
(Camcolit*, Liskonum*, Priadel*) **POM**

Formulations: Oral: 250 mg, 400 mg tablets.

Action: Stimulates bone marrow stem cells, causing an increase in the production of haemopoietic cell lines, particularly granulocytes.

Use:
- Treatment of idiopathic aplastic anaemia, cytotoxic drug-induced neutropenia or thrombocytopenia, oestrogen-induced bone marrow suppression and cyclic haemopoiesis.

There is a lag phase of up to 4 weeks before its effects may be seen. Experimental studies show that lithium may prevent neutropenia associated with cytotoxic drugs when administered concomitantly; clinical trials showing this are lacking. The recommended serum lithium concentration is 0.5–1.8 mmol/l; assess every 3 months if possible.

Safety and handling: Normal precautions should be observed.

Contraindications: Avoid in patients with renal impairment (nephrotoxic at high doses), cardiac disease and conditions with sodium imbalance (e.g. hypoadrenocorticism). Only use in patients that show no signs of dehydration. Do not use in cats.

Adverse reactions: Nausea, diarrhoea, muscle weakness, fatigue, polyuria and polydipsia. Seizures are reported. The release of T3 and T4 may be blocked by lithium; assess thyroid status every 6 months. Lithium is toxic to cats.

Drug interactions: The excretion of lithium may be reduced by ACE inhibitors, loop diuretics, NSAIDs and thiazides, thus increasing the risk of toxicity. Lithium toxicity is made worse by sodium depletion; avoid concurrent use with diuretics. The excretion of lithium may be increased by theophylline. Lithium antagonizes the effects of neostigmine and pyridostigmine. Neurotoxicity may occur if lithium is administered with diltiazem or verapamil.

DOSES
Dogs: 10 mg/kg p.o. q12h. Give with food.
Cats: Do not use.

References
Hall EJ (1992) Use of lithium for treatment of estrogen-induced bone marrow hypoplasia in a dog. *Journal of the American Veterinary Medical Association* **200**, 814–816

Lokivetmab

(Cytopoint [d]) **POM-V**

Formulations: Injectable: 10 mg/ml, 20 mg/ml, 30 mg/ml, 40 mg/ml solutions.

Action: Lokivetmab is a caninized monoclonal antibody (mAb) specifically targeting canine interleukin-31. The blocking of IL-31 by lokivetmab prevents IL-31 from binding to its co-receptor and thereby inhibits IL-31-mediated cell signalling, providing anti-inflammatory activity and relief from pruritus related to atopic dermatitis.

Use:
- Indicated for the treatment of clinical manifestations of atopic dermatitis in dogs.

If the dog does not respond to 2 doses 1 month apart, then alternative treatment should be considered. After repeated doses, the clinical efficacy may persist beyond 1 month.

Safety and handling: Avoid shaking vial. Store in fridge. Do not mix with other injectable products.

Contraindications: Not for use in dogs <3 kg. Lokivetmab may induce anti-drug antibodies which might account for reduced efficacy. Not intended to be used as a long-term maintenance therapy if the offending allergen(s) can be successfully avoided or eliminated.

Adverse reactions: Hypersensitivity reactions (anaphylaxis, facial oedema, urticaria) may occur in rare cases. Clinical signs of immune-mediated diseases, such as haemolytic anaemia or thrombocytopenia, have been reported very rarely.

Drug interactions: None reported.

DOSES

Dogs: 1 mg/kg s.c. monthly.
Cats: Not indicated.

References
Michels GM, Walsh KF, Kryda KA et al. (2016) A blinded, randomized, placebo-controlled trial of the safety of lokivetmab (ZTS-00103289), a caninized anti-canine IL-31 monoclonal antibody in client-owned dogs with atopic dermatitis. *Veterinary Dermatology* **27**, 505–e136

Lomustine (CCNU)

(Lomustine*) **POM**

Formulations: Oral: readily available 40 mg capsules. Available through specialist pharmacies as 5 mg, 10 mg and 20 mg capsules. **VSP**

Action: Interferes with the synthesis and function of DNA, RNA and proteins. Antitumour activity correlates best with formation of interstrand cross-linking of DNA. Exact mechanism of action is not fully understood, it is cell cycle-phase nonspecific. Lomustine is highly lipid-soluble, allowing rapid transport across the blood–brain barrier.

Use:
- Reported to have some efficacy in the treatment of brain tumours, mast cell tumours, refractory lymphoma, histiocytic sarcoma, transmissible venereal tumour (TVT), and epitheliotrophic lymphoma.

- Component of the modified CHOP protocol for treatment of T-cell lymphoma.
- Used in the treatment of primary and metastatic brain tumours in humans.

S-Adenosylmethionine and silybin may be used to prevent or treat lomustine hepatotoxicity.

Safety and handling: Cytotoxic drug: see Appendix and specialist texts for further advice on chemotherapeutic agents.

Contraindications: Bone marrow suppression. Pre-existing liver disease.

Adverse reactions: Myelosuppression is the dose-limiting toxicity, with neutropenia developing 7–14 days after administration (although onset of myelosuppression can range from 1–6 weeks and can be particularly delayed in cats). Neutropenia may be severe and life-threatening at the higher end of the dose range. Thrombocytopenia can also be seen, often with no other concurrent cytopenias. Gastrointestinal and hepatic adverse events also occur; potentially irreversible hepatic toxicities have been reported. Azotaemia is also described.

Drug interactions: Do not use with other myelosuppressive agents. Lomustine requires hepatic microsomal enzyme hydroxylation for the production of antineoplastic metabolites. It should be used with caution in dogs being treated with agents that induce liver enzyme activity, e.g. phenobarbital. In humans, cimetidine enhances the toxicity of lomustine.

DOSES
See Appendix for chemotherapy protocols and conversion of bodyweight to body surface area.
Dogs: All uses: 50–80 mg/m^2 p.o. q3–4wk.
Cats: All uses: A dose of 30–60 mg/m^2 p.o. q4–6wk has been suggested but is not well established. If using this drug in the cat, specialist advice should be sought, as dosing intervals may need to be increased.

References
Kristal O, Rassnick KM, Gliatto JM et al. (2004) Hepatotoxicity associated with CCNU (lomustine) chemotherapy in dogs. *Journal of Veterinary Internal Medicine* **18**, 75–80
Skorupski KA, Hammond GM, Irish AM et al. (2011) Prospective Randomized Clinical Trial Assessing the Efficacy of Denamarin for Prevention of CCNU-Induced Hepatopathy in Tumor-Bearing Dogs. *Journal of Veterinary Internal Medicine* **25**, 838–845

Loperamide
(DiaFix*, Dioraleze*, Entrocalm*, Imodium*, Norimode*)
POM, P, GSL

Formulations: Oral: 2 mg capsules; 2 mg tablets; 0.2 mg/ml syrup.

Action: Opioid agonist that alters GI motility by acting on receptors in the myenteric plexus. Normally has no central action.

Use:
- Management of non-specific acute and chronic diarrhoea, and irritable bowel syndrome.
- Use with care in cats.

Safety and handling: Normal precautions should be observed.

Contraindications: Intestinal obstruction. Do not use in dogs likely to be ivermectin-sensitive, e.g. collies. The mutation of the multiple drug resistance (*ABCB1*) gene in these dogs allows loperamide (a P-glyco-protein substrate) to penetrate the CNS and cause profound sedation.

Adverse reactions: Constipation will occur in some cases. Excitability may be seen in cats.

Drug interactions: Avoid concurrent use with other drugs that reduce GI motility.

DOSES
Dogs, Cats: 0.04–0.2 mg/kg p.o. q8–12h.

Loratadine
(Loratadine*) **GSL**

Formulations: Oral: 10 mg tablets; 1 mg/ml syrup.

Action: Binds to H1 histamine receptors, preventing histamine from binding.

Use:
- Management of allergic disease.

Specific doses for dogs and cats have not been determined by pharmokinetic studies. Use with caution in cases with urinary retention, angle-closure glaucoma and pyloroduodenal obstruction.

Safety and handling: Normal precautions should be observed.

Contraindications: No information available.

Adverse reactions: May cause mild sedation. May reduce seizure threshold

Drug interactions: No information available.

DOSES
Dogs: 5–15 mg p.o. q24h.
Cats: No information available.

Lorazepam
(Ativan*, Intensol*) **POM**

Formulations: Oral: 1 mg tablets; 2 mg/ml suspension.
Injectable: 4 mg/ml solution.

Action: Increases the activity of GABA within the CNS, resulting in anxiolysis.

Use:
- Historically used for short-term management of anxiety disorders in dogs and cats, but there is a lack of controlled studies to support its use.

May be useful during prolonged behavioural therapy programmes to avoid relapses due to exposure to an intensely fear-inducing stimulus during treatment. However, as benzodiazepines may inhibit memory, their routine use as part of a behaviour plan is not recommended except under careful management, and authorized alternative products, e.g. imepitoin, are available. Withdrawal of treatment should be gradual, as acute withdrawal may result in signs of tremor and inappetence.

Safety and handling: Normal precautions should be observed. There is some concern over the risk of acute hepatic necrosis associated with the use of benzodiazepines in cats, but it has not been reported in relation to lorazepam.

Contraindications: Glaucoma, significant liver or kidney disease, hypersensitivity to benzodiazepines. Not recommended in pregnant or lactating animals.

Adverse reactions: A general concern with benzodiazepines concerns disinhibition and the theoretical subsequent emergence of aggression. Drowsiness and mild transient incoordination may develop.

Drug interactions: Caution is advised if used in association with antifungals such as itraconazole, which inhibit its metabolism.

DOSES
Dogs, Cats: 0.02–0.1 mg/kg p.o. q12–24h; start at lower dose and gradually increase.

References
Hughes D, Moreau RE, Overall KL and Winkle TV (1996) Acute hepatic necrosis and liver failure associated with benzodiazepine therapy in six cats, 1986–1995. *Journal of Veterinary Emergency and Critical Care* **6**, 13–20.

Lotilaner
(Credelio [c,d], Credelio Plus [d]) **POM-V**

Formulations: Oral: 56.25 mg, 112.5 mg, 225 mg, 450 mg and 900 mg chewable tablets for dogs; 12 mg and 48 mg chewable tablets for cats. Lotilaner + milbemycin tablets (Credilio Plus).

Action: Inhibits GABA-gated chloride channels leading to death of parasites.

Use:
- Prophylaxis and treatment of fleas and ticks.
- Prevention of heartworm (*Dirofilaria immitis*) and lungworm (*Angiostrongylus vasorum*) (Credilio Plus).
- Likely to be active against other ectoparasites such as *Sarcoptes scabiei, Demodex canis*.

Safety and handling: Normal precautions should be observed.

Contraindications: Do not use in dogs <8 weeks or <1.4 kg, kittens <8 weeks or <0.5 kg, pregnant or lactating animals.

Adverse reactions: None known.

Drug interactions: Lotilaner and milbemycin oxime have been shown to be a substrate for P-glycoprotein (P-gp) and therefore could interact with other P-gp substrates.

DOSES
See Appendix for guidelines on responsible parasiticide use.
Dogs: 20–43 mg/kg p.o. monthly.
Cats: 6–24 mg/kg p.o. monthly.

Lufenuron

(Program [c,d], Program Plus [d]) **POM-V, AVM-GSL**

Formulations: Oral: 67.8 mg, 204.9 mg, 409.8 mg tablets (Program); 133 mg, 266 mg suspensions (Program for cats); 46 mg, 115 mg, 230 mg, 460 mg lufenuron + milbemycin (ratio of 20 mg lufenuron:1 mg milbemycin) (Program Plus). Injectable: 40 mg, 80 mg pre-filled syringes containing 100 mg/ml suspension (Program).

Action: Inhibition of chitin synthetase leading to a failure of chitin production, which means that flea eggs fail to hatch.

Use:
- Prevention of flea infestation (*Ctenocephalides felis*, *C. canis*).
- Lufenuron has an additional antifungal action, but specific doses for the effective treatment of dermatophytosis are currently unknown.

For treatment of flea infestations, the additional use of an approved adulticide is recommended. All animals in the household should be treated. Tablets/suspension should be administered with food. Can be administered during pregnancy and lactation (Program, Program Plus). Can be administered to puppies from 2 weeks or >1 kg (Program Plus), weaned puppies (Program). **See Milbemycin for further details**.

Safety and handling: Normal precautions should be observed.

Contraindications: Should not be administered to unweaned kittens.

Adverse reactions: On very rare occasions, nervous signs, itching, vomiting or diarrhoea have been reported in dogs following treatment with Program tablets. Rarely, lethargy may be seen after injection in cats.

Drug interactions: No information available.

DOSES
See Appendix for guidelines on responsible parasiticide use.
Dogs: Fleas: 10 mg/kg p.o., s.c. q1month (equivalent to a dose of 0.5 mg/kg milbemycin in combined preparations).
Cats: Fleas: 10 mg/kg s.c. q6months or 30 mg/kg p.o. q1month.

Lysine (L-Lysine)

(Enisyl) **general sale**

Formulations: Oral: 250 mg/ml paste in 100 ml bottle; 250 mg, 500 mg capsules.

Action: Antagonizes arginine, which is required for viral replication.

Use:
- Has been used in the management of feline herpesvirus-1 infection. Dietary lysine supplementation is used in an attempt to suppress FHV-1 infection and reactivation.

Oral lysine is safe and may reduce viral shedding in latently infected cats and clinical signs in cats undergoing primary exposure. However, there is limited clinical evidence regarding its efficacy in treating FHV-1. Cats are very sensitive to arginine deficiency and dietary arginine must not be reduced.

Safety and handling: Normal precautions should be observed.

Contraindications: Do not use preparations containing propylene glycol as they may be toxic to cats.

Adverse reactions: Diarrhoea may be seen (mild, reversible).

Drug interactions: No information available.

DOSES
Cats: Adults: 500 mg p.o. q12–24h (equivalent to 2 ml/2 pumps q12h); Kittens: 250 mg p.o. q12–24h (equivalent to 1 ml/1 pump q12h).

Dogs: Not applicable.

References
Thomasy SM and Maggs DJ (2016) A review of antiviral drugs and other compounds with activity against feline herpesvirus type 1. *Veterinary Ophthalmology* **19(S1)**, 119–130

Magnesium salts

(Magnesium sulphate injection BP (Vet) 25% w/v)
POM-VPS, POM

Formulations: Injectable: 25% w/v, 50% w/v solutions containing 1 mEq/ml, 2 mEq/ml magnesium. Dilute to a 20% or lower solution prior to use.

Action: Critical role in muscular excitement and neurological transmission. It is a cofactor in a variety of enzyme systems and maintenance of ionic gradients.

Use:
- Treatment of unresponsive ventricular arrhythmias, especially in the presence of hypokalaemia (when hypomagnesaemia may be present).

Used as infusions and orally to treat hypomagnesaemia.
Reduce i.v. potassium supplementation to avoid hyperkalaemia.
Monitoring of serum magnesium is essential: 30–35% is bound to protein and the remainder is free as the ionized form. Magnesium is compatible in solution with 5% dextrose and calcium gluconate. Treatment of potential overdose or complications should be anticipated and ventilatory support and i.v. calcium gluconate may be required. Product information should be consulted on an individual case basis.

Safety and handling: Normal precautions should be observed.

Contraindications: Do not use in patients with heart block or myocardial damage. Do not use in renal impairment or failure (magnesium is excreted by the kidneys at a rate proportional to serum levels).

Adverse reactions: Somnolence, CNS depression and possibly coma, muscular weakness, bradycardia, hypotension, respiratory depression and prolonged QT intervals have been seen, typically following overdosage. Very high levels can cause neuromuscular blockade and cardiac arrest.

Drug interactions: Additive effects can be seen with other CNS depressants, including barbiturates and general anaesthetics. Do not use with non-depolarizing neuromuscular blocking agents because of the risk of severe neuromuscular blockage. Because serious conduction disturbances can occur, use with extreme caution with digitalis glycosides.

DOSES

Dogs, Cats:
- **Life-threatening ventricular arrhythmia:** 0.15–0.3 mEq/kg i.v. administered over 5–15 min.
- **Magnesium replacement:** 0.75–1.0 mEq/kg/day by CRI in 5% dextrose has been advocated for the first 24–48 hours, followed by a lower dose of 0.3–0.5 mEq/kg/day for 3–5 days to allow complete repletion of magnesium stores.

References
Simmon EE. Alwood AJ and Costello MF (2011) Magnesium sulfate as an adjunct therapy in the management of severe generalized tetanus in a dog. *Journal of Veterinary Emergency and Critical Care* **21**, 542 546

Mannitol (Cordycepic acid)

(Mannitol*) **POM**

Formulations: Injectable: 50 g/500 ml (10%), 75 g/500 ml (15%), 100 g/500 ml (20%) solutions.

Action: Mannitol is an inert sugar alcohol that acts as an osmotic diuretic.

Use:
- Reduction of intracranial pressure (ICP); most effective in acute increases.
- Treatment of acute glaucoma.
- May also be used in the treatment of oliguric renal failure.

Reduction in intracranial and intraocular fluid pressure occurs within 15 minutes of the start of a mannitol infusion and lasts for 3–8 hours after the infusion is discontinued; diuresis occurs after 1–3 hours. There is some evidence that bolus administration (over 20–30 minutes) may be more effective for reduction of intracranial pressure than continuous administration. When used as treatment for raised intracranial pressure, hypovolaemia should be avoided to maintain cerebral perfusion pressure.

Safety and handling: Any crystals that have formed during storage should be dissolved by warming prior to use. The formation of crystals is a particular problem with the 20% formulations, which are supersaturated. An in-line filter should be used when infusing mannitol.

Contraindications: Severe dehydration, severe pulmonary congestion or pulmonary oedema. Mannitol is labelled 'use with care' in intracranial haemorrhage (except during intracranial surgery), but there appears to be little evidence to support this and it is used commonly in humans with traumatic brain injury and cerebral bleeds. There is some evidence for accumulation of mannitol where there has been breakdown of the blood–brain barrier and this may cause rebound increases in ICP following administration or raised ICP with prolonged therapy.

Adverse reactions: The most common adverse reactions seen are fluid and electrolyte imbalances. Infusion of high doses may result in circulatory overload and acidosis. Thrombophlebitis may occur and extravasation of the solution may cause oedema and skin necrosis. Mannitol causes diarrhoea if given orally. Rarely, mannitol may cause acute renal failure in human patients.

Drug interactions: Diuretic-induced hypokalaemia may occur when used with potassium-depleting diuretics. Concurrent potassium-depleting diuretics should be used with care in conjunction with beta-blockers. Nephrotoxicity has been described with concurrent use of mannitol and ciclosporin in human patients. Mannitol may result in temporary impairment of the blood–brain barrier for up to 30 minutes after administration of high doses. Mannitol should never be added to whole blood for transfusion or given through the same set by which blood is being infused. Do not add KCl or NaCl to concentrated mannitol solutions (20% or 25%), as a precipitate may form.

DOSES

Dogs, Cats:
- **Raised intracranial pressure:** 0.25–2 g/kg i.v. infusion of 15–20% solution. There is some evidence that higher doses have greater

clinical effect, but lower doses allow for repeated boluses. Doses of 0.25–1 g/kg are recommended. The dose is given over 20–30 min. The dose may be repeated once or twice after 4–8 hours as long as hydration and electrolyte levels are monitored.

- **Acute glaucoma (if refractory to topical treatments):** 0.5–2 g/kg i.v. infusion over 30 min. Withholding water for the first few hours after administering is recommended. May repeat 2–4 times over next 48 hours; monitor for dehydration.
- **Early oliguric or anuric renal failure (as an alternative to furosemide):** 0.25–0.5 g/kg i.v. infusion over 5–10 min. If successful can repeat in 4 hours. Rehydrate the patient prior to the use of mannitol.

References

Ballocco I, Evangelisti MA, Deiana R *et al.* (2019) A pilot study evaluating the effect of mannitol and hypertonic saline solution in the treatment of increased intracranial pressure in 2 cats and 1 dog naturally affected by traumatic brain injury. *Journal of Veterinary Emergency and Critical Care (San Antonio)* **29**, 578–584

DiFazio J and Fletcher DJ (2013) Updates in the management of the small animal patient with neurologic trauma. *Veterinary Clinics of North America: Small Animal Practice* **43**, 915–940

Marbofloxacin

(Aurizon ^d, Boflox Flavour ^{c,d}, Efex ^{c,d}, Marbocare ^{c,d}, Marbocyl ^{c,d}, Marbodex ^d, Marfloquin ^{c,d}, Quiflor ^{c,d}) **POM-V**

Formulations: Injectable: 200 mg powder for reconstitution giving 10 mg/ml when reconstituted. **Oral:** 5 mg, 10 mg, 20 mg, 40 mg, 80 mg, 100 mg tablets. **Topical:** 3 mg/ml marbofloxacin + clotrimazole + dexamethasone (aural use).

Action: Broad-spectrum antibiotic inhibiting bacterial DNA gyrase via a concentration-dependent mechanism particularly against Gram-negative bacteria. Low urinary pH may reduce the activity.

Use:
- Should be used based on antimicrobial susceptibility testing, wherever possible, and where lower tier antimicrobials would not be effective.
- Active against *Mycoplasma* and many Gram-positive and particularly Gram-negative organisms, including *Pasteurella*, *Staphylococcus*, *Pseudomonas aeruginosa*, *Klebsiella*, *Escherichia coli*, *Mycobacterium*, *Proteus* and *Salmonella*. Fluoroquinolones are effective against beta-lactamase-producing bacteria. Relatively ineffective against obligate anaerobes.

Fluoroquinolones are highly lipophilic drugs that attain high concentrations within cells in many tissues and are particularly effective in the management of soft tissue, urogenital (including pyelonephritis and prostatitis) and skin infections. May allow clearance of *Mycoplasma haemofelis* in cats persistently infected after doxycycline treatment. May be useful in the treatment *Leishmania*, particularly where concurrent chronic kidney disease is present. Used in combination therapy for treatment of mycobacterial infections.

Safety and handling: Normal precautions should be observed.

Contraindications: 20 mg and higher tablets should not be administered to cats.

Adverse reactions: Some animals show GI signs (nausea, vomiting). Use with caution in epileptics until further information is available, as fluoroquinolones potentiate adverse CNS effects when administered with NSAIDs in humans. Enrofloxacin, particularly at high doses, has caused retinal blindness in cats; although not reported with marbofloxacin, caution should be exercised before using dose rates above those recommended by the manufacturer in cats. Cartilage abnormalities have been reported following the use of other fluoroquinolones in growing animals. Such abnormalities have not been specifically reported following the use of marbofloxacin, but the drug is not authorized for use in dogs <12 months or cats <16 weeks. Should not be administered to giant-breed animals <18 months.

Drug interactions: Absorbents and antacids containing cations (Mg^{2+}, Al^{3+}) may bind fluoroquinolones, preventing their absorption from the GI tract. Their absorption may also be inhibited by sucralfate and zinc salts; separate dosing by at least 2 hours. Fluoroquinolones increase plasma theophylline concentrations. Cimetidine may reduce the clearance of fluoroquinolones and so should be used with caution with these drugs. Some fluoroquinolones may decrease the metabolism and increase nephrotoxicity of ciclosporin and tacrolimus in humans and therefore concurrent use in animals is best avoided until more research has been performed. May increase the action of orally administered anticoagulants.

DOSES

Classified as category B (Restrict) by the EMA.

See Appendix for guidelines on responsible antibiotic use.

Dogs:
- **Oral and parenteral:** 2 mg/kg i.v., s.c., p.o. q24h. Higher doses should be considered for certain sites, including in prostatitis, and for certain isolates of *Pseudomonas aeruginosa*.
- **Topical:** 10 drops per ear q24h.

Cats: 2 mg/kg i.v., s.c., p.o. q24h.

References

Federico S, Carrano R, Capone D et al. (2006) Pharmacokinetic interaction between levofloxacin and ciclosporin or tacrolimus in kidney transplant recipients: ciclosporin, tacrolimus and levofloxacin in renal transplantation. *Clinical Pharmacokinetics* **45**, 169–175

Hirt RA, Teinfalt M, Dederichs D et al. (2003) The effect of orally administered marbofloxacin on the pharmacokinetics of theophylline. *Journal of Veterinary Medicine: A Physiology, Pathology and Clinical Medicine* **50**, 246–250

Maropitant

(Cerenia [c,d], Prevomax [c,d], Vetemex [c,d]) **POM-V**

Formulations: Injectable: 10 mg/ml solution. Oral: 16 mg, 24 mg, 60 mg, 160 mg tablets.

Action: Inhibits vomiting reflex by blocking NK-1 receptors in medullary vomiting centre. Highly protein bound, with a long duration of activity (24 hours). Maropitant is not known to have any prokinetic effect. Has an antinociceptive effect in animals undergoing surgery, although not all studies support this.

Use:
- Treatment and prevention of vomiting in dogs, including that caused by chemotherapy and motion sickness (although not all preparations are specifically authorized for these purposes).
- Maropitant is well tolerated and has potent antiemetic activity in cats.

In cases of frequent vomiting, treatment by injection is recommended. Treatment by injection and/or tablets can be given for up to 5 days. In some individual dogs, repeat treatment at a lower dose may be adequate. For motion sickness, treatment for up to 2 days can be given. If longer periods of treatment are required, the recommended interval between the last dose of one course and the first dose of a subsequent course is 72 hours. It should be used in combination with investigation into the cause of vomiting and with other supportive measures and specific treatments. Tablets best given with food; avoid prolonged fasting before administration.

Safety and handling: Normal precautions should be observed. Do not attempt to remove the tablet by pushing through the blister packing as this will damage the tablet.

Contraindications: No specific contraindications but it would be sensible not to use maropitant where GI obstruction or perforation could be present or for longer than 48 hours without a definitive diagnosis. Metabolized by the liver, so use with caution in patients with hepatic disease.

Adverse reactions: Transient pain reaction during injection is reported as a very common occurrence, especially in cats, but no significant lasting adverse reactions. Very high doses in cats may cause haemolysis. Pain on injection can be reduced by injecting the product at refrigerated temperatures.

Drug interactions: No compatibility studies exist, and therefore the injection should not be mixed with any other agent. Should not be used concurrently with calcium-channel antagonists as maropitant has an affinity to calcium-channels. Highly bound to plasma proteins and may compete with other highly bound drugs.

DOSES
Dogs:
- **Vomiting:** 1 mg/kg i.v. or s.c. q24h or 2 mg/kg p.o. q24h.
- **Motion sickness:** tablets at a dose rate of 8 mg/kg q24h for a maximum of 2 days given 1 hour before journey.
- **Prevention of chemotherapy-induced emesis:** 1 mg/kg s.c. q24h or 2 mg/kg p.o. q24h, given at least 1 hour in advance.

Cats: Vomiting: 1 mg/kg i.v., s.c. or p.o. q24h.

References
de la Puente-Redondo VA, Siedek EM, Benchaoui HA *et al.* (2007) The anti-emetic efficacy of maropitant (*Cerenia*) in the treatment of ongoing emesis caused by a wide range of underlying clinical aetiologies in canine patients in Europe. *Journal of Small Animal Practice* **48**, 93–98

Hickman MA, Cox SR, Mahabir S *et al.* (2008) Safety, pharmacokinetics and use of the novel NK-1 receptor antagonist maropitant (*Cerenia*) for the prevention of emesis and motion sickness in cats. *Journal of Veterinary Pharmacology and Therapeutics* **31**, 220–229

Kinobe RT and Miyake Y (2020) Evaluating the anti-inflammatory and analgesic properties of maropitant: A systematic review and meta-analysis. *The Veterinary Journal* **259–260**, 105471

Masitinib mesylate

(Masivet [d]) **POM-V**

Formulations: Oral: 50 mg, 150 mg film-coated tablets.

Action: Protein tyrosine kinase inhibitor, which showed *in vitro* selectively and effectively highest affinity for mutated forms of the c-KIT tyrosine kinase receptor. Tyrosine kinase inhibitors block the TK receptor pathways essential for cell replication.

Use:

- Treatment of dogs with non-resectable mast cell tumours (Patnaik grade 2 or 3), preferably with a confirmed mutated c-KIT tyrosine kinase receptor.
- Studies indicate that masitinib may be useful for the treatment of some dogs with atopic dermatitis, chronic enteropathy, osteosarcoma, anal sac adenocarcinoma and haemangiosarcoma.
- Early studies have investigated the use of masitinib in cats with injection site sarcoma and asthma.

Preliminary studies have investigated safety in healthy cats, but this drug is not authorized in this species and further clinical trials are required. Patients should be monitored closely during treatment. Blood pressure, urinalysis, haematology and biochemistry should be assessed before starting therapy, and then at least once a month (clinicians may also check these parameters 1–2 weeks after drug initiation). Full coagulation profiles and faecal occult blood tests should be undertaken if adverse clinical signs are observed. It is good practice to contact owners weekly for the first 6 weeks of therapy to check for side effects. Use with caution if pre-existing renal or hepatic dysfunction is present.

Safety and handling: Cytotoxic drug; see Appendix or specialist texts for further advice on chemotherapeutic agents.

Contraindications: Do not use in pregnant or lactating bitches, in dogs <24 months or <7 kg, if there are any pre-existing signs of myelosuppression or if the patient has shown previous hypersensitivity to masitinib.

Adverse reactions: Mild to moderate GI reactions (diarrhoea, vomiting) and hair coat changes/hair loss are common. Renal toxicity, anaemia, protein loss, myelosuppression, increased liver enzyme activity, lethargy, cough and lymphadenomegaly have also been described.

Drug interactions: Concurrent use of drugs that are highly protein bound or interact with the cytochrome P450 enzyme pathway may increase the risk of adverse side effects.

DOSES

See Appendix for chemotherapy protocols.

Dogs: All uses: 11–14 mg/kg p.o. q24h (usually 12.5 mg/kg p.o. q24h).

Cats: 50 mg per cat p.o. q24–48h has been administered to healthy cats (limited evidence).

References

Daly M, Sheppard S, Cohen N *et al.* (2011) Safety of masitinib mesylate in healthy cats. *Journal of Veterinary Internal Medicine* **25**, 297–302

Hahn KA, Oglivie G, Rusk T *et al.* (2008) Masitinib is safe and effective for the treatment of canine mast cell tumours. *Journal of Veterinary Internal Medicine* **22**, 1301–1309

A
B
C
D
E
F
G
H
I
J
K
L
M
N
O
P
Q
R
S
T
U
V
W
X
Y
Z

Mavacoxib

(Trocoxil [d]) **POM-V**

Formulations: Oral: 6 mg, 20 mg, 30 mg, 75 mg, 95 mg chewable tablets.

Action: Selectively inhibits COX-2 enzyme, thereby limiting the production of prostaglandins involved in inflammation. The prolonged duration of action of mavacoxib means that animals should be carefully evaluated for their suitability for NSAID therapy before the onset of treatment.

Use:
- Treatment of pain and inflammation associated with degenerative joint disease in dogs at least 12 months old in cases where continuous treatment exceeding 1 month is indicated.

Continuous treatment may have the potential to reduce central sensitization and breakthrough pain. Approximately 5% of dogs are poor metabolizers of mavacoxib. The treatment regimen recommended below is designed to prevent drug accumulation in this sub-population of animals. Preliminary clinical evidence suggests that treatment can be re-started after a 1-month break from dosing. No recommendations have yet been made regarding whether to give a loading dose (first and second doses separated by 14 days) each time treatment is re-started. If necessary, analgesia should be provided in the 1-month break from treatment using a different class of drug.

Safety and handling: Normal precautions should be observed.

Contraindications: Do not give to dehydrated, hypovolaemic or hypotensive patients or those with GI disease or blood clotting problems. Administration of mavacoxib to animals with renal disease must be carefully evaluated. Liver disease prolongs the metabolism of mavacoxib, leading to the potential for drug accumulation and overdose with repeated dosing; use is not recommended. Do not give to pregnant animals or animals <12 months or <5 kg.

Adverse reactions: Should an animal require anaesthesia or develop any illness while receiving mavacoxib, then care must be taken to avoid dehydration, hypotension and hypovolaemia, and prompt intervention to manage these conditions should be implemented if they occur. Although the duration of action of mavacoxib is prolonged, symptomatic management of any side effects associated with drug administration is recommended only until the clinical signs resolve. There is a small risk that NSAIDs may precipitate cardiac failure in humans and this risk in animals is unknown.

Drug interactions: Do not administer concurrently with other NSAIDs or glucocorticoids. Do not administer another NSAID within 1 month of dosing with mavacoxib. Do not administer with other potentially nephrotoxic agents, e.g. aminoglycosides.

DOSES

Dogs: 2 mg/kg p.o. q14d for 2 doses then q1month for a maximum of 7 doses. Should be given immediately before or with the dog's main meal.

Cats: Do not use.

References

Cox SR, Lesman SP, Boucher JF *et al.* (2010) The pharmacokinetics of mavacoxib, a long-acting COX-2 inhibitor, in young adult laboratory dogs. *Journal of Veterinary Pharmacology and Therapeutics* **33**, 461–470

Cox SR, Liao S, Payne-Johnson M *et al.* (2011) Population pharmacokinetics of mavacoxib in osteoarthritic dogs. *Journal of Veterinary Pharmaology and Therapeutics* **34**, 1–11

Medetomidine

(Domitor [c,d], Dorbene [c,d], Dormilan [c,d], Medetor [c,d], Sedastart [c,d], Sedator [c,d], Sededorm [c,d]) **POM-V**

Formulations: Injectable: 1 mg/ml solution.

Action: Agonist at peripheral and central alpha-2 adrenoreceptors producing dose-dependent sedation, muscle relaxation and analgesia.

Use:

- Provides sedation and premedication when used alone or in combination with opioid analgesics.
- Medetomidine combined with ketamine is used to provide a short duration (20–30 min) of surgical anaesthesia.

Specificity for the alpha-2 receptor is greater than that of xylazine, but lower than that of dexmedetomidine. Medetomidine is a potent drug that causes marked changes in the cardiovascular system, including an initial peripheral vasoconstriction that results in an increase in blood pressure and a compensatory bradycardia. After 20–30 min, vasoconstriction wanes while blood pressure returns to normal values. Heart rate remains low due to the central sympatholytic effect of alpha-2 agonists. These cardiovascular changes result in a fall in cardiac output; central organ perfusion is well maintained at the expense of redistribution of blood flow away from the peripheral tissues. Respiratory system function is well maintained; respiration rate may fall but is accompanied by an increased depth of respiration. Oxygen supplementation is advisable in all animals. The duration of analgesia from a 10 μg (micrograms)/kg dose is approximately 1 hour. Combining medetomidine with an opioid provides improved analgesia and sedation. Lower doses of medetomidine should be used in combination with other drugs. Reversal of sedation or premedication with atipamezole shortens the recovery period, which may be advantageous. Analgesia should be provided with other classes of drugs before administering atipamezole. The authorized dose range of medetomidine for dogs and cats is very broad. High doses (>20 μg/kg) are associated with greater physiological disturbances than doses between 5–20 μg/kg. Using medetomidine in combination with other drugs in the lower dose range can provide good sedation and analgesia with minimal side effects. Similarly to dexmedetomidine, medetomidine may be used in low doses to manage excitation during recovery from anaesthesia and to provide perioperative analgesia when administered by CRI.

Safety and handling: Normal precautions should be observed.

Contraindications: Do not use in animals with cardiovascular or other systemic disease. Use in geriatric patients is not advisable. Do not use in pregnant animals. Do not use when vomiting is contraindicated (e.g. foreign body, raised intraocular pressure). Due to effects on blood glucose, use in diabetic animals is not recommended.

Adverse reactions: Causes diuresis by suppressing arginine vasopressin secretion, a transient increase in blood glucose by decreasing endogenous insulin secretion, mydriasis and decreased intraocular pressure. Vomiting after i.m. administration is common. Spontaneous arousal from deep sedation following stimulation can occur with all alpha-2 agonists; aggressive animals sedated with medetomidine must still be managed with caution.

Drug interactions: When used for premedication, medetomidine will significantly reduce the dose of all other anaesthetic agents required to maintain anaesthesia. Drugs for induction of anaesthesia should be given slowly and to effect to avoid inadvertent overdose; the dose of volatile agent required to maintain anaesthesia can be reduced by up to 70%. Do not use in patients receiving or likely to require sympathomimetic amines.

DOSES
When used for sedation is generally given as part of a combination. See Appendix for sedation protocols in cats and dogs.
Dogs, Cats:
- **Premedication:** 5–20 µg (micrograms)/kg i.v., i.m, s.c. in combination with an opioid. Use lower end of dose range i.v.
- Doses of 1–2 µg/kg i.v. can be used to manage excitation in the recovery period, although animals must be monitored carefully following administration.
- A CRI of 2–4 µg/kg/h can be used to provide perioperative analgesia and rousable sedation, particularly when administered as an adjunct to opioid-mediated analgesia.

Meglumine antimonate

(Glucantime*) **POM**

Formulations: Injectable: 300 mg/ml solution.

Action: Reported to interfere with glucose metabolism of *Leishmania* parasites.

Use:
- Treatment of canine leishmaniosis.

Animals may be clinically normal after treatment but parasitological cure is extremely difficult to achieve. Concurrent treatment with allopurinol may be appropriate depending on disease severity/clinical condition. It is advisable to consult specialist texts or seek expert advice when treating leishmaniosis.

Safety and handling: Normal precautions should be observed.

Contraindications: Do not use in animals with severe liver dysfunction, renal dysfunction or heart disease.

Adverse reactions: Limited information available. Pain at injection site has been reported.

Drug interactions: Use with care with agents that can also cause QT interval prolongation.

DOSES
See Appendix for guidelines on responsible parasiticide use.

Dogs: Leishmaniosis: 75–100 mg/kg s.c. q24h or 40–75 mg/kg s.c. q12h until clinical remission achieved. Treat for at least 28 days.

Cats: No information available.

References
Manna L, Corso R, Galiero G *et al.* (2015) Long-term follow-up of dogs with leishmaniosis treated with meglumine antimoniate plus allopurinol *versus* miltefosine plus allopurinol. *Parasites and Vectors* **28**, 289

Noli C and Saridomichelakis MN (2014) An update on the diagnosis and treatment of canine leishmaniosis caused by *Leishmania infantum* (syn. *L. chagasi*). *Veterinary Journal* **202**, 425–435

Solano-Gallego L, Miró G, Koutinas A *et al.* (2011) LeishVet guidelines for the practical management of canine leishmaniosis. *Parasites and Vectors* **4**, 86–102

Melatonin
(Circadin) **POM**

Formulations: Oral: 2 mg and 3 mg tablets. Melatonin is also available in many over-the-counter formulations of various sizes and often with other drugs added.

Action: Hormone which is involved in the neuroendocrine control of seasonal hair loss, although the exact mechanism is not known.

Use:
* Treatment of hair cycling disorders in dogs; in particular the treatment of alopecia X and seasonal flank alopecia.

A 4 6 week trial is recommended, if no growth is noted then treatment should be discontinued. For seasonal flank alopecia, treatment may have to be repeated the following year. The effect of melatonin on hair regrowth in dogs with non-pruritic alopecia of unknown aetiology is variable and every effort should be made to identify the underlying disorder before starting this therapy. Oral bioavailability of melatonin in dogs is unknown

Safety and handling: Normal precautions should be observed.

Contraindications: No information available.

Adverse reactions: No information available.

Drug interactions: No information available.

DOSES
Dogs: Hair cycling disorders: 3–6 mg (total dose) p.o. q8h.

Cats: No information available.

References
Frank LA, Hnilica KA and Oliver JW (2006) Adrenal steroid hormone concentrations in dogs with hair cycle arrest (Alopecia X) before and during treatment with melatonin and mitotane. *Veterinary Dermatology* **1**, 278–284

Meloxicam
(Inflacam [c,d], Loxicom [c,d], Meloxidolor [c,d], Meloxidyl [c,d], Metacam [c,d], Rheumocam [c,d]) **POM-V**

Formulations: Oral: 0.5 mg/ml suspension for cats, 1.5 mg/ml suspension for dogs; 1 mg, 2.5 mg tablets for dogs. **Injectable:** 2 mg/ml solution for cats, 5 mg/ml solution.

Action: Preferentially inhibits COX-2 enzyme thereby limiting the production of prostaglandins involved in inflammation.

Use:
- Alleviation of inflammation and pain in both acute and chronic musculoskeletal disorders and the reduction of postoperative pain and inflammation following orthopaedic and soft tissue surgery.

All NSAIDs should be administered cautiously in the perioperative period as they may adversely affect renal perfusion during periods of hypotension. If hypotension during anaesthesia is anticipated, delay meloxicam administration until the animal is fully recovered from anaesthesia and normotensive. Liver disease will prolong the metabolism of meloxicam, leading to the potential for drug accumulation and overdose with repeated dosing. The oral dose (standard liquid preparation) may be administered directly into the mouth or mixed with food. In the cat, due to the longer half-life and narrower therapeutic index of NSAIDs, particular care should be taken to ensure the accuracy of dosing and not to exceed the recommended dose. Administration to animals with renal disease must be carefully evaluated.

Safety and handling: After first opening a bottle of liquid oral suspension, use contents within 6 months. Shake the bottle of the oral suspension well before dosing. The shelf-life of a broached bottle of injectable solution is 28 days.

Contraindications: Do not give to dehydrated, hypovolaemic or hypotensive patients or those with GI disease or blood clotting problems. Administration of meloxicam to animals with renal disease must be carefully evaluated and is not advisable in the perioperative period. Do not give to pregnant animals or animals <6 weeks.

Adverse reactions: GI signs may occur in all animals after NSAID administration. Stop therapy if this persists beyond 1–2 days. Some animals develop signs with one NSAID and not another. A 3–5 day wash-out period should be allowed before starting another NSAID after cessation of therapy. Stop therapy immediately if GI bleeding is suspected. There is a small risk that NSAIDs may precipitate cardiac failure in humans and this risk in animals is not known.

Drug interactions: Different NSAIDs should not be administered within 24 hours of each other. The optimal wash-out period between NSAID administration and glucocorticoid administration is unknown – allowing 3–5 days between the two classes of drugs is recommended. Do not administer with other potentially nephrotoxic agents, e.g. aminoglycosides.

DOSES

Dogs: Initial dose is 0.2 mg/kg s.c., p.o.; effects last for 24 hours if given as a single preoperative injection. Can be followed by a maintenance dose of 0.1 mg/kg p.o q24h.

Cats:
- Initial injectable dose is 0.2 mg/kg s.c.; effects last for 24 hours if given as a single preoperative injection. To continue treatment for up to 5 days, may be followed 24 hours later by the oral suspension for cats at a dosage of 0.05 mg/kg p.o.
- **Postoperative pain/inflammation:** single injection of 0.3 mg/kg s.c. has been shown to be safe and efficacious. It is not recommended to follow this with oral meloxicam 24 hours later.

- **Chronic pain:** initial oral dose is 0.1 mg/kg p.o. q24h, which can be followed by a maintenance dose of 0.05 mg/kg p.o q24h. Treatment should be discontinued after 14 days if no clinical improvement is apparent.

References
Aragon CL, Hofmeister EH and Budsberg SC (2007) Systematic review of clinical trials of treatments for osteoarthritis in dogs. *Journal of the American Veterinary Medical Association* **230**, 514–521

Leece EA, Brearley JC and Harding EF (2005) Comparison of carprofen and meloxicam for 72 h following ovariohysterectomy in dogs. *Veterinary Anaesthesia and Analgesia* **32**, 184–192

Melphalan

CIL

(Alkeran*) **POM**

Formulations: Oral: 2 mg tablets. **Injectable:** 50 mg powder in vial plus diluent.

Action: Forms inter- and intrastrand cross-links with DNA, resulting in inhibition of DNA synthesis and function. Effects on both resting and dividing cells.

Use:
- Treatment of multiple myeloma.
- May also be used as a substitute for cyclophosphamide in the treatment of canine lymphoma and in some rescue protocols for lymphoma.
- Treatment of some solid tumours (e.g. ovarian carcinoma, osteosarcoma, pulmonary and mammary neoplasia).

Take care in dosing small dogs using their body surface area as there is a risk of overdose due to tablet sizes (tablets should not be split). Give tablets on an empty stomach.

Safety and handling: Cytotoxic drug; see Appendix and specialist texts for further advice on chemotherapeutic agents. Tablets should be stored in a closed, light-protected container under refrigeration (2–8°C).

Contraindications: Bone marrow suppression, concurrent infection and impaired renal function.

Adverse reactions: Myelosuppression is dose-limiting toxicity with leucopenia, thrombocytopenia, anaemia; effect may be prolonged and cumulative. GI adverse reactions include anorexia, nausea and vomiting. Pulmonary infiltrates or fibrosis and neurotoxicosis can also occur. Oral ulceration is seen in humans.

Drug interactions: Cimetidine decreases the oral bioavailability of melphalan. Steroids enhance the antitumour effects of melphalan. In humans, ciclosporin enhances the risk of renal toxicity.

DOSES
See Appendix for chemotherapy protocols and conversion of bodyweight to body surface area.
Dogs:
- **Myeloma:** 2 mg/m^2 p.o. q24h for 1–2 weeks then reduce to 2–4 mg/m^2 p.o. q48h; 0.1 mg/kg p.o. q24h for 10 days then 0.05 mg/kg p.o. q24–48h thereafter; 7 mg/m^2/day (rounded to the nearest whole 2 mg tablet) for 5 consecutive days every 21 days.

Often used with prednisolone, see specialist texts for regimes and alternative doses.

- **Lymphoma:** 20 mg/m^2 q14d, usually as part of a multidrug chemotherapy protocol; it is advised to seek specialist veterinary oncology advice before using this drug.
- **Adjunctive treatment of ovarian carcinoma, lymphoreticular neoplasms, osteosarcoma, mammary/pulmonary neoplasia:** 2–4 mg/m^2 p.o. q48h.

Cats:
- **Chronic lymphocytic leukaemia:** 1.5–2 mg/m^2 p.o. q48h, with or without prednisolone.
- **Multiple myeloma:** 0.1 mg/kg p.o. q24h for 14 days then q48h until improvement or leucopenia detected. Cats with leucopenia and anaemia should be treated q72h. Often used with prednisolone, see specialist texts for regimes.

References
Fernandez R and Chon E (2018) Comparison of two melphalan protocols and evaluation of outcome and prognostic factors in multiple myeloma in dogs. *Journal of Veterinary Internal Medicine* **32**, 1060–1069

Mastromauro ML, Suter SE, Hauck ML and Hess PR (2018) Oral melphalan for the treatment of relapsed canine lymphoma. *Veterinary Comparative Oncology* **16**, 123–129

Memantine
(Maxura*, Nemdatine*) **POM**

Formulations: Oral: 10 mg, 20 mg tablets; 10 mg/ml solution.

Action: Provides analgesia through NMDA antagonist action which may potentiate the effects of other analgesics. It is also an agonist at the dopamine D2 receptor and acts as a non-competitive antagonist at the serotonin 5-HT$_3$ and nicotinic acetylcholine receptors.

Use:
- Used as an adjunctive analgesic for the management of chronic pain in dogs.
- Has been used to treat canine compulsive disorders either alone or with fluoxetine.

Has a similar mechanism of action to amantadine but is significantly cheaper and therefore may be useful for patients where administration of amantadine is cost prohibitive. Anecdotal experience of using memantine in cats is lacking. Memantine is authorized for the management of Alzheimer's disease in humans.

Safety and handling: Normal precautions should be observed.

Contraindications: No information available.

Adverse reactions: In humans, minor CNS effects have been reported (balance impairment, dizziness, drowsiness). Memantine is renally excreted and is likely to accumulate in animals with renal dysfunction, therefore, it should be used cautiously in this patient population.

Drug interactions: No information available.

DOSES
Dogs: 0.3–1.0 mg/kg p.o. q24h. There is a limited evidence base to support this dose recommendation. Start at the low end and titrate upwards.
Cats: No information available.

Mepivacaine

(Intra-epicaine, Mepidor) **POM-V**

Formulations: Injectable: 2% solution (only authorized for horses).

Action: Local anaesthetic action is dependent on reversible blockade of the sodium channel, preventing propagation of an action potential along the nerve fibre. Sensory nerve fibres are blocked before motor nerve fibres, allowing a selective sensory blockade at low doses.

Use:
- Blockade of sensory nerves to produce analgesia following perineural or local infiltration.
- Instillation into joints to provide intra-articular analgesia.

Mepivacaine has less intrinsic vasodilator activity than lidocaine and is thought to be less irritant to tissues. It is of equivalent potency to lidocaine but has a slightly longer duration of action (100–120 min). It does not require addition of adrenaline to prolong its effect.

Safety and handling: Normal precautions should be observed.

Contraindications: Mepivacaine should not be injected i.v.

Adverse reactions: Inadvertent i.v. injection may cause convulsions and/or cardiac arrest.

Drug interactions: No information available.

DOSES

Dogs, Cats: Inject the minimal volume required to achieve effect. 2 mg/kg of the 2% solution injected into the elbow joint prior to arthroscopy has been found to decrease the haemodynamic response to surgery in dogs. Toxic doses of mepivacaine have not been established in companion animals.

References
Dutton TA, Gurney MA and Bright SR (2014) Intra-articular mepivacaine reduces interventional analgesia requirements during arthroscopic surgery in dogs. *Journal of Small Animal Practice* **55**, 405–408

Lamont LA and Lemke KA (2007) The effects of medetomidine on radial nerve blockade with mepivacaine in dogs. *Veterinary Anaesthesia and Analgesia* **35**, 62–68

Methadone

(Comfortan [c,d], Insistor [c,d], Synthadon [c,d]) **POM-V**
CD SCHEDULE 2

Formulations: Injectable: 10 mg/ml solution (generic preservative-free preparations are also available). **Oral:** 10 mg tablets.

Action: Analgesia mediated by the mu opioid receptor.

Use:
- Management of moderate to severe pain in the perioperative period.
- Incorporation into sedative and pre-anaesthetic medication protocols to provide improved sedation and analgesia.
- Methadone may be administered epidurally to provide analgesia; the duration of analgesia following methadone at a dose of 0.1–0.3 mg/kg epidurally is approximately 8 hours in dogs.

Methadone has similar pharmacological properties to morphine. It provides profound analgesia with a duration of action of 3–4 hours in dogs and cats. Accumulation is likely to occur after prolonged repeated dosing which may allow the dose to be reduced or the dose interval extended. Methadone can be given i.v. without causing histamine release and does not cause vomiting when given to animals preoperatively. Transient excitation may occur when methadone is given i.v. Oral methadone is rarely used in cats and dogs due to a high first-pass metabolism leading to low plasma concentrations after administration. Methadone is absorbed into the systemic circulation after oral transmucosal (OTM) administration to cats and provides pain relief when administered by this route. However, the authorized preparations contain preservative and cause salivation when given by the OTM route. Respiratory function should be monitored when given i.v. to anaesthetized patients. The response to all opioids appears to vary between individual patients, therefore, assessment of pain after administration is imperative. Methadone is metabolized in the liver, and some prolongation of effect may be seen with impaired liver function.

Safety and handling: Normal precautions should be observed.

Contraindications: No information available.

Adverse reactions: In common with other mu agonists, methadone can cause respiratory depression, although this is unlikely when used at clinical doses in conscious cats and dogs. Respiratory depression may occur when given i.v. during general anaesthesia due to increased depth of anaesthesia. Vomiting is rare, although methadone will cause constriction of GI sphincters (such as the pyloric sphincter) and may cause a reduction in GI motility when given over a long period. Methadone crosses the placenta and may exert sedative effects in neonates born to bitches treated prior to parturition. Severe adverse effects can be treated with naloxone.

Drug interactions: Other CNS depressants (e.g. anaesthetics, antihistamines, barbiturates, phenothiazines, tranquillizers) may cause increased CNS or respiratory depression when used concurrently with narcotic analgesics.

DOSES
When used for sedation is generally given as part of a combination. See Appendix for sedation protocols in cats and dogs.

Dogs: Analgesia: 0.1–0.5 mg/kg i.m. or 0.1–0.3 mg/kg i.v. prn.

Cats: Analgesia: 0.1–0.5 mg/kg i.m. or 0.1–0.3 mg/kg i.v. prn. Doses of around 0.6 mg/kg are appropriate for oral transmucosal administration in cats.

References
Ferreira TH, Rezende ML, Mama KR et al. (2011) Plasma concentrations and behavioural, antinociceptive and physiological effects of methadone after intravenous or oral transmucosal administration in cats. *American Journal of Veterinary Research* **72**, 764–771

Hunt JR, Attenburrow PM, Slingsby LS et al. (2013) Comparison of premedication with buprenorphine or methadone with meloxicam for postoperative analgesia in dogs undergoing orthopaedic surgery. *Journal of Small Animal Practice* **54**, 418–424

Methenamine (Hexamine hippurate)

(Hiprex*) **POM**

Formulations: Oral: 1 g methenamine hippurate (Hiprex) tablets.

Action: Urinary antiseptic.

Use:
- Long-term control of recurrent urinary tract infections (UTIs).

Evidence for efficacy is currently lacking in animals. Requires acidic urine.

Safety and handling: Normal precautions should be observed.

Contraindications: Severe renal or hepatic impairment, dehydration and metabolic acidosis.

Adverse reactions: Methenamine may cause GI disturbances, bladder irritation or a rash. Often poorly tolerated by cats.

Drug interactions: Efficacy is reduced when drugs that alkalinize urine (e.g. potassium citrate) are used concurrently.

DOSES

Dogs: Management of recurrent UTI: 500 mg/dog p.o. q12h (methenamine).

Cats: Management of recurrent UTI: 250 mg/cat p.o. q12h (methenamine).

References
Olin SJ and Bartges JW (2015) Urinary tract infections. *Veterinary Clinics of North America: Small Animal Practice* **45**, 721–756

Methimazole see Thiamazole

Methionine

(Methionine*) **general sale**

Formulations: Oral: 500 mg tablets.

Action: Urinary acidifier.

Use:
- Treatment of struvite urolithiasis.

There is an increased risk of acidosis if used with other urinary acidifying treatments. Used to be recommended for paracetamol poisoning, but alternative anti-oxidants are now preferred (e.g. acetylcysteine, *S*-adenosylmethionine).

Safety and handling: Normal precautions should be observed.

Contraindications: Renal failure or severe hepatic disease. Young age.

Adverse reactions: Overdosage may lead to metabolic acidosis.

Drug interactions: No information available.

DOSES

Dogs: Urine acidification: 100 mg/kg p.o. q12h. Adjust dose until urine pH $\leq$6.5.

Cats: Urine acidification: 200 mg/cat p.o. q8h. Adjust dose until urine pH $\leq$6.5.

References
Raditic DM (2015) Complementary and integrative therapies for lower urinary tract diseases. *Veterinary Clinics of North America: Small Animal Practice* **45**, 857–878

Methocarbamol

(Robaxin*) **POM**

`CIL`

Formulations: Oral: 500 mg, 750 mg tablets.

Action: Carbamate derivative of guaifenesin that is a CNS depressant with sedative and musculoskeletal relaxant properties. The mechanism of action has not been fully established; it has no direct action on the contractile mechanism of skeletal muscle, the motor endplate or the nerve fibre.

Use:
- Treatment of tetanus and some toxicities (e.g. pyrethroid, strychnine).
- General muscle relaxant for muscular spasms.

The clearance of methocarbamol is significantly impaired in human patients with renal and hepatic disease. There is very limited literature on the use of methocarbamol in cats; case reports describing the use of methocarbamol by intravenous bolus injection and CRI in dogs and cats have been published.

Safety and handling: Normal precautions should be observed.

Contraindications: No information available.

Adverse reactions: Salivation, emesis, lethargy, weakness and ataxia.

Drug interactions: As methocarbamol is a CNS depressant, additive depression may occur when given with other CNS depressants.

DOSES

Dogs, Cats: 20–45 mg/kg p.o. q8h. Very high doses may be required for tetanus. It is recommended that the dose does not exceed 330 mg/kg, although serious toxicity or death has not been reported after overdoses.

References

Draper WE, Bolfer L, Cottam E *et al.* (2013) Methocarbamol CRI for symptomatic treatment of pyrethroid intoxication: a report of three cases. *Journal of the American Animal Hospital Association* **49**, 325–328

Nielsen C and Pluhar GE (2005) Diagnosis and treatment of hindlimb muscle strain injuries in 22 dogs. *Veterinary and Comparative Orthopaedics and Traumatology* **18**, 247–253

Methoprene (*S*-Methoprene)

(Amflee combo [c,d], Bob Martin Clear plus [c,d], Broadline [c], Chanonil plus [c,d], Dadektin Combo [c,d], Duoflect [c,d], Eziflea plus [c,d], Fipnil plu [c,d], Fiproclear [c,d], Fiprotec [c,d], Fleanil Duo [c,d], Fleascreen Combo [c,d], Frontline Combo/Plus [c,d], Fyperix Combo [c,d], Itch Flea [c,d], Joii flea and tick [c,d], On Defence flea and tick [d], Pestigon Combo [c,d], Strecti [c,d], Vetbo [c,d], VetUK flea and Tick treatment Plus [c,d], Zeronil Plus [c,d], Zerotal plus [c,d])
POM-V, AVM-GSL

Formulations: Usually in combination with other agents.
Topical: 9% *S*-methoprene + fipronil in spot-on pipettes of various sizes; *S*-methoprene + eprinomectin + fipronil + praziquantel.
Environmental: *S*-methoprene + permethrin or tetramethrine + permethrin household sprays.

Action: Juvenile hormone analogue that inhibits larval development.

Use:
- Treatment and prevention of flea infestations (*Ctenocephalides canis* and *C. felis*).
- Environmental sprays also have some efficacy against house dust mites *Dermatophagoides farinae* and *D. pteronyssinus*.

For treatment of flea infestations the topical products should be applied every 4 weeks to all in-contact cats and dogs (Spot-on products). Bathing is not recommended between 48 hours before and 24 hours after topical application. Minimum treatment interval 4 weeks. Can be used in pregnant and lactating females. Treat infested household as directed with spray; keep away from birds and fish.

Safety and handling: Normal precautions should be observed.

Contraindications: None (but see entries for other active agents).

Adverse reactions: Local pruritus or alopecia may occur at the site of application. May be harmful to aquatic organisms.

Drug interactions: No information available.

DOSES
See Appendix for guidelines on responsible parasiticide use.
Dogs, Cats: Fleas: 1 pipette per animal monthly according to weight.

References
Curtis C (2004) Current trends in the treatment of *Sarcoptes*, *Cheyletiella* and *Otodectes* mite infestations in dogs and cats. *Veterinary Dermatology* **15**, 108–114

Methotrexate
(Matrex*, Methotrexate*) **POM**

Formulations: Oral: 2.5 mg, 10 mg tablets.

Action: An S-phase-specific antimetabolite antineoplastic agent; competitively inhibits folic acid reductase which is required for purine synthesis, DNA synthesis and cellular replication. This results in inhibition of DNA synthesis and function.

Use:
- Treatment of lymphoma, although its use in animals is often limited by toxicity.
- Also reports of use in canine atopic dermatitis.

In humans, it is used to treat refractory rheumatoid arthritis; however, data are lacking with regards to its use in canine and feline immune-mediated polyarthritides. Monitor haematological parameters regularly.

Safety and handling: Cytotoxic drug; see Appendix and specialist texts for further advice on chemotherapeutic agents.

Contraindications: Pre-existing myelosuppression, severe hepatic or renal insufficiency, or hypersensitivity to the drug.

Adverse reactions: Adverse GI effects (vomiting, diarrhoea, anorexia, nausea) appear the most prevalent. Particularly with high doses, GI ulceration, mucositis, hepatotoxicity, nephrotoxicity, alopecia, depigmentation, pulmonary infiltrates and haemopoietic toxicity may be seen. Low blood pressure and skin reactions are seen in humans. Rarely, anaphylaxis can be seen.

Drug interactions: Methotrexate is a substrate of the ABCG-2 drug transporter and, therefore, may have clinicaly significant interactions with many other drugs. Methotrexate is highly bound to serum albumin and thus may be displaced by phenylbutazone, phenytoin, salicylates, sulphonamides and tetracycline, resulting in increased blood levels and toxicity. Folic acid supplements may inhibit the response to methotrexate (but folate deficiency increases toxicity). Methotrexate increases the cytotoxicity of cytarabine. Cellular uptake is decreased by hydrocortisone, methylprednisolone and penicillins, and is increased by vincristine. Concurrent use of NSAIDs increases the risk of haematological, renal and hepatic toxicity.

DOSES

See Appendix for chemotherapy protocols and conversion of bodyweight to body surface area. It is advised to seek specialist veterinary oncology advise before using this drug.

Dogs: All uses: 2.5–5 mg/m^2 p.o. twice weekly. Adjust the frequency of dosing according to toxic effects. Usually as part of a multidrug chemotherapy protocol.

Cats: All uses: 2.5 mg/m^2 p.o. twice weekly or 0.5–0.6 mg/kg i.v. every 14 days. Adjust the frequency of dosing according to toxic effects. Usually as part of a multidrug chemotherapy protocol.

References

Intile JL, Rassnick KM, Al-Sarraf R and Chretin JD (2019) Evaluation of the tolerability of combination chemotherapy with mitoxantrone and dacarbazine in dogs with lymphoma. *Journal of the American Animal Hospital Association* **55**, 101–109

Methylene blue see Methylthioninium chloride

Methylprednisolone

(Depo-Medrone [c,d], Medrone [c,d], Solu-Medrone [c,d]) **POM-V**

Formulations: Injectable: 40 mg/ml depot suspension of methylprednisolone acetate (Depo-Medrone); 125 mg, 500 mg methylprednisolone sodium succinate powder for reconstitution (Solu-Medrone). **Oral:** 2 mg, 4 mg tablets (Medrone).

Action: Alters the transcription of DNA leading to alterations in cellular metabolism which result in anti-inflammatory, immunosuppressive and antifibrotic effects. Also acts in dogs as an arginine vasopressin antagonist.

Use:
- Anti-inflammatory agent with five times the anti-inflammatory potency of hydrocortisone and 20% more potency than prednisolone.

On a dose basis, 0.8 mg methylprednisolone is equivalent to 1 mg prednisolone. The oral formulation of methylprednisolone is suitable for alternate-day use. The use of steroids in shock and acute spinal cord injury is controversial and many specialists do not use them. Any value in administering steroids declines rapidly after the onset of shock or injury, while the side effects remain constant and may be substantial. Doses should be tapered to the lowest effective dose. Animals receiving chronic therapy should be tapered off steroids when discontinuing them.

Safety and handling: Normal precautions should be observed.

Contraindications: Do not use in pregnant animals. Systemic corticosteroids are generally contraindicated in patients with renal disease and diabetes mellitus.

Adverse reactions: Prolonged use suppresses the hypothalamic–pituitary–adrenal axis and causes adrenal atrophy. Catabolic effects of glucocorticoids lead to weight loss and cutaneous atrophy. Iatrogenic hypercortisolism may develop with long-term use. Vomiting and diarrhoea may be seen and GI ulceration may develop. Glucocorticoids may increase urine glucose levels and decrease serum T3 and T4. Impaired wound healing and delayed recovery from infections may be seen.

Drug interactions: There is an increased risk of GI ulceration if used concurrently with NSAIDs. Hypokalaemia may develop if amphotericin B or potassium-depleting diuretics (furosemide, thiazides) are administered concomitantly with corticosteroids. Insulin requirements are likely to increase in patients taking glucocorticoids. The metabolism of corticosteroids may be enhanced by phenobarbital or phenytoin and decreased by antifungals (e.g. itraconazole).

DOSES
Dogs:
- **Inflammation:** initially 1–2 mg/kg i.m. (methylprednisolone acetate depot injection) q1–3wk or 0.2–0.5 mg/kg p.o. q12h.
- **Hypoadrenocorticism (acute crisis):** 1 mg/kg i.v. (meythprednisolone sodium succinate) followed by 0.5–1 mg/kg i.v. q8–12h until oral supplementation started
- **Immunosuppression:** 1–3 mg/kg p.o. q12h, reducing to 1–2 mg/kg p.o. q48h.

Cats:
- **Asthma:** 1–2 mg/kg i.m. (depot injection) q1–3wk.
- **Inflammation/flea allergy:** 1–2 mg/kg i.m. (depot injection) every 2 months or 1 mg/kg p.o. q24h reducing to 2–5 mg/cat p.o. q48h. Some sources propose 1–20 mg per cat although the risk of iatrogenic diabetes mellitus may be greater with higher doses (unpublished data).

Methylthioninium chloride (Methylene blue)

(Methylthioninium chloride*) **POM**

Formulations: Injectable: 10 mg/ml (1% solution).

Action: Acts as an electron donor to methaemoglobin reductase.

Use:
- Treatment of methaemoglobinaemia.

Use an in-line filter if possible.

Safety and handling: Normal precautions should be observed.

Contraindications: Do not use unless adequate renal function is demonstrated.

Adverse reactions: May cause a Heinz body haemolytic anaemia, especially in cats (relatively contraindicated in this species), and renal failure.

Drug interactions: No information available.

DOSES

Dogs: Methaemoglobinaemia: 1–1.5 mg/kg i.v. slowly once; can be repeated if necessary.

Cats: Methaemoglobinaemia: Use with extreme caution (many consider contraindicated in this species): 1–1.5 mg/kg i.v. slowly once only.

References

Wray JD (2008) Methaemoglobinaemia caused by hydroxycarbamide (hydroxyurea) ingestion in a dog. *Journal of Small Animal Practice* **49**, 211–215

Metoclopramide

(Emeprid [c,d], Metomotyl [c,d], Vomend [c,d]) **POM-V**

Formulations: Injectable: 5 mg/ml solution. **Oral:** 1 mg/ml solution.

Action: Has an antiemetic effect via central dopamine (D2) receptor antagonism and, at higher doses, $5HT_3$ antagonism at the chemoreceptor trigger zone. Dopamine receptors are more important in the vomiting reflex in dogs than in cats, so metoclopramide is less likely to be effective in cats. Gastric prokinetic effect is a result of local D2 antagonism and stimulation of muscarinic acetylcholine and $5HT_4$ receptors leading to increases in oesophageal sphincter pressure, the tone and amplitude of gastric contractions and peristaltic activity in the duodenum and jejunum, and relaxation of the pyloric sphincter. Prokinetic effects appear to be weak and distal intestinal motility is not significantly affected.

Use:
*   Treatment of vomiting of many causes.
*   Prokinetic effect may be beneficial in gastro-oesophageal reflux disease.

Safety and handling: Injection is light sensitive. Obscure fluid bag if used in a CRI.

Contraindications: Do not use where GI obstruction or perforation is present or for >48 hours without a definitive diagnosis. Do not use in the case of gastrointestinal haemorrhage. Do not use in epileptic patients. Reduce dose by 50% in animals with reduced kidney or liver function. Avoid in dogs with pseudopregnancy. In animals with phaeochromo-cytoma, metoclopramide may induce a hypertensive crisis.

Adverse reactions: Unusual, although more common in cats than dogs, and probably relate to relative overdosing and individual variations in bioavailability. The observed effects are transient and disappear when treatment is stopped. They include changes in mentation and behaviour (agitation, ataxia, abnormal positions and/or movements, prostration, tremors, aggression and vocalization). It may also cause sedation. Cats may exhibit signs of frenzied behaviour or disorientation. Very rarely, allergic reactions may occur.

Drug interactions: The activity of metoclopramide may be inhibited by antimuscarinic drugs (e.g. atropine) and narcotic analgesics. The effects of metoclopramide may decrease (e.g. cimetidine, digoxin) or increase (e.g. oxytetracycline) drug absorption. The absorption of nutrients may be accelerated, thereby altering insulin requirements and/or timing of its effects in diabetics. Phenothiazines may potentiate the extrapyramidal effects of metoclopramide. The CNS effects of metoclopramide may be enhanced by narcotic analgesics or sedatives.

DOSES

Dogs, Cats: All uses: 0.25–0.5 mg/kg i.v., i.m., s.c., p.o. q12h; 0.17–0.33 mg/kg i.v., i.m., s.c., p.o. q8h; 1–2 mg/kg i.v. over 24 hours as a CRI.

References

Husnik R, Gaschen FP, Fletcher JM and Gaschen L (2020) Ultrasonographic assessment of the effect of metoclopramide, erythromycin, and exenatide on solid-phase gastric emptying in healthy cats. *Journal of Veterinary Internal Medicine* **34**, 1440–1446

Kempf J, Lewis F, Reusch CE *et al.* (2013) High-resolution manometric evaluation of the effects of cisapride and metoclopramide hydrochloride administered orally on lower esophageal sphincter pressure in awake dogs. *American Journal of Veterinary Research* **75**, 361–366

Metronidazole `CIL`

(Metrobactin [c,d], Metrovis [c,d], Stomorgyl [c,d], Metronidazole*) **POM-V, POM**

Formulations: Injectable: 5 mg/ml i.v. infusion. Oral: 100 mg, 250 mg, 500 mg, 750 mg tablets; 25 mg metronidazole + 46.9 mg spiramycin, 125 mg metronidazole + 234.4 mg spiramycin, 250 mg metronidazole + 469 mg spiramycin tablets (Stomorgyl 2, 10 and 20, respectively); 40 mg/ml oral solution.

Action: Synthetic nitroimidazole with antibacterial and antiprotozoal activity. Its mechanism of action on protozoans is unknown but in bacteria it appears to be reduced spontaneously under anaerobic conditions to compounds that bind to DNA and cause cell death. Spiramycin is a macrolide antibacterial that inhibits bacterial protein synthesis.

Use:
- Treatment of anaerobic infections, including GI infections caused by *Clostridial* spp.
- Management of hepatic encephalopathy.
- No longer recommended to treat chronic enteropathy. Evidence of potential effects on the immune system (modulation of cell-mediated immune responses) in cats and dogs is limited while a negative impact on the canine microbiome has been documented.

Absorbed well from the GI tract and diffuses into many tissues including bone, CSF and abscesses. Spiramycin (a constituent of Stomorgyl) is active against Gram-positive aerobes including *Staphylococcus*, *Streptococcus*, *Bacillus* and *Actinomyces*. Metronidazole is frequently used in combination with penicillin or aminoglycoside antimicrobials to extend the spectrum of activity. There is a greater risk of adverse effects with rapid i.v. infusion or high total doses. It is no longer used in dogs and cats for the treatment of giardiasis as fenbendazole and others are preferred.

Safety and handling: Normal precautions should be observed. Impervious gloves should be used when handling metronidazole and hands washed thoroughly to avoid skin contact.

Contraindications: Avoid use during pregnancy (may be a teratogen especially in early pregnancy). Reduce dose if used in animals with hepatic disease.

Adverse reactions: Adverse effects are generally limited to vomiting, CNS toxicity (nystagmus, ataxia, knuckling, head tilt and seizures), hepatotoxicity, neutropenia and haematuria. Excessive salivation/foaming is noted in some cats. Impaired sense of smell has been reported in explosive detection dogs (resolved following withdrawal of drug). Prolonged therapy or the presence of pre-existing hepatic disease may predispose to CNS toxicity.

Drug interactions: Phenobarbital or phenytoin may enhance metabolism of metronidazole. Cimetidine may decrease the metabolism of metronidazole and increase the likelihood of dose-related adverse effects. Spiramycin should not be used concurrently with other antibiotics of the macrolide group as the combination may be antagonistic.

DOSES

Classified as category D (Prudence) by the EMA.

See Appendix for guidelines on responsible antibiotic use.

Dogs, Cats:
- Metronidazole:
  - **Hepatic encephalopathy:** 7.5 mg/kg p.o. q8−12h.
  - **Antibiosis:** 10−15 mg/kg p.o., s.c., slow i.v. infusion q12h. Label doses are 25 mg/kg q12h p.o. but doses >30 mg/kg per day may increase the risk of neurotoxicosis.
- Stomorgyl: 12.5 mg metronidazole + 23.4 mg spiramycin/kg p.o. (equivalent to 1 tablet/2 kg of Stomorgyl 2, 1 tablet/10 kg of Stomorgyl 10 and 1 tablet/20 kg of Stomorgyl 20) q24h for 5−10 days.

References

Cerquetella M, Rossi G, Suchodolski JS *et al.* (2020) Proposal for rational antibacterial use in the diagnosis and treatment of dogs with chronic diarrhoea. *Journal of Small Animal Practice* **61**, 211−215

Ortiz V, Klein L, Channell S *et al.* (2018) Evaluating the effect of metronidazole plus amoxicillin-clavulanate *versus* amoxicillin-clavulanate alone in canine haemorrhagic diarrhoea: a randomised controlled trial in primary care practice. *Journal of Small Animal Practice* **59**, 398−403

Tauro A, Beltran E, Cherubini GB *et al.* (2018) Metronidazole-induced neurotoxicity in 26 dogs. *Australian Veterinary Journal* **96**, 495−501

Mexiletine

CIL

(Mexitil*, Ritalmex*) **POM**

Formulations: Oral: 50 mg, 100 mg, 200 mg capsules. Only available by Special Import Certificate in the UK. Alternative special reformulations available: 50 mg and 100 mg tablets. **VSP**

Action: Class 1b antiarrhythmic agent similar to lidocaine. It is an inhibitor of the inward sodium current (fast sodium channel), which reduces the rate of rise of the action potential. In the Purkinje fibres it decreases automaticity, the action potential duration and the effective refractory period.

Use:
- Management of rapid or haemodynamically significant ventricular arrhythmias such as frequent complex ventricular premature complexes or ventricular tachycardia.
- Also proven to be effective in some dogs with supraventricular tachycardia due to the presence of an accessory conduction pathway (bypass tract).

Often effective if there has been a response to i.v. lidocaine. Has been combined with sotalol in dogs not fully responsive to sotalol alone, with enhanced effect. Can be given orally at the same time as beta blockers, such as atenolol at 0.5–1 mg/kg q12–24h. Not proven to prevent sudden death in dogs with severe ventricular arrhythmias. Use cautiously in patients with severe CHF, sinus node dysfunction, hepatic dysfunction and seizure disorders. Administer oral dose with food to alleviate adverse GI effects.

Safety and handling: Normal precautions should be observed.

Contraindications: 2nd or 3rd degree AV block not treated by pacemaker therapy.

Adverse reactions: Nausea, anorexia, vomiting, depression, convulsions, tremor, nystagmus, bradycardia, hypotension, jaundice and hepatitis.

Drug interactions: The absorption of mexiletine may be delayed by atropine and opioid analgesics. Mexiletine excretion may be reduced by acetazolamide and alkaline urine, and increased by urinary acidifying drugs (e.g. methionine). The action of mexiletine may be antagonized by hypokalaemia. Cimetidine decreases the rate of mexiletine elimination.

DOSES
Dogs: 4–8 mg/kg p.o. q8–12h; i.v. dose not established.
Cats: No information available.

References
Gelzer ARM, Kraus MS, Rishniw M *et al.* (2010) Combination therapy with mexiletine and sotalol suppresses inherited ventricular arrhythmias in German Shepherd Dogs better than mexiletine or sotalol monotherapy: a randomized cross-over study. *Journal of Veterinary Cardiology* **12**, 93–106

Miconazole

(Adaxio [d], Aurimic [c,d], Easotic [d], Malaseb [c,d], Surolan [c,d], Daktarin*) **POM-V, P**

Formulations: Topical: 2% shampoo (Adaxio); 23 mg/ml suspension (Aurimic); 2% cream/powder (Daktarin); 15.1 mg/ml with hydrocortisone and gentamicin (Easotic); 2% shampoo (Malaseb); 23 mg/ml suspension with prednisolone and polymyxin (Surolan).

Action: Inhibits cytochrome P450-dependent synthesis of ergosterol in fungal cells causing increased cell wall permeability and allowing leakage of cellular contents. Miconazole has activity against *Malassezia*, *Cryptococcus*, *Candida* and *Coccidioides*.

Use:
- Treatment of fungal skin and ear infections, including dermatophytosis.
- Miconazole shampoo is useful in the treatment of dermatophytosis in cats but concurrent itraconazole administration is required.

Safety and handling: Normal precautions should be observed.

Contraindications: No information available.

Adverse reactions: No information available.

Drug interactions: No information available.

DOSES
Dogs:
- Fungal otitis: 2–12 drops in affected ear q12–24h (Surolan). 1 ml per ear q24h for 5 days (Easotic). 5 drops in affected ear q12h (Aurimic).

- **Dermatophytosis:** apply a thin layer of cream topically to affected area twice daily. Continue for 2 weeks after a clinical cure and negative fungal cultures.
- *Malassezia* **dermatitis:** shampoo twice weekly until the clinical signs subside and weekly thereafter or as necessary to keep the condition under control (Malaseb, Adaxio).
- **Small localized skin infections:** apply a few drops to affected skin q12h (Aurimic).

Cats:
- **Fungal otitis:** doses as for dogs.
- **Dermatophytosis:** doses as for dogs.
- *Microsporum canis:* shampoo twice weekly while administering itraconazole for 6–10 weeks or until coat brushings are negative for the culture of *M. canis*, whichever is the longer (Malaseb). The maximum length of the treatment period should not exceed 16 weeks.
- **Small localized skin infections:** doses as for dogs.

References

Moriello KA (2004) Treatment of dermatophytosis in dogs and cats: review of published studies. *Veterinary Dermatology* **15**, 99–107

Mueller RS, Bergvall K, Bensignor E *et al.* (2012) A review of topical therapy for skin infections with bacteria and yeast. *Veterinary Dermatology* **23**, 330–341

Midazolam

(Dormazolam, Buccolam*, Epistatus*, Hypnovel* and several others) **POM-V, POM**

Formulations: Injectable: 1 mg/ml, 2 mg/ml, 5 mg/ml solutions. **Oromucosal solution:** 5 mg/ml in pre-filled syringes of 0.5 ml, 1 ml, 1.5 ml, 2 ml; 10 mg/ml pre-filled syringe. Dormazolam is authorized in horses.

Action: Causes neural inhibition by increasing the effect of GABA on the GABAA receptor, resulting in sedation, anxiolytic effects, hypnotic effects, amnesia, muscle relaxation and anticonvulsive effects. Compared with diazepam, it is more potent, has a shorter onset and duration of action (<1 hour in dogs) and is less irritant to tissues.

Use:
- Provides sedation with amnesia; as part of a premedication regime or as part of combined anaesthetic protocols.
- Emergency control of epileptic seizures (including status epilepticus).

Provides unreliable sedation as a sole agent, although it will sedate depressed animals. It is often used to offset muscle hypertonicity caused by ketamine. It is used with opioids and/or acepromazine for pre-anaesthetic medication in the critically ill. If used at induction it may reduce propofol or alfaxalone requirement. Midazolam can be diluted with saline, but avoid fluids containing calcium as this may result in precipitation of midazolam. Use with caution in severe hypotension, cardiac disease and respiratory disease. As it is metabolized by the cytochrome P450 enzyme system, care should be taken in animals with hepatic impairment. Flumazenil (a benzodiazepine antagonist) will reverse the effects of midazolam.

Safety and handling: Normal precautions should be observed.

Contraindications: Avoid in neonates.

Adverse reactions: In human patients, i.v. administration of midazolam has been associated with respiratory depression and severe hypotension. Excitement may occasionally develop.

Drug interactions: Midazolam potentiates the effect of some anaesthetic agents, including propofol and some inhalation agents, reducing the dose required. Concurrent use of midazolam with NSAIDs (in particular diclofenac), antihistamines, barbiturates, opioid analgesics or CNS depressants may enhance the sedative effect. Opioid analgesics may increase the hypnotic and hypotensive effects of midazolam. Erythromycin inhibits the metabolism of midazolam.

DOSES
When used for sedation is generally given as part of a combination. See Appendix for sedation protocols in cats and dogs.
Dogs, Cats:
- Emergency management of seizures including status epilepticus: bolus dose of 0.2–0.3 mg/kg i.v. Time to onset of clinical effect is rapid for i.v. use, therefore, repeat q10min if there is no clinical effect (up to 3 times).
- Can be given rectally if venous access is not available, although it has been shown to be more effective at controlling status epilepticus if given intranasally in dogs.
- Midazolam may be used in conjunction with diazepam for emergency control of seizures. In dogs, additional doses may be administered if appropriate supportive care facilities are available (for support of respiration). Once the seizures have been controlled, the dog can be maintained on a CRI of 0.3 mg/kg/h.

References
Charalambous M, Bhatti S, Van Ham L *et al.* (2017) Intranasal Midazolam versus Rectal Diazepam for the Management of Canine Status Epilepticus: A Multicenter Randomized Parallel-Group Clinical Trial. *Journal of veterinary internal medicine* **31**, 1149–1158
Minghella E, Auckburally A, Pawson P *et al.* (2016) Clinical effects of midazolam or lidocaine co-induction with a propofol target-controlled infusion (TCI) in dogs. *Veterinary Anaesthesia and Analgesia* **43**, 472–481
Schwartz M, Muñana KR, Nettifee-Osborne JA *et al.* (2013) The pharmacokinetics of midazolam after intravenous, intramuscular, and rectal administration in healthy dogs. *Journal of Veterinary Pharmacology and Therapeutics* **36**, 471–477

Milbemycin
(Credelio Plus [d], Milbactor [c,d], Milbemax [c,d], Milprazon [c,d], Milpro [c,d], Milquantel [c,d], Nexgard Spectra [d], Program plus [d], Trifexis) **POM-V**

Formulations: Always in combination with other agents. **Oral:** 2.5 mg, 12.5 mg milbemycin with praziquantel tablets (Milbemax for dogs and several others); 4 mg, 16 mg with praziquantel tablets (Milbemax for cats); 2.3 mg, 5.75 mg, 11.5 mg, 23 mg milbemycin with lufenuron tablets (20 mg lufeneron:1 mg milbemycin; Program plus); 1.875 mg, 3.75 mg, 7.5 mg, 15 mg, 30 mg milbemycin with afoxolaner (Nexgard Spectra); 4.5 mg, 7.1 mg, 11.1 mg, 17.4 mg, 27 mg milbemycin with spinosad (Trifexis).

Action: Interacts with GABA and glutamate-gated channels, leading to flaccid paralysis of parasites.

Use:
- Treatment of adult nematode infestation; roundworms (*Toxocara canis*, *T. cati*), hookworms (*Ancylostoma caninum*, *A. tubaeforme*), whipworms (*Trichuris vulpis*) and cestodes (*Dipylidium caninum*, *Taenia* spp., *Echinococcus* spp., *Mesocestoides* spp.).
- Prevention of heartworm disease (*Dirofilaria immitis*) in countries where this parasite is endemic.
- Can also be used to treat nasal mite infestations by weekly administration for 3 weeks.
- Treatment of *Angiostrongylus vasorum* infections, milbemycin oxime should be given 4 times at weekly intervals. Reduction of the level of infection of *Crenosoma vulpis*.
- Treatment of *Thelazia callipaeda*, milbemycin oxime should be given in 2 treatments, 7 days apart.
- Some efficacy against adult fleas.

Can be used in pregnant and lactating females.

Safety and handling: Normal precautions should be observed.

Contraindications: Do not use in animals suspected of having heartworm disease. Not for use in dogs <2 weeks, cats <6 weeks or any animal <0.5 kg.

Adverse reactions: No information available. The safety of milbemycin in dogs with an *ABCB1* mutation has not been demonstrated and these dogs may be at increased risk of adverse effects.

Drug interactions: No information available.

DOSES
See Appendix for guidelines on responsible parasiticide use.
Dogs: Nematodes: 0.5 mg milbemycin/kg p.o. q30d. For *Angiostrongylus vasorum*, administer same dose 4 times at weekly intervals.
Cats: Nematodes: 2 mg milbemycin/kg p.o. q30d.

Miltefosine
(Milteforan) **POM-V**

Formulations: Oral: 20 mg/ml solution.

Action: Directly toxic to *Leishmania* and also enhances T cell and macrophage activation.

Use:
- Treatment of canine leishmaniosis leading to a substantial reduction in the parasitic load without complete elimination (similar to other treatment strategies).

Nearly as effective as the allopurinol/meglumine antimonate protocol with fewer serious side effects. A Special Treatment Authorization is required to obtain this product (it is authorized for veterinary use in Spain and Germany). It is recommended to pour the product on to the animal's food to reduce digestive side effects. Allopurinol is recommended as an adjunctive treatment and should be continued after the course of miltefosine is complete.

Safety and handling: May cause eye and skin irritation and sensitization: personal protective equipment consisting of gloves and glasses should be worn when handling. To avoid foaming, do not shake the vial.

Contraindications: Do not use during pregnancy, lactation or in breeding animals.

Adverse reactions: Moderate and transient vomiting and diarrhoea are very common and can last up to 7 days. The side effects do not affect the efficacy of the product and do not require discontinuation of treatment or dose change. Overdoses may produce uncontrollable vomiting.

Drug interactions: No information available.

DOSES
See Appendix for guidelines on responsible parasiticide use.

Dogs: Leishmaniosis: 2 mg/kg p.o. q24h for 28 days (it is particularly important that the full course is completed and given with allopurinol).

Cats: No information available.

References
Iarussi F, aradies P, Manzillo VF *et al.* (2020) Comparison of Two Dosing Regimens of Miltefosine, Both in Combination With Allopurinol, on Clinical and Parasitological Findings of Dogs With Leishmaniosis: A Pilot Study. *Frontiers in veterinary science* **7**, 577395

Manna L, Corso R, Galiero G *et al.* (2015) Long-term follow-up of dogs with leishmaniosis treated with meglumine antimoniate plus allopurinol *versus* miltefosine plus allopurinol. *Parasites and Vectors* **28**, 289

Miró G, Oliva G, Cruz I *et al.* (2009) Multicentric, controlled clinical study to evaluate effectiveness and safety of miltefosine and allopurinol for canine leishmaniosis. *Veterinary Dermatology* **20**, 397–404

Mineral oil see **Paraffin**

Minocycline
(Aknemin*, Minocin*) **POM**

Formulations: Oral: 50 mg, 100 mg capsules or tablets.

Action: Inhibition of bacterial protein synthesis by binding to the 30S subunit of the bacterial ribosome. Minocycline is the most lipid-soluble tetracycline with a broad spectrum of antibacterial activity in addition to antirickettsial, antimycoplasmal and antichlamydial activity. Due to its superior lipid solubility it tends to have greater clinical efficacy compared with other tetracyclines.

Use:
- Treatment of bacterial, rickettsial, mycoplasmal and chlamydial diseases.
- Often recommended in treatment protocols for heartworm disease (dirofilariasis).

Appears to be an effective alternative to doxycycline for the treatment of non-acute *Ehrlichia canis*. Its rate of excretion is not affected by renal function as it is cleared by hepatic metabolism and is therefore recommended when tetracyclines are indicated in animals with renal impairment. Use with care in animals with hepatic disease. Being extremely lipid-soluble, it penetrates well into prostatic fluid and bronchial secretions. If oral dosing in cats, avoid dry pilling as for doxycycline and follow with a water bolus to reduce the risk of oesophageal erosions. Recommended doses for veterinary species have not been clearly defined and recommendations are made on anecdote and a small number of studies.

Safety and handling: Normal precautions should be observed.

Contraindications: No specific information available. Should not be used in pregnant or young animals.

Adverse reactions: Nausea, vomiting and diarrhoea. In common with other tetracyclines may cause bone and teeth abnormalities if used in developing animals.

Drug interactions: Absorption of minocycline is reduced by antacids, calcium, magnesium and iron salts, and sucralfate. Phenobarbital and phenytoin may increase its metabolism, decreasing plasma levels.

DOSES
Classified as category D (Prudence) by the EMA.
See Appendix for guidelines on responsible antibiotic use.
Dogs, Cats: 5–10 mg/kg p.o. q12h.

References
Maaland MG, Guardabassi L and Papich MG (2014) Minocycline pharmacokinetics and pharmacodynamics in dogs: Dosage recommendations for treatment of meticillin-resistant *Staphylococcus pseudintermedius* infections. *Veterinary Dermatology* **25**, 182–190
Tynan BE, Papich MG, Kerl ME *et al.* (2015) Pharmacokinetics of minocycline in domestic cats. *Journal of Feline Medicine and Surgery* **18**, 257–263

Mirtazapine
(Mirataz^c, Zispin) **POM-V, POM**

Formulations: Oral: 15 mg tablets, 15 mg/ml solution. **Topical:** 20 mg/g transdermal ointment.

Action: Tricyclic antidepressant that acts on central alpha-2 receptors, increasing noradrenaline levels within the brain. Also inhibits several types of serotonin and histamine (H1) receptors.

Use:
- Appetite stimulation. Efficacy in cats with stable chronic kidney disease has been demonstrated.
- Antiemetic role in conjunction with other drugs, but authorized preparations should be used.
- Anecdotal evidence beginning to appear concerning its use in the management of anxiety in dogs, including those being treated with antiepileptic medication, but no controlled studies published.

Monitor animal carefully, particularly if there is also cardiac, hepatic or renal disease.

Safety and handling: Normal precautions should be observed.

Contraindications: Do not use in patients with pre-existing haematological disease.

Adverse reactions: Sedation is common and can be profound. Can affect behaviour in many different ways, increased vocalization and interaction with others. Has been associated with blood dyscrasias in humans.

Drug interactions: Several interactions known in humans, principally involving other behaviour-modifying drugs. Avoid concommittant use with other serotonergic agents.

DOSES
Dogs: 1.1–1.3 mg/kg p.o. q24h (do not exceed 30 mg total dose per day).
Cats: 2 mg/cat p.o. or administered topically on inner pinna of ear q24–48h.

Misoprostol

CIL

(Angusta*, Cytotec*, Topogyne*) **POM**

Formulations: Oral: 25 μg (microgram), 200 μg, 400 μg tablets.

Action: Cytoprotection of the gastric mucosa: it inhibits gastric acid secretion and increases bicarbonate and mucus secretion, epithelial cell turnover and mucosal blood flow. It prevents, and promotes healing of, gastric and duodenal ulcers, particularly those associated with the use of NSAIDs. Some reports suggest it may not prevent gastric bleeding associated with high doses of methylprednisolone. It may also be useful in the management of canine atopy, although other treatments are likely safer.

Use:
- Protection against NSAID-induced gastric ulceration.
- Has been used in combination with aglepristone to induce abortion in dogs and cats.

Give with food. Combinations with diclofenac are available for humans, but are not suitable for small animals because of different NSAID pharmacokinetics. In humans, higher doses (20 μg (micrograms)/kg p.o. q6–12h) are used to manage pre-existing NSAID-induced gastric ulceration, while doses of 2–5 μg/kg p.o. q6–8h are used prophylactically to prevent ulceration.

Safety and handling: People who are or may become pregnant should not handle this drug.

Contraindications: Do not use in pregnant animals.

Adverse reactions: Diarrhoea, abdominal pain, nausea, vomiting and abortion.

Drug interactions: Use of misoprostol with gentamicin may exacerbate renal dysfunction.

DOSES

Dogs:
- **Protection against NSAID-induced gastric ulceration:** 2–5 μg (micrograms)/kg p.o. q8–12h.
- **Atopic dermatitis:** 3–6 μg/kg p.o. q8h has been suggested.

Cats: **Protection against NSAID-induced gastric ulceration:** 5 μg (micrograms)/kg p.o. q8h.

Mitotane (o,p'-DDD)

CIL

(Lysodren*) **POM**

Formulations: Oral: 500 mg tablets or capsules.

Action: Necrosis of the adrenal cortex reducing the production of adrenal cortical hormones.

Use:
- Management of pituitary-dependent hypercortisolism in dogs. However, other medications are authorized for this condition (see Trilostane).
- Has been used in the management of adrenal-dependent hypercortisolism with variable success.

Mitotane is available from Europe for animals that have failed to respond to trilostane therapy. It should be given with food high in fat/oil to improve its absorption. Closely monitor for any decrease in appetite (typically seen within 3–10 days of therapy); an ACTH response test should be performed to monitor treatment efficacy. In diabetic animals, the insulin dose should be reduced by 30%. The addition of prednisolone is generally not recommended. If switching from trilostane to mitotane, then post-ACTH cortisol concentrations should be >200 nmol (nanomoles)/l before starting mitotane. Not recommended in cats as trilostane is more likely to be effective.

Safety and handling: Drug crosses skin and mucous membrane barriers. Wear gloves when handling this drug and avoid inhalation of dust.

Contraindications: No information available.

Adverse reactions: Anorexia, vomiting, diarrhoea and weakness, generally associated with too rapid a drop in plasma cortisol levels. They usually resolve with steroid supplementation. Acute-onset of neurological signs may be seen 2–3 weeks after initiation of therapy, possibly due to rapid growth of a pituitary tumour. Provide supplemental glucocorticoids during periods of stress. Approximately 5% of dogs require permanent glucocorticoid and mineralocorticoid replacement therapy if given mitotane overdose.

Drug interactions: Barbiturates and corticosteroids increase the hepatic metabolism of mitotane. There may be enhanced CNS depression with concurrent use of CNS depressants. Spironolactone blocks the action of mitotane. Diabetic animals may have rapidly changing insulin requirements during the early stages of therapy.

DOSES
Dogs: 30–50 mg/kg p.o. (with/after food) q24h to effect (generally 3–10 days) then 50 mg/kg p.o. q7–14 days in 2–3 divided doses as required. Higher doses (50–150 mg/kg p.o. q24h) may become necessary for adrenal carcinomas.

Cats: Similar dose to dogs but efficacy is very variable, with many showing no response at non-toxic levels.

Mitoxantrone
(Novantrone*) **POM**

Formulations: Injectable: 2 mg/ml.

Action: Antitumour antibiotic which inhibits topoisomerase II. It is cell cycle non-specific, but most active during S phase.

Use:
- Treatment of canine and feline lymphoma, squamous cell carcinoma (SCC) and transitional cell carcinoma.
- Its use has also been described in many other cancers, including renal adenocarcinoma, fibroid sarcoma, anal gland adenocarcinoma, thyroid carcinoma, prostate carcinoma, mammary gland adenocarcinoma, feline injection site sarcoma, haemangiopericytoma and as a radiosensitizer in cats with oral SCC.

Renal excretion is minimal, so it is far safer to administer to cats with renal insufficiency than doxorubicin, although anecdotally acute renal failure in cats can occur following administration.

Safety and handling: Potent cytotoxic drug that should only be prepared and administered by trained personnel. See Appendix and specialist texts for further advice on chemotherapeutic agents. Mitoxantrone should be stored at room temperature. While the manufacturer recommends against freezing, one study demonstrated that the drug maintained cytotoxic effects when frozen and thawed at various intervals over a 12-month period.

Contraindications: Avoid in patients with myelosuppression, concurrent infection, hepatic disease or impaired cardiac function (although it is likely to be much less cardiotoxic than doxorubicin). Cardiotoxicity is not yet reported in dogs and only very rarely reported in humans.

Adverse reactions: GI signs (vomiting, anorexia, diarrhoea) and bone marrow suppression are the most common signs of toxicity. White blood cell counts are generally lowest 10 days after administration. Seizure activity in cats has been reported. In very rare cases, there may be discoloration of the urine and sclera (blue tinge).

Drug interactions: Use with extreme caution if administering other myelosuppressive or immunosuppressive agents. Chemically incompatible with heparin.

DOSES
See Appendix for chemotherapy protocols and conversion of bodyweight to body surface area.
Dogs:
- All uses: 5–6 mg/m^2 i.v. once every 3 weeks. It should be diluted with up to 50 ml of 0.9% NaCl.
- Intrapleural/intraperitoneal dose: 5–5.5 mg/m^2 diluted in 0.9% NaCl over a 5–10 min period. In one report this dose was diluted 1:1 in 0.9% NaCl then again in 1 ml/4.5 kg bodyweight (it is advised to consult a veterinary oncology specialist before administering via this route).

Cats: All uses: 5.5–6.5 mg/m^2 i.v. once every 3 weeks. It should be diluted with up to 50 ml of 0.9% NaCl.

References
Allstadt SD, Rodriguez CO, Boostrom B *et al.* (2015) Randomized phase III trial of piroxicam in combination with mitoxantrone or carboplatin for first-line treatment of urogenital tract transitional cell carcinoma in dogs. *Journal of Veterinary Internal Medicine* **29**, 261–267
Marquardt TM, Lindley SES, Smith AN *et al.* (2019) Substitution of mitoxantrone for doxorubicin in a multidrug chemotherapeutic protocol for first-line treatment of dogs with multicentric intermediate- to large-cell lymphoma. *Journal of the American Veterinary Medical Association* **254**, 236–242

Morphine
`CIL`

(Morphine*, Oramorph*) **POM CD SCHEDULE 2**

Formulations: Injectable: 10 mg/ml, 15 mg/ml, 20 mg/ml, 30 mg/ml solution. Oral: 10 mg, 30 mg, 60 mg, 100 mg tablets; suspensions, slow-release capsules and granules in a wide range of strengths. Rectal: suppositories in a wide range of strengths.

Action: Analgesia mediated by the mu opioid receptor.

Use:
- Management of moderate to severe pain in the perioperative period.
- Morphine can be given by CRI to provide analgesia intraoperatively and in the postoperative period.

- Incorporation into sedative and pre-anaesthetic medication protocols to provide improved sedation and analgesia.
- Preservative-free morphine can be administered into the epidural space where it will provide analgesia for up to 24 hours.

Methadone should be used in preference to morphine as the authorized alternative for single or repeated bolus administration to dogs and cats. The greater availability of data describing morphine by CRI may justify its use over methadone for this method of administration. Morphine is the reference opioid with which all others are compared. It provides profound analgesia and forms the mainstay of postoperative analgesic protocols in humans. In dogs, it has a short duration of action and needs to be given frequently to be effective. CRI can also be used to overcome this limitation. The duration of action in cats has not been rigorously evaluated, but appears to be 3–4 hours. Accumulation is likely to occur after prolonged repeated dosing, which may allow the dose to be reduced or the dose interval extended. Morphine causes histamine release when given rapidly i.v., so it should be diluted and given slowly i.v. Transient excitation may occur when morphine is given i.v. Oral morphine is rarely used in cats and dogs due to a high first-pass metabolism, leading to a low plasma concentration after oral administration. Respiratory function should be monitored when morphine is given to anaesthetized patients. The response to all opioids appears to vary between individual patients; assessment of pain after administration is imperative. As morphine is metabolized in the liver, some prolongation of effect may be seen with impaired liver function.

Safety and handling: Normal precautions should be observed.

Contraindications: Commonly causes vomiting when given to animals that are not in pain preoperatively, therefore should be avoided when vomiting is contraindicated (e.g. raised intraocular pressure).

Adverse reactions: In common with other mu agonists, morphine can cause respiratory depression, although this is unlikely when used at clinical doses in awake cats and dogs. Respiratory depression may occur due to increased depth of anaesthesia when given i.v. during general anaesthesia. Vomiting is common after morphine administration and it causes constriction of GI sphincters (such as the pyloric sphincter) and may cause a reduction in GI motility when given over a long period. Morphine crosses the placenta and may exert sedative effects in neonates born to bitches treated prior to parturition. Severe adverse effects can be treated with naloxone.

Drug interactions: Other CNS depressants (e.g. anaesthetics, antihistamines, barbiturates, phenothiazines, tranquillizers) may cause increased CNS or respiratory depression when used concurrently with narcotic analgesics.

DOSES
When used for sedation is generally given as part of a combination. See Appendix for sedation protocols in cats and dogs.
Dogs:
- **Analgesia:** 0.5 mg/kg i.v., i.m. q2h is required to produce analgesia in experimental models. Pain should be assessed frequently and the dose adjusted based on requirement for analgesia.
- **CRI:** 0.15–0.2 mg/kg/h i.v.

- **Epidural morphine (use a preservative-free preparation):** 0.1–0.2 mg/kg diluted with 0.2 ml/kg of sterile saline (up to a total maximum volume of 6 ml in all dogs) or bupivacaine. There is a latent period of 30–60 minutes following epidural administration; duration of action is 18–24 hours.

Cats:
- **Analgesia:** 0.1–0.4 mg/kg i.v., i.m. q3–4h. Pain should be assessed frequently and the dose adjusted based on requirement for analgesia.
- CRI use has not been widely evaluated in cats.
- **Epidural morphine:** dose as for dogs.

References

Guedes AGP, Papich MG, Rude EP *et al.* (2007) Pharmacokinetics and physiological effects of two intravenous infusion rates of morphine in conscious dogs. *Journal of Veterinary Pharmacology and Therapeutics* **30**, 224–233

Muir WW, Wiese A and March PA (2003) Effects of morphine, lidocaine, ketamine, and morphine-lidocaine-ketamine drug combination on minimum alveolar concentration in dogs anaesthetized with isoflurane. *American Journal of Veterinary Research* **64**, 1155–1160

Moxidectin

(Advocate [c,d], Bravecto plus [c], Endectrid [c,d], Imidamox [c,d], Moxiclear [c,d], Prevensa [c,d], Prinocate [c,d], Prinovox [c,d], Simparica Trio [d]) **POM-V**

Formulations: Topical: 2.5 mg/kg moxidectin + 10 mg/kg imidacloprid spot-on for dogs; 1.0 mg/kg moxidectin + 10 mg/kg imidacloprid spot-on for cats; 14 mg/ml moxidectin + 280 mg/ml fluralaner spot-on for cats (Bravecto Plus). **Oral:** 0.024–0.048 mg/kg moxidectin + 1.2–2.4 mg/kg sarolaner + 5–10 mg/kg pyrantel chewable tablets (Simparica Trio).

Action: Interacts with GABA- and glutamate-gated channels, leading to flaccid paralysis of parasites.

Use:
- Treatment and prevention of flea infestation (*Ctenocephalides felis*), canine biting lice (*Trichodectes canis*), ear mite infestation (*Otodectes cyanotis*), notoedric mange (*Notoedres cati*), sarcoptic mange (*Sarcoptes scabiei* var. *canis*) demodicosis caused by *Demodex canis*, *Eucoleus* (syn. *Capillaria*) *boehmi*, *Eucoleus aerophilus* (syn. *Capillaria aerophila*), *Thelazia callipaeda*, *Spirocerca lupi* and gastrointestinal nematodes.
- Also used for the prevention of heartworm disease (*Dirofilaria immitis*), cutaneous dirofilariosis (*Dirofilaria repens*), angiostrongylosis, *Crenosoma vulpis* and spirocercosis.
- Product containing fluralaner: flea and tick control 12 weeks, treatment of infestations with ear mites (*Otodectes cynotis*), heartworm (*Dirofilaria immitis*) prevention 8 weeks, treatment of *Toxacara cati* and *Ancylostoma tubaeforme*.
- Product containing sarolaner: flea and tick control 5 weeks, treatment of gastrointestinal nematodes, prevention of heartworm (*Dirofilaria immitis*) and angiostrongylosis (*Angiostrongylus vasorum*)

For effective treatment of canine sarcoptic mange the product should be applied on 3 occasions at 2-week intervals. Although approved for the treatment of canine demodicosis, this product is not uniformly efficacious. Frequent shampooing may reduce the efficacy of the product.

Safety and handling: Normal precautions should be observed. Highly toxic to aquatic organisms.

Contraindications: Not for use in cats <9 weeks or dogs <7 weeks. Do not use in dogs with class 4 heartworm disease. Moxidectin/fluralaner: not for use in breeding males, cats <9 weeks or <1.2 kg. Moxidectin/sarolaner/pyrantel: not for use in dogs <8 weeks or <1.25 kg.

Adverse reactions: Transient pruritus and erythema at the site of application may occur. Severe effects may be seen if applied to cats with adult heartworm disease. Fluralaner/moxidectin: uncommonly, dyspnoea after licking the application site, hypersalivation, emesis, haematemesis, diarrhoea, lethargy, pyrexia, tachypnoea, mydriasis. Sarolaner/moxidectin/pyrantel: GI upset, lethargy, anorexia, rarely neurological signs.

Drug interactions: Do not use concurrently with other P-glycoprotein substrates or macrocyclic lactones.

DOSES
See Appendix for guidelines on responsible parasiticide use.
Dogs:
- **Parasites:** 2.5 mg/kg moxidectin. Apply once every month. Minimum dose recommendation 0.1 ml/kg.
- **Demodicosis (severe):** apply product weekly.

Cats:
- **Parasites:** 1.0 mg/kg moxidectin. Apply once every month. Minimum dose recommendation 0.1 ml/kg.
- **Product containing fluralaner:** apply once every 3 months.

Mycophenolate mofetil (MMF, Mycophenolic acid)

(CellCept* (MMF), Myfortic* (MPA)) **POM**

Formulations: Oral: 180 mg, 360 mg tablets; 250 mg capsules, 500 mg tablets, 1 g/5 ml powder for oral suspension (MMF). **Injectable:** 500 mg powder for reconstitution and slow i.v. infusion (mycophenolic acid).

Action: Inhibits the enzyme that controls the rate of synthesis of guanine monophosphate in the *de novo* pathway of purine synthesis. This pathway is important in the proliferation of B and T lymphocytes. This action is similar to that of azathioprine.

Use:
- Management of immune-mediated disease including immune-mediated haemolytic anaemia, immune-mediated polyarthritis, immune-mediated skin disease, immune-mediated thrombocytopenia and myasthenia gravis.

In humans, mycophenolate is more lymphocyte specific and less bone marrow suppressive than azathioprine.

Safety and handling: Cytotoxic drug; see Appendix and specialist texts for further advice on chemotherapeutic agents.

Contraindications: Bone marrow suppression, pre-existing infections.

Adverse reactions: Adverse GI effects were seen in up to 25% of dogs in one study. Neutropenia, anaemia, thrombocytopenia and dermatological signs were also seen but were much less common. Hepatopathy and pancreatitis have been reported in one cat receiving MMF. In humans, headache, hypertension, peripheral oedema, confusion, coughs, tremors and an increased risk of lymphoma have been reported.

Drug interactions: Competes with other drugs that undergo active renal tubular secretion, resulting in increased concentration of either drug. Concomitant administration of antacids (such as omeprazole) may decrease absorption.

DOSES
See Appendix for immunosuppression protocols.
Dogs:
- **Immune-mediated disease:** 8–12 mg/kg (typically 10 mg/kg) p.o., i.v. (give slowly over at least 2 hours) q12h (MMF), the dose can be reduced or given q24h if adverse effects are observed.
- **Pemphigus:** 7–13 mg/kg p.o. q8h (MMF).

Cats: **Immune-mediated disease:** 10 mg/kg p.o. q12h based on limited experience. Other immunosuppressants may be preferable.

References
Bacek LM and Macintire DK (2011) Treatment of immune-mediated hemolytic anemia with mycophenolate mofetil in two cats. *Journal of Veterinary Emergency and Critical Care* **21**, 45–49

Wang A, Smith JR and Creevy KE (2013) Treatment of canine idiopathic immune-mediated haemolytic anaemia with mycophenolate mofetil and glucocorticoids: 30 cases (2007 to 2011). *Journal of Small Animal Practice* **54**, 399–404

A
B
C
D
E
F
G
H
I
J
K
L
M
N
O
P
Q
R
S
T
U
V
W
X
Y
Z

Naloxone

(Naloxone*, Narcan*) **POM**

Formulations: Injectable: 0.02 mg/ml, 0.4 mg/ml solutions.

Action: Competitive antagonist for opioid receptors, reversing the effects of opioid agonists.

Use:
- Treatment of opioid overdose.
- Also used to identify persistent activity of opioid drugs.

Onset of action is very rapid when given i.v., but duration is short (30–40 min). Repeated doses or CRI may be required to manage overdose of longer acting opioids such as morphine and methadone or high-dose fentanyl. Naloxone will also antagonize the effects of endogenous opioids; therefore, it can cause antanalgesic effects in opioid naïve subjects. Administration to animals that could be in pain must therefore be considered carefully. Low dose naloxone i.v. will cause a transient elevation of unconsciousness when persistent opioid activity contributes to an unexpectedly long recovery from anaesthesia.

Safety and handling: Normal precautions should be observed.

Contraindications: No information available.

Adverse reactions: Indiscriminate use in animals that have undergone major surgery or trauma will expose the recipient to acute severe discomfort. In such cases, the effects of opioid overdose (respiratory depression) should be managed by endotracheal intubation and artificial ventilation. Naloxone should be reserved for emergency situations when the effects of opioid overdose are severe.

Drug interactions: No information available.

DOSES

Dogs, Cats: 0.01–0.02 mg/kg i.v.; 0.04 mg/kg i.m., s.c., intratracheal. Naloxone can be administered as a CRI at 0.02 mg/kg/h i.v. if a longer duration of opioid antagonism is required.

References
Golder FJ, Wilson J, Larenza FP *et al.* (2010) Suspected acute meperidine toxicity in a dog. *Veterinary Anaesthesia and Analgesia* **37**, 471–477

Nandrolone

(Laurabolin[c,d], Decadurabolin*) **POM-V, POM**

Formulations: Injectable: 25 mg/ml, 50 mg/ml (in oil).

Action: Binds to testosterone receptors and stimulates protein synthesis.

Use:
- In cases where excessive tissue breakdown or extensive repair processes are taking place.
- Management of aplastic anaemia.
- Management of anaemia associated with renal failure; however, may also have adverse effects on renal failure by increasing protein turnover.

Monitor haematology to determine the efficacy of treatment and liver enzyme activities to assess for hepatotoxicity.

Safety and handling: Normal precautions should be observed.

Contraindications: Do not use in breeding bitches or queens, in pregnant animals or in those with diabetes mellitus.

Adverse reactions: Androgenic effects may develop. Use in immature animals may result in early closure of epiphyseal growth plates.

Drug interactions: The concurrent use of anabolic steroids with adrenal steroids may potentiate the development of oedema.

DOSES
Dogs: 1–5 mg/kg i.m., s.c. q21d. Maximum dose 40–50 mg/dog.
Cats: 1–5 mg/kg i.m., s.c. q21d. Maximum dose 20–25 mg/cat.

Neomycin
(Neopen [c,d], Maxitrol*, Nivemycin*) **POM-V, POM**

Formulations: Oral: 500 mg tablets (Nivemycin). **Injectable:** 100 mg/ml neomycin + 200 mg/ml penicillin G (Neopen). **Topical:** many dermatological, ophthalmic and otic preparations contain 0.25–0.5% neomycin.

Action: A concentration-dependent antimicrobial agent that inhibits bacterial protein synthesis once it has gained access to the bacterial cell via an oxygen-dependent carrier mechanism. As other aminoglycosides, the concentration-dependent cell killing mechanism confers a marked post antibiotic effect.

Use:
- Active primarily against Gram-negative bacteria, although some *Staphylococcus* and *Enterococcus* species are sensitive. All obligate anaerobic bacteria and many haemolytic streptococci are resistant.
- Since parenteral neomycin is extremely nephrotoxic and ototoxic; it is used topically for infections of the skin, ear or mucous membranes.
- Used orally to reduce the intestinal bacterial population in the management of hepatic encephalopathy.

As with other aminoglycosides, it is not absorbed after oral administration unless GI ulceration is present. Neomycin is more active in an alkaline environment.

Safety and handling: Normal precautions should be observed.

Contraindications: For systemic use, do not use in animals with pre-existing renal disease. Do not use ear preparations if the tympanum is ruptured.

Adverse reactions: Systemic toxicity, ototoxicity and nephrotoxicity may very occasionally occur following prolonged high-dose oral therapy or where there is severe GI ulceration/inflammatory bowel disease, as sufficient neomycin may be absorbed. Nephrotoxicity and ototoxicity are potential side effects associated with parenteral use. Some patients may develop a severe diarrhoea/malabsorption syndrome and bacterial or fungal superinfections. Topical ophthalmic preparation may cause local irritation.

Drug interactions: Absorption of digoxin, methotrexate, potassium and vitamin K may be decreased. Other ototoxic and nephrotoxic drugs, e.g.

furosemide, should be used with caution in patients receiving oral neomycin therapy as the combinations are likely to have synergistic toxicity.

DOSES

Classified as category C (Caution) by the EMA.

See Appendix for guidelines on responsible antibiotic use.

Dogs, Cats:
- **Parenteral:** Not recommended due to nephrotoxicity.
- **Oral:** 20 mg/kg p.o. q6–8h; or per rectum as a retention enema for management of acute hepatic encephalopathy only. As the drug is not absorbed, it is not an effective treatment for other sites of infection. In stable animals, decrease frequency to q12h.
- **Ophthalmic:** 1 drop per eye q6–8h.
- **Otic:** 2–12 drops per ear or apply liberally to skin q4–12h.

Neostigmine

(Neostigmine*, Neostigmine/Glycopyrronium bromide*) **POM**

Formulations: Injectable: 2.5 mg/ml solution (on special order); 0.5 mg/ml glycopyrronium bromide + 2.5 mg/ml neostigmine metilsulfate solution. **Oral:** 15 mg tablets.

Action: Prolongs the action of acetylcholine at the neuromuscular junction, but with low CNS penetration due to its polar structure. In comparison with edrophonium, it has a slower onset but a longer duration of action of approximately 30 minutes to 2 hours.

Use:
- Treatment of acute myasthenic crises if oral dosing with pyridostigmine is not possible.
- A safe and viable alternative to the previously utilized edrophonium challenge, particularly when weak positive responses are considered negative for acquired myasthenia gravis.
- Also used to antagonize non-depolarizing neuromuscular blocking agents.

Historically, a dose of 0.05 mg neostigmine has been suggested but there is a more recent report of this dose causing a cholinergic crisis. To reduce the risk, it is recommended that the combined formulation with glycopyrronium is used. If neostigmine is being used to diagnose myasthenia gravis then atropine (0.05 mg/kg i.v.) should be available for immediate administration to control cholinergic side effects (e.g. salivation, urination). Improvement should be noted within 5–10 minutes, with the effects dissipating within 2–4 hours. Due to its longer duration of effect, it is used in the diagnosis of myasthenia gravis when the collapse episodes are brief. In these cases, instead of injecting the anticholinesterase drug after the collapse episodes, the dog is pretreated with neostigmine and then exercised to assess whether the collapse episodes have been abolished. If an overdose of neostigmine has been administered, maintenance of respiration should take priority. Atropine does not antagonize the nicotinic effects, including muscle weakness and paralysis. If muscle twitching is severe, it can be controlled with small doses of a competitive neuromuscular blocker. The cholinesterase reactivator pralidoxime can be used as an adjunct to atropine. Supportive treatment should be provided as required. Use with extreme caution in patients with bronchial disease (especially feline asthma), bradycardia (and other arrhythmias), hypotension, renal impairment or epilepsy.

Safety and handling: Normal precautions should be observed.

Contraindications: Contraindicated in mechanical GI or urinary tract obstruction and in peritonitis.

Adverse reactions: Primarily due to excessive cholinergic stimulation and most commonly include nausea, vomiting, increased salivation and diarrhoea. Overdosage may lead to muscle fasciculations and paralysis. Severe bradyarrhythmias, even asystole, may occur if neostigmine is used to antagonize neuromuscular block without the co-injection of atropine. Overdosage may lead to a 'cholinergic crisis', with both muscarinic and nicotinic effects. These effects may include lacrimation, defecation and urination, miosis, nystagmus, bradycardia and other arrhythmias, hypotension, muscle cramps, fasciculations, weakness and paralysis, respiratory signs and increased bronchial secretion combined with bronchoconstriction. CNS side effects include ataxia, seizures and coma.

Drug interactions: Effect may be antagonized by drugs with neuromuscular blocking activity, including aminoglycosides, clindamycin and halogenated inhalational anaesthetics. Drugs that may increase the clinical severity of myasthenia gravis, including quinine and related compounds and beta-blockers, may reduce the effectiveness of neostigmine treatment in these cases. Concurrent use of neostigmine and beta-blockers may result in bradycardia. Neostigmine, as well as other anticholinesterases, inhibits the metabolism of suxamethonium, thereby prolonging and enhancing its clinical effect; combined use is not recommended. Neostigmine antagonizes the effect of non-depolarizing muscle relaxants. Antimuscarinic drugs such as atropine antagonize the muscarinic effects of neostigmine.

DOSES

Dogs:
- **Diagnosis of myasthenia gravis:** 0.02 mg/kg i.v of neostigmine. If no response within 4 hours and no apparent side effects, the test can be repeated using 0.03 mg/kg. A positive response may be seen with some myopathies.
- **Treatment of myasthenia gravis if pyridostigmine is not available or oral medication cannot be given due to regurgitation:** 0.04 mg/kg i.m, s.c. q6h.
- **Myasthenic crisis:** 0.01–0.1 mg/kg i.v., i.m., s.c., interval dependent upon duration of response. For longer term use 0.1–0.25 mg/kg p.o. q4h (total daily dose not to exceed 2 mg/kg).
- **Antagonism of non-depolarizing neuromuscular blocking agents:** neostigmine (0.05 mg/kg) is mixed with glycopyrronium (0.01 mg/kg) and injected i.v. over 2 min once signs of spontaneous recovery from 'block', e.g. diaphragmatic 'twitching', are present. Continued ventilatory support should be provided until full respiratory muscle activity is restored. If glycopyrronium is unavailable, atropine (0.04 mg/kg) is given i.v., followed by neostigmine (0.02–0.04 mg/kg) as soon as heart rate rises.

Cats:
- **Myasthenic crisis:** use not reported in cats but extrapolation from dogs seems reasonable.
- **Antagonism of non-depolarizing neuromuscular blocking agents:** doses as for dogs.

References

Cridge H, Little A, José-López R *et al.* (2001) The clinical utility of neostigmine administration in the diagnosis of acquired myasthenia gravis. *Journal of Veterinary Emergency and Critical Care (San Antonio)* **31**, 647–655

Jones RS, Auer U and Mosing M (2015) Reversal of neuromuscular block in companion animals. *Veterinary Anaesthesia and Analgesia* **42**, 455–471

Niacinamide see Nicotinamide

Nicotinamide (Niacinamide, Vitamin B3)

(Numerous trade names) **general sale**

Formulations: Oral: 50 mg, 250 mg tablets.

Action: Blocks antigen-induced histamine release, inhibits phosphodiesterase activity and protease release.

Use:
- Used historically in combination with oxytetracycline/tetracycline or doxycycline in the management of certain immune-mediated dermatoses such as lupoid onychodystrophy, discoid lupus erythematosus and pemphigus foliaceus. Long term use of antibiotics is not recommended.

Safety and handling: Normal precautions should be observed.

Contraindications: Do not use nicotinic acid (niacin) as it causes vasodilation.

Adverse reactions: May cause mild GI irritation.

Drug interactions: No information available.

DOSES

Dogs: Immunomodulation: 250 mg/dog q8h (dogs up to 25 kg), 500 mg/dog q8h (dogs >25 kg). Taper to effect.

Cats: No information available.

References

Rosenkrantz W (2004) Pemphigus: current therapy. *Veterinary Dermatology* **15**, 90–98

Wiemelt SP, Goldschmidt MH, Greek JS *et al.* (2004) A retrospective study comparing the histopathological features and response to treatment in two canine nasal dermatoses, DLE and MCP. *Veterinary Dermatology* **15**, 341–348

Nitenpyram

(Bob Martin Clear Flea [c,d], Capstar [c,d], Johnson's 4Fleas [c,d]) **AVM-GSL**

Formulations: Oral: 11.4 mg, 57 mg tablets.

Action: Post-synaptic binding to insect nicotinic receptors leads to insect paralysis and death. Kills fleas on animal within 30 minutes.

Use:
- Treatment of fleas on dogs and cats.

Should be used as part of a fully integrated flea control programme. All animals in the affected household should be treated. Safe in pregnancy and lactation.

Safety and handling: Normal precautions should be observed.

Contraindications: Do not use 11.4 mg tablets in animals <1 kg or <4 weeks. Do not use 57 mg tablets in dogs <11 kg.

Adverse reactions: Transient increase in pruritus may be seen after administration due to fleas reacting to the product. Rarely, neurological signss such as tremors, convulsions

Drug interactions: No information available.

DOSES
See Appendix for guidelines on responsible parasiticide use.
Dogs, Cats: Fleas: 1 mg/kg once (minimum dose) or q24h.

Nitrofurantoin
(Furadantin*, Nitrofurantoin*) **POM**

Formulations: Oral: 50 mg, 100 mg tablets; 25 mg/5 ml suspension.

Action: Reacts with bacterial nitroreductase enzymes to form products that interact with bacterial DNA and cause strand breakage.

Use:
- Exclusively for treatment of urinary tract infections especially those confirmed-sensitive to nitrofurantoin.
- Active against many Gram-positive and Gram-negative bacteria. Well absorbed following oral administration but rapidly excreted in urine.

Therapeutic levels are only attained in the urinary tract and not in serum or tissues (not appropriate for treatment of pyelonephritis or any infections outside of the urinary tract). The concentration of nitrofurantoin is highest in alkaline urine; however, urine should not be alkalinized as the activity of nitrofurantoin is significantly decreased. Use is limited due to toxicity and concerns about mutagenicity and carcinogenicity.

Safety and handling: Mutagenic – wear gloves when handling.

Contraindications: Do not use in patients with significant renal impairment, as serum levels will rise and give an increased risk of serious toxicity. Since nitrofurans are mutagenic, they should not be given to pregnant animals.

Adverse reactions: In humans, may rarely cause a peripheral neuritis, pulmonary complications, hepatotoxicity, emesis, diarrhoea and GI bleeding. High oral doses may cause thrombocytopenia, anaemia and leucopenia, with prolonged bleeding times.

Drug interactions: The bioavailability of nitrofurantoin may be increased by antimuscarinic drugs and food as they delay gastric emptying time and increase absorption of this weak acid from the stomach. Antagonism may be observed with fluoroquinolones. May increase the hyperkalaemic effects of spironolactone.

DOSES

Classified as category D (Prudence) by the EMA.

See Appendix for guidelines on responsible antibiotic use.

Dogs, Cats: For urinary tract infections only: 4.4–5 mg/kg p.o. q8h.

References

Leuin AS, Hartmann F and Viviano K (2021) Administration of nitrofurantoin in dogs with lower urinary tract infections: 14 cases (2013–2019). *Journal of Small Animal Practice* **62**, 42–48

Weese JS, Blondeau J, Boothe D *et al.* (2019). International society for companion animal infectious diseases (ISCAID) guidelines for the diagnosis and management of bacterial urinary tract infections in dogs and cats. *The Veterinary Journal* **247**, 8–25

Nitroglycerin(e) see Glyceryl trinitrate

Nitrous oxide

(Entonox*, Nitrous oxide*) **POM**

Formulations: Inhalational: 100% nitrous oxide (N_2O) gas. Entonox is N_2O plus oxygen.

Action: Causes CNS depression.

Use:
- Used with oxygen to carry volatile anaesthetic agents such as isoflurane for the induction and maintenance of anaesthesia.
- N_2O reduces the concentration of inhalant agent required to maintain anaesthesia.

Administration of N_2O at the beginning of volatile agent anaesthesia increases the speed of uptake of volatile agent from the alveoli (via the 2nd gas effect and concentration effect), hastening attainment of a stable plane of volatile agent anaesthesia. Oxygen must be supplemented for 5–10 minutes after N_2O is discontinued to prevent diffusion hypoxia. N_2O causes minimal respiratory and cardiovascular effects and is a useful addition to a balanced anaesthesia technique. A minimum oxygen concentration of 30% is required during anaesthesia. The inspired concentration of oxygen may fall to critically low levels when N_2O is used in rebreathing circuits during low flow rates. Do not use in such systems unless the inspired oxygen concentration can be measured on a breath-by-breath basis.

Safety and handling: Prolonged exposure can have serious adverse effects on human health. Scavenging is essential. N_2O is not absorbed by charcoal in passive scavenging systems utilizing activated charcoal. Nitrous oxide is a potent greenhouse gas and is ozone-depleting. Nitrous oxide confers the largest carbon footprint of the anaesthetic gases within the acute sector, accounting for at least 80% of the total anaesthetic gas footprint of the NHS in 2019/2020. The negative environmental impact of nitrous oxide brings into question its continued use in veterinary medicine.

Contraindications: Do not give to patients with air-filled spaces within the body, e.g. pneumothorax or gastric dilatation. N_2O will cause a rapid expansion of any gas-filled space, increasing volume or pressure. Do not give to animals with marked respiratory compromise, due to the risks of hypoxaemia. Do not give to animals with raised intracranial pressure due to an increase in cerebral blood flow associated with administration.

Adverse reactions: The cobalt ion present in vitamin B12 is oxidized by N_2O so that it is no longer able to act as the cofactor for methionine synthase. The result is reduced synthesis of methionine, thymidine, tetrahydrofolate and DNA. Exposure lasting only a few hours may lead to megaloblastic changes in bone marrow and more prolonged exposure (a few days) may result in agranulocytosis.

Drug interactions: No information available.

DOSES

Dogs, Cats: Inspired concentrations of 50–70%.

References

Duke T, Caulkett NA and Tataryn JM (2006) The effect of nitrous oxide on halothane, isoflurane and sevoflurane requirements in ventilated dogs undergoing ovariohysterectomy. *Veterinary Anaesthesia and Analgesia* **33**, 343–350

Nystatin

(Canaural [c,d], Nystan*, Nystatin*) **POM-V, POM**

Formulations: Oral: 100,000 IU/ml suspension. **Topical:** Various products.

Action: Binds to ergosterol, a major component of the fungal cell membrane, and forms pores in the membrane that lead to potassium leakage and death of the fungus.

Use:
* Antifungal agent with a broad spectrum of activity but noted for its activity against *Candida*, particularly *C. albicans*.

Not absorbed from the GI tract.

Safety and handling: Normal precautions should be observed.

Contraindications: No information available.

Adverse reactions: No information available.

Drug interactions: No information available.

DOSES

Dogs, Cats: Topical antifungal therapy: apply to affected areas q8–12h.

References

Paterson S (2016) Topical ear treatment – options, indications and limitations of current therapy. *Journal of Small Animal Practice* **57**, 668–678

Oclacitinib

(Apoquel[d]) **POM-V**

Formulations: Oral: 3.6 mg, 5.4 mg, 16 mg tablets (including chewable tablets)

Action: Inhibits janus-kinases (preferentially JAK1), thereby inhibiting the function of a variety of cytokines, particularly proinflammatory cytokines associated with the allergic response.

Use:
- For the treatment of pruritus associated with allergic dermatitis in dogs.

Dogs receiving long-term oclacitinib should be monitored regularly with complete blood counts and serum biochemistry.

Safety and handling: Normal precautions should be observed.

Contraindications: Do not use in dogs <12 months or <3 kg. Not to be used during pregnancy or lactation or in animals intended for breeeding. Do not use in dogs with evidence of immune suppression, such as hypercortisolism, or with evidence of progressive malignant neoplasia as the active substance has not been evaluated in these cases.

Adverse reactions: Diarrhoea, vomiting, anorexia, new cutaneous or subcutaneous swellings, interdigital furunculosis, lethargy, polyphagia, polydipsia, otitis, cystitis, lyphadenopathy and increased aggression. May increase susceptibility to infection, papillomas and demodicosis. May increase the incidence of histiocytomas. Hypercholesterolaemia, hypoproteinaemia , proteinuria, leucopenia, elevated liver enzyme activities have been reported in dogs receiving chronic therapy.

Drug interactions: No information available.

DOSES

Dogs: Atopic dermatitis: 0.4–0.6 mg/kg p.o. q12h for 14 days, then q24h for maintenance.

Cats: Not approved for use in this species. The safety profile of oclacitinib in cats has not been established.

References

Cosgrove SB, Wren JA, Cleaver DM et al. (2013) A blinded, randomized, placebo-controlled trial of the efficacy and safety of the Janus kinase inhibitor oclacitinib (Apoquel®) in client-owned dogs with atopic dermatitis. *Veterinary Dermatology* **24**, 587–597
Ortalda C, Noli C, Colombo S et al. (2015) Oclacitinib in feline nonflea-, nonfood-induced hypersensitivity dermatitis: results of a small prospective pilot study of client-owned cats. *Veterinary Dermatology* **26**, 235–e52
Simpson AC, Schissler JR, Rosychuk RAW and Moore AR (2017) The frequency of urinary tract infection and subclinical bacteriuria in dogs with allergic dermatitis treated with oclacitinib: a prospective study. *Veterinary Dermatology* **28**, 485–e113

Octreotide

(Sandostatin*, Sandostatin LAR*) **POM**

Formulations: Injectable: 50 µg (micrograms)/ml, 100 µg/ml, 200 µg/ml, 500 µg/ml solutions; depot preparation: 10 mg, 20 mg, 30 mg vials.

Action: Somatostatin analogue that inhibits hormone release from the anterior pituitary (thyroid-stimulating hormone (TSH) and growth hormone (GH)), and hormones of the gastroenteropancreatic endocrine system (insulin and glucagon).

Use:
- Management of pancreatic endocrine tumours (e.g. insulinoma, gastrinoma).
- Management of acromegaly.
- Anecdotal reports of use to manage protein-losing enteropathy (PLE), extrapolated from use in humans.

Research suggests that octreotide is not useful in most insulinomas. Tumours not expressing somatostatin receptors will not respond. In humans, doses up to 200 µg (micrograms)/person q8h are used. Similar doses of the aqueous preparation may be required in animals, but dosages for the depot preparation are not known. Newer somatostatin analogues such as pasireotide hold more promise for treatment of acromegaly but are expensive.

Safety and handling: Normal precautions should be observed.

Contraindications: No information available.

Adverse reactions: GI disturbances (anorexia, vomiting, abdominal pain, bloating, diarrhoea and steatorrhoea), hepatopathy and pain at injection sites have been recorded in humans.

Drug interactions: No information available.

DOSES
Dogs, Cats:
- 10–50 µg (micrograms)/animal s.c. q8–12h.
- **Proposed dose for management of refractive PLE:** 10 µg/kg s.c. q8h.

References
Gostelow R, Scudder C, Keyte S *et al.* (2017) Pasireotide long-acting release treatment for diabetic cats with underlying hypersomatotropism. *Journal of Veterinary Internal Medicine* **31**, 355–364

Lane M, Larson J, Hecht S and Tolbert MK (2016) Medical management of gastrinoma in a cat. *JFMS Open Reports* **2**, doi: 10.1177/2055116916646389

Oestriol see Estriol

Ofloxacin `CIL`
(Exocin*) **POM**

Formulations: Topical: 0.3% solution in 5 ml bottle.

Action: Concentration-dependent antimicrobial which works by inhibiting the bacterial DNA gyrase enzyme, causing damage to the bacterial DNA.

Use:
- For ophthalmic use where lower tier antimicrobials would not be effective and based on antimicrobial susceptibility testing wherever possible.
- Active against many ocular pathogens, including *Staphylococcus* and *Pseudomonas aeruginosa*, although there is increasing resistance among some staphylococcal and streptococcal organisms. Better corneal penetration than ciprofloxacin.

Safety and handling: Normal precautions should be observed.

Contraindications: No information available.

Adverse reactions: May cause local irritation after application.

Drug interactions: No information available.

DOSES

Classified as category B (Restrict) by the EMA.
See Appendix for guidelines on responsible antibiotic use.
Dogs, Cats: 1 drop to affected eye q6h; intensive therapy q30–120min for short-term use (1–2 days).

Olopatadine hydrochloride

(Opatanol*) **POM**

Formulations: Ophthalmic: 1 mg/ml olopatadine hydrochloride solution in a 5 ml bottle.

Action: Mast cell stabilizer. A selective histamine H1 antagonist that inhibits *in vitro* type-1 immediate hypersensitivity reaction. Inhibits the release of mast cell inflammatory mediators.

Use:
- Treatment of juvenile follicular conjunctivitis in dogs.
- Treatment of seasonal allergic conjunctivitis in dogs.

Safety and handling: Discard bottle 4 weeks after opening. Normal precautions should be observed.

Contraindications: None.

Adverse reactions: Olopatadine eye drops contain benzalkonium chloride which may cause eye irritation. The most frequent treatment-related adverse reaction in humans is eye pain, reported at an overall incidence of 0.7%. Prolongation of the QT interval in dogs has been observed only at exposures considered sufficiently in excess of the maximum human exposure, indicating little relevance to clinical use.

Drug interactions: None reported.

DOSES

Dogs: Apply 1 drop q12h to affected eye(s), reduce to q24h once an improvement in clinical signs has been observed.
Cats: Not applicable.

Omeprazole `CIL`

(Gastrogard*, Losec*, Mepradec*, Mezzopram*, Pyrocalm*, Zanprol*) **POM-V, POM**

Formulations: Oral: 10 mg, 20 mg, 40 mg gastro-resistant capsules, gastro-resistant tablets, multiple unit pellet system (MUPS) tablets. 2 mg/ml or 4 mg/ml oral suspension; numerous oral paste products authorized for use in horses. **Injectable:** 40 mg vial for reconstitution for i.v. injection; powder for solution for infusion must be dissolved in 100 ml of either 0.9% NaCl or 5% dextrose and should be initially dissolved in 5 ml of liquid then immediately diluted to 100 ml. Do not use if any particles are present in the reconstituted solution. Once reconstituted, stability has been demonstrated for 12 hours when dissolved in NaCl 0.9% solution and for 6 hours in 5% glucose when reconstituted under controlled aseptic conditions and stored below 25°C. Chemical and physical in-use stability has also been demonstrated for 24 hours at 2–8°C in both NaCl 0.9% solution and 5% glucose.

Action: Proton-pump inhibitor.

Use:
- Management of gastric and duodenal ulcers, oesophagitis, and hypersecretory conditions secondary to gastrinoma (Zollinger–Ellison syndrome) or mast cell neoplasia.
- Preoperative administration of omeprazole reduces the incidence of gastro-oesophageal reflux during anaesthesia in dogs.

Several products are authorized for use in equids, but the formulation (370 mg/g paste) makes accurate dosing of small animals impossible. Lansoprazole, rabeprazole and pantoprazole are similar drugs but have no known clinical advantage over omeprazole. Esomeprazole is a newer preparation containing only the active isomer of omeprazole. Studies have shown that omeprazole produces mild increases in canine gastric pH but that the effects are significantly greater than that produced by famotidine, cimetidine or ranitidine. Twice-daily administration of omeprazole raises intragastric pH enough to suggest potential therapeutic efficacy for acid-related disease when assessed by criteria used for human patients, but once-daily administration does not. Omeprazole was not helpful in reducing frequency or severity of gastrointestinal adverse effects in dogs receiving piroxicam and was in fact associated with more frequent and severe gastrointestinal adverse effects. Omeprazole prophylaxis induced faecal dysbiosis and increased intestinal inflammatory markers when coadministered with carprofen to otherwise healthy dogs with no other risk factors for GI bleeding, compared to carprofen alone. Omeprazole is probably overprescribed in hospitalized animals.

Safety and handling: Normal precautions should be observed.

Contraindications: No information available.

Adverse reactions: Chronic suppression of acid secretion has caused hypergastrinaemia in laboratory animals, leading to mucosal cell hyperplasia, rugal hypertrophy and the development of carcinoids, and so treatment for a maximum of 8 weeks has been recommended. However, such problems have not been reported in companion animals. Adverse effects do include nausea, diarrhoea, constipation, skin rashes and tooth fractures. An i.v. preparation of rabeprazole causes pulmonary oedema in dogs at high doses.

Drug interactions: Omeprazole may enhance the effects of phenytoin. There is a risk of interaction with tacrolimus, mycophenolate mofetil, clopidogrel, digoxin and itraconazole.

DOSES
Dogs: All uses: 0.5–1.5 mg/kg i.v., p.o. q12–24h.
Cats: All uses: 0.75–1 mg/kg p.o. q24h.

References
Jones SM, Gaier A, Enomoto H *et al.* (2020) The effect of combined carprofen and omeprazole administration on gastrointestinal permeability and inflammation in dogs. *Journal of Veterinary Internal Medicine* **34**, 1886–1893

Shaevitz MH, Moore GE and Fulkerson CM (2021) A prospective, randomized, placebo-controlled, double-blinded clinical trial comparing the incidence and severity of gastrointestinal adverse events in dogs with cancer treated with piroxicam alone or in combination with omeprazole or famotidine. *Journal of the American Veterinary Medical Association* **259**, 385–391

Ondansetron

CIL

(Setofilm*, Zofran*) **POM**

Formulations: Injectable: 2 mg/ml solution in 2 ml and 4 ml ampoules. Oral: 4 mg, 8 mg tablets; 4 mg/5 ml syrup.

Action: Potent antiemetic effects through action on the GI tract and the chemoreceptor trigger zone. It was developed for, and is particularly useful in, the control of emesis induced by chemotherapeutic drugs. Its mechanism of action makes it a suitable choice as part of the management of vomiting caused by peripheral emetogenic stimuli (e.g. irritation of the GI tract).

Use:
- Indicated for the management of nausea and vomiting in patients whose signs are not controlled by other drugs (e.g. maropitant, metoclopramide).
- Management of obstructive sleep apnoea.

Dolasetron, granisetron, palanosetron and tropisetron are similar drugs but have yet to be extensively used in companion animals. Oral bioavailability considered to be low. Subcutaneous administration of ondansetron to healthy cats is more bioavailable and results in a more prolonged exposure than oral administration.

Safety and handling: Normal precautions should be observed.

Contraindications: Intestinal obstruction.

Adverse reactions: Well tolerated. In humans, constipation, headaches, occasional alterations in liver enzymes and, rarely, hypersensitivity reactions have been reported.

Drug interactions: Ondansetron may reduce the effectiveness of tramadol and so the dose of tramadol may need to be increased.

DOSES

Dogs, Cats: All uses: 0.5 mg/kg i.v. loading dose followed by 0.5 mg/kg/h CRI for 6 hours or 0.5–1 mg/kg p.o. q12–24h.

References

Sedlacek HS, Ramsey DS, Boucher JF *et al.* (2008) Comparative efficacy of maropitant and selected drugs in preventing emesis induced by centrally or peripherally acting emetogens in dogs. *Journal of Veterinary Pharmacology and Therapeutics* **31**, 533–537
Yalcin E and Keser GO (2017) Comparative efficacy of metoclopramide, ondansetron and maropitant in preventing parvoviral enteritis-induced emesis in dogs. *Journal of Veterinary Pharmacology and Therapeutics* **40**, 599–560

Orbifloxacin

(Posatex [d]) **POM-V**

Formulations: Oral: 30 mg/ml suspension. Otic: Ear drops containing 8.5 mg/ml orbifloxacin combined with mometasone (steroid) and posaconazole (antifungal).

Action: Concentration-dependent inhibition of DNA gyrase, meaning that pulse dosing regimens may be effective.

Use:
- Use should be based on antimicrobial susceptibility testing, wherever possible, and where lower tier antimicrobials would not be effective.
- Particularly active against mycoplasmas, many Gram-negative

organisms and some Gram-positives including *Pasteurella*, *Staphylococcus*, *Pseudomonas*, *Escherichia coli*, *Proteus* and *Salmonella*. Fluoroquinolones are effective against beta-lactamase-producing bacteria. Orbifloxacin is ineffective in treating obligate anaerobic infections.

Safety and handling: Normal precautions should be observed.

Contraindications: Do not use the otic preparation in animals <4 months or if the tympanum is not intact.

Adverse reactions: No information available.

Drug interactions: No information available.

DOSES
Classified as category B (Restrict) by the EMA.
See Appendix for guidelines on responsible antibiotic use.
Dogs: For the otic preparation: 2–8 drops per ear q24h. The number of drops is determined by the weight of the dog.
Cats: Not recommended.

Osaterone

(Ypozane [d]) **POM-V**

Formulations: Oral: 1.875 mg, 3.75 mg, 7.5 mg, 15 mg tablets.

Action: Competitively prevents the binding of androgens to their prostatic receptors and blocks the transport of testosterone into the prostate.

Use:
* Treatment of benign prostatic hypertrophy (BPH) in male dogs.

In dogs with BPH associated with prostatitis, osaterone can be administered concurrently with antimicrobials. Quick onset of decrease in size (40% reduction within 2 weeks) without loss of fertility. Non-invasive treatment that can be used in dogs that are not fit for surgical castration or that are still used as stud dogs. Effects of treatment last for about 6 months. Use with caution in dogs with a history of liver disease.

Safety and handling: People who are or may become pregnant should not handle this drug.

Contraindications: No information available.

Adverse reactions: A transient reduction of plasma cortisol concentration may occur; this may continue for several weeks after administration. Appropriate monitoring should be implemented in dogs under stress (e.g. following surgery) or those with hypoadrenocorticism. The response to an ACTH stimulation test may also be suppressed for several weeks after administration of osaterone. Transient increases in appetite and changes in behaviour occur commonly. Other adverse reactions include transient vomiting and/or diarrhoea, polyuria/polydipsia, lethargy and feminization syndrome including mammary gland hyperplasia. Treatment of some dogs with liver disease has resulted in reversible increases in alanine aminotransferase (ALT) and alkaline phosphatase (ALP).

Drug interactions: No information available.

DOSES

Dogs: Benign prostatic hypertrophy: 0.25–0.5 mg/kg p.o. q24h for 7 days.

Cats: No indication.

References

Albouy M, Sanquer A, Maynard L *et al.* (2008) Efficacies of osaterone and delmadinone in the treatment of benign prostatic hyperplasia in dogs. *Veterinary Record* **163**, 179–183

Niżański W, Orchota M, Fontaine C and Pasikowska J (2020) Comparison of Clinical Effectiveness of Deslorelin Acetate and Osaterone Acetate in Dogs with Benign Prostatic Hyperplasia. *Animals: an open access journal from MDPI* **10**, 1936

Oxantel see Pyrantel

Oxybutynin hydrochloride

(Ditropan*, Lyrinel*, Oxybutynin*) **POM**

Formulations: Oral: 2.5 mg, 3 mg, 5 mg tablets; 5 mg, 10 mg modified-release tablets; 2.5 mg/5 ml, 5 mg/5 ml solution.

Action: Works as a urinary antispasmodic with antimuscarinic and spasmolytic effects on smooth muscle.

Use: May be useful for the treatment of detrusor hyperreflexia/overactive bladder in cats and dogs.

Safety and handling: Normal precautions should be observed.

Contraindications: Limited animal data but in humans contraindications include obstructive GI disease/ileus, gastro-oesophageal reflux/hiatal hernia, glaucoma, cardiac disease, myasthenia gravis and obstructive urinary disease.

Adverse reactions: Diarrhoea, constipation, urinary retention and sedation have all been reported in small animals. In humans, other reported adverse effects include dry mouth/eyes, skin reactions, tachycardia, vomiting, palpitations and confusion.

Drug interactions: Use with caution in patients receiving other anticholinergic agents, azole antifungals, CNS depressants and macrolide antibiotics.

DOSES

Dogs: Detrusor hyperreflexia (refractory incontinence): 0.2 mg/kg p.o. q8–12h.

Cats: Detrusor hyperreflexia: 0.5–1.25 mg/cat p.o. q8–12h.

Oxypentifylline see Pentoxifylline

Oxytetracycline

(Engemycin [c,d], Oxycare [d]) **POM-V**

Formulations: Injectable: 100 mg/ml solution. Oral: 50 mg, 100 mg, 250 mg tablets.

Action: Time-dependent antimicrobial agent inhibiting protein synthesis by inhibiting the 30S ribosomal subunit in bacteria.

Use:
- Active against many Gram-positive and Gram-negative bacteria, rickettsiae, mycoplasmas, spirochaetes and other microbes.
- Has been used in combination with nicotinamide in the management of immune-mediated conditions, including discoid lupus erythematosus and lupoid onychodystrophy.

Long term use for management of chronic enteropathy is not recommended.

Safety and handling: Normal precautions should be observed.

Contraindications: Only use in cats when no other agent is suitable. The concentrated injectable depot formulations used for cattle and sheep should never be given to small animals.

Adverse reactions: Include vomiting, diarrhoea, depression, hepatotoxicity (rare), fever, hypotension (following i.v. administration) and anorexia (cats). Prolonged use may lead to development of superinfections. Oral tetracyclines may cause GI disturbances. Although not well documented in veterinary medicine, tetracyclines induce dose-related functional changes in renal tubules in several species, which may be exacerbated by dehydration, haemoglobinuria, myoglobinuria or concomitant administration of other nephrotoxic drugs. Severe tubular damage has occurred following the use of outdated or improperly stored products and occurs due to the formation of a degradation product. Tetracyclines stain the teeth of children when used in the last 2–3 weeks of pregnancy or the first month of life. Although this phenomenon has not been well-documented in animals, it does occur in dogs and it is prudent to restrict the use of tetracyclines in all young animals.

Drug interactions: The bactericidal action of penicillins may be inhibited by oxytetracycline. Antacids containing divalent or trivalent cations (Mg^{2+}, Ca^{2+}, Al^{3+}), food or milk products bind tetracycline, reducing its absorption. Tetracyclines may increase the nephrotoxic effects of methoxyflurane. The GI effects of tetracyclines may be increased if administered concurrently with theophylline products.

DOSES

Classified as category D (Prudence) by the EMA.
See Appendix for guidelines on responsible antibiotic use.
Dogs: 10 mg/kg i.m., s.c. q24h; 20–25 mg/kg p.o. q6–8h for 5–21 days (dependent on indication). Give oral dose on an empty stomach.
Cats: 10 mg/kg i.m., s.c. q24h or once and repeat once after 48–60 hours if required.

Oxytocin

(Oxytocin S [c,d]) **POM-V**

Formulations: Injectable: 10 IU/ml solution.

Action: Synthetic oxytocin.

Use:
- Induces contractions during parturition and up to 24 hours postpartum, facilitating evacuation of uterine contents.
- Decreases haemorrhage following parturition by improving involution.

- Promotes milk 'let-down' for feeding of young or treatment of mastitis.

Before oxytocin is used, it is important to ensure that there is no evidence of obstructive dystocia and that blood calcium levels are adequate. If calcium deficiency is the cause of inertia, calcium borogluconate should be administered 20 minutes before oxytocin. Can also be used i.v. diluted in water for injection.

Safety and handling: Store in refrigerator.

Contraindications: Closed cervix.

Adverse reactions: Overstimulation of the uterus can be hazardous to the bitch/queen and fetuses.

Drug interactions: Severe hypertension may develop if used with sympathomimetic pressor amines.

DOSES

Dogs:
- **Obstetric indications:** 2–6 IU/dog i.v., i.m. q30min for up to 3 doses.
- **Milk let-down:** 2–10 IU/dog i.v., i.m., s.c. once.

Cats:
- **Obstetric indications:** 2–4 IU/cat i.v., i.m. q30min for up to 2 doses.
- **Milk let-down:** 1–10 IU/cat i.v., i.m. once.

Pamidronate

(Aredia*, Pamidronate*) **POM**

Formulations: Injectable: 15 mg, 30 mg, 90 mg powders in vials for reconstitution and i.v. infusion.

Action: Inhibits osteoclast activity and induces osteoclast apoptosis.

Use:
- Treatment of hypercalcaemia (especially associated with vitamin D toxicosis and hypercalcaemia of malignancy).
- Some studies support the use of pamidronate as an adjunctive analgesic for pain associated with bone tumours in dogs.
- In human medicine, it is also used to treat osteolytic lesions and bone pain due to bone metastases associated with breast cancer, multiple myeloma and Paget's disease.

Safety and handling: Normal precautions should be observed.

Contraindications: Renal dysfunction.

Adverse reactions: Can cause renal toxicity, nausea, diarrhoea, hypocalcaemia, hypophosphataemia, hypomagnesaemia and hypersensitivity reactions. In humans, ophthalmic syndromes, bone pain, electrolyte abnormalities and blood dyscrasias have also been reported.

Drug interactions: Concurrent use of aminoglycosides may result in severe hypocalcaemia. Use with caution with NSAIDs.

DOSES

Dogs: 0.65–2 mg/kg (typically 1 mg/kg) i.v. slow infusion with NaCl 0.9% over 2–4 hours, can be repeated q28d if required. Some clinicans advocate 0.9% NaCl i.v. for 2 hours before and after the infusion. For cholecalciferol-induced toxicosis, give on days 1 and 4 post ingestion.
Cats: 1.0–2.0 mg/kg i.v. slow infusion over 4 hours.

References
Fan TM (2009) Intravenous Aminobisphosphonates for Managing Complications of Malignant Osteolysis in Companion Animals. *Topics in Companion Animal Medicine* **24**, 151–156
Hostutler RA, Chew DJ, Jaeger JQ *et al.* (2005) Uses and effectiveness of pamidronate disodium for treatment of dogs and cats with hypercalcemia. *Journal of Veterinary Internal Medicine* **19**, 29–33

Pancreatic enzyme supplements

(Lypex, Pancreatic Enzyme for cats and dogs, Panzym, Pro-Enzorb) **AVM-GSL**

Formulations: Oral: formulations vary in the amount and type of enzyme present. Non-enteric-coated powders and enteric-coated granules and tablets are available. Readers are referred to individual products for further details.

Action: Exogenous replacement enzymes.

Use:
- Pancreatic enzymes (lipase, protease, amylase) are used to control signs of EPI.

Efficacy may be augmented by vitamin B12 therapy for any associated hypocobalaminaemia. Concomitant administration of acid blockers is not cost-effective and there is no requirement for pre-incubation with food. Fresh raw, or fresh-frozen pig pancreas (approximately 100 g per meal) can also be an effective treatment (and is not a Specified Risk Material) but availability is limited and there is a risk of pathogen ingestion by this method.

Safety and handling: Powder spilled on hands should be washed off or skin irritation may develop. Avoid inhaling powder as it causes mucous membrane irritation and may trigger asthma attacks in susceptible individuals. These risks are not associated with enteric-coated pancreatic granules.

Contraindications: No information available.

Adverse reactions: Contact dermatitis of the lips is occasionally seen with powdered non-coated enzyme and some dogs develop an offensive odour. Non-coated pancreatic enzymes may cause oral or oesophageal ulcers, and so dosing should be followed with food or water. High doses may cause diarrhoea and signs of GI cramping.

Drug interactions: The effectiveness may be diminished by antacids (magnesium hydroxide, calcium carbonate).

DOSES

Dogs, Cats: Use the manufacturer's recommendations to determine the minimum required initial dose. Lypex capsules must be opened and the contents sprinkled in with food for every meal. The dose should be adjusted to obtain faeces of normal consistency and will thus be variable. When signs are controlled, it is advisable to reduce the dose gradually over a 7-day period in order to determine the minimum effective dose.

References
Batchelor DJ, Noble PJ, Taylor RH *et al.* (2007) Prognostic factors in canine exocrine pancreatic insufficiency: prolonged survival is likely if clinical remission is achieved. *Journal of Veterinary Internal Medicine* **21**, 54–60

Papaveretum

(Omnopon*, Papaveretum*) **POM CD SCHEDULE 2**

Formulations: Injectable: 7.7 mg/ml, 15.4 mg/ml solutions; 15.4 mg/ml papaveretum + 0.4 mg/ml hyoscine (scopolamine) solution. 7.7 mg/ml and 15.4 mg/ml solutions provide the equivalent of 5 mg/ml and 10 mg/ml anhydrous morphine, respectively.

Action: Analgesia mediated by the mu opioid receptor.

Use:
- Management of moderate to severe pain in the perioperative period.
- Incorporation into sedative and pre-anaesthetic medication protocols to provide improved sedation and analgesia.

Papaveretum is a mixture of the alkaloids of opium containing the equivalent of anhydrous morphine 85.5%, anhydrous codeine 6.8% and papaverine 7.8%. It has a similar effect to morphine and is thought to have a 4-hour duration of action. Papaveretum is not widely used to provide postoperative analgesia in dogs and cats and tends to be used in combination with acepromazine to provide good sedation in aggressive dogs. The comparative sedation produced by papaveretum and other mu agonists combined with acepromazine has not been evaluated in rigorous clinical studies. It has not been widely evaluated in experimental or clinical analgesia studies. Methadone should be used in preference to papaveretum as the authorized alternative for single or repeated bolus administration to dogs and cats.

Safety and handling: Normal precautions should be observed.

Contraindications: No information available.

Adverse reactions: In common with other mu agonists, papaveretum can cause respiratory depression, although this is unlikely when used at clinical doses in conscious cats and dogs. Respiratory depression may occur when papaveretum is given i.v. during general anaesthesia, due to the increased depth of anaesthesia that accompanies administration. Respiratory function should be monitored using capnometry when given to anaesthetized patients. Vomiting is common after papaveretum administration. It causes constriction of GI sphincters (such as the pyloric sphincter) and may cause a reduction in GI motility when given over a long period. The response to all opioids appears to be very variable between individual patients, therefore, assessment of pain after administration is imperative. Papaveretum is metabolized in the liver; some prolongation of effect may be seen with impaired liver function. Papaveretum crosses the placenta and may exert sedative effects in neonates born to bitches treated prior to parturition. Severe adverse effects can be treated with naloxone.

Drug interactions: Other CNS depressants (e.g. anaesthetics, antihistamines, barbiturates, phenothiazines and tranquillizers) may cause increased CNS or respiratory depression when used concurrently with narcotic analgesics.

DOSES
When used for sedation is generally given as part of a combination. See Appendix for sedation protocols in cats and dogs.
Dogs: Analgesia: 0.2–0.8 mg/kg i.v., i.m., s.c.; use lower doses i.v.; only use higher doses when deep sedation is required.
Cats: Analgesia: 0.2–0.3 mg/kg i.v., i.m., s.c.

Paracetamol (Acetaminophen) CIL
(Pardale-V [d], Paracetamol*, Perfalgan*) **POM-V, POM, P**

Formulations: Oral: 500 mg tablets; 120 mg/5 ml, 250 mg/5 ml suspensions; 400 mg paracetamol + 9 mg codeine phosphate tablets (Pardale-V). Injectable: 10 mg/ml solution.

Action: It has been proposed that its antipyretic and analgesic actions are due to decreased prostaglandin synthesis within the CNS, possibly via indirect actions on the cannabinoid system; however, its exact mechanism of action is unclear.

Use:
- Control of mild to moderate pain.
- Antipyretic action.
- Injectable paracetamol may be useful to provide adjunctive analgesia in dogs during the perioperative period.

There are limited data describing the analgesic efficacy of paracetamol in dogs. Paracetamol has poor anti-inflammatory effects. It is believed to produce few GI side effects and therefore is commonly administered if traditional NSAIDs are contraindicated; however, there are limited clinical data to support this practice. Although common practice in human anaesthesia, the combination of an NSAID and paracetamol to provide perioperative analgesia has not undergone rigorous investigation in dogs in terms of either safety or efficacy. The authorized oral preparation of paracetamol contains codeine; however, due to a high first-pass metabolism of opioids, this codeine is not bioavailable and therefore is unlikely to contribute to analgesia.

Safety and handling: Normal precautions should be observed.

Contraindications: Do not use in cats as they lack the glucuronyl transferase enzymes required to metabolize the drug.

Adverse reactions: Overdose of paracetamol causes liver damage through the production of N-acetyl-p-aminobenzoquinonimine during metabolism, which causes hepatocyte cell death and centrilobular hepatic necrosis. Treatment of overdose with oral methionine or i.v. acetylcysteine is directed at replenishing hepatic glutathione, though this treatment is not backed by clinical data. Fatal toxicosis has been recognized in cats due to methaemoglobinaemia.

Drug interactions: Metoclopramide may increase absorption of paracetamol, thereby enhancing its effects.

DOSES
Dogs: 10–20 mg/kg p.o., i.v. q8h. Authorized dose of Pardale-V preparation is 1 tablet per 12 kg (equivalent to 33 mg/kg) q8h for 5 days, although longer term adminsitration of Pardale-V is widely used clinically without apparent side effects. For acute pain management, doses of 20–33 mg/kg q8h, for a period not exceeding 5–7 days, have been advocated. However there are limited data describing the pharmaco-dynamics of paracetamol in dogs and it is difficult to make evidence-based dose recommendations. Recent studies have shown a lack of efficacy of paracetamol when used as a monotherapy for acute and chronic pain.

Cats: Do not use.

References
Leung J, Beths T, Carter JE *et al.* (2021) Intravenous acetaminophen does not provide adequate postoperative analgesia in dogs following ovariohysterectomy. *Animals* **11**, 3609
Pacheco M, Knowles TG, Hunt J *et al.* (2020) Comparing paracetamol/codeine and meloxicam for postoperative analgesia in dogs: a non inferiority trial. *Veterinary Record* **187**, e61

Paraffin (Liquid paraffin, Mineral oil)
(Katalax, Lacri-Lube*, Liquid paraffin oral emulsion*, Simple Eye Ointment*) **P, GSL**

Formulations: Oral: white soft paraffin paste (Katalax); liquid paraffin (50/50 oil/water mix). **Topical:** 3.5 g, 4 g or 5 g ophthalmic ointment.

Action: Paraffin is a laxative; it softens stools by interfering with intestinal water resorption. It is also a lipid-based tear substitute that mimics the lipid portion of the tear film and helps prevent evaporation of tears.

Use:
- Used to manage constipation.
- It is beneficial in the management of keratoconjunctivitis sicca, during general anaesthesia and for eyelid paresis. It is a long-acting ocular lubricant and is used when frequent application is difficult.

Safety and handling: Normal precautions should be observed.

Contraindications: Do not give orally in patients with a reduced gag reflex.

Adverse reactions: As paraffin is tasteless, normal swallowing may not be elicited if syringing orally; thus, inhalation and subsequent lipoid pneumonia are a significant risk. Paraffin ointment may blur vision, although this is not often a problem in dogs or cats.

Drug interactions: Reduced absorption of fat-soluble vitamins may follow prolonged use.

DOSES

Dogs:
- **Constipation:** 1–2 tablespoons per meal prn.
- **Ocular:** apply to eye at night or q6–12h prn.

Cats:
- **Constipation:** adults 25 mm Katalax paste p.o. q12–24h; kittens 10 mm Katalax paste p.o. q12–24h.
- **Ocular:** apply to eye at night or q6–12h prn.

Paroxetine CIL

(Paxil*, Seroxat*) **POM**

Formulations: Oral: 20 mg, 30 mg tablets; 2 mg/ml liquid suspension.

Action: Blocks serotonin reuptake in the brain, resulting in antidepressive activity and a raising in motor activity thresholds.

Use:
- Treatment of generalized anxiety and impulsivity in dogs.
- Treatment of urine marking in cats, especially when accompanied with overt aggression.

The selective serotonin reuptake inhibitor fluoxetine and non-selective serotonin reuptake inhibitor clomipramine are authorized and available for use in dogs. Accordingly, these may be preferable to use for these indications as there is no empirical evidence to support the use of paroxetine over these agents.

Safety and handling: Normal precautions should be observed.

Contraindications: Known sensitivity to paroxetine or other SSRIs, history of seizures. Do not use alongside other serotonergic agents due to risk of serotonin syndrome.

Adverse reactions: Possible reactions include lethargy, decreased appetite and vomiting. Trembling, restlessness, GI disturbance and an apparent paradoxical increase in anxiety may occur in some cases. Owners should be warned of a potential increase in aggression in response to medication and frequency of urination should be monitored when used in cats.

Drug interactions: Paroxetine should not be used within 2 weeks of treatment with an MAOI (e.g. selegiline) and an MAOI should not be used within 6 weeks of treatment with paroxetine. Paroxetine, like other SSRIs, antagonizes the effects of anticonvulsants and so is not recommended for use with epileptic patients or in association with other agents which lower seizure threshold, e.g. phenothiazines. Caution is warranted if paroxetine is used concomitantly with aspirin or other anticoagulants, since the risk of increased bleeding in the case of tissue trauma may be increased. Should not generally be used alongside other serotonergic agents given the risk of serotonin syndrome, although use alongside trazodone may be considered in exceptional cases, so long as patient carefully monitored for signs of serotonin syndrome.

DOSES
Dogs: 1–2 mg/kg p.o. q24h.
Cats: 0.5–1 mg/kg p.o. q24h; can be increased to 2 mg/kg p.o. q24h but close monitoring is required.

References
Peremans K, Audenaert K, Hoybergs Y *et al.* (2005) The effect of citalopram hydrobromide on 5-HT 2A receptors in the impulsive–aggressive dog, as measured with 123 I-5-I-R91150 SPECT. *European Journal of Nuclear Medicine and Molecular Imaging* **32**, 708–716

Penicillamine
(Pendramine*, Penicillamine*) **POM**

Formulations: Oral: 125 mg, 250 mg tablets.

Action: Penicillamine is an orally administered chelating agent that binds copper, mercury, lead and cystine to form stable complexes which are excreted via the kidney.

Use:
- Management of copper-associated hepatitis in susceptible breeds. Penicillamine is not helpful in an acute crisis as copper chelation can take weeks to months.
- Used in cystinuria as it decreases cystine excretion by combining with cystine to form the soluble complex, cystine-D-penicillamine disulphide.
- May be used in the management of lead toxicity, when injecting ethylenediaminetetraacetic acid (EDTA) is too difficult or long-term chelation is required.

Dogs that fail to tolerate even the lower dose regimes may be pretreated with antiemetic drugs (phenothiazines or antihistamines) 30–60 minutes before penicillamine. Penicillamine is used for treating rheumatoid arthritis in humans, but has not yet been used in immune-mediated erosive arthropathies in companion animals.

Safety and handling: Normal precautions should be observed.

Contraindications: Moderate to marked renal impairment or a history of penicillamine-related blood dyscrasias. Penicillamine can reduce GI absorption of dietary minerals, including zinc, iron, copper and calcium and, therefore, cause deficiencies with long-term use. Contraindicated in pregnant or lactating animals and in patients receiving cytotoxic drugs or phenylbutazone. Has inhibitory effects on collagen and elastin synthesis; use with caution prior to elective surgery or during wound healing.

Adverse reactions: Anorexia, vomiting, pyrexia and nephrotic syndrome are seen in dogs. Serious adverse effects that have been described in humans given penicillamine include leucopenia, thrombocytopenia, fever, lymphadenopathy, skin hypersensitivity reactions and lupus-like reactions. Weekly initial monitoring including a full blood count and urinalysis is advised. In humans, patients who are allergic to penicillin may react similarly to penicillamine, but cross-sensitivity appears to be rare.

Drug interactions: The absorption of penicillamine is decreased if administered with antacids, food, or iron or zinc salts. An increase in the renal and haematological effects of penicillamine have been recorded in humans receiving cytotoxic drugs. Concomitant use of NSAIDs and other nephrotoxic drugs may increase the risk of renal damage.

DOSES

Dogs:
- **Copper-associated hepatitis:** 10 mg/kg p.o. q12h given on an empty stomach at least 1 hour before feeding.
- **Cystinuria:** 10–15 mg/kg p.o. q12h.
- **Lead poisoning:** patients commonly receive CaEDTA before receiving penicillamine 30 minutes before feeding at 30 mg/kg p.o. q6–8h for 1–2 weeks. Dose may then be reduced to 5 mg/kg p.o. q6–8h if serum lead levels remain high despite the resolution of clinical signs.

Cats: **Lead poisoning:** patients commonly receive CaEDTA before receiving penicillamine 30 minutes before feeding at 15 mg/kg p.o. q6–8h for 1 week. Dose may then be reduced to 5 mg/kg p.o. q6–8h if serum lead levels remain high despite the resolution of clinical signs.

References

Dirksen K and Fieten H (2017) Canine copper-associated hepatitis. *Veterinary Clinics of North America: Small Animal Practice* **47**, 631
Fieten H, Dirksen K, van den Ingh TS *et al.* (2013) D-penicillamine treatment of copper-associated hepatitis in Labrador Retrievers. *Veterinary Journal* **196**, 522–527

Penicillin G (Benzyl penicillin)

(Crystapen, Depocillin [c,d], Neopen [c,d], Norocillin) **POM-V**

Formulations: Injectable: comes in a variety of salts (sodium, procaine and benzathine), which affect solubility. Penicillin G sodium (highly soluble): 3 g powder for reconstitution for i.v. use; procaine penicillin (less soluble): 300 mg/ml suspension for s.c. use, slower release. 200 mg/ml penicillin G + 100 mg/ml neomycin for i.m use; 15% w/v procaine penicillin + 11.5% w/v benzathine penicillin long-acting preparation.

Action: Binds to penicillin-binding proteins involved in cell wall synthesis, decreasing bacterial cell wall strength and rigidity, and affecting cell division, growth and septum formation. As animal cells lack a cell wall, the beta-lactam antibiotics are safe. Kills bacteria in a time-dependent fashion.

Use:
- A beta-lactamase-susceptible antimicrobial. Narrow spectrum of activity and susceptible to acid degradation in the stomach.
- Used parenterally to treat infections caused by sensitive organisms (e.g. *Streptococcus, Clostridium, Borrelia burgdorferi,* fusospirochaetes).

The sodium salt is absorbed well from s.c. or i.m. sites. Procaine penicillin is sparingly soluble, providing a 'depot' from which it is slowly released. As penicillin kills in a time-dependent fashion, it is important to maintain tissue concentrations above the MIC for the target organism throughout the interdosing interval. Patients with significant renal or hepatic dysfunction may need dosage adjustment.

Safety and handling: After reconstitution, penicillin G sodium is stable for 24 hours when refrigerated.

Contraindications: Do not use in animals sensitive to beta-lactam antimicrobials.

Adverse reactions: 600 mg of penicillin G sodium contains 1.7 mEq of Na$^+$. This may be clinically important for patients on restricted sodium intakes. Administration of >600 mg/ml i.m. may cause discomfort.

Drug interactions: Aminoglycosides may inactivate penicillins when mixed in parenteral solutions *in vitro*, but they act synergistically when administered at the same time *in vivo*. Procaine can antagonize the action of sulphonamides and so procaine penicillin G should not be used with them.

DOSES

Classified as category D (Prudence) by the EMA.
See Appendix for guidelines on responsible antibiotic use.
Dogs, Cats: Penicillin G sodium: 15–25 mg/kg i.v., i.m. q4–6h; Penicillin G procaine: 30 mg/kg s.c. q24h; Penicillin G procaine and benzathine combined: 15 mg/kg procaine penicillin with 11.25 mg/kg benzathine penicillin (equivalent to 1 ml/10 kg).

Pentamidine isethionate

(Pentacarinat*) **POM**

Formulations: Injectable: 300 mg vials of powder for reconstitution.

Action: Kills protozoans by interacting with DNA. It is rapidly taken up by the parasites by a high-affinity energy-dependent carrier.

Use:
- Treatment of leishmaniosis when resistance to the pentavalent antimony drugs (meglumine antimonate and sodium stibogluconate) has occurred.

Pentamidine is a toxic drug and the potential to cause toxic damage to kidney and liver in particular should be carefully considered prior to use. Seek expert advice before using it.

Safety and handling: Care should be taken by staff handling this drug as it is a highly toxic agent. Similar precautions to those recommended when handling cytotoxic agents used in chemotherapy (**see Appendix**) should be taken.

Contraindications: Impaired liver or kidney function. Never administer by rapid i.v. injection due to cardiovascular effects.

Adverse reactions: Pain and necrosis at the injection site, hypotension, nausea, salivation, vomiting and diarrhoea. Hypoglycaemia and blood dyscrasias are also reported in humans.

Drug interactions: No information available.

DOSES

See Appendix for guidelines on responsible parasiticide use.
Dogs: Leishmaniosis: 4 mg/kg i.m. q48–72h (seek expert advice on treatment duration).
Cats: No information available.

References
Noli C and Auxilia ST (2005) Treatment of canine Old World visceral leishmaniasis: a systematic review. *Veterinary Dermatology* **16**, 213–232

Pentobarbital (Pentobarbitone)

(Dolethal [c,d], Euthanimal [c,d], Euthasol [c,d], Euthatal [c,d], Euthoxin [c,d], Lethobarb [c,d], Pentobarbital for euthanasia [c,d], Pentoject [c,d]) **POM-V CD SCHEDULE 3**

Formulations: Injectable: 200 mg/ml, 400 mg/ml, 500 mg/ml as either a blue, yellow or pink non-sterile aqueous solution.

Action: CNS depressant: direct action on the medulla results in rapid depression of the respiratory centre followed by cardiac arrest.

Use:

- For euthanasia.

When it is predicted that euthanasia may be problematical (e.g. aggressive patients), it is recommended that premedication with an appropriate sedative is given. The animal should be restrained in order to forestall narcotic excitement until anaesthesia supervenes. This is particularly important with cats. The route of choice is i.v. if possible, but alternatives such as intraperitoneal (preferred) or intrathoracic are possible when venepuncture is difficult to achieve. The intrathoracic route is usually the last resort; there is a risk of injection into the lungs, which causes coughing and distress. Direct injection into a chamber of the heart is rapid, but it may be difficult to locate the heart chambers accurately and repeated attempts could cause unnecessary pain and distress. There is no authorized pentobarbital product in the UK that is suitable for the emergency control of seizures and there are several other, more suitable, products available for this use.

Safety and handling: Normal precautions should be observed.

Contraindications: Should not be given i.m. as it is painful and slow to act. Do not use solutions intended for euthanasia to try to control seizures.

Adverse reactions: Narcotic excitement may be seen with agitated animals. Agonal gasping is sometimes seen.

Drug interactions: Antihistamines and opioids increase the effect of pentobarbital.

DOSES

Dogs, Cats: Euthanasia: 80 mg/kg in debilitated animals, up to 120–160 mg/kg in younger and fitter animals, rapid i.v. injection.

Pentosan polysulphate

(Cartrophen [d], Osteopen [d]) **POM-V**

Formulations: Injectable: 100 mg/ml solution.

Action: Semi-synthetic polymer of pentose carbohydrates with heparin-like properties that binds to damaged cartilage matrix comprising aggregated proteoglycans and stimulates the synthesis of new aggregated glycosaminoglycan (GAG) molecules. Ability to inhibit a range of proteolytic enzymes may be of particular importance. Modulates cytokine action, stimulates hyaluronic acid secretion, preserves proteoglycan content and stimulates articular cartilage blood flow, resulting in analgesic and regenerative effects.

Use:
- In dogs, authorized as a disease-modifying agent that reduces the pain and inflammation associated with osteoarthritis.
- It has been suggested that pentosan polysulphate may be of benefit in the management of cats suffering from chronic idiopathic, non-obstructive, lower urinary tract disease because cats suffering from this condition have been shown to have reduced concentrations of GAGs within the protective mucosal layer of the bladder; however, there is currently no evidence to support this contention. There is good evidence to suggest that this drug is of minimal value in acute cases.

Administered by aseptic s.c. injection, using an insulin syringe for accurate dosing. The manufacturer recommends monitoring haematocrit and total solids.

Safety and handling: Normal precautions should be observed.

Contraindications: Do not use if septic arthritis is present or if renal or hepatic impairment exists. As it may induce spontaneous bleeding, do not use in animals with bleeding disorders.

Adverse reactions: Pain at the injection site has been reported. Because of its fibrinolytic action, the possibility of bleeding from undiagnosed tumours or vascular abnormalities exists.

Drug interactions: The manufacturers state that pentosan polysulphate should not be used concurrently with steroids or non-steroidal drugs, including aspirin, or used concomitantly with coumarin-based anticoagulants or heparin. However, many dogs suffering from osteoarthritis that might benefit from pentosan polysulphate treatment are concurrently receiving NSAID therapy. The risk of bleeding associated with concurrent administration of pentosan polysulphate and COX-2 preferential and COX-2 selective NSAIDs is probably low in animals with no history of blood clotting disorders.

DOSES

Dogs: 3 mg/kg (0.3 ml/10 kg) s.c. q5–7d on four occasions. Avoid i.m. injection due to risk of haematoma formation.

Cats: Oral formulations available in other countries have been used in cats for osteoarthritis and for chronic refractory cases of feline lower urinary tract disease (FLUTD). The use of the injectable form has not been well reported in this species, one study reports the use of 3 mg/kg s.c. in cats with FLUTD.

References

Budsberg SC, Bergh MS, Reynolds LR *et al.* (2007) Evaluation of pentosan polysulfate sodium in the postoperative recovery from cranial cruciate injury in dogs: a randomized, placebo-controlled clinical trial. *Veterinary Surgery* **36**, 234–244

Wallius BM and Tidholm AE (2009) Use of pentosan polysulphate in cats with idiopathic, non-obstructive, lower urinary tract disease: a double-blind, randomized, placebo-controlled trial. *Journal of Feline Medicine and Surgery* **11**, 409–412

Pentoxifylline (Oxypentifylline)

CIL

(Trental*) **POM**

Formulations: Oral: 400 mg tablets.

Action: Reduces blood viscosity. Anti-inflammatory through reduction of TNF-alpha production.

Use:
- Treatment of vasculitis and vasculopathies.
- Modest effect in the treatment of atopic dermatitis and contact dermatitis.

Dose adjustment may be required in patients with renal impairment.

Safety and handling: Normal precautions should be observed.

Contraindications: No information available.

Adverse reactions: GI irritation. Decreased platelet function has been seen in humans given this drug although this has not been demonstrated in dogs or cats.

Drug interactions: There is a possible increased risk of bleeding when pentoxifylline is given with NSAIDs.

DOSES

Dogs: Vasculopathies: 15 mg/kg p.o. q8–12h.

Cats: No information available.

References

Morris DO (2013) Ischaemic Dermatopathies. *Veterinary Clinics of North America: Small Animal Practice* **43**, 99–111

Singh SK, Dimri U, Saxena SK *et al.* (2010) Therapeutic management of canine atopic dermatitis by combination of pentoxifylline and PUFAs. *Journal of Veterinary Pharmacology and Therapeutics* **33**, 495–498

Permethrin

(Activyl Tick Plus [d], Advantix [d], Ataxxa [d], Frontect, Indorex, Vectra 3D [d]) **POM-V, general sale**

Formulations: Topical: 480 mg/ml permethrin and indoxacarb (Activyl Tick Plus); 500 mg/ml permethrin and imidacloprid (Advantix); 500 mg/ml permethrin with imidacloprid (Ataxxa); 504 mg/ml permethrin with fipronil (Frontect); 397 mg/ml permethrin with dinotefuran and pyriproxyfen (Vectra 3D), all in spot-on pipettes of various sizes. Environmental: permethrin and pyriproxyfen/piperonyl butoxide spray (Indorex). Also found in many proprietary products.

Action: Acts as a sodium 'open-channel blocker' resulting in muscular convulsions and death in arthropods. It also repels ticks and insects.

Use:
- Treatment and prevention of flea (*Ctenocephalides felis*, *C. canis*) infestations.
- Has acaricidal (killing) and repellent (anti-feeding) efficacy against tick infestations (*Ixodes ricinus*, *Rhipicephalus sanguineus*, *Dermacentor reticulatus*).
- Also used for the treatment of canine biting/chewing lice (*Trichodectes canis*) infestation.

Safety and handling: Normal precautions apply. Toxic to aquatic organisms; dogs should not be allowed to swim for 48 hours after application. Dispose of carefully.

Contraindications: Do not use on cats.

Adverse reactions: Transient pruritus and erythema at the site of application may occur.

Drug interactions: No information available.

DOSES
See Appendix for guidelines on responsible parasiticide use.
Dogs: Flea control: apply 1 pipette per dog according to weight. Treatment should be repeated not more frequently than every 4 weeks. Check individual product details.
Cats: Do not use.

References
Boland LA and Angles JM (2010) Feline permethrin toxicity: retrospective study of 42 cases. *Journal of Feline Medicine and Surgery* **12**, 61–71
Pfister K and Armstrong R (2016) Systemically and cutaneously distributed ectoparasiti-cides: a review of the efficacy against ticks and fleas on dogs. *Parasites and Vectors* **9**, 436

Pethidine (Meperidine)

(Pethidine [c,d], Demerol*, Meperidine*) **POM CD SCHEDULE 2**

Formulations: Injectable: 10–50 mg/ml solutions. 50 mg/ml solution is usually used in veterinary practice.

Action: Analgesia mediated by the mu opioid receptor.

Use:
- Management of mild to moderate pain.
- Incorporation into sedative and pre-anaesthetic medication protocols to provide improved sedation and analgesia.

Pethidine has a fast onset (10–15 min) and short duration (45–60 min) of action. Frequent redosing is required for analgesia. The short duration of action may be desirable in some circumstances (e.g. when a rapid recovery is required or in animals with compromised liver function). It shares common opioid effects with morphine but also has anticholinergic effects, producing a dry mouth and sometimes an increase in heart rate. It causes less biliary tract spasm than morphine, suggesting that it may be useful for the management of pain in dogs and cats with pancreatitis. Due to the concentration of commercially available solutions, the injection volume can be 2–3 ml in large dogs, which can cause pain on i.m. injection.

Safety and handling: Normal precautions should be observed.

Contraindications: Do not give i.v. due to histamine release. Not advisable to use at all in animals at risk from histamine release (e.g. some skin allergies, asthma, mast cell tumours).

Adverse reactions: Histamine released during i.v. injection causes hypotension, tachycardia and bronchoconstriction. Histamine-mediated reactions may also occur after i.m. injection, resulting in local urticaria. Pethidine crosses the placenta and may exert sedative effects in neonates born to animals treated prior to parturition. Severe adverse effects can be treated with naloxone.

Drug interactions: Other CNS depressants (e.g. anaesthetics, antihistamines, barbiturates, phenothiazines and tranquillizers) may cause increased CNS or respiratory depression when used concurrently with narcotic analgesics. Pethidine may produce a serious interaction if administered with monoamine oxidase inhibitors (MAOIs). The mechanism of this interaction is not clear but effects include coma, convulsions and hyperpyrexia.

DOSES
When used for sedation is generally given as part of a combination. See Appendix for sedation protocols in cats and dogs.
Dogs: Analgesia: 2–10 mg/kg i.m., s.c. q1–2h depending on pain assessment.
Cats: Analgesia: 5–10 mg/kg i.m., s.c. q1–2h depending on pain assessment.

Phenobarbital (Phenobarbitone)
(Epiphen[d], Epityl[d], Phenoleptil[d], Soliphen[d], Phenobarbital*)
POM-V, POM CD SCHEDULE 3

Formulations: Oral: 12.5 mg, 30 mg, 50 mg, 60 mg, 100 mg tablets; 4% (40 mg/ml) oral solution. Injectable: 15 mg/ml, 30 mg/ml, 60 mg/ml, 200 mg/ml solutions (phenobarbital sodium BP).

Action: Thought to mediate its antiepileptic effect through affinity for the GABA$_A$ receptor, resulting in a GABA-ergic effect; GABA being the major inhibitory mammalian neurotransmitter with prolonged opening of the chloride channel. Phenobarbital also blocks the AMPA receptor, inhibiting release of the excitatory neurotransmitter glutamate. This combined potentiation of GABA and inhibition of glutamate leads to reduced neuronal excitability.

Use:
- Phenobarbital and imepitoin are the initial medications of choice for the management of epileptic seizures due to idiopathic epilepsy in dogs. The choice of initial medication is guided by patient requirements: phenobarbital is more efficacious, while imepitoin has a more rapid onset of action than phenobarbital (does not need to achieve a steady state), does not require the determination of serum concentrations and has a less severe adverse effect profile.
- Also authorized for the management of epileptic seizures due to structural brain disease in dogs.
- Used for the management of epileptic seizures in cats, although not authorized.

Phenobarbital may also be used in dogs in combination with propranolol and a behaviour modification programme for the control of fears and anxieties, especially those with a large physiological component which may be antagonizing the condition through biofeedback processes. Phenobarbital is rapidly absorbed after oral administration in dogs; maximal plasma concentrations reached within 4–8 hours. Wide range of elimination half-life (40–90 hours) in dogs. Steady state serum concentrations are not reached until 7–10 days after treatment is initiated and the full clinical effect of a dose cannot be ascertained until this point. Serum concentrations should be determined once a steady state has been reached; if <15 μg (micrograms)/ml, the dose should be increased accordingly. If seizures are not adequately controlled, the dose may be increased up to a maximum serum concentration of 45 μg/ml. Plasma concentrations above this level are associated with increased hepatotoxicity. Blood samples for serum concentration determination should be collected at the same time of day relative to the time of dose administration in dogs on higher daily doses, but timing is not normally important in dogs on a total daily dose of <8 mg/kg. For accuracy of dosing, dogs <4 kg should commence therapy with the oral solution. With chronic therapy, induction of the hepatic microsomal enzyme system results in a decreased half-life, particularly during the first 6 months of therapy in dogs. As a result, the dose may need to be increased. Phenobarbital levels should be assessed every 6–12 months. Any termination of phenobarbital therapy should be performed gradually (recommended protocol: reduce the dose by 25% of the original dose each month).

Safety and handling: Normal precautions should be observed.

Contraindications: Do not administer to animals with impaired hepatic function. Not for use in pregnant animals and nursing bitches, although the risk associated with uncontrolled seizures may be greater than the risk associated with phenobarbital. Do not use to control seizures resulting from hepatic disease (e.g. portosystemic shunt), hypoglycaemia or toxic causes where the clinical signs are mediated through the GABA channels (ivermectin and moxidectin toxicity) as this may exacerbate the seizures. Do not administer high doses in animals with marked respiratory depression.

Adverse reactions: Sedation, ataxia, polyphagia and polyuria/polydipsia (PU/PD). Polyphagia and PU/PD are likely to persist throughout therapy. Ataxia and sedation occur commonly following initiation of therapy but usually resolve within 1 week, although they may continue if high doses are used. Hepatic toxicity is rare but may occur at high serum concentrations (or as a rare idiosyncratic reaction within 2 weeks of starting treatment). Hyperexcitability has been reported in dogs receiving subtherapeutic doses. Haematological abnormalities, including neutropenia, anaemia and thrombocytopenia, may occur. Rarely, it may cause a superficial necrolytic dermatitis. Long-term administration is associated with significant increases in alkaline phosphatase and, to a lesser extent, alanine aminotransferase and gamma-glutamyl transferase activity without evidence of morphological liver damage on histology. A transient decrease in serum albumin (up to 6 months after starting therapy) may be seen but there are no changes in aspartate aminotransferase, bilirubin or fasting bile acids. Therefore, liver function should be assessed by dynamic bile acid assay. Phenobarbital treatment does not affect adrenal function tests (ACTH response test and low-dose dexamethasone test) despite acceleration of dexamethasone metabolism. Phenobarbital significantly decreases total thyroxine and free thyroxine, and cholesterol levels tend to increase towards the upper limits of the normal range. Additional adverse effects documented in cats include facial pruritus and pseudolymphoma.

Drug interactions: The effect of phenobarbital may be increased by other CNS depressants (antihistamines, narcotics, phenothiazines). Phenobarbital may enhance the metabolism of, and therefore decrease the effect of, corticosteroids, beta-blockers, metronidazole and theophylline. Chronic administration of phenobarbital has been found to alter the binding, bioavailability, metabolism and pharmacokinetics of propranolol, and so long-term use of this combination for the control of anxiety needs to be monitored carefully. It also increases the clearance of levetiracetam and zonisamide. Barbiturates may enhance the effects of other antiepileptics. Cimetidine, itraconazole and chloramphenicol increase serum phenobarbital concentration through inhibition of the hepatic microsomal enzyme system.

DOSES

Dogs:
- **Initial therapy:** 1–2.5 mg/kg p.o. q12h (authorized dose). However, in one study only 40% of dogs started on this dose achieved therapeutic serum concentrations. Therefore, initial dose recommendation is usually 2.5–3 mg/kg p.o. q12h. Incremental modifications of the initial dose, based on serum concentrations, are essential.
- **Emergency management of status epilepticus or severe cluster seizures in dogs that have not been receiving maintenance phenobarbital:** aim for a total loading dose of 18–24 mg/kg, followed by a maintenance dose of 2–3 mg/kg q12h. The loading dose is given as an initial 12 mg/kg slow i.v. and then after 20 minutes, two further doses of 4–6 mg/kg slow i.v. 20 minutes apart. Always wait 20 minutes before giving additional doses as CNS levels take 20 minutes to respond, and do not administer if the dog is excessively sedated or has evidence of respiratory depression. Higher doses may be required in very small dogs.
- **Emergency management in dogs that have been receiving maintenance phenobarbital:** 4–6 mg/kg i.v. or i.m. to increase the blood levels slightly in case these were subtherapeutic. Always take a serum sample for phenobarbital level determination first, before giving the top-up dose.
- **Control of fear and anxiety:** 2–3 mg/kg p.o. q12h with propranolol also at 2–3 mg/kg p.o. q12h.

Cats:
- **Initial therapy:** 1.5–3 mg/kg p.o. q12h.
- **Emergency management:** doses as for dogs.

References

Charalambous M, Brodbelt D and Volk HA (2014) Treatment in canine epilepsy – a systematic review. *BMC Veterinary Research* **10**, 257

Finnerty KE, Barnes Heller HL, Mercier MN *et al.* (2014) Evaluation of therapeutic pheno-barbital concentrations and application of a classification system for seizures in cats: 30 cases (2004–2013). *Journal of the American Veterinary Medical Association* **244**, 195–199

Phenoxybenzamine `CIL`

(Dibenyline*, Phenoxybenzamine*) **POM**

Formulations: Oral: 10 mg capsules. Injectable: 50 mg/ml solution.

Action: An alpha-adrenergic antagonist that irreversibly blocks pre-synaptic and post-synaptic receptors, producing a chemical sympathectomy (interruption of the sympathetic nervous pathway).

Use:
- Treatment of reflex dyssynergia or functional urethral obstruction due to urethral spasm, although recent studies have questioned the

use of alpha-adrenergic antagonists in management of feline urethral obstruction.
- Treatment of severe hypertension in animals with phaeochromocytoma prior to surgery to reduce mortality. If concurrent beta-blockers are also used (for severe tachycardia/arrhythmias), only start these once alpha blockade is in place (to avoid a hypertensive crisis).

Use with extreme caution in animals with pre-existing cardiovascular disease.

Safety and handling: Normal precautions should be observed.

Contraindications: No information available.

Adverse reactions: Adverse effects associated with alpha-adrenergic blockade include hypotension, miosis, tachycardia and nasal congestion.

Drug interactions: There is an increased risk of a first dose hypotensive effect if administered with beta-blockers or diuretics. Phenoxybenzamine will antagonize effects of alpha-adrenergic sympathomimetic agents (e.g. phenylephrine).

DOSES
Dogs:
- **Reflex dyssynergia:** 0.25–1 mg/kg p.o. q8–24h for a minimum of 5 days.
- **Hypertension associated with phaeochromocytoma:** 0.25–0.5 mg/kg p.o. q12h for 10–14 days prior to surgery, titrating up to an effective dose (maximum of 2.5 mg/kg q12h) as required or administer long term for medical management if adrenalectomy not possible.

Cats: 0.5–1 mg/kg p.o. q12h for 5 days before evaluating efficacy.

Phenylephrine
(Phenylephrine hydrochloride*) **POM**

Formulations: Injectable: 1% (10 mg/ml) solution. **Ophthalmic:** 2.5%, 10% solution (single-dose vials).

Action: Alpha-1 selective adrenergic agonist that causes peripheral vasoconstriction when given i.v., resulting in increased diastolic and systolic blood pressure, a small decrease in cardiac output and an increased circulation time. Directly stimulates the alpha-adrenergic receptors in the iris dilator musculature.

Use:
- Used in conjunction with fluid therapy to treat hypotension secondary to drugs or vascular failure.
- When applied topically to the eye, causes vasoconstriction and mydriasis (pupil dilation).
- Ophthalmic uses include mydriasis prior to intraocular surgery (often in conjunction with atropine), differentiation of involvement of superficial conjunctival vasculature from deep episcleral vasculature (by vasoconstriction) and reduction of haemorrhage during ophthalmic surgery.
- It is also used in the diagnosis of Horner's syndrome (HS) (denervation hypersensitivity), by determining the time to pupillary dilation following administration of 1% phenylephrine topically to

both eyes. Essentially, the shorter the time to pupillary dilation, the closer the lesion to the iris: <20 minutes suggests third-order HS; 20–45 minutes suggests second-order HS; 60–90 minutes suggests first-order HS or no sympathetic denervation of the eye. If 10% phenylephrine is used, mydriasis occurs in 5–8 minutes in post-ganglionic (third-order neuron) lesions.

Phenylephrine is not a cycloplegic in the dog, so its use in uveitis is limited to mydriasis to reduce posterior synechiae formation. It is inappropriate for diagnostic mydriasis because its onset of action is too slow (2 hours in the dog). Vasoconstrictors should be used with care; although they raise blood pressure, they do so at the expense of perfusion of vital organs. In many patients with shock, peripheral resistance is already high and raising it further is unhelpful. Has minimal effects on cardiac beta-adrenergic receptors.

Safety and handling: Normal precautions should be observed.

Contraindications: No information available. Use lower concentrate solutions in cats and small dogs. Do not apply once ophthalmic surgery has started (to avoid direct arterial absorption).

Adverse reactions: These include hypertension, tachycardia, and reflex bradycardia. Extravasation injuries can be serious (necrosis and sloughing).

Drug interactions: There is a risk of arrhythmias if phenylephrine is used in patients receiving digoxin or with volatile anaesthetic agents. The pressor effects may be enhanced when used concurrently with oxytocic agents, leading to severe hypertension.

DOSES
Dogs:
- **Hypotension:** correct blood volume then infuse 0.01 mg/kg very slowly i.v. q15min. Continuously monitor blood pressure if possible.
- **Ophthalmic use:** 1 drop approximately 2 hours before intraocular surgery (for mydriasis). 1 drop as a single dose for vasoconstriction. 1 drop of 1% solution to both eyes for diagnosis of Horner's syndrome.

Cats: Ophthalmic use: as for dogs (**NB:** ineffective for mydriasis as sole agent).

References
Franci P, Leece EA and McConnell JF (2011) Arrhythmias and transient changes in cardiac function after topical administration of one drop of phenylephrine 10% in an adult cat undergoing conjunctival graft. *Veterinary Anaesthesia and Analgesia* **38**, 208–212

Phenylpropanolamine (Diphenylpyraline)
(Continence[d], Proin[d], Propalin[d], Urilin[d]) **POM-V**

Formulations: Oral: 40 mg/ml phenylpropanolamine syrup (equivalent to 50 mg/ml phenylpropanolamine hydrochloride); 15 mg, 50 mg phenylpropanolamine hydrochloride tablets (equivalent to 12 mg, 40 mg phenylpropanolamine, respectively).

Action: Sympathomimetic – increases urethral outflow resistance and has some peripheral vasoconstrictive effects.

Use:
- Treatment of urinary incontinence secondary to urethral sphincter incompetence.

Incontinence may recur if doses are delayed or missed. The onset of action may take several days.

Safety and handling: Normal precautions should be observed.

Contraindications: Use with caution in the presence of cardiovascular disease, renal or hepatic insufficiency, glaucoma, diabetes mellitus or hyperthyroidism.

Adverse reactions: May include restlessness, aggressiveness, irritability, gastrointestinal signs and hypertension. Cardiotoxicity has been reported.

Drug interactions: Concurrent administration with estriol may potentiate efficacy.

DOSES
Dogs, Cats: 0.8 mg/kg (equivalent to 1 mg/kg phenylpropanolamine hydrochloride) p.o. q8h or 1.2 mg/kg (equivalent to 1.5 mg/kg phenylpropanolamine hydrochloride) p.o. q12h.

References
Byron JK (2015) Micturition Disorders. *Veterinary Clinics of North America: Small Animal Practice* **45**, 769–782

Phenytoin (Diphenylhydantoin)
(Epanutin*, pro-Epanutin*) **POM**

Formulations: Oral: 25 mg, 50 mg, 100 mg, 300 mg capsules; 100 mg tablets, 50 mg chewable tablets; 30 mg/5 ml suspension. **Injectable:** 50 mg/ml; 75 mg/ml fosphenytoin (equivalent to 50 mg/ml phenytoin).

Action: Diminishes the spread of focal neural discharges by promoting sodium efflux from neurons via the voltage-gated sodium channels, thereby stabilizing the membrane and threshold against hyperexcitability.

Use:
- Used to control most forms of epilepsy in humans. In dogs, it is metabolized very rapidly so that high doses need to be given often, and is associated with hepatic toxicity; cats metabolize the drug very slowly and toxicity easily develops. These undesirable pharmacokinetic properties mean that the drug is not recommended for use in dogs and cats as a maintenance therapy as there are alternative drugs with a better efficacy and fewer adverse effects.
- Recent evidence suggests that it may be effective as treatment for status epilepticus especially when used as the fosphenytoin preparation which has less risk of cardiac, blood-pressure and infusion-site adverse effects.
- Has been employed as an oral or i.v. antiarrhythmic agent in cats and dogs.
- Described in various case reports in both species as a treatment of myokymia (undulating vermiform movements of the overlying skin due to contraction of small bands of muscle fibres) with variable success.

Safety and handling: Normal precautions should be observed.

Contraindications: Do not use as an anticonvulsant in cats. No longer recommended for long-term treatment of epilepsy in dogs.

Adverse reactions: Adverse effects include ataxia, vomiting, hepatic toxicity, peripheral neuropathy, toxic epidermal necrolysis and pyrexia.

Drug interactions: A large number of potential drug interactions are reported in human patients, in particular complex interactions with other antiepileptics. The plasma concentration of phenytoin may be increased by cimetidine, diazepam, metronidazole, phenylbutazone, sulphonamides and trimethoprim. The absorption, effects or plasma concentration of phenytoin may be decreased by antacids, barbiturates and calcium. The metabolism of corticosteroids, doxycycline, theophylline and thyroxine may be increased by phenytoin. The analgesic properties of pethidine may be reduced by phenytoin, whereas the toxic effects may be enhanced. Concomitant administration of two or more antiepileptics may enhance toxicity without a corresponding increase in antiepileptic effect.

DOSES
Dogs:
- **For treatment of ventricular arrhythmias:** 10 mg/kg i.v. slowly; 30–50 mg/kg p.o. q8h.
- **For treatment of status epilepticus:** following a benzodiazepine, 22.5 mg/kg fosphenytoin (equivalent to 15 mg/kg phenytoin) i.v. slowly (1 ml/min).
- **For treatment of myokymia:** 50–100 mg/kg p.o. q24h sustained-release phenytoin.

Cats: Do not use.

References
Bhatti SF, Vanhaesebrouck AE, Van Soens I *et al.* (2011) Myokymia and neuromyotonia in 37 Jack Russell terriers. *The Veterinary Journal* **89**, 284–288
Patterson EE, Leppik IE, Coles LD *et al.* (2015) Canine status epilepticus treated with fosphenytoin: a proof of principle study. *Epilepsia* **56**, 882–887

Pheromones see Dog appeasing pheromone, Feline facial fraction F3

Pholcodine
(Benylin Children's Dry Cough Mixture*, Galenphol*)
general sale

Formulations: Oral: 2 mg/5 ml, 5 mg/5 ml, 10 mg/5 ml solutions. Note that many adult cough mixtures contain dextromethorphan (another opiate derivative about which little is known in dogs) and/or guaifenesin (an expectorant).

Action: A derivative of codeine that acts as an antitussive and has mild sedating but no analgesic properties. It depresses the cough reflex by acting on the cough centre in the CNS. It has a lower potential than codeine for inducing dependence.

Use:
- Cough suppression where the cause of the cough cannot be removed and the coughing is becoming detrimental to the animal's health (e.g. in chronic bronchitis, tracheal or mainstem bronchial collapse).

It is not effective in respiratory tract infections in humans and would be unlikely to be effective in kennel cough in dogs. In humans, it is effective in reducing coughs associated with lung tumours. Do not use unless cause of cough has been identified and any other inciting cause treated/managed.

Safety and handling: Normal precautions should be observed.

Contraindications: Respiratory depression, raised intracranial pressure.

Adverse reactions: Sedation, constipation (although less than codeine). Has been associated with anaphylaxis in humans.

Drug interactions: Likely to interact with other opiates (including tramadol).

DOSES
Dogs: 0.1–0.2 mg/kg up to 4 times daily (anecdotal).
Cats: No information available.

Phosphate (Toldimphos)

(Phosphate-Sandoz*) **GSL**

Formulations: Injectable: 40 mmol phosphate + 30 mmol potassium + 30 mmol sodium in 20 ml vials. Oral: Effervescent tablets containing 1.936 g sodium acid phosphate + 350 mg sodium bicarbonate + 315 mg potassium bicarbonate (500 mg (16.1 mmol) phosphate + 468.8 mg (20.4 mmol) sodium + 123 mg (3.1 mmol) potassium).

Action: Phosphate is essential for intermediary metabolism, adenosine triphosphate production, DNA and RNA synthesis, nerve, muscle and red blood cell function. Phosphate is filtered by the kidneys but 80% is resorbed.

Use:
- To correct hypophosphataemia.
- To supplement patients on large-volume i.v. fluid therapy that have inadequate intake or patients that become hypophosphataemic following administration of insulin therapy or parenteral nutrition.
- In diabetic ketoacidotic patients, a combination of potassium chloride and potassium phosphate in equal parts may be indicated to meet the patient's potassium needs and to treat or prevent significant hypophosphataemia.

Safety and handling: Normal precautions should be observed.

Contraindications: Hyperphosphataemia, hypocalcaemia, oliguric renal failure or significant tissue necrosis.

Adverse reactions: May result in hypotension, renal failure or metastatic calcification of soft tissue. Hyperkalaemia or hypernatraemia may result in patients predisposed to these abnormalities and monitoring of electrolyte profiles is required. Overdose or administration to patients with renal compromise may lead to hyperphosphataemia.

Drug interactions: Phosphates are incompatible with metals, including calcium and magnesium.

DOSES
Dogs:
- Acute severe hypophosphataemia: 0.06–0.18 mmol/kg of potassium phosphate i.v. over 6 hours, adjust according to response.
- Chronic hypophosphataemia: 140–280 mg (1–2 ml) i.m., s.c. q48h for 5–10 doses; 0.5–2 mmol/kg/day p.o.

Cats:
- Acute severe hypophosphataemia: 0.06–0.18 mmol/kg of potassium phosphate i.v. over 6 hours, adjust according to response.
- Chronic hypophosphataemia: 0.5–2 mmol/kg/day p.o.

Phytomenadione see Vitamin K1

Pilocarpine
(Pilocarpine hydrochloride*) **POM**

Formulations: Ophthalmic: 1%, 2%, 4% solutions in 10 ml bottles, single-use vials (2%). Most common concentration used in dogs is 1%.

Action: Direct-acting parasympathomimetic that stimulates cholinergic receptors. It lowers intraocular pressure by causing ciliary body muscle contraction, miosis and improved aqueous humour outflow.

Use:
- Used in the management of glaucoma, although this role has been superseded by other topical drugs such as carbonic anhydrase inhibitors and prostaglandin analogues. Pilocarpine produces miosis in 10–15 minutes for 6–8 hours in the dog.
- Oral pilocarpine increases lacrimation and can be used in the management of neurogenic keratoconjunctivitis sicca (KCS) in the dog; topical ophthalmic pilocarpine can also be used but can be irritant.

Pilocarpine is rarely used for ophthalmic purposes in the cat because of potential toxicity.

Safety and handling: Normal precautions should be observed.

Contraindications: Avoid in uveitis and anterior lens luxation.

Adverse reactions: Conjunctival hyperaemia (vasodilation) and local irritation (due to low pH). Signs of systemic toxicity include salivation, lacrimation, urinary incontinence, gastrointestinal disturbances and cardiac arrhythmias.

Drug interactions: No information available.

DOSES
Dogs:
- **Open-angle glaucoma:** 1 drop per eye of 1% solution q8–12h.
- **Neurogenic KCS:** 1 drop of 1–2% solution/10 kg p.o. q12h (with food) as initial dose. Dose is increased by 1 drop q2–3d until Schirmer tear test values improve or signs of systemic toxicity are observed (see Adverse reactions) and then lowered to previously tolerated dose.

Cats: No information available.

References
Galley AP, Beltran E and Tetas Pont R (2022) Neurogenic keratoconjunctivitis sicca in 34 dogs: A case series. *Veterinary Ophthalmology* **25**, 140–152

Matheis FL, Walser-Reinhardt L and Spiess BM (2012) Canine neurogenic kerato-conjunctivitis sicca: 11 cases (2006–2010). *Veterinary Ophthalmology* **15**, 288–290

Sarchahi AA, Abbasi N and Gholipour MA (2012) Effects of an unfixed combination of latanoprost and pilocarpine on the intraocular pressure and pupil size of normal dogs. *Veterinary Ophthalmology* **15(S1)**, 64–70

Pimobendan

(Cardisure [d], Fortekor-Plus [d], Pimocard [d], Vetmedin [d])
POM-V

Formulations: Injectable: 0.75 mg/ml solution (5 ml vial, Vetmedin). Oral: 5 mg hard capsules; 1.25 mg, 5 mg, 10 mg chewable tablets (Vetmedin); 1.25 mg, 2.5 mg, 5 mg, 10 mg flavoured tablets (Cardisure, Pimocard); 1.25 mg pimobendan + 2.5 mg benazepril, 5 mg pimobendan + 10 mg benazepril tablets (Fortekor-Plus).

Action: Inodilator producing both positive inotropic and vasodilatory effects. Inotropic effects are mediated via sensitization of the myocardial contractile apparatus to intracellular calcium and by phosphodiesterase (PDE) III inhibition. Calcium sensitization allows for a positive inotropic effect without an increase in myocardial oxygen demand. Vasodilation is mediated by PDE III and V inhibition, resulting in arterio- and venodilation. It is also a positive lusitrope and has a mild inhibitory action on platelet aggregation in dogs at standard doses.

Use:
- Management of congestive heart failure due to valvular insufficiency (mitral and/or tricuspid regurgitation) or dilated cardiomyopathy (DCM) in the dog. Indicated for use with concurrent congestive heart failure therapy (e.g. furosemide, ACE inhibitors).
- Has been shown to delay the onset of heart failure or sudden death in Dobermanns with preclinical DCM and dogs weighing 4–15 kg, aged 6 years or over with myxomatous mitral valve disease (MMVD). Authorized for use in preclinical DCM in Dobermanns (Vetmedin) and MMVD.
- There is evidence of efficacy in the treatment of pulmonary hypertension secondary to mitral valve disease in dogs.
- Has also been used in cats with heart failure associated with systolic dysfunction, although it is not authorized; the pharmacokinetics in cats may differ from in dogs.

The presence of food may reduce bioavailability.

Safety and handling: Normal precautions should be observed.

Contraindications: Do not use in hypertrophic cardiomyopathy and in cases where augmentation of cardiac output via increased contractility is not possible (e.g. aortic stenosis).

Adverse reactions: A moderate positive chronotropic effect and vomiting may occur in some cases, which may be avoided by dose reduction.

Drug interactions: The positive inotropic effects are attenuated by drugs such as beta-blockers and calcium-channel blockers (especially verapamil). No interaction with digitalis glycosides has been noted.

DOSES

Dogs, Cats: 0.1–0.3 mg/kg p.o. q12h 1 hour before food. In dogs, it is advised to use a minimum dose of 0.2 mg/kg p.o. q12h.

Dogs: 0.15 mg/kg i.v. single dose. Oral pimobendan can be continued 12 hours after administration of the injection.

References
Häggström J, Boswood A, O'Grady MR *et al.* (2008) Effect of pimobendan or benazepril hydrochloride on survival times in dogs with congestive heart failure caused by naturally

occurring myxomatous mitral valve disease: the QUEST Study. *Journal of Veterinary Internal Medicine* **22**, 1124–1135

Summerfield NJ, Boswood A, O'Grady MR *et al.* (2012) Efficacy of pimobendan in the prevention of congestive heart failure or sudden death in Doberman Pinschers with preclinical dilated cardiomyopathy (The PROTECT Study). *Journal of Veterinary Internal Medicine* **26**, 1337–1349

Piperazine

(Various authorized proprietary products) **AVM-GSL**

Formulations: Oral: 500 mg tablets. There are a variety of different formulations.

Action: An anti-ascaridial anthelmintic that blocks acetylcholine, thus affecting neurotransmission and paralysing the adult worm; has no larvicidal activity.

Use:
- Active against *Toxocara cati*, *T. canis*, *Toxascaris leonine* and *Uncinaria stenocephala*.

Ineffective against tapeworms and lung worms. High doses are required to treat hookworm infection. Puppies and kittens may be wormed from 6–8 weeks of age and should be weighed accurately to prevent overdosing. Fasting is not necessary. Piperazine may be used in pregnant animals.

Safety and handling: Normal precautions should be observed.

Contraindications: No information available.

Adverse reactions: Uncommon but occasionally vomiting or muscle tremors and ataxia have been reported.

Drug interactions: Piperazine and pyrantel have antagonistic mechanisms of action; do not use together.

DOSES
See Appendix for guidelines on responsible parasiticide use.
Dogs, Cats:
- **Puppies and kittens:** 200 mg/kg as a single dose. Repeat every 2 weeks until 3 months of age and then at 3-monthly intervals.
- **Adult dogs and cats:** 200 mg/kg as a single dose. Repeat at 3-monthly intervals.

Piroxicam `CIL`

(Brexidol*, Feldene*, Piroxicam*) **POM**

Formulations: Oral: 10 mg, 20 mg capsules; 20 mg dissolving tablets. Injectable: 20 mg/ml solution. Rectal: Suppositories.

Action: Inhibition of COX enzymes limits the production of prostaglandins involved in inflammation. Also limits tumour growth but the exact mechanism is still to be determined.

Use:
- In veterinary medicine, piroxicam has been used to treat certain tumours, e.g. urothelial cell carcinoma of the bladder, prostatic carcinoma, colonic-rectal carcinoma and polyps.

Piroxicam suppositories are available and are useful in the management of colorectal polyps/neoplasia in humans. Other NSAIDs are authorized for veterinary use in various inflammatory conditions but there is limited information on the effect of these drugs in neoplastic conditions.

Safety and handling: Normal precautions should be observed.

Contraindications: Gastric ulceration, bleeding disorders, renal disease, concurrent use of corticosteroids.

Adverse reactions: As a non-specific COX inhibitor it may cause general adverse effects associated with NSAIDs, including GI toxicity, gastric ulceration and renal papillary necrosis (particularly if patient is dehydrated). There is a small risk that NSAIDs may precipitate cardiac failure in humans and this risk in animals is unknown. Ulcerative skin lesions have been reported in the cat.

Drug interactions: Do not use with corticosteroids or other NSAIDs and use with caution with bisphosphonates (increased risk of gastric ulceration). Concurrent use with diuretics or aminoglycosides may increase risk of nephrotoxicity. Piroxicam is highly protein bound and may displace other protein-bound drugs. The clinical significance of this is not well established.

DOSES
See Appendix for chemotherapy protocols.
Dogs: All uses: 0.3 mg/kg p.o. q24–72h; start at least frequent administration and slowly increase if no side effects observed. Suppositories: usually 20 mg/dog per rectum q2–3d (dose equivalent to 0.24–0.4 mg/kg/day).
Cats: All uses: 0.3 mg/kg p.o. q24–96h; start at least frequent administration and slowly increase if no side effects observed.

References
Bulman-Fleming JC, Turner TR and Rosenberg MP (2010) Evaluation of adverse events in cats receiving long-term piroxicam therapy for various neoplasms. *Journal of Feline Medicine and Surgery* **12**, 262–268
Knapp DW, Richardson RC, Chan TC *et al.* (1994) Piroxicam therapy in 34 dogs with transitional cell carcinoma of the urinary bladder. *Journal of Veterinary Internal Medicine* **8**, 273–278

Polymyxin B
(Surolan [c,d], Polyfax*) **POM-V, POM**

Formulations: Topical: 5,500 IU polymyxin/ml + miconazole + prednisolone suspension for dermatological and otic use (Surolan). 10,000 IU polymyxin/g + bacitracin ointment for dermatological and ophthalmic use (Polyfax).

Action: Concentration-dependent disruption of the outer membrane of Gram-negative bacteria through its action as a cationic surface acting agent.

Use:
- Use should be based on antimicrobial susceptibility testing wherever possible and where lower tier antimicrobials would not be effective.
- Effective against Gram-negative organisms; Gram-positive organisms usually resistant. Particularly effective in the treatment of external pseudomonal infections, e.g. keratoconjunctivitis, otitis externa.

Polymyxins are too toxic for systemic use and because of their strongly basic nature are not absorbed from the GI tract.

Safety and handling: Normal precautions should be observed.

Contraindications: Do not use if the tympanum is ruptured.

Adverse reactions: Should not be used systemically as it is nephrotoxic. Potentially ototoxic.

Drug interactions: Acts synergistically with a number of other antibacterial agents as it disrupts the outer and cytoplasmic membranes, thus improving penetration of other agents into bacterial cells. Cationic detergents (e.g. chlorhexidine) and chelating agents (e.g. EDTA) potentiate the antibacterial effects of polymyxin B against *Pseudomonas aeruginosa*.

DOSES

Classified as category B (Restrict) by the EMA.

See Appendix for guidelines on responsible antibiotic use.

Dogs, Cats:
- **Otic:** clean ear and apply a few drops into affected ear q12h.
- **Dermatological:** apply a few drops and rub in well q12h.

Polyvinyl alcohol
(Liquifilm Tears*, Refresh Ophthalmic*, Sno Tears*) **P**

Formulations: Ophthalmic: 1.4% (0.4 ml vials, 15 ml bottle).

Action: Polyvinyl alcohol is a synthetic water-based tear substitute, which mimics the aqueous layer of the trilaminar tear film (lacromimetic).

Use:
- Used for lubrication of dry eyes.
- In cases of keratoconjunctivitis sicca it will improve ocular surface lubrication, tear retention and patient comfort while lacrostimulation therapy (e.g. topical ciclosporin) is initiated.

It is more adherent and less viscous than hypromellose. Patient compliance is poor if administered >q4h; consider using a longer-acting tear replacement.

Safety and handling: Normal precautions should be observed.

Contraindications: No information available.

Adverse reactions: No information available.

Drug interactions: No information available.

DOSES

Dogs, Cats: 1 drop per eye q1h.

Potassium bromide
(Epilease [d], K-BroVet, Libromide [d], Vetbromide [d]) **POM-V**

Formulations: Oral: 325 mg, 600 mg tablets; 250 mg capsules; 250 mg/ml oral solution (K-BroVet).

Action: Competes with transmembrane chloride transport and inhibits sodium within the CNS, resulting in membrane hyperpolarization and elevation of the seizure threshold. Bromide competes with chloride in post-synaptic anion channels following activation by inhibitory neurotransmitters and therefore potentiates the effect of GABA.

Use:
- Control of seizures that are refractory to treatment with phenobarbital or where the use of phenobarbital or imepitoin is contraindicated. Usually used in conjunction with phenobarbital. Although not authorized for this use, potassium bromide (KBr) has been used in conjunction with imepitoin.

Bromide has a long half-life (>20 days) and steady state plasma concentrations may not be achieved for 3–4 months. Monitor serum drug concentrations and adjust dose levels accordingly. The serum KBr concentration should reach 0.8–1.5 mg/ml to be therapeutic. In some cases, the dog may need to be started on a loading dose to raise levels in the blood rapidly to therapeutic levels. Loading doses of KBr are associated with an increased incidence of adverse effects (primarily sedation and ataxia) and should only be used in dogs with poorly controlled severe seizures. The loading dose can be administered via enema if an animal is not conscious enough to receive oral medication, but side effects of increased sedation and transient diarrhoea may be seen. Serum samples should be taken after the end of loading to check the serum concentration. The slow rise of plasma bromide levels after enteral administration limits its usefulness in status epilepticus. Bromide is well absorbed from the GI tract and eliminated slowly by the kidney in competition with chloride. High levels of dietary salt increase renal elimination of bromide. Consequently, it is important that the diet be kept constant once bromide therapy has started. Bromide will be measured in assays for chloride and will therefore produce falsely high 'chloride' results. Use with caution in dogs with renal disease.

Safety and handling: Normal precautions should be observed.

Contraindications: Do not use in the cat; severe coughing develops due to eosinophilic bronchitis, which may be fatal. Avoid use in dogs with a history of, or a predisposition for the development of, pancreatitis.

Adverse reactions: Ataxia, sedation and somnolence are seen with overdosage and loading doses. Skin reactions have been reported in animals with pre-existing skin diseases, e.g. flea bite dermatitis. Vomiting may occur after oral administration, particularly if high concentrations (>250 mg/ml) are used. Polyphagia, polydipsia and pancreatitis have also been reported. In the case of acute bromide toxicity, 0.9% NaCl i.v. is the treatment of choice. Less commonly, behavioural changes, including irritability or restlessness, may be evident.

Drug interactions: Bromide competes with chloride for renal resorption. Increased dietary salt, administration of fluids or drugs containing chloride, and use of loop diuretics (e.g. furosemide) may result in increased bromide excretion and decreased serum bromide concentrations. Acts synergistically with other therapeutic agents that have GABA-ergic effects (such as phenobarbital).

DOSES

Dogs: The initial daily maintenance dose is 20–40 mg/kg p.o q24h. It is not necessary to dose more frequently, but more frequent dosing is not detrimental. The loading dose is 200 mg/kg/day p.o. divided into 4–6 doses for 5 days, after which the dose is decreased to the maintenance dose (20–40 mg/kg p.o. q24h). If seizures resolve sooner, it is advisable to decrease the loading dose to maintenance levels earlier to reduce adverse effects. A single loading dose of 600–1000 mg/kg p.o. can be given but this is likely to result in excessive sedation, ataxia and potentially vomiting. Intrarectal bromide can be loaded over a 24-hour period. The loading schedule for liquid bromide (250 mg/ml) by rectum is 100 mg/kg q4h for 6 doses (total 600 mg/kg).

Cats: Do not use.

References

Baird-Heinz HE, Van Schoick AL, Pelsor FR *et al.* (2012) A systematic review of the safety of potassium bromide in dogs. *Journal of the American Veterinary Medical Association* **240**, 705–715
Charalambous M, Brodbelt D and Volk HA (2014) Treatment in canine epilepsy—a systematic review. *BMC Veterinary Research* **10**, 257

Potassium chloride see Potassium salts

Potassium citrate

(Cystopurin*, Potassium citrate BP*) **AVM-GSL**

Formulations: Oral: 30% solution. Various preparations are available.

Action: Enhances renal tubular resorption of calcium and alkalinizes urine.

Use:
* Management of calcium oxalate and urate urolithiasis, and fungal urinary tract infections.
* May be used to treat hypokalaemia, although potassium chloride or gluconate is preferred.
* Used to treat some forms of metabolic acidosis.

Safety and handling: Normal precautions should be observed.

Contraindications: Renal impairment or cardiac disease.

Adverse reactions: Rare, but may include GI signs and hyperkalaemia.

Drug interactions: No information available.

DOSES

Dogs, Cats: Urinary alkalinization: 75 mg/kg or 2 mmol/kg p.o. q12h.

References

Bartges JW, Kirk C and Lane IF (2004) Update: management of calcium oxalate uroliths in dogs and cats. *Veterinary Clinics of North America: Small Animal Practice* **34**, 969–987

Potassium gluconate see Potassium salts
Potassium phosphate see Phosphate

Potassium salts (Potassium chloride, Potassium gluconate)

(Kaminox, Tumil-K) **general sale**

Formulations: Injectable: 20% KCl solution (2 g KCl/10 ml; 26 mmol K^+). Before use, dilute the solution with at least 70 times its volume of sodium chloride intravenous fluid. **Oral:** tablets containing 2 mEq potassium gluconate; powder (2 mEq per ¼ teaspoon) (Tumil-K); 1 mEq/ml potassium gluconate liquid formulated with a range of amino acids, B vitamins and iron (Kaminox). **NB:** 1 mmol/l = 1 mEq/l.

Action: Replacement of potassium.

Use:

- Treatment or prevention of known hypokalaemic states; prolonged anorexia and chronic renal failure are the most common, but can also use with diuretics that are not potassium sparing. Table below outlines supplementation guidance based on patient's serum potassium and outlines the amount of potassium to be added to fluid bag of saline and infused at maintenance fluid rates.

Serum potassium	Amount to be added to 250 ml 0.9% NaCl
<2 mmol/l	20 mmol
2–2.5 mmol/l	15 mmol
2.5–3 mmol/l	10 mmol
3–3.5 mmol/l	7 mmol
3.5–5.5 mmol/l	5 mmol (minimum daily need in anorectic patients)

If rapid correction is not necessary, may be added to s.c. fluids but do not exceed 30 mEq/l as higher levels are irritating. As potassium is primarily an intracellular electrolyte, serum concentrations may not immediately reflect clinical effect. Do not give rapid i.v. injections. Concentrated solutions must be diluted before i.v. use.

Safety and handling: Normal precautions should be observed.

Contraindications: Hyperkalaemia, acute or obstructive renal failure, untreated Addison's disease, acute dehydration and diseases with impaired or obstructed GI motility. Use with caution in any patient with renal failure as 80–90% of excretion is renal. Use with caution in digitalized patients.

Adverse reactions: Primarily development of hyperkalaemia when administered too rapidly or to patients with impaired renal function. Varied clinical signs include muscle weakness, GI disturbances, cardiac arrhythmias and cardiac arrest. Concentrations >60 mmol/l can cause pain and peripheral vein sclerosis, and increase the risk of overdose.

Drug interactions: Potassium retention leading to severe hyperkalaemia may develop when used with ACE inhibitors (e.g. captopril, enalapril) or potassium-sparing diuretics (e.g. spironolactone). Potassium chloride is not compatible with many drugs, especially those in sodium salt form.

DOSES

Dogs:

- **Correction of hypokalaemia:** intravenous doses must be titrated for each patient; dilute concentrated solutions prior to use (normally to 20–60 mmol/l). Rate of i.v. infusion should not exceed 0.5 mmol/kg/h, especially when concentration in replacement fluid is >60 mmol/l. Use of fluid pumps is recommended.
- **Oral:** replacement dose needs to be titrated to effect to maintain mid-range normal values in each individual patient. Starting doses are 2 mEq/4.5 kg in food q12h or 2.2 mEq per 100 kcal required energy intake.

Cats:
- **Correction of hypokalaemia:** intravenous doses as for dogs.
- **Oral:** replacement dose needs to be titrated to effect to maintain mid-range normal values in each individual patient. Starting doses are 2.2 mEq per 4.5 kg in food q12h or 2–6 mEq/cat/day p.o. in divided doses q8–12h.

Potentiated sulphonamides see Trimethoprim/Sulphonamide

Pradofloxacin

(Veraflox [c,d]) **POM-V**

Formulations: Oral: 15 mg, 60 mg, 120 mg tablets; 25 mg/ml solution.

Action: 3rd generation fluoquinolone. Broad-spectrum, concentration-dependent antibiotic that inhibits DNA gyrase and topoisomerase IV, blocking bacterial replication.

Use:
- Use should be based on antimicrobial susceptibility testing, wherever possible and where lower tier antimicrobials would not be effective.
- Active against many Gram-negative and Gram-positive organisms. Improved activity *versus* anaerobes compared with earlier generation fluoroquinolones. Lipid solubility enables pradofloxacin to attain high concentrations, especially in the urogenital tract including the prostate gland.
- Specific indications include superficial and deep pyodermas and wound infections associated with susceptible organisms such as *Staphylococcus pseudintermedius*, urinary tract infections associated with susceptible organisms such as *Escherichia coli* and *S. pseudintermedius*, severe periodontal disease associated with anaerobes such as *Porphyromonas* spp. and *Prevotella* spp. and acute severe upper respiratory tract infections associated with organisms such as *E. coli*, *Staphylococcus* spp. and *Pasteurella multocida*.

Safety and handling: Normal precautions should be observed.

Contraindications: Do not use in pregnant or lactating animals. Do not use in dogs <12 months (<18 months for giant-breeds) or cats <6 weeks due to potential adverse effects on cartilage. Do not use in animals with persistent cartilage lesions. Do not use in dogs or cats with neurological disease, especially epilepsy.

Adverse reactions: Most common is mild GI upset.

Drug interactions: Absorbents and antacids containing cations (Mg^{2+}, Al^{3+}) may bind fluoroquinolones, preventing their absorption from the GI tract. Their absorption may also be inhibited by sucralfate and zinc salts; separate dosing by at least 2 hours. Fluoroquinolones increase plasma theophylline concentrations. Cimetidine may reduce the clearance of fluoroquinolones and so should be used with caution with these drugs. Some fluoroquinolones may decrease the metabolism and increase nephrotoxicity of ciclosporin and tacrolimus in humans; concurrent use in animals is best avoided. May increase the action of orally administered anticoagulants.

DOSES

Classified as category B (Restrict) by the EMA.

See Appendix for guidelines on responsible antibiotic use.

Dogs: 3–5 mg/kg p.o. q24h. Dose from the high end of the approved range.

Cats: 3–5 mg/kg p.o. q24h (tablet); 5.0 mg/kg p.o. q24h (suspension).

References

Boothe DM, Bush KM, Boothe HW and Davis HA (2018) Pharmacokinetics and pharmaco-dynamics of oral pradofloxacin administration in dogs. *American Journal of Veterinary Research* **79**, 1268–1276. *Erratum in American Journal of Veterinary Research* **80**, 504 (2019)

Sykes JE and Blondeau JM (2014) Pradofloxacin: a novel veterinary fluoroquinolone for treatment of bacterial infections in cats. *Veterinary Journal* **201**, 207–214

Pralidoxime

(Pralidoxime*) **POM**

Formulations: Powder for reconstitution: 1 g vial which produces 50 mg/ml solution.

Action: Reactivates the cholinesterase enzyme damaged by organophosphate (OP) and allows the destruction of accumulated acetylcholine at the synapse to be resumed. In addition, pralidoxime detoxifies certain OPs by direct chemical inactivation and retards the 'ageing' of phosphorylated cholinesterase to a non-reactive form.

Use:

- Management of OP toxicity.

Most effective if given within 24 hours Pralidoxime does not appreciably enter the CNS, thus CNS toxicity is not reversed. If given within 24 hours of exposure, treatment is usually only required for 24–36 hours. Respiratory support may be necessary. Treatment of OP toxicity should also include atropine. Use at a reduced dose with renal failure.

Safety and handling: Normal precautions should be observed.

Contraindications: Do not use for poisoning due to carbamate or OP compounds without anticholinesterase activity.

Adverse reactions: Nausea, tachycardia, hyperventilation and muscular weakness are reported in humans.

Drug interactions: Aminophylline, morphine, phenothiazines and theophylline should be avoided in these patients.

DOSES

Dogs, Cats: Organophosphate toxicity: dilute to a 20 mg/ml solution and administer 20–50 mg/kg slowly i.v. (over at least 2 min – 500 mg/min max.), i.m., s.c. Repeat after 1 hour if signs still severe, then q8–12h.

References

Bahri LE (2002) Pralidoxime. *Compendium on Continuing Education for the Practising Veterinarian* **24**, 884–886

Praziquantel

(Anthelmin [c,d], Broadline Spot-on [c], Cazitel [c,d], Cestem [d], Droncit [c,d], Dronspot [c], Drontal [c,d], Endoguard [d], Felpreva [c], Milbactor [c,d], Milbemax [c,d], Milprazon [c,d], Milpro [c,d], NexGard Combo [c], Prazitel [c,d], Profender [c,d], Veloxa [d], WormCat [c], WORMclear [c], various other authorized proprietary preparations) **POM-V, NFA-VPS, AVM-GSL**

Formulations: Oral: 10 mg, 20 mg, 25 mg, 30 mg, 40 mg, 50 mg, 125 mg, 144 mg, 150 mg, 175 mg tablets. **Topical:** 20 mg, 25 mg, 30 mg, 60 mg, 75 mg, 96 mg in spot-on pipettes.

Action: Cestocide that increases cell membrane permeability of susceptible worms, resulting in loss of intracellular calcium and paralysis. This allows the parasites to be phagocytosed or digested.

Use:
*   Treatment of *Dipylidium caninum*, *Taenia*, *Echinococcus granulosus* and *Mesocestoides* in dogs and cats.

As it kills all intestinal forms of *Echinococcus*, it is the preferred drug in most *Echinococcus* control programmes. The PETS travel scheme requires animals to be treated with praziquantel prior to entry into the UK. The inclusion of pyrantel and febantel in some preparations increases the spectrum of efficacy. Drontal plus can be used from 2 weeks of age. Drontal cat tablets can be used from 6 weeks of age. Retreatment is usually unnecessary unless reinfection takes place.

Safety and handling: Normal precautions should be observed. Solutions containing emodepside should not be handled by people who are or may become pregnant.

Contraindications: Do not use in unweaned puppies or kittens, as they are unlikely to be affected by tapeworms. Do not use the spot-on preparation in animals <1 kg.

Adverse reactions: Injection may cause localized tissue sensitivity, particularly in cats. Can cause transient hypersalivation if a cat licks the site of spot-on application. Oral administration can occasionally result in anorexia, vomiting, lethargy and diarrhoea.

Drug interactions: No information available.

DOSES
See Appendix for guidelines on responsible parasiticide use.
Dogs, Cats: Varies with preparation. Approximately 5.0 mg/kg p.o.; 8 mg/kg spot-on.

Prazosin

CIL

(Hypovase*, Prazosin*) **POM**

Formulations: Oral: 0.5 mg, 1 mg, 2 mg, 5 mg tablets.

Action: Prazosin is a post-synaptic alpha-1 blocking agent causing arterial and venous vasodilation. This leads to reduction in blood pressure and systemic vascular resistance.

Use:
- Promoting urine flow in patients with functional urethral obstruction, although evidence supporting this is limited.
- Management of systemic or pulmonary hypertension.
- Adjunctive therapy of congestive heart failure secondary to mitral or aortic regurgitation in cases refractory to standard therapy (not often used for this indication).

Efficacy may decline over time.

Safety and handling: Normal precautions should be observed.

Contraindications: Hypotension, renal failure.

Adverse reactions: Hypotension, syncope, drowsiness, weakness, GI upset. An increased risk of urethral re-obstruction has been shown in one study.

Drug interactions: Concomitant use of beta-blockers (e.g. propranolol) or diuretics (e.g. furosemide) may increase the risk of a first-dose hypotensive effect. Calcium-channel blockers may cause additive hypotension. Prazosin is highly protein-bound and so may be displaced by, or displace, other highly protein-bound drugs (e.g. sulphonamide) from plasma proteins.

DOSES
Dogs:
- **To decrease urethral resistance in idiopathic vesico-urethral reflex dyssynergia:** 1 mg/15 kg p.o. q12h.
- **For adjunctive treatment for heart failure:** 1 mg/dog p.o. q8–12h (dogs up to 15 kg); 2 mg/dog p.o. q8–12h (dogs >15 kg). Monitor efficacy by measuring blood pressure and clinical response.

Cats: 0.25–1 mg/cat p.o. q8–12h given initially for 5–7 days then wean off if possible.

References
Conway DS, Rozanski EA and Wayne AS (2022) Prazosin administration increases the rate of recurrent urethral obstruction in cats: 388 cases. *Journal of the American Veterinary Medical Association* **260** (S2), S7–S11

Fischer JR, Lane IF and Cribb AE (2003) Urethral pressure profile and hemodynamic effects of phenoxybenzamine and prazosin in non-sedated male Beagle dogs. *Canadian Journal of Veterinary Research* **67**, 30–38

Prazosin

Prednisolone

(Prednicare [c,d], Prednidale [c,d], Pred-forte*) **POM-V, POM**

Formulations: Ophthalmic: prednisolone acetate 0.5%, 1% suspensions in 5 ml, 10 ml bottles (Pred-forte). **Topical:** prednisolone is a component of many topical dermatological, otic and ophthalmic preparations. Oral: 1 mg, 5 mg, 25 mg tablets.

Action: Binds to specific cytoplasmic receptors which then enter the nucleus and alter the transcription of DNA, leading to alterations in cellular metabolism which result in anti-inflammatory, immunosuppressive and antifibrotic effects. Also has glucocorticoid activity and acts in dogs as an arginine vasopessin antagonist.

Use:
- Management of chronic allergic/inflammatory conditions (e.g. atopy, chronic enteropathy).

- Management of immune-mediated conditions.
- Management of hypoadrenocorticism.
- Management of lymphoproliferative and other neoplasms.

Prednisolone has approximately 4 times the anti-inflammatory potency and half the relative mineralocorticoid potency of hydrocortisone. Like methylprednisolone, it is considered to have an intermediate duration of activity and is suitable for alternate-day use. Animals receiving chronic therapy should be tapered off their steroids when discontinuing the drug. There are no studies comparing protocols for tapering immuno-suppressive or anti-inflammatory therapy; it is appropriate to adjust the therapy according to laboratory or clinical parameters. For example, cases with immune-mediated haemolytic anaemia should have their therapy adjusted following monitoring of their haematocrit. There is no evidence that long-term low doses of glucocorticoids do, or do not, prevent relapse of immune-mediated conditions. Impaired wound healing and delayed recovery from infections may be seen. The use of steroids in most cases of shock and spinal cord injury is of no benefit and may be detrimental.

Safety and handling: Shake suspensions before use.

Contraindications: Do not use in pregnant animals. Systemic cortico-steroids are generally contraindicated in patients with renal disease and diabetes mellitus. Topical corticosteroids are contraindicated in ulcerative keratitis.

Adverse reactions: Prolonged use of glucocorticoids suppresses the hypothalamic pituitary–adrenal axis, causing adrenal atrophy, and may cause significant proteinuria and glomerular changes in the dog. Catabolic effects of glucocorticoids lead to weight loss and muscle atrophy. Iatrogenic hypercortisolism may develop with chronic use. Vomiting, diarrhoea and GI ulceration may develop; the latter may be more severe when corticosteroids are used in animals with neurological injury. Hyperglycaemia and decreased serum T4 values may be seen in patients receiving prednisolone.

Drug interactions: There is an increased risk of GI ulceration if used concurrently with NSAIDs. Hypokalaemia may develop if acetazolamide, amphotericin B or potassium-depleting diuretics (e.g. furosemide, thiazides) are administered concurrently with corticosteroids. Glucocorticoids may antagonize the effect of insulin. The metabolism of corticosteroids may be enhanced by phenytoin or phenobarbital and decreased by antifungals (e.g. itraconazole).

DOSES
See Appendix for chemotherapy and immunosuppression protocols.
Dogs:
- **Ophthalmic:** dosage frequency and duration of therapy is dependent upon type of lesion and response to therapy. Usually 1 drop in affected eye(s) q4–24h, tapering in response to therapy.
- **Hypoadrenocorticism:** starting dose 0.2 mg/kg p.o. q24h with desoxycortone pivalate (DOCP); 0.1 mg/kg p.o. q24h with fludrocortisone. The dose of prednisolone may be reduced considerably in most cases once the animal is stable; in cases with fludrocortisone it may be discontinued but in cases with DOCP it should be continued at a low dose.
- **Allergy:** 0.5–1 mg/kg p.o. q12h initially, tapering to lowest dose q48h.
- **Anti-inflammatory:** 0.5 mg/kg p.o. q12–24h; taper to 0.25–0.5 mg/kg q48h.

- **Immunosuppression:** 1–2 mg/kg p.o. q24h, tapering slowly to 0.5 mg/kg q48h (for many conditions this will take 4–6 months).
- **Lymphoma: see Appendix**.

Cats:
- **Ophthalmic, hypoadrenocorticism, allergy:** doses as for dogs.
- **Anti-inflammatory:** 0.5–1 mg/kg p.o. q12–24h; taper to 0.5 mg/kg q48h.
- **Immunosuppression:** 1–2 mg/kg p.o. q12–24h, tapering slowly to 0.5–1 mg/kg q48h (for many conditions this will take 6 months).
- **Lymphoma: see Appendix**.

Pregabalin `CIL`

(Bonqat^c, Alzain*, Axalid*, Lyrica*, Pregabalin*) **POM-V, POM CD SCHEDULE 3**

Formulations: Oral: 25 mg, 50 mg, 75 mg, 100 mg, 150 mg, 200 mg, 225 mg, 300 mg tablets or capsules; 20 mg/ml oral solution; 50 mg/ml oral solution for cats (Bonqat).

Action: Similar mechanism of action to gabapentin; binds to voltage-dependent calcium channels in the CNS, reducing calcium influx and release of excitatory neurotransmitters such as glutamate and substance P. Also increases neuronal GABA levels. Pregabalin is 3–10 times more potent than gabapentin, owing to a greater affinity for the binding site, and generally has a longer duration of action.

Use:
- Authorized veterinary use is for reduction of acute anxiety and fear asociated with transportation and veterinary visits in cats.
- Adjunctive therapy in the treatment of epileptic seizures refractory to conventional treatment.
- Treatment of neuropathic pain.

Pregabalin seems to be well absorbed after oral administration in dogs. and cats and can reach serum levels shown to be effective in humans with neuropathic pain. The longer half-life of pregabalin in cats suggests that a dosing schedule of every 12 hours or more may be appropriate, which may be an advantage compared with gabapentin but might lead to long term accumulation with continued use.

Safety and handling: Normal precautions should be observed.

Contraindications: Avoid use in pregnant animals as toxicity has been demonstrated in experimental studies. Do not discontinue abruptly if using on a longer term basis, e.g. epilepsy. Use with care in patients with renal impairment as the majority is excreted by the kidneys. Safety of the authorized form for use in cats has not been established in cats <2 kg, <5 months or >15 years, or with anything more than mild systemic illness. It is recommended that the cat's health status be established prior to use. In the main clinical trial used to support authorization in cats, approximately 50% of subjects had a good or better result, so a careful risk–benefit analysis is required before prescription.

Adverse reactions: Many dogs develop sedation or ataxia, although not usually severe enough to warrant cessation of therapy. Mild increases in hepatic enzyme activities may also occur following prolonged therapy. Sedation, ataxia and vomiting are common side effects in cats (between 1–10% of cases), other side effects, e.g muscle tremor, are recognized but uncommon.

Drug interactions: No information available.

DOSES

Dogs:
- **For refractory epilepsy:** 3–4 mg/kg p.o. q8h, starting at 2 mg/kg and gradually increasing.
- **For neuropathic pain:** 4 mg/kg p.o. q12h (limited evidence).

Cats: For anxiolytic properties, the recommended dose is 5 mg/kg approximately 1.5 hours before the event (approximately 50% of cats have a good or better response). This is considerably higher than the longer term 'off licence' use of 1–3 mg/kg p.o. q12h (limited evidence).

References

Kukanich B (2013) Outpatient oral analgesics in dogs and cats beyond non-steroidal anti-inflammatory drugs: an evidence-based approach. *Veterinary Clinics of North America: Small Animal Practice* **43**, 1109–1125

Lamminen T, Korpivaara M, Suokko M *et al.* (2021) Efficacy of a single dose of pregabalin on signs of anxiety in cats during transportation-a pilot study. *Frontiers in veterinary science* **8**, 711816

Muñana KR (2013) Management of refractory epilepsy. *Topics in Companion Animal Medicine* **28**, 67–71

Procaine hydrochloride with epinephrine bitartrate

(Willcain [c,d]) **POM-VPS**

Formulations: Injectable: 5% w/v procaine hydrochloride + 0.0036% w/v epinephrine bitartrate solution.

Action: Local anaesthetic action is dependent on reversible blockade of the sodium channel, preventing propagation of an action potential along the nerve fibre. Sensory nerve fibres are blocked before motor nerve fibres, allowing a selective sensory blockade at low doses. Addition of epinephrine (adrenaline) to procaine increases the duration of action by reducing the rate of systemic absorption.

Use:
- To provide local anaesthesia via perineural injection.

Procaine has a shorter duration of action than lidocaine or bupivacaine (50 minutes in humans), although the addition of epinephrine will prolong the duration of action compared to the administration of procaine alone.

Safety and handling: Take care to avoid accidental self-injection.

Contraindications: Do not administer intravenously, intra-articularly or epidurally. Do not use for i.v. regional anaesthesia. Vasoconstrictors such as epinephrine should be used with caution in lower limb blocks due to the risk of digital ischaemia or when significant systemic absorption of the drug is expected.

Adverse reactions: Inadvertent intravascular injection may precipitate severe cardiac arrhythmias that are refractory to treatment.

Drug interactions: Procaine may inhibit the action of sulphonamides and their concurrent administration should be avoided.

DOSES

Dogs, Cats: 0.25–1.0 ml s.c.

Proligestone

(Delvosteron [c,d]) **POM-V**

Formulations: Injectable: 100 mg/ml suspension.

Action: Alters the transcription of DNA, leading to alterations in cellular metabolism which mimic those caused by progesterone.

Use:
- Postponement of oestrus in the bitch and queen.

As coat colour changes may occasionally occur, injection into the medial side of the flank fold is recommended for thin-skinned or show animals. Although authorized for use in miliary dermatitis in cats, specific glucocorticoids are preferred.

Safety and handling: Normal precautions should be observed.

Contraindications: Best avoided in diabetic animals, as insulin requirements are likely to change unpredictably. Do not give to bitches before or at first oestrus.

Adverse reactions: The time the animal will stay in anoestrus cannot be predicted reliably and some bitches will remain in anoestrus for up to 3 years. Proligestone does not appear to be associated with as many or as serious adverse effects as other progestogens (e.g. megestrol acetate, medroxyprogesterone acetate). However, adverse effects associated with long-term progestogen use, e.g. temperament changes (listlessness and depression), increased thirst or appetite, cystic endometrial hyperplasia/pyometra, diabetes mellitus, acromegaly, adrenocortical suppression, mammary enlargement/neoplasia and lactation, may be expected. Irritation at site of injection may occur and calcinosis circumscripta at the injection site has been reported.

Drug interactions: No information available.

DOSES

Dogs: 10–33 mg/kg depending on bodyweight:

Bodyweight (kg)	Dose (mg)
<5	100–150
5–10	150–250
10–20	250–350
20–30	350–450
30–45	450–550
45–60	550–600
>60	10 mg/kg

This dose should be given once for the suppression of oestrus. If permanent postponement of oestrus is required, dose is given preferably before onset of pro-oestrus, a second dose 3 months later, a third dose 4 months after the second, and subsequent doses every 5 months thereafter. Once dosing ceases, bitches may come into oestrus, on average 6–7 months later, but it may take longer in some cases. Doses for treatment of acromegaly are as above, given monthly by injection until signs of hair growth are evident.

Cats:
- **Oestrus postponement:** 100 mg/cat s.c.
- **Miliary dermatitis:** 33–50 mg/kg s.c. repeated once after 14 days if the response is inadequate.

Promethazine
(Phenergan*) **POM**

Formulations: Oral: 10 mg, 20 mg, 25 mg tablets; 1 mg/ml syrup. Injectable: 25 mg/ml solution.

Action: Binds to H1 histamine receptors and prevents histamine from binding.

Use:
- Management of allergic disease.
- Early treatment of anaphylaxis.

Specific doses for dogs and cats have not been determined by pharmokinetic studies. Not widely used. Use with caution in cases with urinary retention, angle-closure glaucoma and pyloroduodenal obstruction.

Safety and handling: Normal precautions should be observed.

Contraindications: No information available.

Adverse reactions: May cause mild sedation. May reduce seizure threshold.

Drug interactions: No information available.

DOSES
Dogs, Cats: 0.2–0.4 mg/kg i.v., i.m. q6–8h; 12.5–25 mg/dog p.o. q24h.

Propantheline
(Pro-Banthine*) **POM**

Formulations: Oral: 15 mg tablets.

Action: Quarternary antimuscarinic agent.

Use:
- Treatment of anticholinergic-responsive bradycardia.
- Management of incontinence caused by detrusor hyperreflexia.
- Peripherally acting antiemetic.
- Adjunctive therapy to treat GI disorders associated with smooth muscle spasm.

Safety and handling: Normal precautions should be observed.

Contraindications: No information available.

Adverse reactions: Antimuscarinics may cause constipation and paralytic ileus with resultant dysbiosis. Other adverse effects include sinus tachycardia, ectopic complexes, mydriasis, photophobia, cycloplegia, increased intraocular pressure, vomiting, abdominal distension, urinary retention and drying of bronchial secretions.

Drug interactions: Antihistamines and phenothiazines may enhance the activity of propantheline and its derivatives. Chronic corticosteroid use may potentiate the adverse effects of propantheline (and its derivatives) on intraocular pressure. Propantheline and its derivatives may enhance the actions of sympathomimetics and thiazide diuretics. Propantheline and its derivatives may antagonize the actions of metoclopramide.

DOSES
Dogs:
- **Bradycardia:** 0.25–0.5 mg/kg p.o. q8–12h.
- **Urge incontinence:** 0.2 mg/kg p.o. q6–8h.
- **GI indications:** 0.25 mg/kg p.o. q8–12h (round dose to nearest 3.75 mg).

Cats:
- **Urge incontinence:** 0.25–0.5 mg/kg p.o. q12–24h.
- **GI indications:** doses as for dogs.

References
Forrester D and Roudebush P (2007) Evidence-based management of feline lower urinary tract disease. *Veterinary Clinics of North America: Small Animal Practice* **37**, 533–558

Proparacaine see Proxymetacaine

Propentofylline
(Canergy[d], Vitofyllin[d], Vivitonin[d]) **POM-V**

Formulations: Oral: 50 mg, 100 mg tablets.

Action: Propentofylline is a xanthine derivative that increases blood flow to the heart, muscle and CNS via inhibition of phosphodiesterase. It also has an antiarrhythmic action, bronchodilator effects, positive inotropic and chronotropic effects on the heart, inhibitory effects on platelet aggregation and reduces peripheral vascular resistance.

Use:
- Improvement of demeanour in animals.
- Treatment of age-related behaviour problems, in particular in combination with selegiline and dietary management for canine cognitive dysfunction.

Use with care in patients with cardiac disease.

Safety and handling: Normal precautions should be observed.

Contraindications: Do not administer to pregnant bitches or breeding animals, as it has not yet been evaluated in this class of animal.

Adverse reactions: May increase myocardial oxygen demand.

Drug interactions: No information available.

DOSES
Dogs: 2.5–5 mg/kg p.o. q12h. Administer 30 min before food.
Cats: Cognitive dysfunction: 12.5 mg/cat p.o. q24h.

References
Siwak CT, Gruet P, Woehrlé F *et al.* (2000) Comparison of the effects of adrafinil, propentofylline, and nicergoline on behavior in aged dogs. *American Journal of Veterinary Research* **61**, 1410–1414

Propofol

(Norofol [c,d], PropoFlo Plus [c,d], Propofol Lipuro Vet [c,d], Propomitor [c,d], Proposure [c,d]) **POM-V**

Formulations: Injectable: 10 mg/ml lipid emulsion available both with and without a preservative (benzyl alcohol) in 20 ml bottles.

Action: The mechanism of action is not fully understood but it is thought to involve modulation of the inhibitory activity of GABA at $GABA_A$ receptors.

Use:
- Induction of anaesthesia and maintenance of anaesthesia using intermittent boluses or CRI.

The solution containing benzyl alcohol preservative should not be used for maintenance of anaesthesia by CRI due to the risk of toxicity caused by prolonged administration. Injection i.v. produces a rapid loss of consciousness as the CNS takes up the highly lipophilic drug. Over the next few minutes propofol distributes to peripheral tissues and the concentration in the CNS falls such that, in the absence of further doses, the patient wakes up. In dogs, propofol is rapidly metabolized in the liver and other extrahepatic sites, although the clinical relevance of extrahepatic metabolism in animals is not established and may be species-dependent. In cats, recovery is less rapid due to the phenolic nature of the compound. Propofol does not have analgesic properties, therefore, it is better used in combination with other drugs to maintain anaesthesia; for example, a CRI of a potent opioid. Considerable care must be taken with administration in hypovolaemic animals and those with diminished cardiopulmonary, hepatic and renal reserves.

Safety and handling: Shake the lipid emulsion well before use and do not mix with other therapeutic agents or therapeutic fluids prior to administration. If using a preparation that contains no bacteriostat, opened bottles should be stored in a refrigerator and used within 8 hours or discarded. Once broached, the lipid preparation with a preservative has a shelf-life of 28 days.

Contraindications: No information available.

Adverse reactions: The rapid injection of large doses causes apnoea, cyanosis, bradycardia and severe hypotension. Problems are less likely when injected over 30–60 seconds. Muscle rigidity, paradoxical muscle movements and tremors can sometimes occur in dogs immediately after i.v. administration. The muscle movements are unresponsive to management with diazepam, and further doses of propofol compound the problem. The tremors and movements wane with time without treatment. One study associated repeated daily administration (for 5 days) of the lipid preparation with Heinz body anaemia in cats, although more recent studies have found conflicting results. Propofol is not irritant to tissues but a pain reaction may be evident during i.v. injection; the underlying mechanism causing pain is unknown.

Drug interactions: No information available.

DOSES

Dogs:
- **Unpremedicated:** 6–7 mg/kg i.v.
- **Premedicated:** 1–4 mg/kg i.v.

- **CRI for sedation or maintenance of anaesthesia:** 0.1–0.4 mg/kg/min. Lower doses are required when propofol is combined with other drugs for maintenance of anaesthesia.

Cats:
- **Unpremedicated:** 8 mg/kg i.v.
- **Premedicated:** 2–5 mg/kg i.v.
- **CRI for maintenance of anaesthesia:** 0.1–0.4 mg/kg/min depending on other agents given in combination. Likely to result in prolonged recovery in cats.

References
Bley CR, Roos M, Price J *et al.* (2007) Clinical assessment of repeated propofol associated anaesthesia in cats. *Journal of the American Veterinary Medical Association* **231**, 1347–1353

Propranolol

(Propranolol*, Syprol*) **POM**

Formulations: Injectable: 1 mg/ml solution. **Oral:** 10 mg, 40 mg, 80 mg, 160 mg tablets; 5 mg/5 ml, 10 mg/5 ml, 40 mg/5 ml, 50 mg/5 ml oral solution.

Action: Non-selective beta blocker. Blocks the chronotropic and inotropic effects of beta-1 adrenergic stimulation on the heart, thereby reducing myocardial oxygen demand. Blocks the dilatory effects of beta-2 adrenergic stimulation on the vasculature and bronchial smooth muscle, leading to vaso- and bronchoconstriction. The antihypertensive effects are mediated through reducing cardiac output, altering the baroreceptor reflex sensitivity and blocking peripheral adrenoceptors.

Use:
- Management of cardiac arrhythmias (sinus tachycardia, atrial fibrillation or flutter, supraventricular tachycardia, ventricular arrhythmias).
- Treatment of hypertrophic cardiomyopathy or obstructive cardiac disease (severe aortic or pulmonic stenosis).
- Potential efficacy as an additional antihypertensive drug.
- Can be used following introduction of alpha blockade in management of phaeochromocytoma.
- Used to reverse some of the clinical features of thyrotoxicosis prior to surgery in patients with hyperthyroidism.
- May be used in behavioural therapy to reduce somatic signs of anxiety and is therefore useful in the management of situational anxieties and behavioural problems where contextual anxiety is a component. Some authors suggest using propranolol in combination with phenobarbital for the management of fear- and phobia-related behaviour problems.

There is a significant difference between i.v. and oral doses. This is a consequence of propranolol's lower bioavailability when administered orally as a result of decreased absorption and a high first-pass effect. Wean off slowly when using chronic therapy.

Safety and handling: Normal precautions should be observed.

Contraindications: Do not use in patients with bradyarrhythmias, acute or decompensated CHF. Relatively contraindicated in animals with medically controlled congestive heart failure as is poorly tolerated. Do not administer concurrently with alpha-adrenergic agonists (e.g. adrenaline). Care in cats with lower airway disease.

Adverse reactions: Bradycardia, AV block, myocardial depression, heart failure, syncope, hypotension, hypoglycaemia, bronchospasm, diarrhoea and peripheral vasoconstriction. Depression and lethargy are occasionally seen as a result of CNS penetration. Propranolol may exacerbate any pre-existing renal impairment. Sudden withdrawal of propranolol may result in exacerbation of arrhythmias or the development of hypertension.

Drug interactions: The hypotensive effect of propranolol is enhanced by many agents that depress myocardial activity including anaesthetic agents, phenothiazines, antihypertensive drugs, diuretics and diazepam. There is an increased risk of bradycardia, severe hypotension, heart failure and AV block if propranolol is used concurrently with calcium-channel blockers. Concurrent digoxin administration potentiates bradycardia. The metabolism of propranolol is accelerated by thyroid hormones, thus reducing its effect. The dose of propranolol may need to be decreased when initiating carbimazole therapy. Oral aluminium hydroxide preparations reduce propranolol absorption. Cimetidine may decrease the metabolism of propranolol, thereby increasing blood levels. Propranolol enhances the effects of muscle relaxants (e.g. suxa-methonium, tubocurarine). Hepatic enzyme induction by phenobarbital or phenytoin may increase the rate of metabolism of propranolol. There is an increased risk of lidocaine toxicity if administered with propranolol due to a reduction in lidocaine clearance. The bronchodilatory effects of theophylline may be blocked by propranolol. Although the use of propranolol is not contraindicated in patients with diabetes mellitus, insulin requirements should be monitored as propranolol may enhance the hypoglycaemic effect of insulin.

DOSES
Dogs:
- **Cardiac indications:** 0.02–0.08 mg/kg i.v. slowly over 5 min q8h; 0.1–1.5 mg/kg p.o. q8h. Start at the lower doses if myocardial function is poor and titrate upwards cautiously.
- **Phaeochromocytoma:** 0.15–0.5 mg/kg p.o. q8h in conjunction with an alpha-blocker.
- **Behavioural modification:** 0.5–3.0 mg/kg p.o. as required up to q12h.

Cats:
- **Cardiac indications and severe thyrotoxicosis (thyroid storm):** 0.02–0.06 mg/kg i.v. slowly (i.e. dilute 0.25 mg in 1 ml of saline and administer 0.1–0.2 ml boluses i.v. to effect); 2.5–5 mg/cat p.o. q8h.
- **Behavioural modification:** 0.2–1.0 mg/kg p.o. as required up to q8h.

References
Eason BD, Fine DM, Leeder D *et al.* (2014) Influence of beta blockers on survival in dogs with severe subaortic stenosis. *Journal of Veterinary Internal Medicine* **28**, 857–862

Prostaglandin F2 see Dinoprost tromethamine

Protamine sulphate

(Protamine sulphate*) **POM**

Formulations: Injectable: 10 mg/ml solution.

Action: An anticoagulant that, when administered in the presence of heparin, forms a stable salt, causing the loss of anticoagulant activity of both compounds.

Use:
- Treatment of heparin overdose.

The effects of heparin are neutralized within 5 minutes of protamine administration, with the effect persisting for approximately 2 hours. In humans, protamine is also used for low molecular weight heparin (LMWH) overdose, however anti-Xa activity is not completely inhibited and no information is available for LMWH neutralization in cats and dogs.

Safety and handling: Do not store diluted solutions.

Contraindications: No information available.

Adverse reactions: Anaphylaxis, hypotension, bradycardia, nausea, vomiting, pulmonary hypertension and lethargy are seen in humans.

Drug interactions: No information available.

DOSES

Dogs, Cats: Heparin overdosage: 1 mg of protamine inactivates 80–100 IU of heparin. Heparin disappears rapidly from the circulation. Decrease the dose of protamine by half for each 30-minute period since the heparin was administered. Give protamine i.v. very slowly over 1–3 minutes. Do not exceed 50 mg in any 10-minute period. Dilute protamine in 5% dextrose or normal saline.

Proxymetacaine (Proparacaine)

(Proxymetacaine*) **POM**

Formulations: Ophthalmic: 0.5% solution in single-use vials.

Action: Local anaesthetic action is dependent on reversible blockade of the sodium channel, preventing propagation of an action potential along the nerve fibre. Sensory nerve fibres are blocked before motor nerve fibres, allowing a selective sensory blockade at low doses.

Use:
- Proxymetacaine is used on the ocular surface (cornea and conjunctival sac), the external auditory meatus and the nares. It acts rapidly (within 1 minute) and provides anaesthesia for 25–55 minutes in the conjunctival sac depending on the species.

Serial application increases duration and depth of anaesthesia. Topical anaesthetics block reflex tear production and should not be applied before a Schirmer tear test.

Safety and handling: Store in refrigerator and in the dark; reduced efficacy if stored at room temperature for >2 weeks.

Contraindications: Do not use for therapeutic purposes.

Adverse reactions: Conjunctival hyperaemia is common; local irritation manifested by chemosis may occasionally occur for several hours after administration (less likely than with tetracaine). All topical anaesthetics are toxic to the corneal epithelium and repeated application delays healing of ulcers.

Drug interactions: No information available.

DOSES

Dogs:
- **Ophthalmic:** 1–2 drops per eye; maximal effect at 15 min, duration 45–55 min.
- **Aural/nasal:** 5–10 drops per ear or nose every 5–10 min (maximum 3 doses if used intranasally).

Cats: Ophthalmic: 1–2 drops per eye; maximal effect at 15 min, duration 25 min.

Pyrantel

(Anthelmin [c,d], Cazitel [c,d], Cestem [d], Dolpac, Drontal [c,d], Endoguard [d], Prazitel [c,d], Simparica Trio [d], Veloxa [d], WORMclear [c], various authorized proprietary products)
POM-V

Formulations: Oral: 10 mg, 50 mg, 80 mg, 87 mg, 120 mg, 125 mg, 175 mg tablets; 5 mg/ml liquid. **NB:** some formulations and doses give content of pyrantel (febantel, oxantel) in terms of pyrantel embonate/ pamonate (50 mg pyrantel is equivalent to 144 mg pyrantel embonate/ pamonate).

Action: A pyrimidine anthelmintic that kills worms by agonizing nicotinic acetylcholine receptors and causing contraction paralysis. Febantel and oxantel are derivatives of pyrantel with increased activity against whipworms.

Use:
- Control of *Toxocara canis*, *Toxascaris leonina*, *Trichuris vulpis*, *Uncinaria stenocephala* and *Ancylostoma caninum*.

Safety and handling: Normal precautions should be observed.

Contraindications: Do not use in puppies <2 months or <1 kg. Safety has not been established in pregnant or lactating animals and therefore its use is not recommended. Not recommended for use in debilitated animals due to potential for pronounced cholinergic effects.

Adverse reactions: Vomiting and diarrhoea may be observed.

Drug interactions: The addition of febantel or oxantel has a synergistic effect. Do not use with levamisole, piperazine or cholinesterase inhibitors. Concurrent use with cholinergic drugs may result in enhanced cholinergic effects.

DOSES

See Appendix for guidelines on responsible parasiticide use.

Dogs: Varies with preparation. Approximately 5 mg/kg pyrantel + 15 mg/kg febantel or 20 mg/kg oxantel p.o., repeat as required.

Cats: Varies with preparation. Approximately 57.5 mg/kg pyrantel embonate.

Pyridostigmine

(Mestinon*, Pyridostigmine bromide*) **POM**

Formulations: Oral: 60 mg tablets; 12 mg/ml solution (pharmceutical company will make a lower dose solution (1 mg/ml) upon request).

Action: Reversible inhibitor of cholinesterase activity, with a similar mechanism of action to neostigmine but a slower onset of activity and longer duration of action. Inhibits the enzymatic hydrolysis of acetylcholine by acetylcholinesterase and other cholinesterases, thereby prolonging and intensifying the physiological actions of acetylcholine. It may also have direct effects on skeletal muscle.

Use:
- Treatment of myasthenia gravis.
- Also used to reverse the neuromuscular blockade produced by competitive neuromuscular blockers, but in general is less effective than neostigmine.
- May also have a role in the treatment of paralytic ileus.

Pyridostigmine is specifically used to increase the activity of acetylcholine at nicotinic receptors and thereby stimulate skeletal muscle, the autonomic ganglia and the adrenal medulla. However, it also prolongs the effect of acetylcholine released from postganglionic parasympathetic nerves, and from some postganglionic sympathetic nerves, to produce peripheral actions which correspond to those of muscarine. The muscarinic actions primarily comprise vasodilation, cardiac depression, stimulation of the vagus and parasympathetic nervous system, and increases in lacrimal, salivary and other secretions. The dosage should be reduced by 25% if muscarinic adverse effects appear. Overdose in myasthenic patients can be difficult to distinguish from the effects associated with myasthenic crisis. Treat muscarinic adverse effects with atropine. Animals with megaoesophagus should receive injectable therapy until able to swallow liquid or tablets.

Safety and handling: Normal precautions should be observed.

Contraindications: Do not use in patients with mechanical GI or urinary tract obstructions or peritonitis. Use with caution in patients with bronchial disease (especially feline asthma), bradycardia (and other arrhythmias), hypotension, renal impairment or epilepsy.

Adverse reactions: Vomiting, increased salivation, diarrhoea and abdominal cramps. Clinical signs of overdose are related to muscarinic adverse effects and are generally less severe for pyridostigmine than for other parasympathomimetics (particularly neostigmine), but may include bronchoconstriction, increased bronchial secretions, lacrimation, involuntary defecation and micturition, miosis, nystagmus, bradycardia, heart block, arrhythmias, hypotension, agitation and weakness eventually leading to fasciculation and paralysis.

Drug interactions: Aminoglycosides, clindamycin, lincomycin and propranolol may antagonize the effect of pyridostigmine. Pyridostigmine may enhance the effect of depolarizing muscle relaxants (e.g. suxamethonium) but antagonize the effect of non depolarizing muscle relaxants (e.g. pancuronium and vecuronium).

DOSES

Dogs: 0.5–3 mg/kg p.o. q8–12h. Dose should be incrementally adjusted to maximize muscle strength and minimize adverse effects.

Cats: 0.1–0.5 mg/kg p.o. q8–12h. Titrate dose as above.

References
Dickinson PJ and LeCouteur RA (2004) Feline neuromuscular disorders. *Veterinary Clinics of North America: Small Animal Practice* **34**, 1307–1359

Khorzad R, Whelan M, Sisson A and Shelton GD (2011) Myasthenia gravis in dogs with an emphasis on treatment and critical care management. *Journal of Veterinary Emergency and Critical Care (San Antonio)* **21**, 193–208

Pyrimethamine

(Daraprim*) **P**

Formulations: Oral: 25 mg tablets.

Action: Interference with folate metabolism of parasites, preventing purine synthesis (and therefore DNA synthesis).

Use:
- Treatment of infections caused by *Toxoplasma gondii* and *Neospora caninum*.

Should not be used in pregnant or lactating animals without adequate folate supplementation.

Safety and handling: Normal precautions should be observed.

Contraindications: No information available.

Adverse reactions: Depression, anorexia and reversible bone marrow suppression (within 6 days of the start of therapy). Folate supplementation (5 mg/day) may prevent bone marrow suppression.

Drug interactions: Increased antifolate effect if given with phenytoin or sulphonamides. Folate supplementation for the host will reduce the efficacy of the drug if given concomitantly and should thus be given a few hours before pyrimethamine.

DOSES
See Appendix for guidelines on responsible parasiticide use.

Dogs, Cats: Toxoplasmosis/neosporosis: 1 mg/kg p.o. q24h or divided q12h for 4 weeks, alongside sulphonamides.

References
Foster SF and Martin P (2011) Lower respiratory tract infections in cats: reaching beyond empirical therapy. *Journal of Feline Medicine and Surgery* **13**, 313–332

Pyriprole

(Prac-tic [d]) **NFA-VPS (Northern Ireland)**

Formulations: Topical: 125 mg/ml spot-on pipettes of various sizes.

Action: Interaction with ligand-gated (GABA) chloride channels, blocking pre- and post-synaptic transfer of chloride ions, leads to death of parasites.

Use:
- Treatment and prevention of flea infestations (*Ctenocephalides canis, C. felis*) and tick prevention in dogs >8 weeks and >2 kg.

For treatment of flea infestations, the additional use of an approved insect growth regulator is recommended. For large dogs, the 5 ml dose should be applied in 2–3 spots. Bathing is not recommended for 48 hours prior to and 24 hours after application.

Safety and handling: Normal precautions should be observed. May be harmful to aquatic organisms.

Contraindications: Safety has not been established in pregnant or lactating bitches. Do not use on cats.

Adverse reactions: Pruritus/dermatitis at application site, lethargy, ataxia, convulsions, emesis, diarrhoea.

Drug interactions: No information available.

DOSES
See Appendix for guidelines on responsible parasiticide use.
Dogs: Fleas and ticks: minimum dose 12.5 mg/kg topically q4wk.
Cats: Do not use.

References
Barnett S, Luempert L, Schuele G *et al.* (2008) Efficacy of pyriprole topical solution against the cat flea, *Ctenocephalides felis*, on dogs. *Veterinary Therapeutics: Research in Applied Veterinary Medicine* **9**, 4–14

Pyriproxyfen
(Duowin [d], Effipro [c,d], Fipralone Duo [c,d], Indorex household spray, Johnson's 4 Fleas [c,d], Pyriproxyfen 1% premix for dog [d], Vectra 3D [d], Vectra felis [c]) **POM-V, AVM-GSL**

Formulations: Environmental: Spray with permethrin/piperonyl butoxide. **Topical:** Spot-on products (various sizes) with fipronil (cats, dogs) or permethrin (dogs). Also available as a combination with dinotefuran (an insecticide of the neonicotinoid class) and permethrin (Vectra 3D). **Oral:** 1% premix feed in 1.5 kg and 22.5 kg bags or barrels.

Action: Juvenile hormone analogue. Arrests the development of flea larvae in the environment.

Use:
- Use as part of a comprehensive flea control programme in conjunction with on-animal adulticide products.

Safety and handling: Normal precautions should be observed. The product should not enter watercourses as this may be dangerous for fish and other organisms.

Contraindications: Do not use environmental spray directly on animals. Products also containing permethrin should not be used on cats.

Adverse reactions: None reported.

Drug interactions: None reported.

DOSES
See Appendix for guidelines on responsible parasiticide use.
Dogs, Cats:
- **Fleas:** apply spot-on/spray products monthly.
- **Feed mix:** 100 g/10 kg bodyweight (equivalent to 500 µg (micrograms) pyriproxyfen/kg) per day.
- **Household spray:** one can covers 79 m^2. Use in the environment as directed.

Quinalbarbitone/Cinchocaine see **Secobarbital**

Rabacfosadine
(Tanovea-CA1) **POM-V**

Formulations: Injectable: Sterile lyophilized powder for reconstitution before use. After reconstitution with 2 ml 0.9% NaCl, the reconstituted solution contains 8.2 mg/ml of rabacfosadine.

Action: Prodrug of the nucleotide analogue PMEG; causes cytotoxicity in dividing cells due to inhibition of DNA polymerases.

Use:
- Rabacfosadine has been trialled in canine lymphoma (B and T cell) and multiple myeloma.

Safety and handling: Potent cytotoxic drug that should only be prepared and administered by trained personnel. See Appendix and specialist texts for further advice on chemotherapeutic agents.

Contraindications: Contraindicated in patients with known hypersensitivity. Do not use in patients with pre-existing bone marrow suppression or liver dysfunction. Do not use in patients with known pulmonary disease or those susceptible to pulmonary fibrosis.

Adverse reactions: May cause myelosuppression and GI adverse events (including haemorrhagic gastroenteritis). Liver enzyme activity elevation, azotaemia, fever, weight loss, lethargy, dermatological signs, pulmonary fibrosis, injected sclera and urinary signs/proteinuria/glycosuria are also reported. There is the possibility for enhanced acute adverse events related to radiotherapy if used concurrently.

Drug interactions: Not known at present.

DOSES
Dogs: 0.82–1 mg/kg i.v. over 30 min q21d, usually up to 5 doses. Has been used in combination with doxorubicin at weeks 0, 6, 12 as part of an alternating protocol.

Cats: No information available.

References
DeClerq E (2018) Tanovea® for the treatment to lymphoma in dogs. *Biochemical Pharmacology* **154**, 265–269
Saba CF, Vickery KR, Clifford CA *et al.* (2017) Rabacfosadine for relapsed canine B-cell lymphoma: efficacy and adverse event profiles of 2 different doses. *Veterinary and Comparative Oncology* **16**, 76–82

Ramipril
(Vasotop [d]) **POM-V**

Formulations: Oral: 1.25 mg, 2.5 mg, 5 mg tablets.

Action: ACE inhibitor. Inhibits conversion of angiotensin I to angiotensin II and inhibits the breakdown of bradykinin. Overall effect is a reduction in preload and afterload via venodilation and arteriodilation, decreased salt and water retention via reduced aldosterone production and inhibition of the angiotensin-aldosterone-mediated cardiac and vascular remodelling. Efferent arteriolar dilation in the kidney can reduce intraglomerular pressure and therefore glomerular filtration. This may decrease proteinuria.

Use:

- Treatment of CHF in dogs. Often used in conjunction with diuretics when heart failure is present as most effective when used in these cases. Can be used in combination with other drugs to treat heart failure (e.g. pimobendan, spironolactone, digoxin).
- Can also be used for heart failure in cats. The use of ACE inhibitors in cats with cardiac disease stems from extrapolation from theoretical benefits and studies showing a benefit in other species with heart failure and different cardiac diseases (mainly dogs and humans).
- Management of proteinuria associated with chronic renal insufficiency, glomerular disorders and protein-losing nephropathies.
- May reduce blood pressure in hypertension. ACE inhibitors are more likely to cause or exacerbate prerenal azotaemia in hypotensive animals and those with poor renal perfusion (e.g. acute, oliguric renal failure). Use cautiously if hypotension, hyponatraemia or outflow tract obstruction are present.

Regular monitoring of blood pressure, serum creatinine, urea and electrolytes is strongly recommended with ACE inhibitor treatment.

Safety and handling: Normal precautions should be observed.

Contraindications: Do not use in cases of haemodynamically relevant outflow tract obstruction (e.g. valvular stenosis, obstructive hypertrophic cardiomyopathy).

Adverse reactions: Potential adverse effects include hypotension, hyperkalaemia and azotaemia. Monitor blood pressure, serum creatinine and electrolytes when used in cases of heart failure. Dosage should be reduced if there are signs of hypotension (weakness, disorientation). Anorexia, vomiting and diarrhoea are rare. It is not recommended for breeding, pregnant or lactating bitches, as safety has not been established.

Drug interactions: Concomitant use of potassium-sparing diuretics (e.g. spironolactone) or potassium supplements could result in hyperkalaemia. However, in practice, spironolactone and ACE inhibitors appear safe to use concurrently. There may be an increased risk of nephrotoxicity and decreased clinical efficacy when used with NSAIDs. There is a risk of hypotension with concomitant administration of diuretics, vasodilators (anaesthetic agents, antihypertensive agents) or negative inotropes (beta blockers).

DOSES

Dogs: 0.125 mg/kg p.o. q24h increasing to 0.25 mg/kg p.o. q24h after 2 weeks depending on the severity of pulmonary congestion.

Cats: 0.125 mg/kg p.o. q24h increasing to 0.25 mg/kg p.o. q24h for systemic arterial hypertension.

References

Lefebvre HP, Jeunesse E, Laroute V et al. (2006) Pharmacokinetic and pharmacodynamic parameters of ramipril and ramiprilat in healthy dogs and dogs with reduced glomerular filtration rate *Journal of Veterinary Internal Medicine* **20**, 499–507

Van Israel N, Desmoulins PO, Huyghe B et al. (2009) Ramipril as a First Line Monotherapy for the Control of Feline Hypertension and Associated Clinical Signs. *Proceedings of the 19th ECVIM-CA Congress, Porto*

Ranitidine

`CIL`

(Ranicalm*, Ranitidine*, Zantac*) **POM**

Formulations: Injectable: 25 mg/ml solution. **Oral:** 75 mg tablets; 15 mg/ml syrup.

Action: Ranitidine is an H2 receptor antagonist blocking histamine-induced gastric acid secretion. It is more potent than cimetidine but has lower bioavailability (50%) and undergoes hepatic metabolism. It also has some prokinetic effects through stimulation of local muscarinic acetylcholine receptors, which may be of benefit when gastric motility is impaired by gastritis or ulceration, and in feline idiopathic megacolon.

Use:
- Management of gastric and duodenal ulcers, idiopathic, uraemic or drug-related erosive gastritis, oesophagitis, and hypersecretory conditions secondary to gastrinoma, mast cell neoplasia or short bowel syndrome.
- GI prokinetic effect.

Studies show minimal increases in gastric pH in healthy dogs given ranitidine. Ranitidine was not an effective acid suppressant in healthy cats. If used for the treatment of ulceration, then treatment should continue for 2 weeks after remission of clinical signs which typically means a 1-month course. Absorption is not clinically significantly affected by food intake, anticholinergic agents or antacids.

Safety and handling: Normal precautions should be observed.

Contraindications: No information available.

Adverse reactions: Rarely reported but include cardiac arrhythmias and hypotension, particularly if administered rapidly i.v.

Drug interactions: It is advisable, although not essential, that sucralfate is administered 2 hours before H2 blockers. Stagger oral doses of ranitidine when used with other antacids, digoxin or metoclopramide by 2 hours as it may reduce their absorption or effect.

DOSES

Dogs: All uses: 2 mg/kg slow i.v., s.c., p.o. q8–12h.
Cats: All uses: 2 mg/kg/day CRI; 2.5 mg/kg i.v. slowly q12h; 3.5 mg/kg p.o. q12h.

References
Favarato ES, Souza MV, Costa PR *et al.* (2012) Evaluation of metoclopramide and ranitidine on the prevention of gastroesophageal reflux episodes in anesthetized dogs. *Research in Veterinary Science* **93**, 466–467
Šutalo S, Ruetten M, Hartnack S *et al.* (2015) The effect of orally administered ranitidine and once-daily or twice-daily orally administered omeprazole on intragastric pH in cats. *Journal of Veterinary Internal Medicine* **29**, 840–846

Remdesivir

`CIL`

(Veklury*) **POM**

Formulations: Injectable: intravenous or subcutaneous. **VSP**

Action: A nucleoside analogue that terminates the RNA chain of the viral RNA-dependent RNA polymerase. It acts as an alternative substrate for viral RNA synthesis, resulting in RNA chain termination during viral RNA transcription.

Use:
- Treatment of confirmed or strongly suspected feline infectious peritonitis (FIP).

Safety and handling: Store in refrigerator. The vial should be brought to room temperature prior to injection.

Contraindications: Use with care in animals with significant renal or hepatic disease.

Adverse reactions: Transient stinging and/or injection site reactions are possible. Cats may also appear depressed or show signs of nausea (restlessness, lip licking, hypersalivation) for a few hours after i.v. administration. Raised renal parameters (e.g. symmetric dimethylarginine) have been reported as have raised liver enzyme activities (e.g. alanine aminotransferase). Effusions, especially pleural effusion, can worsen for 1 to 2 days, especially after i.v. administration. Neurological signs may appear or worsen during the first few days of treatment. There may be a transient increase in serum globulins but this should resolve before 6 weeks of treatment as any effusions are resorbed.

Drug interactions: There are no known drug interactions.

DOSES
Dogs: Not applicable.

Cats: Minimum doses:
- **Effusive (wet) FIP without ocular or neurological signs:** 10 mg/kg q24h
- **Dry/effusive FIP with ocular signs:** 15 mg/kg q24h
- **Dry FIP with neurological signs:** 20 mg/kg q24h
- **Routes:** i.v. or s.c. Protocols differ according to disease severity but typically continue for 3–14 days before transitioning to oral GS‑441524

References
Barker E and Taylor S (2021) FIP: Hope on the horizon for cats with FIP. *Vet Times* **51**, 32
Gunn-Moore D, Barker E, Taylor S, Tasker S and Sorrell S (2021) An update on treatment of cats with FIP. *Vet Times* **51**, 50

Retinol see Vitamin A

Rifampin (Rifampicin)
(Rifadin*, Rifampicin*, Rimactane*) **POM**

Formulations: Oral: 150 mg, 300 mg capsules; 20 mg/ml syrup; 35 mg rifampicin + 30 mg azithromycin capsules (veterinary special). **VSP**

Action: Binds to the beta subunit of RNA polymerase causing abortive initiation of RNA synthesis.

Use:
- Use **must be** based on culture results and antimicrobial susceptibility testing and where lower tier antimicrobials would not be effective.
- Used as part of a combination of treatments for tuberculous and non-tuberculous mycobacterial infections and for lesions in cats associated with *Rhodococcus equi*. Various combinations of clarithromycin, enrofloxacin, clofaxamine and doxycycline have been used with rifampin in the management of mycobacteriosis. Until controlled studies are conducted to investigate the value of rifampin in these infections, recommendations remain empirical.

Exact indications for small animal veterinary practice remain to be fully established. Wide spectrum of antimicrobial activity including bacteria (particularly Gram-positive), *Chlamydia*, *Rickettsia*, some protozoans and poxviruses. Active against *Staphylococcus aureus*, *S. pseudintermedius* and mycobacteria. Gram-negative aerobic bacteria are usually innately resistant. Obligate anaerobes (Gram-positive or Gram-negative) are usually susceptible. Chromosomal mutations readily lead to resistance; rifampin should be used in combination with other antimicrobial drugs to prevent the emergence of resistant organisms.

Safety and handling: People who are or may become pregnant should not handle this drug.

Contraindications: Rifampin may be teratogenic at high doses and should not be administered to pregnant animals. It should not be administered to animals with liver disease.

Adverse reactions: In dogs, increases in serum levels of hepatic enzymes are commonly seen and this can progress to clinical hepatitis. Rifampin metabolites may colour urine, saliva and faeces orange-red. GI disturbances (vomiting, diarrhoea, anorexia) are commonly reported. May rarely be associated with thrombocytopenia, haemolytic anaemia and acute kidney injury.

Drug interactions: Rifampin is a potent hepatic enzyme inducer and increases the rate of metabolism of other drugs in humans, including barbiturates, theophylline and itraconazole. Increased dosages of these drugs may be required if used in combination with rifampin.

DOSES

Classified as category A (Avoid) by the EMA.

See Appendix for guidelines on responsible antibiotic use.

Dogs, Cats: 5 mg/kg p.o. q12h; 10–15 mg/kg p.o. q24h.

References

De Lucia M, Bardagi M, Fabbri E *et al.* (2017) Rifampicin treatment of canine pyoderma due to multidrug-resistant meticillin-resistant staphylococci: a retrospective study of 32 cases. *Veterinary Dermatology* **28**, 171–e36

Gunn-Moore DA (2014) Feline mycobacterial infections. *The Veterinary Journal* **201**, 230–238

Rivaroxaban

(Xarelto*) **POM**

Formulations: Oral: 2.5 mg, 10 mg, 15 mg, 20 mg tablets.

Action: Direct inhibitor of activated clotting factor X (factor Xa) and of prothrombinase activity. The inhibition of Xa decreases thrombin generation and explains its anticoagulant effects.

Use:

* Prevention and management of thrombosis in dogs and cats.

Animals at particular risk of thrombosis include dogs with immune-mediated haemolytic anaemia (IMHA), protein-losing nephropathy and heartworm disease, and cats with hypertrophic cardiomyopathies.

Safety and handling: Normal precautions should be observed.

Contraindications: Anticoagulants should not be used in patients that are actively bleeding or at high risk of bleeding. Use with caution in patients with significant kidney and hepatic dysfunction.

Adverse reactions: Can increase risk of bleeding when other risk factors exist.

Drug interactions: Coadministration with antithrombotics or other anticoagulants such as aspirin, clopidogrel, heparins or warfarin increase risk of bleeding. Agents that inhibit cytochrome P450 and P-glycoprotein (e.g. ketoconazole) can decrease efficacy of rivaroxaban.

DOSES

Dogs: 1–2 mg/kg p.o. q24h has been proposed.

Cats: 0.5–1 mg/kg p.o. q24h has been proposed.

References

Blais M-C, Bianco D, Goggs R *et al.* (2019) Consensus on the rational use of antithrombotics in veterinary critical care (CURATIVE): domain 3-defining antithrombotic protocols. *Journal of Veterinary Emergency and Critical Care* **29**, 60–74

Morassi A, Bianco D, Park E, Nakamura RK and White GA (2016) Evaluation of the safety and tolerability of rivaroxaban in dogs with presumed primary immune-mediated hemolytic anemia. *Journal of Veterinary Emergency and Critical Care* **26**, 488–494

Robenacoxib

(Onsior [c,d]) **POM-V**

Formulations: Oral: 5 mg, 10 mg, 20 mg, 40 mg flavoured tablets for dogs; 6 mg flavoured tablets for cats. Injectable: 20 mg/ml solution.

Action: Selectively inhibits COX-2 enzyme, thereby limiting the production of prostaglandins involved in inflammation. Robenacoxib is tissue selective, defined as being preferentially distributed and concentrated at sites of inflammation combined with having a short half-life in plasma (approximately 2 hours). This may confer advantages in terms of reducing exposure of target side effect organs (e.g. liver and kidneys) to robenacoxib in a 24-hour dose interval, although there are currently no clinical data to support this contention.

Use:
- Alleviation of inflammation and pain in both acute and chronic musculoskeletal disorders in dogs and cats.
- Reduction of postoperative pain and inflammation following orthopaedic and soft tissue surgery in dogs and cats.

Administer injectable preparation s.c. approximately 30 minutes before the start of surgery in order to provide perioperative analgesia. One injection provides pain control for up to 24 hours. All NSAIDs should be administered cautiously in the perioperative period as they may adversely affect renal perfusion during periods of hypotension. If hypotension during anaesthesia is anticipated, delay robenacoxib administration until the animal is fully recovered and normotensive. The oral dose may be administered directly into the mouth or, for cats, mixed with a small amount of food. It is recommended not to administer to dogs with food as this has been shown to reduce efficacy. In the cat, due to the longer half-life and narrower therapeutic index of NSAIDs, particular care should be taken to ensure the accuracy of dosing and not to exceed the recommended dose. The tablets are very palatable to cats and many cats will eat spontaneously, facilitating dosing. In dogs, treatment with the oral preparation should be discontinued after 10 days if no clinical improvement is apparent. In cats with chronic musculoskeletal conditions, treatment should be discontinued after 6 weeks if no clinical improvement is seen.

Safety and handling: Normal precautions should be observed.

Contraindications: Do not give to dehydrated, hypovolaemic or hypotensive patients, or those with GI disease or blood clotting problems. Administration of robenacoxib to animals with renal disease must be carefully evaluated and is not advisable in the perioperative period. Do not give to pregnant animals, dogs <12 weeks, cats <16 weeks or animals <2.5 kg.

Adverse reactions: GI signs are commonly reported, but most cases are mild and recover without treatment. Stop therapy if signs persist beyond 1–2 days. Some animals develop signs with one NSAID and not another. A 3–5 day wash-out period should be allowed before starting therapy with another NSAID. Stop therapy immediately if GI bleeding is suspected. There is a small risk that NSAIDs may precipitate cardiac failure in humans and this risk in animals is unknown. Liver disease will prolong the metabolism of robenacoxib, leading to the potential for drug accumulation and overdose with repeated dosing.

Drug interactions: Different NSAIDs should not be administered within 24 hours of each other. The optimal wash-out period between NSAID administration and glucocorticoid administration is unknown, but allowing 3–5 days between the two classes of drugs is recommended. Do not administer with other potentially nephrotoxic agents, e.g. aminoglycosides.

DOSES

Dogs, Cats: 2 mg/kg s.c. q24h for a maximum of 2 doses; 1–2 mg/kg p.o. q24h. Monitoring of long term treatment (>12 weeks) is recommended.

References

Edamura K, King JN, Seewald W *et al.* (2012) Comparison of oral robenacoxib and carprofen for the treatment of osteoarthritis in dogs: a randomized clinical trial. *Journal of Veterinary Medical Science* **74**, 1121–131

Kamata M, King JN, Seewald W *et al.* (2012) Comparison of injectable robenacoxib *versus* meloxicam for perioperative use in cats: results of a randomized clinical trial. *Veterinary Journal* **193**, 14–18

Rocuronium

(Esmeron*) **POM**

Formulations: Injectable: 10 mg/ml solution.

Action: Inhibits the actions of acetylcholine at the neuromuscular junction by binding competitively to the nicotinic acetylcholine receptor on the postjunctional membrane.

Use:
- Provision of neuromuscular blockade during anaesthesia.
- Improve surgical access through muscle relaxation, facilitate positive pressure ventilation or intraocular surgery.

Rocuronium is very similar to vecuronium but it has a more rapid onset of action and shorter duration to spontaneous recovery in dogs. Its availability in aqueous solution and longer shelf life increase convenience. Monitoring (using a nerve stimulator) and reversal of the neuromuscular blockade is recommended to ensure complete recovery before the end of anaesthesia. The neuromuscular blockade caused by rocuronium can be rapidly reversed using sugammadex (a cyclodextrin developed to reverse aminosteroidal neuromuscular blocking agents) at a dose of 8 mg/kg i.v. in dogs. Hypothermia, acidosis and hypokalaemia will prolong the duration of action of neuromuscular blockade. Hepatic disease may prolong duration of action of rocuronium; atracurium is preferred in this group of patients. The effects of renal disease on duration of action of rocuronium require further investigation; in an experimental study in cats, recovery from rocuronium was found to be independent of renal perfusion.

Safety and handling: Normal precautions should be observed.

Contraindications: Do not administer unless the animal is adequately anaesthetized and facilities to provide positive pressure ventilation are available.

Adverse reactions: Causes an increase in heart rate and a mild hypertension when used at high doses.

Drug interactions: Neuromuscular blockade is more prolonged when rocuronium is given in combination with volatile anaesthetics, aminoglycosides, clindamycin and lincomycin.

DOSES

Dogs: 0.4 mg/kg i.v. followed, when required, by a maintenance dose of 0.16 mg/kg i.v. prn or CRI of 0.2 mg/kg/h. Considerably lower doses are required to centralize the globe for ophthalmic surgery (0.05–0.1 mg/kg i.v.).

Cats: Doses of 0.3–0.6 mg/kg i.v. have been evaluated in cats. 0.6 mg/kg had a rapid onset and short duration of action (20 min). Rocuronium has been evaluated to improve conditions for endotracheal intubation in cats at a dose of 0.6 mg/kg; however, this strategy requires prompt successful intubation and ventilation until the effects of the neuromuscular blockade wane (or the effects are reversed) and spontaneous respiration resumes.

Romiplostim

(Nplate*) **POM**

Formulations: Injectable: 125 µg (micrograms) powder for solution in vials; 250 µg powder and solvent for solution in pre-filled disposable devices.

Action: Fc-peptide fusion protein that binds and activates thrombopoietin receptors (as a mimetic agent) to stimulate platelet production in functional bone marrow.

Use:
- Treatment of chronic immune-mediated (idiopathic) thrombocytopenia that is poorly responsive to standard immunosuppressive therapy in patients deemed at particular risk of spontaneous bleeding.

Safety and handling: Normal precautions should be observed.

Contraindications: Not for use in patients with myelodysplastic syndromes or thrombocytopenias due to causes other than immune-mediated destruction. Use with caution in patients at risk of thromboembolism.

Adverse reactions: Significant thrombocytosis was noted in a dog treated for immune-mediated thrombocytopenia when treatment also included vincristine, prednisolone and mycophenolate mofetil. In humans, adverse reactions include anaemia, headache, fatigue, arthralgia, bone marrow fibrosis, thrombocytosis, constipation, diarrhoea, nausea and skin reactions.

Drug interactions: No information available.

DOSES

Dogs: Chronic immune-mediated (idiopathic) thrombocytopenia: the extrapolated dose described for dogs is 3–5 µg (micrograms)/kg s.c. q1wk initially, adjusted based on response. Most of the dogs reported in the literature were maintained on doses of 2–4 µg/kg s.c. per week until remission (3–35 weeks post initiation of therapy). In one report, a dog was initiated on 10 µg/kg s.c. followed by 5 µg/kg s.c. a week later and showed an adequate response in platelet numbers. Typical response in platelet numbers is seen 3–6 days post initiation of therapy.

Cats: No reported use in cats.

References

Kohn B, Bal G, Chirek A Rehbein S and Salama A (2016) Treatment of 5 dogs with immune-mediated thrombocytopenia using Romiplostim. *BMC Veterinary Research* **12**, 96
Polydoros T, Ioannidi OM, Korsavvidis I *et al.* (2021) Romiplostim as Adjunctive Treatment of Refractory Amegakaryocytic Immune Thrombocytopenia in a Dog. *Topics in Companion Animal Medicine* **42**, 100488

Ronidazole `CIL`

(Ronidazole)

Formulations: Chemical grade formulated for the treatment of an individual animal. **VSP**

Action: A nitroimidazole antimicrobial drug that induces DNA strand breakage and organelle damage within bacteria and protozoa.

Use:
- Treatment of *Tritrichomonas foetus* infections in cats.

Although authorized for use in pigeons, the formulation is not suitable for cats. However, as ronidazole is currently considered to be the treatment of choice for *T. foetus*, a special order on a named patient basis can be reformulated and prescribed under the cascade.

Safety and handling: Embryotoxic and potentially teratogenic and carcinogenic. Care must be taken to avoid exposure. People who are or may become pregnant should not handle this drug. Wear impervious gloves when handling and pilling and wash hands carefully after use.

Contraindications: Do not use in patients with hypersensitivity to nitroimidazoles such as metronidazole. Avoid use in pregnancy and use milk replacer if used in nursing cats.

Adverse reactions: Neurotoxicity has been reported in cats and signs may include lethargy, ataxia, nystagmus, seizures, agitation, tremors and anorexia. Neurological side effects may occur with doses of 30 mg/kg and above.

Drug interactions: Likely to see similar interactions to metronidazole. Cimetidine and ketoconazole may decrease the metabolism and increase toxicity of ronidazole. Ronidazole may increase serum levels of ciclosporin and fluorouracil. Oxytetracycline may antagonize the efficacy of ronidazole. Phenobarbital, rifampin and phenytoin may increase the metabolism and decrease the efficacy of ronidazole. Ronidazole may potentiate the anticoagulant effects of warfarin.

DOSES

Classified as category D (Prudence) by the EMA.

See Appendix for guidelines on responsible antibiotic use.
See Appendix for guidelines on responsible parasiticide use.

Dogs: No indication.

Cats:
- For treatment of *T. foetus*: 30–50 mg/kg p.o. q12–24h for 14 days. Dose given once daily in majority of reports.
- **Kittens and cats with hepatopathy:** use reduced dose of 10 mg/kg p.o. q24h.

References

Morgan GB (2019) An evaluation of the use of ronidazole for the treatment of Tritrichomonas foetus in cats. *Veterinary Evidence* **4**, DOI: 10.18849/VE.V4I4.263

Ropinirole

(Clevor [d]) **POM-V**

Formulations: Ophthalmic: 30 mg/ml eye drop solution in single-dose container.

Action: Dopamine agonist. Induces emesis by activating D2-like receptors in the chemoreceptor trigger zone.

Use:
- Induction of vomiting. >90% of dogs respond to a single dose.

In healthy dogs, time to first vomit was 3–37 minutes (median 10 minutes). The median duration of vomiting was 16 minutes. Some dogs will require a second dose. A very small proportion of dogs may fail to respond to the second dose; it is not recommended to administer further doses to these dogs.

Safety and handling: Can cause eye irritation to humans. The product should not be administered by pregnant or breast-feeding people as ropinirole might reduce the level of prolactin.

Contraindications: Do not use in dogs with CNS depression, seizures or reduced gag reflex. Do not use in dogs that are hypoxic or dyspnoeic. Do not use in cases of ingestion of sharp foreign objects, corrosives, volatile substances or organic solvents. Safety has not been studied in dogs with cardiac disease/dysfunction, liver dysfunction or in dogs with clinical signs due to the ingestion of foreign materials. Safety and efficacy have not been studied in dogs with ocular disease. In cases of a pre-existing ocular condition with clinical signs, use the product only according to risk–benefit assessment. Not recommended in pregnant or lactating bitches.

Adverse reactions: Mild ocular irritation is common. May cause a transient increase in heart rate for up to 2 hours. May cause extended vomiting (>60 minutes). Administer antiemetic treatment if vomiting persists – metoclopramide is recommended.

Drug interactions: Dopamine antagonists (such as metoclopramide), chlorpromazine, acepromazine and other drugs with antiemetic properties (e.g. maropitant or antihistamines) may reduce effectiveness.

DOSES

Dogs: 2–15 µl (microlitres)/kg in dogs, i.e. 1–8 drops given into the eye. Each eye drop is 27 µl and contains 810 µg (micrograms) of ropinirole. Dogs weighing 1.8–5 kg: 1 drop; 5.1–10 kg: 2 drops; 10.1–20 kg: 3 drops; 20.1–35 kg: 4 drops; 35.1–60 kg: 6 drops; 60.1–100 kg: 8 drops. When 2–4 drops are to be administered, divide between both eyes. When 6–8 drops are to be administered, the dose should be divided into two administrations given 1–2 minutes apart. If the dog does not vomit within 15 minutes, a second dose may be given. The second dose should be the same as the initial dose.

Cats: No information available. Unlikely to be effective.

References

Suokko M, Saloranta L, Lamminen T, Laine T and Elliott J (2020) Ropinirole eye drops induce vomiting effectively in dogs: a randomised, double-blind, placebo-controlled clinical study. *Veterinary Record* **186**, 283

Ropivacaine

(Naropin*) **POM**

Formulations: Injectable: 2 mg/ml, 5 mg/ml, 7.5 mg/ml, 10 mg/ml solutions.

Action: Reversible blockade of the sodium channel in nerve fibres produces local anaesthesia.

Use:
- Provision of analgesia by perineural nerve blocks, regional and epidural techniques.

Onset of action (10–20 minutes for epidural analgesia) is slower than lidocaine but quicker than bupivacaine, duration of action is still relatively prolonged (3–8 hours). Ropivacaine is less cardiotoxic than bupivacaine and is more selective for sensory nerves than bupivacaine, decreasing the degree of associated motor blockade following administration. Lower doses should be used when systemic absorption is likely to be high (e.g. intrapleural analgesia). Small volumes of ropivacaine can be diluted with normal saline to enable wider distribution of the drug for perineural blockade. Doses of ropivacaine up to 4 mg/kg q8h are unlikely to be associated with systemic side effects if injected perineurally, epidurally or intrapleurally in dogs. The toxic dose has not been established in cats; it is recommended not to exceed 2 mg/kg.

Safety and handling: Normal precautions should be observed.

Contraindications: Do not give i.v. or use for i.v. regional anaesthesia.

Adverse reactions: Inadvertent intravascular injection may precipitate cardiac arrhythmias that are refractory to treatment.

Drug interactions: All local anaesthetics share similar side effects; therefore, the dose of ropivacaine should be reduced when used in combination with other local anaesthetics. The addition of adrenaline does not appear to alter the duration of the block.

DOSES

Dogs:

- **Perineural:** volume of injection depends on the site of placement and size of the animal. As a guide: 0.1 ml/kg per injection site for femoral and sciatic nerve blocks; 0.1 ml/kg for each of the three injection sites for the combined radial, ulnar, musculocutaneous and median nerve blocks; 0.3 ml/kg for brachial plexus nerve block; 0.25–1 ml total volume for blockade of the infraorbital, mental, maxillary and mandibular nerves. Choose an appropriate concentration of ropivacaine to achieve a 2–3 mg/kg dose within these volume guidelines.
- **Epidural:** 1–2 mg/kg ropivacaine combined with preservative-free morphine 0.1–0.2 mg/kg. Limit the total volume of solution injected into the epidural space to 1 ml/4.5 kg up to a maximum volume of 6 ml in order to limit the cranial distribution of drugs in the epidural space and prevent adverse pressure effects.
- **Interpleural:** 1 mg/kg diluted with normal saline to a total volume of 5–20 ml depending on the size of the animal. The solution can be instilled via a thoracotomy tube. Dilution reduces pain on injection caused by the acidity of ropivacaine.

Cats: Do not exceed 2 mg/kg total dose; accurate dosing in cats is essential to prevent overdose.

References

Lewis KA, Bednarski RM, Aarnes TK *et al.* (2014) Postoperative comparison of four perioperative analgesia protocols in dogs undergoing stifle joint surgery. *Journal of the American Veterinary Medical Association* **244**, 1041–1046

S-Adenosylmethionine (SAMe)
(Denamarin, Denosyl, Doxion, Hepaticare, Hepatosyl Plus, MaxxiSAMe, Novifit, Nutramarin+, Samylin, Zentonil Advanced, various proprietary products)
GSL, general sale

Formulations: Oral: 90 mg, 100 mg, 200 mg, 225 mg, 400 mg, 425 mg tablets; 50 mg, 100 mg, 200 mg capsules; 75 mg, 150 mg, 300 mg, 400 mg powder. Also included in some nutraceutical mixtures that may help cognitive functioning or reduce cognitive decline.

Action: SAMe is an endogenous molecule synthesized by cells throughout the body and is a component of several biochemical pathways. SAMe is especially important in hepatocytes because of their central role in metabolism. SAMe is required for the production of glutathione (GSH), which is important in many metabolic processes and cell detoxification and is a potent antioxidant which protects hepatocytes from toxins and death. In liver disease, the level of GSH may be reduced; SAMe has been shown to increase hepatic GSH levels. SAMe also appears to have mood elevating effects in older animals, although the mechanism is unclear, since the evidence for neuronal penetration from oral administration is limited, but it may affect monoamine metabolism and membrane fluidity resulting in improved cell functioning. Supplementation with SAMe may also improve signs of age-related mental decline in dogs. In humans, antidepressant effects of SAMe are also documented.

Use:
- Adjunctive treatment for liver disease, especially for acute hepatotoxin-induced liver disease.
- Can also be used in patients receiving long-term therapy with potentially hepatotoxic drugs including lomustine (CCNU).
- May improve bile flow in cats.
- Used as an aid in the management of age-related behaviour problems and cognitive dysfunction in dogs and cats.

Administration should begin at the first signs of age-related behaviour problems. Tablets should be given whole. Use as an antidepressant in animals has yet to be established. The safety of exogenous SAMe has not been proven in pregnancy; therefore, it should be used with caution.

Safety and handling: Normal precautions should be observed.

Contraindications: No information available.

Adverse reactions: GI signs (nausea, vomiting, diarrhoea), dry mouth, headache, sweating and dizziness are occasionally reported in humans. Paradoxical increase in anxiety may occur.

Drug interactions: Concurrent use of SAMe with tramadol, meperidine, pentazocine, monoamine oxidase inhibitors (MAOIs) including selegiline, selective serotonin reuptake inhibitors (SSRIs) such as fluoxetine, or other antidepressants (e.g. clomipramine, amitriptyline) could cause additive serotonergic effects. SAMe may increase the clearance of drugs that undergo hepatic glucuronidation, including paracetamol, diazepam and morphine.

DOSES
Dogs: All uses: At least 100 mg/10 kg p.o. q24h.
Cats: All uses: 100 mg/cat p.o. q24h.

Refer to individual products for dosing advice as regimens vary. Suggested starting dose in absence of other information is 20 mg/kg p.o. q24h. Administer on an empty stomach at least 1 hour before food.

References

Skorupski KA, Hammond GM, Irish AM et al. (2011) Prospective randomized clinical trial assessing the efficacy of Denamarin for prevention of CCNU-induced hepatopathy in tumor-bearing dogs. Journal of Veterinary Internal Medicine **25**, 838–845

Vandeweerd JM, Cambier C and Gustin P (2013) Nutraceuticals for canine liver disease: assessing the evidence. Veterinary Clinics of North America: Small Animal Practice **43**, 1171–1179

Salbutamol

CIL

(Ventolin*) **POM**

Formulations: Inhalational: 100 µg (micrograms) per metered inhalation.

Action: Selective beta-2 stimulation causes smooth muscle relaxation and bronchodilation.

Use:

- Treatment of bronchospasm in inflammatory airway disease and irritation in cats and dogs.

Experimental studies have shown chronic use in cats can exacerbate airway inflammation, leading to recommendations that salbutamol be reserved for acute/short-term management in this species.

Safety and handling: Normal precautions should be observed.

Contraindications: No information available.

Adverse reactions: In humans, side effects of the beta-2 agonists include headache, muscle cramps and palpitation. Other side effects include tachycardia, arrhythmias, peripheral vasodilation, and disturbances of sleep and behaviour. Shivering and agitation is occasionally seen in dogs.

Drug interactions: In humans, there is an increased risk of side effects if salbutamol is used by patients also taking diuretics, digoxin, theophylline or corticosteroids.

DOSES

Administer via spacer device and count 7–10 breaths per treatment.

Dogs: Bronchodilation: 100–300 µg (micrograms)/dog q4–6h or as needed for relief of bronchospasm.

Cats: Bronchodilation: 100 µg (micrograms)/cat q4–6h or as needed for relief of bronchospasm.

References

Reinero CR (2009) Enantiomer-specific effects of albuterol on airway inflammation in healthy and asthmatic cats. International Archives of Allergy and Immunology **150**, 43–50

Sarolaner

(Simparica [d], Simparica Trio [d], Stronghold Plus [c]) **POM-V**

Formulations: Oral: 5 mg, 10 mg, 20 mg, 40 mg, 80 mg, 120 mg tablets; with pyrantel embonate and moxidectin (Simparica Trio). **Topical:** spot-on solution for cats with selamectin: 3 sizes (Stronghold Plus).

Action: Sarolaner acts at ligand-gated chloride channels, in particular those gated by GABA, thereby blocking pre- and post-synaptic transfer of chloride ions across cell membranes.

Use:

- Treatment of fleas, ticks, ear mite infestations (*Otodectes cynotis*) in dogs and cats, demodicosis (*Demodex canis*) and *Sarcoptes scabiei* in dogs. Parasites need to start feeding on the host to become exposed to sarolaner; therefore, the transmission of infectious parasite-borne diseases cannot be excluded.
- Treatment of biting lice infestations (*Felicola subrostratus*), adult roundworms (*Toxocara cati*) and adult intestinal hookworms (*Ancylostoma tubaeforme*) (spot-on for cats).
- Treatment of roundworm and hookworms, and prevention of *Dirofilariasis* (heartworm) and *Angiostrongylus vasorum* (lungworm) infestation in dogs (Simparica Trio).

Safety and handling: Normal precautions should be observed.

Contraindications: Do not use in dogs <8 weeks or <1.3 kg. Do not use in cats <8 weeks or <1.25 kg.

Adverse reactions: Mild GI signs may occur. Mild pruritus at site of application of spot-on product. Rarely, tremors, ataxia, convulsions.

Drug interactions: Sarolaner is highly bound to plasma proteins and might compete with other highly bound drugs such as NSAIDs and the cumarin derivative warfarin.

DOSES

See Appendix for guidelines on responsible parasiticide use.

Dogs: 2–4 mg/kg. Administer monthly.

Cats: 6 mg/kg selamectin and 1 mg/kg sarolaner. Administer monthly.

References

Crosaz O, Chapelle E, Cochet-Faivre N *et al.* (2016) Open field study on the efficacy of oral fluralaner for long-term control of flea allergy dermatitis in client-owned dogs in Ile-de-France region. *Parasites and Vectors* **9**, 174

Secobarbital (Quinalbarbitone/Cinchocaine)

(Somulose [c,d]) **POM-V CD SCHEDULE 2**

Formulations: Injectable: 400 mg/ml secobarbital with 25 mg/ml cinchocaine solution.

Action: Rapidly and profoundly depresses the CNS, including the respiratory centres. Cinchocaine has marked cardiotoxic effects at high doses. When given in combination, the barbiturate produces rapid loss of consciousness and cessation of respiration while the cinchocaine depresses cardiac conduction, resulting in early cardiac arrest. Since cardiac arrest is not dependent on development of profound hypoxia, euthanasia with the secobarbital/cinchocaine combination is generally not accompanied by the gasping that may occur with other agents.

Use:

- For euthanasia of cats and dogs.

Speed of injection is very important. An injection rate that is too slow may induce normal collapse but prolong the period until death. It is always advisable to have an alternative method of euthanasia available.

Perivascular administration of secobarbital may delay the onset of effect, cause pain and result in excitement. Placement of a venous catheter is therefore recommended and care should be taken to ensure that the injection is correctly placed in the vein.

Safety and handling: This is a potent drug that is rapidly and highly toxic to humans. Extreme care should be taken to avoid accidental self-administration. Use an i.v. catheter instead of a needle whenever possible. Only administer in the presence of an assistant/other individual. Wear suitable protective gloves when handling. Wash off splashes from skin and eyes immediately. In the event of accidental self-administration, by injection or skin absorption, do not leave the person unattended, seek urgent medical assistance advising the medical services of barbiturate and local anaesthetic poisoning, and show the label advice to a doctor. Maintain airways in the injured person and give symptomatic and supportive treatment. Cinchocaine can cause hypersensitivity following skin contact; this can lead to contact dermatitis, which can become severe.

Contraindications: Somulose must not be used for anaesthesia as it is non-sterile and cardiotoxic.

Adverse reactions: No information available.

Drug interactions: No information available.

DOSES

Dogs, Cats: 0.25 ml/kg i.v. over 10–15 seconds to minimize premature cardiac arrest.

Selamectin

(Evicto [c,d], Selehold [c,d], Stronghold [c,d], Stronghold plus [c])
POM-V

Formulations: Topical: 6%, 12% selamectin spot-on pipettes, 5 sizes for dogs, 2 sizes for cats; selamectin combined with sarolaner spot-on solution for cats.

Action: Interacts with GABA- and glutamate-gated channels leading to flaccid paralysis of parasites.

Use:
- Treatment and prevention of flea and heartworm infestation (*Dirofilaria immitis*).
- Treatment of roundworms, biting lice, ear mites (cats and dogs), hookworms (cats) sarcoptic acariasis (dogs).

Frequent shampooing may reduce the efficacy of the product. Can be used in lactation and pregnancy. Monthly treatment during pregnancy and lactation can protect litter for up to 7 weeks.

Safety and handling: Highly toxic to aquatic organisms; therefore, take care with disposal and do not let animal into water courses for 2 hours after application.

Contraindications: Not for use in animals <6 weeks.

Adverse reactions: Transient pruritus and erythema at the site of application may occur.

Drug interactions: Avoid use with other P-glycoprotein substrates.

DOSES

See Appendix for guidelines on responsible parasiticide use.

Dogs, Cats: Minimum dose recommendation 6 mg/kg. For flea and heartworm prevention, apply monthly. For the treatment of roundworms, hookworms, lice and ear mites, apply once. For effective treatment of sarcoptic mange, apply product on three occasions at 2-week intervals.

References

Nolan TJ and Lok JB (2012) Macrocyclic lactones in the treatment and control of parasitism in small companion animals. *Current Pharmaceutical Biotechnology* **13**, 1078–1094

Selegiline (L-Deprenyl)

(Selgian [d]) **POM-V**

Formulations: Oral: 4 mg, 10 mg tablets.

Action: Selegiline modifies the concentration of monoaminergic neurotransmitters, especially phenylethylamine and dopamine, by selectively inhibiting the activity of type-B monoamine oxidase (which normally breaks down these chemicals). It also appears to have neuroprotective properties.

Use:

- Authorized for the treatment of behavioural disorders of emotional origin, such as depression and anxiety, and, in association with behaviour therapy, for the treatment of signs of emotional origin observed in behavioural conditions such as overactivity, separation problems, generalized phobia and unsociable behaviour. These emotional disorders are characterized by a modification of feeding, drinking, autostimulatory behaviour, sleep, exploratory behaviour, aggression related to fear and/or irritation, social behaviour and somatic disorders (tachycardia, emotional micturition).
- May also enhance learning in certain contexts and is indicated for the treatment of canine cognitive dysfunction, especially when signs of anxiety and/or social withdrawal are associated with these problems.
- May also be used to treat signs of cognitive decline in older cats.

Treatment can be stopped suddenly without gradual dose reduction.

Safety and handling: Normal precautions should be observed.

Contraindications: Selegiline should not be used in animals with a known sensitivity to the drug or administered to lactating or pregnant bitches as it may act on prolactin secretion.

Adverse reactions: No information available.

Drug interactions: Selegiline should not be administered with alpha-2 antagonists (or within 24 hours before or after their use), pethidine, ephedrine, potential monoamine oxidase inhibitors (e.g. amitraz) or phenothiazines. The effect of morphine is potentiated when used simultaneously. Interactions with metronidazole, prednisolone and trimethoprim may exist. Selegiline should not be used for at least 2–3 weeks after the use of tricyclic antidepressants (e.g. amitriptyline, doxepin, clomipramine) or 6 weeks after the long term use of fluoxetine.

DOSES

Dogs: 0.5–1 mg/kg p.o. q24h for a minimum of 2 months.

Cats: 1 mg/kg p.o. q24h.

References

Pageat P, Lafont C, Falewee C *et al.* (2007) An evaluation of serum prolactin in anxious dogs and response to treatment with selegiline or fluoxetine. *Applied Animal Behaviour Science* **105**, 342–350

Sertraline
(Lustral*, Setraline*, Zoloft* and many others) **POM**

Formulations: Oral: 50 mg, 100 mg tablets.

Action: Selective serotonin reuptake inhibitor (SSRI). Blocks serotonin reuptake in the brain, resulting in antidepressive activity and a rise in motor activity thresholds.

Use:
- Treatment of anxiety-related behaviours, including compulsive type behaviour such as acral lick in dogs.
- Use to increase inhibitory control in cats (e.g. play-related aggressive behaviour) has been suggested, but there are no good empirical studies published to support this.

The SSRI fluoxetine and the non-selective serotonin reuptake inhibitor clomipramine are authorized and available for use in dogs; accordingly, these drugs should generally be used in preference, although there is some anecdotal evidence to suggest sertraline may have less appetite suppressant effects than generic formulations of fluoxetine.

Safety and handling: Normal precautions should be observed.

Contraindications: Known sensitivity to sertraline or other SSRIs, history of seizures.

Adverse reactions: Possible reactions include lethargy, decreased appetite and vomiting. Trembling, restlessness, GI disturbance and an apparent paradoxical increase in anxiety may occur in some cases. Owners should be warned of a potential increase in aggression in response to medication.

Drug interactions: Sertraline should not be used within 2 weeks of treatment with a monoamine oxidase inhibitor (MAOI) (e.g. selegiline) and an MAOI should not be used within 6 weeks of treatment with sertraline. Sertraline, like other SSRIs, antagonizes the effects of anticonvulsants and so is not recommended for use with epileptic patients or in association with other agents that lower seizure threshold, e.g. phenothiazines. Caution is warranted if sertraline is used concomitantly with aspirin or other anticoagulants since the risk of increased bleeding in the case of tissue trauma may be increased. Should not generally be used alongside other serotonergic agents given risk of serotonin syndrome, although use alongside trazodone may be considered in exceptional cases, so long as patient carefully monitored for signs of serotonin syndrome.

DOSES

Dogs: 1–3 mg/kg p.o. q24h, although higher doses are described in the literature.

Cats: 0.5–1.5 mg/kg p.o. q24h.

Sevelamer hydrochloride

(Renagel) **POM**

Formulations: Oral: 800 mg tablets; 0.8 g and 2.4 g oral powder sachets.

Action: Sevelamer is an organic ion-exchange resin that binds intestinal phosphate.

Use:
- Reduction of serum phosphate in azotaemia.

Hyperphosphataemia is implicated in the progression of chronic renal failure. Phosphate-binding agents are usually only used if low phosphate diets are unsuccessful. Monitor serum phosphate levels at 4–6 week intervals and adjust dosage accordingly if trying to achieve target serum concentrations. May inhibit vitamin absorption including vitamin K; consider monitoring prothrombin time.

Safety and handling: Normal precautions should be observed.

Contraindications: GI obstruction.

Adverse reactions: Pills are hygroscopic and will expand. Constipation is possible.

Drug interactions: No information available.

DOSES

Dogs, Cats: Chronic kidney disease: 30–40 mg/kg p.o. q8h, titrated to the desired serum phosphate concentration. Should be given with meals and at least 1 hour before or 3 hours after other medications.

Sevoflurane

(SevoFlo [c,d], Sevohale [c,d], Sevotek [c,d]) **POM-V**

Formulations: Inhalational: 250 ml bottle containing liquid sevoflurane.

Action: The mechanism of action of volatile anaesthetic agents is not fully understood.

Use:
- Induction and maintenance of anaesthesia.

Sevoflurane is potent and highly volatile so should only be delivered from a suitable calibrated vaporizer. It is less soluble in blood than halothane and isoflurane; therefore, induction and recovery from anaesthesia are quicker. Sevoflurane has a less pungent smell than isoflurane and induction of anaesthesia using chambers or masks is usually well tolerated in small dogs and cats. The concentration of sevoflurane required to maintain anaesthesia depends on the other drugs used in the anaesthesia protocol; the concentration should be adjusted according to clinical assessment of anaesthetic depth. The cessation of administration results in rapid recovery, which may occasionally be associated with signs of agitation. Sevoflurane does not sensitize the myocardium to catecholamines to the extent that halothane does.

Safety and handling: Measures should be adopted to prevent contamination of the environment.

Contraindications: No information available.

Adverse reactions: Causes a dose-dependent hypotension that does not wane with time. The effects of sevoflurane on respiration are dose-dependent and comparable to isoflurane, i.e. more depressant than halothane. Sevoflurane crosses the placental barrier and will affect neonates delivered by caesarean section. Sevoflurane is degraded by soda lime to compounds that are nephrotoxic in rats (principally Compound A). Conditions accelerating degradation (i.e. low gas flows, high absorbent temperatures and high sevoflurane concentrations) should be avoided in long operations, although no studies in have demonstrated Compound A to accumulate in concentrations capable of causing renal toxicity in cats and dogs.

Drug interactions: Sedatives, opioid agonists and nitrous oxide reduce the concentration of sevoflurane required to achieve surgical anaesthesia. The effects of sevoflurane on the duration of action of non-depolarizing neuromuscular blocking agents are similar to those of isoflurane, i.e. greater potentiation compared with halothane.

DOSES

Dogs, Cats: The expired concentration required to maintain surgical anaesthesia in 50% of recipients is about 2.5% in animals (minimum alveolar concentration). Administration of other anaesthetic agents and opioid analgesics reduces the dose requirement of sevoflurane; therefore, the dose should be adjusted according to individual requirement. 6–8% sevoflurane concentration is required to induce anaesthesia in unpremedicated patients.

Sildenafil

CIL

(Revatio*, Sildenafil*, Viagra*) **POM**

Formulations: Oral: 20 mg, 25 mg, 50 mg tablets; 10 mg/ml oral suspension (Revatio). **Injectable:** 0.08 mg/ml (Revatio IV). Special reformulations available: 6.25 mg, 10 mg and 12.5 mg tablets. **VSP**

Action: Pulmonary vasculature vasodilation, due to an increase in vascular levels of cGMP caused by inhibition of cGMP-specific phosphodiesterase type V.

Use:
- Indicated for the treatment of pulmonary arterial hypertension.
- Management of congenital megaoesophagus.

Data from clinical studies suggest that while sildenafil therapy in dogs with pulmonary hypertension does not significantly reduce the echocardiographic measurements, patients receiving therapy may have improvements in quality of life.

Safety and handling: Normal precautions should be observed.

Contraindications: Systemic hypotension, significant hepatic or renal impairment or bleeding disorders.

Adverse reactions: Vomiting, dizziness and raised intraocular pressure.

Drug interactions: Cimetidine, erythromycin, itraconazole and phenobarbital increase plasma sildenafil concentration. Sildenafil treatment should not be started at the same time as an alpha-adrenergic blocker. Avoid concomitant use of nitrates, which significantly enhance its hypotensive effect.

DOSES

Dogs: 0.5–2.7 mg/kg p.o. q8–24h; suggested median dose from clinical studies in dogs is 3 mg/kg/day. **For megaoesophagus:** 1 mg/kg p.o. q12h.

Cats: Reported dose of 1.6 mg/kg p.o. q12h tolerated and clinically efficacious.

References

Brown AJ, Davison E and Sleeper MM (2010) Clinical Efficacy of Sildenafil in Treatment of Pulmonary Arterial Hypertension in Dogs. *Journal of Veterinary Internal Medicine* **24**, 850–854

Novo-Matos J, Hurter K, Bektas R *et al.* (2014) Patent ductus arteriosus in an adult cat with pulmonary hypertension and right-sided congestive heart failure: hemodynamic evaluation and clinical outcome following ductal closure. *Journal of Veterinary Cardiology* **16**, 197–203

Silver sulfadiazine

(Flamazine*) **POM**

Formulations: Topical: 50 g, 250 g, 500 g of 1% cream (water soluble).

Action: Slowly releases silver in concentrations that are toxic to bacteria (Gram-positive and negative) and yeasts. The sulfadiazine component also has anti-infective qualities.

Use:
- Topical antibacterial and antifungal drug particularly active against Gram-negative organisms such as *Pseudomonas aeruginosa*.
- Used in the management of second- and third-degree burns to prevent infection.

Up to 10% may be absorbed, depending on the size of area treated.

Safety and handling: Use gloves.

Contraindications: Do not use in neonates or pregnant animals.

Adverse reactions: Patients hypersensitive to sulphonamides may react to silver sulfadiazine. Absorption over large areas of skin may result in leucopenias and anaemia. Inhibits re-epithelialization.

Drug interactions: No information available.

DOSES

Classified as category D (Prudence) by the EMA.
See Appendix for guidelines on responsible antibiotic use.

Dogs, Cats: Localized skin infections: Apply a thin film twice daily after cleaning area with antiseptic.

References

Castellano JJ, Shafii SM, Ko F *et al.* (2007) Comparative evaluation of silver-containing antimicrobial dressings and drugs. *International Wound Journal* **4**, 114–122

Silybin (Milk thistle, Silibinin, Silymarin)

(Denamarin, Doxion, Hepaticare, Hepato Liquid, Hepato Support, Hepatosyl Plus, Nutramarin+, Samylin, Zentonil Advanced, various proprietary products) **AVM-GSL, general sale**

Formulations: Oral: 9 mg, 24 mg, 25 mg, 35 mg, 40 mg, 50 mg, 70 mg, 100 mg tablets; 10 mg, 40 mg, 53 mg powder.

Action: Silybin is the active component of milk thistle or silymarin. It acts as an antioxidant and free radical scavenger, promotes hepatocyte protein synthesis and increases the level of glutathione. It also inhibits leucotriene production, reducing the inflammatory response.

Use:
- Hepatoprotectant in liver disease, especially for acute hepatotoxin-induced liver disease.
- Can also be used in patients on long-term therapy with potentially hepatotoxic drugs including lomustine (CCNU).

Safety and handling: Normal precautions should be observed.

Contraindications: No information available.

Adverse reactions: None reported. GI signs, pruritus and headaches have been recognized in primates.

Drug interactions: Silybin may inhibit microsomal cytochrome P450 isoenzyme 2C9 (CYP2C9). May increase plasma levels of beta-blockers (e.g. propranolol), calcium-channel blockers (e.g. verapamil), diazepam, lidocaine, metronidazole, pethidine and theophylline. Silymarin may increase the clearance of drugs that undergo hepatic glucuronidation, including paracetamol, diazepam and morphine. Clinical significance has not been determined for this interaction and the usefulness of silymarin for treating paracetamol toxicity has not been determined.

DOSES

Dogs, Cats: Therapeutic dosage is unknown, but suggested doses range from 50–250 mg/kg p.o. q24h. Refer to individual products for dosing advice.

References
Vandeweerd JM, Cambier C and Gustin P (2013) Nutraceuticals for canine liver disease: assessing the evidence. *Veterinary Clinics of North America: Small Animal Practice* **43**, 1171–1179

Smectite see **Calcium aluminosilicate**

Sodium bicarbonate

(Sodium bicarbonate*) **POM**

Formulations: Injectable: 1.26%, 4.2%, 8.4% solutions for i.v. infusion (8.4% solution = 1 mmol/ml). Oral: 300 mg, 500 mg, 600 mg tablets.

Action: Provision of bicarbonate ions.

Use:
- Management of severe metabolic acidosis.
- Urine alkalinization.

- Adjunctive therapy in the treatment of hypercalcaemic or hyperkalaemic crisis.

Active correction of acid−base imbalance requires blood gas analysis. Do not attempt specific therapy unless this facility is immediately available. 1 g of sodium bicarbonate provides 11.9 mEq of Na^+ and 11.9 mEq of bicarbonate. Use cautiously and administer slowly in hypocalcaemic patients. As oral sodium bicarbonate (especially at higher doses) may contribute significant amounts of sodium, use with caution in patients on salt-restricted intakes, e.g. those with CHF.

Safety and handling: Normal precautions should be observed.

Contraindications: Should not be used in animals that are unable to effectively expel carbon dioxide (e.g. hypoventilating, hypercapnoeic patients).

Adverse reactions: Excessive use of sodium bicarbonate i.v. can lead to metabolic alkalosis, hypernatraemia, CHF, a shift in the oxygen dissociation curve causing decreased tissue oxygenation and paradoxical CNS acidosis leading to respiratory arrest.

Drug interactions: Sodium bicarbonate is incompatible with many drugs and calcium salts: do not mix unless checked beforehand. Alkalinization of the urine by sodium bicarbonate decreases the excretion of quinidine and sympathomimetic drugs, and increases the excretion of aspirin, phenobarbital and tetracyclines (especially doxycycline).

DOSES
Dogs, Cats:
- **Severe metabolic acidosis:** mmol $NaHCO_3$ required = base deficit × 0.5 × bodyweight (kg) (0.3 is recommended instead of 0.5 in some references). Give half the dose slowly over 3−4 hours, recheck blood gases and clinically re-evaluate the patient. Avoid over-alkalinization.
- **Adjunctive therapy of hypercalcaemia:** 0.5−1 mmol/kg i.v. over 30 min.
- **Adjunctive therapy of hyperkalaemia:** 2−3 mmol/kg i.v. over 30 min.
- **Metabolic acidosis secondary to renal failure or to alkalinize the urine:** initial dose 8−12 mg/kg p.o q8h and then adjust dose to maintain total CO_2 concentration at 18−24 mEq/l. The dose may be increased to 50 mg/kg to adjust urine pH in patients with normal renal, hepatic and cardiac function.

Sodium chloride
(Aqupharm [c,d], Hypertonic saline [c,d], Sodium chloride [c,d], Vetivex [c,d]) **POM-V**

Formulations: Injectable: 0.45−7% NaCl solutions; 0.18% NaCl + 4% glucose, 0.9% NaCl + 5% glucose solutions. **Oral:** 300 mg, 600 mg tablets. **Ophthalmic:** 5% ointment (compounded by an ocular pharmacy).

Action: Isotonic and hypertonic formulations expand plasma volume and replace lost extracellular fluid. Hypotonic formulations provide free water and may promote oedema formation. When used for fluid replacement, NaCl (0.45% and 0.9%) will expand the plasma volume compartment. Compared with colloids, 2.5−3 times as much fluid must be given because the crystalloid is distributed to other fluid compartments.

Use:

- Intravenous fluid replacement, including treatment of choice for patients with hypercalcaemia or hyperchloraemic alkalosis.
- Sodium chloride solutions are often used as a drug diluent.
- Hypertonic saline is used to expand the circulating blood volume rapidly in animals with shock, particularly during the preoperative period.
- The hypertonic ophthalmic ointment is used in the management of corneal oedema.
- Oral sodium supplementation is recommended by some authors in the long-term management of hypoadrenocorticism.

Hypertonic saline solutions have very high sodium concentrations and it is important to monitor serum sodium concentrations before and after their administration; maintenance with an isotonic crystalloid is usually required after administration to correct electrolyte and fluid disturbances.

Safety and handling: Hypertonic saline solutions should be regarded as drugs and not as intravenous fluids and should be stored separately to prevent confusion.

Contraindications: Hypertonic saline should not be administered to dehydrated animals and hypotonic solutions should not be administered to hypovolaemic animals.

Adverse reactions: Peripheral oedema is more likely to occur after crystalloids because muscle and subcutaneous capillaries are less permeable to protein. Normal saline contains higher amounts of chloride than plasma, which will increase the risk of acidosis. The degree of acidosis is not likely to be a problem in a healthy patient but may be exacerbated in a compromised patient. Hypertonic saline administered at fluid rates >1 ml/kg/min can cause a vagally mediated bradycardia, therefore the rate of fluid administration must be carefully controlled. Enteric-coated products for oral use may not be adequately absorbed by dogs and therefore may be of unpredictable efficacy. The ophthalmic ointment may cause a stinging sensation.

Drug interactions: No information available.

DOSES

Dogs, Cats:

- **Fluid therapy:** fluid requirements depend on the degree of dehydration and ongoing losses. In uncomplicated cases 0.45–3% solutions should be administered at a dose of 50–60 ml/kg/day i.v., p.o. Higher doses are required if the animal is dehydrated. Solutions containing 0.9–3% NaCl are suitable for replacing deficits. Solutions containing 0.45% NaCl (with added potassium) are indicated for longer-term maintenance.
- **Hypotension/shock:** 5–7.5% NaCl solutions (hypertonic saline) at doses of 3–8 ml/kg i.v. Hypertonic solutions should be used with caution and with other appropriate fluid replacement strategies. Hypertonic NaCl may be combined with colloid solutions to stabilize the increase in vascular volume provided.
- **Salt-wasting syndromes (hypoadrenocorticism):** 1–5 g p.o. q24h.
- **Corneal oedema:** apply a small amount of ointment q4–24h.

References

Rozanski E and Rondeau M (2002) Choosing fluids in traumatic hypovolaemic shock: the role of crystalloids, colloids and hypertonic saline. *Journal of the American Animal Hospital Association* **38**, 499–501

Sodium chromoglycate see **Sodium cromoglicate**

Sodium citrate
(Micolette*, Micralax*, Relaxit*) **P**

Formulations: Rectal: micro-enemas containing 450 ml sodium citrate + 45 mg sodium alkylsulphoacetate (Micralax) or 45 mg sodium lauryl sulphoacetate (Micolette) or 75 mg sodium lauryl sulphate (Relaxit).

Action: An osmotic laxative that causes water to be retained within the lumen of the GI tract. It is formulated with a stool softener that augments its action.

Use:
- Low-volume enema used to treat constipation and to prepare the lower GI tract for proctoscopy and radiography.

Safety and handling: Normal precautions should be observed.

Contraindications: Not recommended for use in cases with chronic enteropathy.

Adverse reactions: Uncommon. Largely due to water and electrolyte disturbances.

Drug interactions: No information available.

DOSES
Dogs, Cats: 1 enema inserted per rectum to full length of nozzle.

Sodium cromoglicate (Sodium chromoglycate)
(There are >20 OTC products including Allercrom*, Aspire*, Catacrom*, Eycrom*, Intal*, Nalcrom*, Opticrom*, Optrex allergy*, Pollinase*, Sodium cromoglicate*, Vividrin*) **P, POM**

Formulations: Topical: 2% ocular drops (GSL); 5 mg/dose pressurized inhaler (POM). Oral: 100 mg tablets (POM).

Action: Stabilizes mast cell membranes, preventing degranulation.

Use:
- Management of allergic conjunctivitis and rhinitis.

Action is localized to the site of application.

Safety and handling: Normal precautions should be observed.

Contraindications: No information available.

Adverse reactions: May cause local irritation.

Drug interactions: No information available.

DOSES
Dogs, Cats: Allergic reactions: 1–2 drops in eye or nose q6h.

Sodium hypochlorite (Hypochlorous acid)

(Renasan spray, Vetericyn Regular, Vetericyn VF) **GSL**

Formulations: Topical: 250 ml, 500 ml bottles containing 150 ppm free active chlorine (Vetericyn VF (veterinary formulation)); 89 ml, 236 ml, 473 ml bottles containing 80 ppm (Vetericyn Regular); 60 ml, 100 ml, 250 ml, 500 ml, 750 ml bottles containing 140 ppm (Renasan).

Action: Assists in the mechanical removal of cellular debris, senescent cells, necrotic tissue, and foreign material from the skin and wound surface through debridement and has antibacterial and antifungal action. The hypochlorous acid is pH balanced to a physiological range.

Use: For the topical treatment of wounds and skin infections.

Safety and handling: Normal precautions should be observed.

Contraindications: None reported.

Adverse reactions: None reported.

Drug interactions: None reported.

DOSES

Dogs, Cats: Spray affected areas up to twice daily.

References

Pariser M, Gard S, Gram D et al. (2013) An in vitro study to determine the minimal bactericidal concentration of sodium hypochlorite (bleach) required to inhibit meticillin-resistant *Staphylococcus pseudintermedius* strains isolated from canine skin. *Veterinary Dermatology* **24**, 632–634

Sakarya S, Gunay N, Karakulak M et al. (2014) Hypochlorous Acid: an ideal wound care agent with powerful microbicidal, antibiofilm, and wound healing potency. *Wounds* **26**, 342–350

Somatotropin (Growth hormone)

(Genotropin*, Humatrope*, Norditropin*) **POM**

Formulations: Injectable: 2–16 IU vials for reconstitution.

Action: Recombinant human growth hormone that mimics growth hormone action in other species.

Use:
• Treatment of growth hormone deficiency.

Serum IGF-1 measurements may be helpful to monitor therapy. Antibody formation may limit its effectiveness in the long term.

Safety and handling: Normal precautions should be observed.

Contraindications: No information available.

Adverse reactions: Growth hormone is diabetogenic; monitor blood glucose. Local reactions may be seen; rotate injection sites.

Drug interactions: No information available.

DOSES

Dogs, Cats: 0.1–0.2 IU/kg s.c., i.m. (painful) 3–5 times a week. Continue for at least 6 weeks to evaluate response.

Sotalol

CIL

(Sotacor*, Sotalol*) **POM**

Formulations: Oral: 40 mg, 80 mg, 160 mg, 200 mg tablets. Injectable: 10 mg/ml solution. Special reformulations available: 10 mg, 30 mg tablets. **VSP**

Action: Produces a prolongation of action potential duration and refractory period via selective inhibition of potassium channels (Class III antiarrhythmic). Also has non-selective beta-adrenergic blocking effects, but considered a weak beta blocker.

Use:
- Treatment of ventricular arrhythmias, less so supraventricular arrhythmia (most associated with accessory pathway). Used most commonly in dogs with ventricular arrhythmias secondary to myocardial disease.

The beta-blocking activity is about one-third of that of propranolol. Preferable to assess efficacy with repeated Holter ECG monitoring. Can be used successfully in combination with mexilitine for severe ventricular arrhythmia. Use with caution in patients with renal failure or medically controlled CHF.

Safety and handling: Normal precautions should be observed.

Contraindications: Asthma, sinus bradycardia, AV block or decompensated CHF, prolonged QT interval on ECG.

Adverse reactions: The non-selective beta-blocking effects can decrease heart rate, stroke volume and cardiac output in dogs and may precipitate CHF. The drug is eliminated in urine and faeces and elimination half-life may increase with renal insufficiency, leading to accumulation at standard doses. Adverse effects include hypotension, bradyarrhythmias, bronchospasm, depression, nausea, vomiting and diarrhoea. The drug is potentially proarrhythmic and high doses can cause prolonged QT interval and increase the risk of torsades de pointes, especially if hypokalaemia is present.

Drug interactions: Sympathomimetics (e.g. terbutaline, phenylpropanolamine, adrenaline) may have their actions blocked by sotalol and may, in turn, reduce the efficacy of sotalol. Additive myocardial depression may occur with the concurrent use of sotalol and other beta-blockers or myocardial depressant anaesthetic agents. Hypotensive effects may be enhanced by phenothiazines, furosemide, hydralazine and other vasodilators. Sotalol may prolong the hypoglycaemic effects of insulin therapy. Concurrent use of negative inotropics (e.g. calcium-channel blockers) should be done with caution, particularly in patients with pre-existing systolic dysfunction or CHF.

DOSES

Dogs: 0.5–3 mg/kg p.o. q12h. Start with lower doses if myocardial function is reduced. Anecdotal doses starting at 0.5 mg/kg i.v. given over 2 min, up to 3 times (to a total dose of 1.5 mg/kg i.v.).
Cats: 10–20 mg/cat p.o. q12h.

References
Gelzer ARM, Kraus MS, Rishniw M *et al.* (2010) Combination therapy with mexiletine and sotalol suppresses inherited ventricular arrhythmias in German Shepherd Dogs better than mexiletine or sotalol monotherapy: a randomized cross-over study. *Journal of Veterinary Cardiology* **12**, 93–106
Meurs KM, Spier AW, Wright NA *et al.* (2002) Comparison of the effects of four antiarrhythmic treatments for familial ventricular arrhythmias in Boxers. *Journal of the American Veterinary Medical Association* **221**, 522–527

Spinosad

(Comfortis) **POM-V**

Formulations: Oral: 90 mg, 140 mg, 270 mg, 425 mg, 665 mg, 1040 mg, 1620 mg chewable tablets. Also available with milbemycin (Trifexis).

Action: Activation of nicotinic acetylcholine receptors.

Use:
- Treatment and prevention of flea infestations.
- Administer with food.

As it acts on larvae and adults, there will be a short lag phase after administration due to the emergence of adult fleas from pupae already in the environment. If used as part of a treatment programme for flea allergy dermatitis, combine with an insect growth regulator. Give with food.

Safety and handling: Normal precautions should be observed.

Contraindications: Avoid in dogs <1.3 kg and cats < 1.2 kg or <14 weeks as accurate dosing not possible. Use with caution in dogs and cats with pre-existing epilepsy. Safety in pregnancy and lactation unknown.

Adverse reactions: Vomiting occurs occasionally. Rare side effects include lethargy, diarrhoea, anorexia, ataxia and seizures.

Drug interactions: No information available.

DOSES

See Appendix for guidelines on responsible parasiticide use.

Dogs: 45–70 mg/kg p.o. q28d with or immediately after food.

Cats: 50–75 mg/kg p.o. q28d with or immediately after food.

Spiramycin see **Metronidazole**

Spironolactone

(Cardalis[d], Prilactone[d], Aldactone*, Spironolactone*)
POM-V, POM

Formulations: Oral: 10 mg, 40 mg, 50 mg, 80 mg, 100 mg tablets; 20 mg spironolactone + 2.5 mg benazepril; 40 mg spironolactone + 5 mg benazepril; 80 mg spironolactone + 10 mg benazepril (Cardalis).

Action: Aldosterone receptor antagonist that acts on the kidneys as a weak potassium-sparing diuretic (preventing sodium resorption in the distal tubule) via competition with aldosterone for the mineralocorticoid receptor in the principle cells of the collecting duct and acts on the myocardium and vasculature to inhibit aldosterone-mediated fibrosis and remodelling.

Use:
- Treatment of CHF. Authorized for use in combination with standard therapy for treatment of CHF caused by valvular regurgitation in dogs.
- Used in the management of ascites secondary to hepatic failure (when hypokalaemia can exacerbate hepatic encephalopathy).
- Treatment of hyperaldosteronism due to adrenal tumours.

Spironolactone is a weak diuretic and does not have a significant diuretic effect in healthy dogs. Its beneficial effects in heart failure appear to be related to inhibition of myocardial fibrosis, vascular remodelling and endothelial dysfunction. It is particularly useful for hypokalaemic patients with heart failure. Use with caution in patients with renal or hepatic dysfunction.

Safety and handling: Normal precautions should be observed.

Contraindications: Do not use in animals with hypoadrenocorticism, hyperkalaemia or hyponatraemia. Do not give in conjunction with NSAIDs to animals with renal insufficiency. Do not use during pregnancy or lactation, or in animals intended for breeding.

Adverse reactions: Hyponatraemia and hyperkalaemia may develop. Discontinue if hyperkalaemia occurs. Reversible prostatic atrophy may occur in entire male dogs. Severe ulcerative facial dermatitis has been reported in Maine Coon cats. Hepatotoxicity is reported in humans.

Drug interactions: Potentiates thiazide and loop diuretics. Hyperkalaemia may result if ACE inhibitors, NSAIDs, ciclosporin or potassium supplements are administered in conjunction with spironolactone. However, in practice, spironolactone and ACE inhibitors appear safe to use concurrently. Monitor renal function and serum potassium levels in animals receiving spironolactone and ACE inhibitors. There is an increased risk of nephrotoxicity if spironolactone is administered with NSAIDs. The plasma concentration of digoxin may be increased by spironolactone.

DOSES

Dogs, Cats: 2–4 mg/kg p.o. q24h.

References

James RA, Guillot E, Gilmour J et al. (2015) Efficacy of Spironolactone (SP) Following Oral Administration of SP in Cats with Heart Failure: Final Results of the SEISICAT Study. *Proceedings of the 25th ECVIM-CA Congress, Lisbon*

Lefebvre HP, Ollivier E, Atkins CE et al. (2013) Safety of spironolactone in dogs with chronic heart failure because of degenerative valvular disease: a population-based, longitudinal study. *Journal of Veterinary Internal Medicine* **27**, 1083–1091

Sterculia

(Peridale, Normacol*) **AVM-GSL, GSL**

Formulations: Oral: 98% granules (Peridale); 620 mg/g granules (Normacol).

Action: Bulk-forming agent that increases faecal mass and stimulates peristalsis.

Use:
- Management of impacted anal sacs, diarrhoea and constipation, and control of stool consistency after surgery.

Sterculia is inert and not absorbed. During treatment, fluid should be provided or a moist diet given. As the preparations swell in contact with water, they should be administered with plenty of water available.

Safety and handling: Normal precautions should be observed.

Contraindications: Do not use in cases of intestinal obstruction or where enterotomy or enterectomy is to be performed.

Adverse reactions: No information available.

Drug interactions: No information available.

DOSES

Dogs: 1.5 g p.o. q24h (dogs <5 kg); 3 g p.o. q12–24h (5–15 kg); 4 g p.o. q12–24h (>15 kg). Sprinkle over feed or place on tongue.

Cats: Kittens: 118 mg q24h. **Adults:** 118 mg q12h.

Succinylcholine see **Suxamethonium**

Sucralfate   CIL
(Antepsin*, Antepsin suspension*, Carafate*, Sulcrate*)
POM

Formulations: Oral: 1 g tablets; 0.2 g/ml suspension.

Action: In an acidic medium an aluminium ion detaches from the compound, leaving a very polar, relatively non-absorbable ion. This ion then binds to proteinaceous exudates in the upper GI tract, forming a chemical diffusion barrier over ulcer sites, preventing further erosion from acid, pepsin and bile salts. However, its major action appears to relate to stimulation of mucosal defences and repair mechanisms (stimulation of bicarbonate and prostaglandin production and binding of epidermal growth factor). These effects are seen at neutral pH.

Use:
- Treatment of oesophageal, gastric and duodenal ulceration.
- Not recommended as a phosphate binder in chronic kidney disease.

Can be used alongside an H2 receptor antagonist or proton-pump inhibitor but should be given separately.

Safety and handling: Normal precautions should be observed.

Contraindications: Perforated ulcer.

Adverse reactions: Minimal; constipation is the main problem in humans. Bezoar formation and hypophosphataemia are also reported in humans.

Drug interactions: Sucralfate may decrease the bioavailability of H2 antagonists, phenytoin and tetracyclines. It may be a wise precaution to administer sucralfate at least 2 hours before or after these drugs. Sucralfate interferes significantly with the absorption of fluoroquinolones and digoxin.

DOSES

Dogs: All uses: 500 mg/dog p.o. q6–8h (dogs <20 kg); 1–2 g/dog p.o. q6–8h (dogs >20 kg).

Cats: All uses: 250 mg/cat p.o. q8–12h.

References
Bazelle J, Threlfall A and Whitley N (2018) Gastroprotectants in small animal veterinary practice – a review of the evidence. Part 1: cyto-protective drugs. *Journal of Small Animal Practice* **59**, 587–602

Marks SL, Kook PH, Papich MG, Tolbert MK and Willard MD (2018) ACVIM consensus statement: support for rational administration of gastrointestinal protectants to dogs and cats. *Journal of Veterinary Internal Medicine* **32**, 1823–1840

Sulfasalazine

CIL

(Salazopyrin*, Sulphasalazine*) **POM**

Formulations: Oral: 500 mg tablets; 250 mg/5 ml oral suspension.

Action: Sulfasalazine is a prodrug: a diazo bond binding sulfapyridine to 5-ASA is cleaved by colonic bacteria to release free 5-ASA, which acts locally in the colon as an anti-inflammatory.

Use:
- Used in the management of colitis, although evidence of efficacy is lacking. There is a significant risk of keratoconjunctivitis sicca (KCS) and periodic Schirmer tear tests should be performed.

Safety and handling: Normal precautions should be observed.

Contraindications: Dobermanns appear to be sensitive to adverse effects associated with sulfapyridine.

Adverse reactions: Can include KCS, vomiting, allergic dermatitis and cholestatic jaundice. Owners should be made aware of the seriousness of KCS and what signs to monitor. The cause of KCS is not clear; historically, sulfapyridine has been blamed. Olsalazine has been recommended as the incidence of KCS is less with its use, although not completely abolished. It is possible that 5-ASA may sometimes be responsible.

Drug interactions: The absorption of digoxin may be inhibited by sulfasalazine, and the measurement of serum folate concentration may be affected. Sulfasalazine may cause a reduction in serum thyroxine concentrations.

DOSES
Dogs: All uses: 15–30 mg/kg p.o. q8–12h, maximum 6 g/day.
Cats: All uses: 10–20 mg/kg p.o. q8–12h.

Sulphonamide see **Trimethoprim/ Sulphonamide**

Suxamethonium (Succinylcholine)

(Suxamethonium*) **POM**

Formulations: Injectable: 50 mg/ml solution.

Action: Non-competitively binds to the nicotinic acetylcholine receptor. Persistent depolarization prevents the transmission of further action potentials, resulting in muscle relaxation.

Use:
- Used to facilitate intubation in cats.

There are no indications for suxamethonium in dogs. Suxamethonium has a very rapid onset of action (5–15 seconds) and short duration of action (3–5 minutes). However, use of neuromuscular blockade to facilitate intubation is rarely required in small animals and suxamethonium has been largely replaced by non-depolarizing drugs.

Safety and handling: Store in refrigerator.

Contraindications: Do not administer unless the animal is adequately anaesthetized and facilities to provide positive pressure ventilation are available. Do not use in animals exposed to organophosphate compounds. Use with caution in patients with hepatic disease.

Adverse reactions: Can cause arrhythmias (sinus bradycardia, ventricular arrhythmias) via stimulation of muscarinic receptors in the sinus node. A small rise in potassium concentration is expected after suxamethonium; patients with burns and neuromuscular disorders are at severe risk of hyperkalaemia.

Drug interactions: The actions of suxamethonium may be enhanced by beta-adrenergic blockers (e.g. propranolol), furosemide, isoflurane, lidocaine, magnesium salts and phenothiazines. Diazepam may reduce the duration of action of suxamethonium. Neostigmine and pyrido-stigmine should not be administered with suxamethonium as they inhibit pseudocholinesterases, thereby enhancing suxamethonium's effect.

DOSES

Dogs: Do not use.

Cats: 1.0 mg/kg i.v. A total dose of 3.5 mg is satisfactory in cats >3.5 kg.

T3 see **Liothyronine**
T4 see **L-Thyroxine**

Tacrolimus (FK 506)

(Protopic*, Tacrolimus*) **POM**

Formulations: Topical: 0.03%, 0.1% skin ointments (30 g, 60 g tubes); 0.02% eye drop solution (15 ml). **Oral:** various preparations – avoid switching between brands.

Action: T-lymphocyte inhibition.

Use:
- Topical aqueous and oil-based formulations have been used in eyes to treat canine keratoconjunctivitis sicca that is unresponsive to topical ciclosporin.

Prior to availibility of an ophthalmic preparation in the UK, there were anecdotal reports that the skin ointment (0.1%) formulation has been used successfully and without adverse effects. Has also been used for localized autoimmune dermatoses and localized lesions of atopic dermatitis. Long-term effects, potential adverse effects and toxicities are as yet unknown and tacrolimus must be reserved for special cases only. Systemic (oral) administration has been used for a limited number of cases of anal furunculosis where ciclosporin has failed.

Safety and handling: Use gloves.

Contraindications: No information available.

Adverse reactions: Discomfort on application (blepharospasm). Topical treatment may be associated with an increased risk of malignancy (e.g corneal squamous cell carcinoma). May affect circulating levels of insulin and cause hyperglycaemia; in the presence of diabetes mellitus, the effect of treatment on glycaemic control must be monitored.

Drug interactions: Suspected to be similar to ciclosporin.

DOSES

See Appendix for immunosuppression protocols.

Dogs: Apply 1 drop to the affected eye q12h.

Cats: No information available.

References
Dreyfus J, Schobert CS and Dubielzig RR (2011) Superficial corneal squamous cell carcinoma occurring in dogs with chronic keratitis. *Veterinary Ophthalmology* **14**, 161–168

Tamsulosin hydrochloride `CIL`

(Cositam XL*, Flomaxtra*) **POM, P**

Formulations: Oral: 0.4 mg tablets or capsules.

Action: Alpha-1 adrenergic antagonist with selectivity for the urinary tract; relaxes smooth muscle in the prostate, urethra and bladder neck aiding urine flow. Longer acting than prazosin or phenoxybenzamine.

Use:
- Treatment of reflex dyssynergia/urethral spasm. May also aid passage of urethroliths/ureteroliths.

- An alternative to prazosin or phenoxybenzamine in refractory cases of reflex dyssynergia, with less effect on systemic blood pressure.

Safety and handling: No information available.

Contraindications: No information available.

Adverse reactions: Hypotension possible (especially at high doses).

Drug interactions: Concurrent use of other alpha-1 blockers (e.g. prazosin) or sildenafil may exacerbate hypotensive effects.

DOSES
Dogs: Urethral relaxant: 10 μg (micrograms)/kg p.o. q24h (up to 0.4 mg/dog (total dose) q24h), can increase to q12h if necessary. Capsules should not be split and compounding may be required.

Cats: Urethral relaxant: 4–6 μg (micrograms)/kg p.o. q12–24h. Limited clinical experience or safety data exists.

References
Ohtake A, Sato S, Saitoh C *et al.* (2004) Effects of tamsulosin on hypogastric nerve stimulation-induced intraurethral pressure elevation in male and female dogs under anesthesia. *European Journal of Pharmacology* **497**, 327–334

Sato S, Ohtake A, Hatanaka T *et al.* (2007) Relationship between the functional effect of tamsulosin and its concentration in lower urinary tract tissues in dogs. *Biological and Pharmaceutical Bulletin* **30**, 481–486

Tasipimidine
(Tessie [d]) **POM-V**

Formulations: Oral: 0.3 mg/ml solution.

Action: By binding to alpha-2A adrenergic receptors, tasipimidine inhibits the release and action of norepinephrine from the sympathetic nervous system. Within the CNS, this leads to dose-dependent sedation, as well as possible suppression of the cardiovascular and respiratory systems.

Use:
- Short-term alleviation of situational anxiety and fear in dogs triggered by noise or owner departure.

Safety and handling: Normal precautions should be observed. Use graduated syringe supplied with the product.

Contraindications: Should not be used in animals with severe systemic disease affecting liver, kidney or cardiovascular function. Do not use in pregnant or lactating animals, or animals already sedated.

Adverse reactions: In clinical trials, lethargy and vomiting were very common (>10% of animals) adverse reactions. Undesirable behavioural reactions (e.g. barking, avoidance, disorientation, increased reactivity), sedation, ataxia, diarrhoea, urinary incontinence, nausea, gastroenteritis, polydipsia, leucopenia, hypersensitivity reactions, somnolence and anorexia were seen in 1–10% of animals. Decrease in heart rate, blood pressure and body temperature have been reported in non-anxious animals involved in preclinical trials.

Drug interactions: Effects may be potentiated by other CNS depressants.

DOSES
Dogs: 0.1 ml/kg p.o. (equivalent to 30 μg (micrograms)/kg).

Cats: No information available.

Telmisartan

(Semintra[c]) **POM-V**

Formulations: Oral: 4 mg/ml, 10 mg/ml solution.

Action: Angiotensin II receptor (type AT1) antagonist which acts to inhibit the effects of angiotensin (i.e. vasoconstriction, increased aldosterone synthesis, sodium and water retention and renal, vascular and cardiac remodelling). In the kidney, angiotensin II may result in glomerular capillary hypertension and increased protein in the glomerular filtrate, which could trigger or potentiate interstitial fibrosis.

Use:
- Authorized for the reduction of proteinuria associated with chronic kidney disease in cats.
- Treatment of systemic hypertension in cats.

The effects on the long-term prognosis of feline kidney disease are currently not established. Telmisartan would appear to be as effective as benazepril at delaying deterioration in proteinuria over 6 months in cats with chronic kidney disease (IRIS stages II to IV, urine specific gravity <1.035 and no comorbidities). The safety and efficacy of telmisartan for the management of systemic hypertension above 200 mmHg has not been investigated. Monitoring of blood pressure is recommended in cats that develop clinical signs referable to hypotension or cats undergoing general anaesthesia. Both oral solutions seem to be accepted well by most cats. There are case reports of its successful use to treat protein-losing nephropathy and hypertension (in combination with amlodipine) in dogs.

Safety and handling: Normal precautions should be observed.

Contraindications: The safety of telmisartan has not been established in breeding, pregnant or lactating cats or cats <6 months.

Adverse reactions: Mild and transient GI signs (regurgitation, vomiting, diarrhoea). Rare increased alanine aminotransferase activity that resolved within a few days of stopping therapy. Healthy cats administered 5 times the recommended dose for 6 months experienced decreases in blood pressure and red blood cell count and increases in blood urea nitrogen.

Drug interactions: Cats that received concomitant therapy with amlodipine at the recommended dose did not experience clinical evidence of hypotension. Avoid concurrent use of ACE inhibitors.

DOSES

Dogs: 0.5–1 mg/kg p.o. q24h (limited information).

Cats:
- For proteinuria: 1 mg/kg p.o. q24h.
- For hypertension: 2 mg/kg p.o. q24h.

References

Caro-Vadillo A, Daza-González MA, Gonzalez-Alonso-Alegre E *et al.* (2018) Effect of a combination of telmisartan and amlodipine in hypertensive dogs. *Veterinary Record Case Reports* **6**, e000471

Glaus TM, Elliott J, Herberich E *et al.* (2019) Efficacy of long-term oral telmisartan treatment in cats with hypertension: results of a prospective European clinical trial. *Journal of Veterinary Internal Medicine* **33**, 413–422

Sent U, Gössl R, Elliott J *et al.* (2015) Comparison of efficacy of long-term oral treatment with telmisartan and benazepril in cats with chronic kidney disease. *Journal of Veterinary Internal Medicine* **29**, 1479–1487

Temozolomide

(Temcad*, Temodal*, Temodar*) **POM**

Formulations: Oral: 5 mg, 20 mg, 100 mg, 140 mg, 180 mg, 250 mg capsules.

Action: Oral alkylating agent. Has the ability to alkylate or methylate DNA (which most often occurs at the N−7 or O−6 positions of guanine residues). This methylation damages DNA and leads to cell death.

Use:
- Preliminary investigations have evaluated temozolomide in canine lymphoma, melanoma and gliomas.

Safety and handling: Potent cytotoxic drug that should only be prepared and administered by trained personnel. See Appendix and specialist texts for further advice on chemotherapeutic agents.

Contraindications: Contraindicated in patients with known hypersensitivity. Do not use in patients with pre-existing bone marrow suppression. Should be used with caution in patients with reduced hepatic or renal function.

Adverse reactions: May cause myelosuppression and gastrointestinal adverse events. Lethargy, polydipsia, and altered renal and hepatic parameters are also described.

Drug interactions: Not reported at present.

DOSES

Dogs: 60−65 mg/m^2 p.o. q24h for 5 consecutive days q28d for 4 to 6 cycles. 100 mg/m^2 p.o. q24h for 5 consecutive days every 2 weeks is described for relapsed lymphoma.

Cats: Not advised based on early toxicity studies.

References

Cancedda S, Rohrer Bley C, Aresu L et al. (2016) Efficacy and side effects of radiation therapy in comparison with radiation therapy and temozolomide in the treatment of measurable canine malignant melanoma. *Veterinary and Comparative Oncology* **14**, 146−157

Treggiari E, Elliot JW, Baines SJ et al. (2017) Temozolomide alone or in combination with doxorubicin as a rescue agent in 37 cases of canine multicentric lymphoma. *Veterinary and Comparative Oncology* **16**, 194−201

Terbinafine

(Neptra[d], Osurnia[d], Lamisil*) **POM-V, POM, GSL**

Formulations: Oral: 250 mg tablets. Topical: 1% cream, gel, solution and spray; 10 mg terbinafine + florfenicol + betamethasone ear gel (Osurnia); 16.7 mg terbinafine + florfenicol + mometasone ear gel (Neptra).

Action: Inhibits ergosterol synthesis by inhibiting squalene epoxidase, an enzyme that is part of the fungal cell wall synthesis pathway.

Use:
- Management of dermatophytosis, *Malassezia* dermatitis and otitis, subcutaneous and systemic fungal infections in cats and dogs.

The gel is authorized for the treatment of acute otitis externa and acute exacerbation of recurrent otitis externa associated with *Staphylococcus pseudintermedius* and *Malassezia pachydermatis*. Ear gel should be instilled in a cleaned ear. Administer one tube per infected ear. Repeat the administration after 7 days (Osurnia). The maximum clinical response may not be seen until 28 days after the first administration of Osurnia or sole administration of Neptra. Optimal therapeutic regimens for systemic use (e.g. for refractory nasal aspergillosis) are still under investigation: pretreatment and monitoring CBC, renal and liver function tests are advised when using systemic drug long term.

Safety and handling: Normal precautions should be observed. Osurnia ear gel should be stored in a refrigerator.

Contraindications: Do not use ear gel if the eardrum is perforated, in dogs with generalized demodicosis or in pregnant or breeding animals. Do not use Osurnia in animals <2 months or <1.4 kg, Neptra in animals <3 months or <4 kg. Ear gels are not indicated for cats.

Adverse reactions: Vomiting, diarrhoea, increased liver enzymes, pruritus (cats). Topical solutions contain alcohol and may cause irritation. Transient deafness or impaired hearing may occur in elderly dogs after administration of the ear gel. Corneal ulceration and keratoconjunctivitis sicca have rarely been reported in dogs.

Drug interactions: No information available.

DOSES
Dogs, Cats: Antifungal: 30–40 mg/kg p.o. q24h; doses greater than 30 mg/kg may be required to reach therapeutic levels in the skin of dogs. Cream may be used to treat localized *Malassezia* infections.

References
Balda C, Otsuka M, Gambale W *et al.* (2004) P-12 Comparative study of griseofulvin and terbinafine therapy in the treatment of canine and feline dermatophytosis. *Veterinary Dermatology* **15(S1)**, 44
Gimmler JR, White AG, Kennis RA *et al.* (2015) Determining canine skin concentrations of terbinafine to guide the treatment of *Malassezia* dermatitis. *Veterinary Dermatology* **26**, 411–416

Terbutaline
CIL

(Bricanyl*, Monovent*) **POM**

Formulations: Injectable: 0.5 mg/ml solution. **Oral:** 5 mg tablets.

Action: Selective beta-2 adrenergic agonist that directly stimulates bronchodilation.

Use:
* Bronchodilation.
* Maintenance of heart rate in animals with sick sinus syndrome.

Use with caution in patients with diabetes mellitus, hyperthyroidism, hypertension or seizure disorders.

Safety and handling: Normal precautions should be observed.

Contraindications: No information available.

Adverse reactions: Fine tremor, tachycardia, hypokalaemia, hypotension and hypersensitivity reactions. Administration i.m. may be painful.

Drug interactions: There is an increased risk of hypokalaemia if theophylline or high doses of corticosteroids are given with high doses of terbutaline. Use with digitalis glycosides or inhalational anaesthetics may increase the risk of cardiac arrhythmias. Beta-blockers may antagonize its effects. Other sympathomimetic amines may increase the risk of adverse cardiovascular effects.

DOSES

Dogs:
- **Bronchodilation:** 1.25–5 mg/dog p.o. q8–12h, 0.01 mg/kg i.m., s.c., i.v. q4h.
- **Bradyarrhythmias:** 0.2 mg/kg p.o. q8–12h.

Cats:
- **Bronchodilation:** 0.312–1.25 mg/cat p.o. q8–12h, 0.01 mg/kg i.m., s.c., i.v. q4h.
- **Bradyarrhythmias:** 0.625 mg/cat p.o. q8–12h.

References

Foster SF and Martin P (2011) Lower respiratory tract infections in cats: reaching beyond empirical therapy. *Journal of Feline Medicine and Surgery* **13**, 313–332

Tetanus antitoxin

(Tetanus antitoxin Behring[d]) **POM-V**

Formulations: Injectable: 1000 IU/ml solution.

Action: Antibody binds to tetanus toxin.

Use:
- Preventative measure in animals at risk of developing tetanus from wounds.
- Best used in developing cases of tetanus (i.e. immediate clinical signs or when contamination of wound is severe and progression to a severe form of tetanus is possible). It is less effective in established tetanus cases as it does not displace bound toxin.

Risk of tetanus in dogs and cats is very low; routine prophylaxis is not warranted.

Safety and handling: Normal precautions should be observed.

Contraindications: Avoid in cats (cannot metabolize phenol preservative).

Adverse reactions: All antisera have the potential to produce anaphylactoid reactions, particularly if the patient has previously received products containing horse protein. Repeated doses may lead to hypersensitivity reactions. Adrenaline or antihistamines may be used to manage adverse effects.

Drug interactions: No information available.

DOSES

Dogs:
- **Prophylactic:** 80 IU/kg (maximum of 2500 IU/dog) i.m., s.c. once.
- **Therapy of developing tetanus:** 100–1000 IU/kg (maximum 20,000 IU/dog) i.m., s.c. once (off-licence i.v. administration following a s.c./ intradermal test dose is reported).

Cats: Not required.

References

Adamantos S and Boag A (2007) Thirteen cases of tetanus in dogs. *Veterinary Record* **161**, 298–302

Tetracaine (Amethocaine)
(Amethocaine hydrochloride*) **POM**

Formulations: Ophthalmic: 0.5%, 1% solution (single-use vials).

Action: Local anaesthetic action is dependent on reversible blockade of the sodium channel, preventing propagation of an action potential. Sensory nerve fibres are blocked before motor nerve fibres, allowing a selective sensory blockade at low doses.

Use:
- Local anaesthesia of the ocular surface (cornea and conjunctival sac).

Although effective, it is uncommonly used in small animal practice. An alternative topical ophthalmic anaesthetic such as proxymetacaine is advised. Duration of action has not been reported in small animal species. Topical anaesthetics block reflex tear production and should not be applied before a Schirmer tear test.

Safety and handling: Check conditions for storage (unlike proxymetacaine, refrigeration is not required).

Contraindications: Do not use for therapeutic purposes.

Adverse reactions: Tetracaine often causes marked conjunctival irritation, chemosis and pain on application (more so than proxymetacaine). All topical anaesthetics are toxic to the corneal epithelium and repeated administration can delay healing of ulcers.

Drug interactions: No information available.

DOSES
Dogs, Cats: Ophthalmic: 1 drop per eye, single application.

Tetracosactide (Tetracosactrin, ACTH)
(Cosacthen [d], Synacthen*) **POM**

Formulations: Injectable: 0.25 mg/ml solution for intravenous use. A 0.1 mg/ml solution is available on a named patient basis. In the event of availability problems, an alternative lyophilized formulation (0.25 mg/ml) for intramuscular use may be imported on a named patient basis. **VSP**

Action: ACTH analogue that binds to specific receptors on the cell membrane of adrenocortical cells and induces the production of steroids from cholesterol.

Use:
- Diagnosis of hypercortisolism (Cushing's syndrome) or hypoadrenocorticism (Addison's disease).
- See *BSAVA Manual of Canine and Feline Endocrinology* for advice on performance and interpretation of ACTH response test.
- In case of availability problems, supplies should be reserved for diagnosis of hypoadrenocorticism.
- The effect on cortisol production in cats is less dramatic than in dogs, so the same reference ranges cannot be used.

Safety and handling: Normal precautions should be observed. Small aliquots of the intravenous and intramuscular preparations may be frozen and thawed once without undue loss of activity.

Contraindications: No information available.

Adverse reactions: Intramuscular administration tends to produce a pain reaction so i.v. is preferred.

Drug interactions: None reported.

DOSES

Dogs: ACTH response test: 5 μg (micrograms)/kg i.v., i.m. The same doses may be used for the lyophilized product but must be administered i.m.

Cats: ACTH response test: 5 μg (micrograms)/kg or 125 μg/cat. i.v., i.m.

References
Arenas Bermejo C, Pérez Alenza D, García San José P *et al.* (2020) Laboratory assessment of trilostane treatment in dogs with pituitary-dependent hyperadrenocorticism. *Journal of Veterinary Internal Medicine* **34**, 1413–1422

L-Theanine (*N*-ethyl-L-glutamine, suntheanine, green tea leaf extract)
(Anxitane) **GSL**

Formulations: Oral: 50 mg, 100 mg tablets based on green tea extracts. Also included in some other formulations alongside other potentially calming nutraceuticals.

Action: Binds to AMPA, kainate, and *N*-methyl-D-aspartate receptors and blocks the binding of L-glutamic acid to the glutamate receptors in the cerebral cortex. This results in increases in brain serotonin, dopamine and GABA levels which, through diverse mechanisms, result in anxiolysis. May also have neuroprotective effects.

Use:
- Used to aid in the management of mild anxieties and fears, including social anxiety without aggression towards people in dogs.

Clinical evidence to date is largely based on open-label studies. Not intended for use in cases of severe phobia or separation anxiety, or aggressive behaviour.

Safety and handling: Normal precautions should be observed.

Contraindications: No information available.

Adverse reactions: No information available.

Drug interactions: No information available.

DOSES

Dogs, Cats: 5 mg/kg p.o. q12h for maintenance or q6h during event exposure.

References
Pike AL, Horwitz DF and Lobprise H (2015) An open-label prospective study of the use of L-theanine (Anxitane) in storm-sensitive client-owned dogs. *Journal of Veterinary Behavior* **10**, 324–331

Theophylline
(Corvental D[d]) **POM-V**

Formulations: Oral: 100 mg, 200 mg, 500 mg sustained-release capsules.

Action: Causes inhibition of phosphodiesterase, alteration of intracellular calcium, release of catecholamine, and antagonism of adenosine and prostaglandin, leading to bronchodilation and other effects. Spasmolytic agent with a mild diuretic action.

Use:
- Used in the treatment of small airway disease.
- Beneficial effects include bronchodilation, enhanced mucociliary clearance, stimulation of respiratory centre, increased sensitivity to $PaCO_2$, increased diaphragmatic contractility, stabilization of mast cells and a mild inotropic effect.

Theophylline has a low therapeutic index and should be dosed on a lean bodyweight basis. Administer with caution in patients with severe cardiac disease, gastric ulcers, hyperthyroidism, renal or hepatic disease, severe hypoxia or severe hypertension. Therapeutic plasma theophylline values are 5–20 µg (micrograms)/ml.

Safety and handling: Normal precautions should be observed.

Contraindications: Patients with a known history of arrhythmias or seizures.

Adverse reactions: Vomiting, diarrhoea, polydipsia, polyuria, reduced appetite, tachycardia, arrhythmias, nausea, twitching, restlessness, agitation, excitement and convulsions. Hyperaesthesia is seen in cats. Most adverse effects are related to the serum level and may be symptomatic of toxic serum concentrations. The severity of these effects may be decreased by the use of modified-release preparations. They are more likely with more frequent administration.

Drug interactions: Agents that may increase the serum levels of theophylline include cimetidine, diltiazem, erythromycin, fluoro-quinolones and allopurinol. Phenobarbital may decrease the serum concentration of theophylline. Theophylline may decrease the effects of pancuronium. Theophylline and beta-adrenergic blockers (e.g. propranolol) may antagonize each other's effects. Theophylline administration with halothane may cause an increased incidence of cardiac dysrhythmias, and with ketamine an increased incidence of seizures.

DOSES

Dogs: Bronchodilation: 20 mg/kg p.o. q24h or 10 mg/kg p.o. q12h which may be increased to 15 mg/kg p.o. q12h if no side effects on lower dose (**NB:** manufacturer only recommends q24h dosing). Some texts indicate q12h dosing of the sustained-release preparation is required to maintain therapeutic serum levels.

Cats: Bronchodilation: 15–19 mg/kg p.o. q24h (sustained-release preparation).

References
Bach JF, Kukanich B, Papich MG *et al.* (2004) Evaluation of the bioavailability and pharmacokinetics of two extended-release theophylline formulations in dogs. *Journal of the American Veterinary Medical Association* **224**, 1113–1119

Guenther-Yenke CL, McKiernan BC, Papich MG *et al.* (2007) Pharmacokinetics of an extended-release theophylline product in cats. *Journal of the American Veterinary Medical Association* **231**, 900–906

Thiamazole (Methimazole)

(Felimazole [c], Thiafeline [c], Thyronorm [c]) **POM-V**

Formulations: Oral: 1.25 mg, 2.5 mg, 5 mg tablets; 5 mg/ml solution. Also available as a transdermal formulation on a named patient basis.

Action: Interferes with thyroid hormone synthesis by inhibiting thyroid peroxidase. Has no effect on iodine uptake, peripheral de-iodination of thyroxine (T4) to triiodothyronine (T3) or release of stored hormone.

Use:
- Control of thyroid hormone levels in cats with hyperthyroidism.

2–3 weeks of treatment are generally needed to establish euthyroidism. Monitor therapy on the basis of serum thyroxine concentrations (4–6 hours after dosing) and adjust dose accordingly for long-term medical management. Assess haematology, biochemistry and serum total T4 after 3, 6, 10 and 20 weeks and thereafter every 3 months, adjusting dosage as necessary. Transdermal thiamazole gels are also used in hyperthyroid cats, particularly in fractious cats or in those that develop GI side effects from oral formulations. However, this route is not as reliable as oral medication or as safe for humans who apply the gel.

Safety and handling: Oral: normal precautions should be observed. Transdermal formulation: wear gloves when administering or handling the product. Do not touch area of application for at least 2 hours. Thiamazole is a human teratogen and crosses the placenta, concentrating in the fetal thyroid gland.

Contraindications: Do not use in pregnant or lactating queens.

Adverse reactions: Vomiting and inappetence/anorexia may be seen but are often transient. Jaundice, cytopenias, immune-mediated diseases (including myasthenia gravis) and dermatological changes (pruritus, alopecia and self-induced trauma) are reported, but rare; withdrawal of treatment may be necessary. Treatment of hyperthyroidism can decrease glomerular filtration rate, thereby increasing serum urea and creatinine values, and can occasionally unmask occult renal failure. Animals that have an adverse reaction to carbimazole are likely to also have an adverse reaction to thiamazole.

Drug interactions: Phenobarbital may reduce clinical efficacy. Benzimidazole drugs reduce hepatic oxidation and may lead to increased circulating drug concentrations. Thiamazole should be discontinued before iodine-131 treatment. Do not use with low-iodine prescription diets.

DOSES

Dogs: Hyperthyroidism: 2.5–5 mg/dog p.o. q12h depending on size.

Cats: Hyperthyroidism: 2.5 mg/cat p.o. q12h. Apply transdermal gel to pinna. The dose may need to be increased over time.

References

Daminet S, Kooistra HS, Fracassi F *et al.* (2014) Best practice for the pharmacological management of hyperthyroid cats with antithyroid drugs. *Journal of Small Animal Practice* **55**, 4–13

Thiamine see **Vitamin B1**

Thyroid-stimulating hormone
(Thyrotropin alfa, TSH)
(Thyrogen*) **POM**

Formulations: Injectable: 1.1 mg vial. After reconstitution with 1.2 ml sterile water, the TSH concentration is 0.9 mg/ml.

Action: Binds to specific receptors on thyroid follicular cell membranes and stimulates the proteolytic degradation of thyroglobulin and the release of thyroxine (T4) and smaller quantities of triiodothyronine (T3).

Use:
- Diagnosis of canine hypothyroidism (TSH stimulation test).

Not suitable for evaluation of thyroid function in patients receiving L-thyroxine. The diagnostic value in cats has not been fully assessed.

Safety and handling: Normal precautions should be observed.

Contraindications: Repeated administration is not advisable.

Adverse reactions: Chemical grade TSH may be associated with anaphylactic responses; do not use.

Drug interactions: Anabolic or androgenic steroids, carbimazole, barbiturates, corticosteroids, diazepam, heparin, mitotane (o, p'-DDD), phenylbutazone, phenytoin and salicylates may all decrease serum T4 levels. Fluorouracil, insulin, oestrogens, propranolol and prostaglandins may increase T4 levels. These drugs will make the TSH stimulation test hard to interpret.

DOSES

Dogs: TSH stimulation test: 50–150 µg (micrograms)/dog. A study using 75 µg/dog found high discriminatory power. Higher doses may be considered in dogs with comorbidities or those receiving thyroid-suppressing drugs. Blood sample for total T4 taken prior to, and 6 hr after, TSH administration.

Cats: TSH stimulation test: 25–50 µg (micrograms)/cat (sample timing as for dogs).

References
Campos M, van Hoek I, Peremans K et al. (2012) Recombinant human thyrotropin in veterinary medicine: current use and future perspectives. *Journal of Veterinary Internal Medicine* **26**, 853–862

Corsini A, Faroni E, Lunetta F and Fracassi F (2021) Recombinant human thyrotropin stimulation test in 114 dogs with suspected hypothyroidism: a cross-sectional study. *Journal of Small Animal Practice* **62**, 257–264

Wakeling J, Hall T and Williams TL (2020) Correlation of thyroid hormone measurements with thyroid stimulating hormone stimulation test results in radioiodine-treated cats. *Journal of Veterinary Internal Medicine* **34**, 2265–2275

L-**Thyroxine** (T4, Levothyroxine)
(Leventa[d], Soloxine[d], Thyforon[d]) **POM-V**

Formulations: Oral: 0.1 mg, 0.2 mg, 0.3 mg, 0.5 mg, 0.8 mg tablets; 1 mg/ml solution.

Action: Binds to specific intracellular receptors and alters gene expression.

Use:
• Treatment of hypothyroidism.

Cases with pre-existing cardiac disorders require lower initial doses.

Safety and handling: Normal precautions should be observed.

Contraindications: Uncorrected adrenal insufficiency.

Adverse reactions: Clinical signs of overdosage include tachycardia, excitability, nervousness and excessive panting. Can unmask Addison's disease in patients with autoimmune polyglandular syndrome.

Drug interactions: The actions of catecholamines and sympathomimetics are enhanced by thyroxine. Diabetic patients receiving thyroid hormones may have altered insulin requirements; monitor carefully during the initiation of therapy. Oestrogens may increase thyroid requirements by increasing thyroxine-binding globulin. The therapeutic effect of ciclosporin, digoxin and digitoxin may be reduced by thyroid hormones. Tachycardia and hypertension may develop when ketamine is given to patients receiving thyroid hormones. In addition, many drugs may affect thyroid function tests and therefore monitoring of therapy.

DOSES
See Appendix for conversion of bodyweight to body surface area.
Dogs, Cats: Hypothyroidism: 0.02–0.04 mg/kg/day. Dose given with food once, or divided twice, a day. Alternatively, dose at 0.5 mg/m² body surface area daily. Very few dogs will require greater than 1 mg q24h. Monitor serum T4 levels pre-dosing (trough) and 4–8 hours after dosing (peak).

References
Le Traon G, Brennan SF, Burgaud S et al. (2009) Clinical evaluation of a novel liquid formulation of l-thyroxine for once daily treatment of dogs with hypothyroidism. *Journal of Veterinary Internal Medicine* **23**, 43–49
Lewis VA, Morrow CMK, Jacobsen JA et al. (2018) A pivotal field study to support the registration of levothyroxine sodium tablets for canine hypothyroidism. *Journal of the American Animal Hospital Association* **54**, 201–208

Tigilanol tiglate
(Stelfonta[d]) **POM-V**

Formulations: Injectable: 1 mg/ml solution.

Action: Stimulates the action of protein kinase C enzymes involved in cell growth and survival, interrupting blood supply and resulting in cell death.

Use:
• For use in non-resectable, non-metastatic mast cell tumours.

If dermal, tumours can be located anywhere on the body; if subcutaneous they must be located at or below the elbow or hock. Tumours must be ≤8 cm³ in volume and must be accessible for intratumoural injection. Treatment causes a change in the tissue architecture, it is therefore unlikely that an accurate histological tumour grading can be obtained after treatment. The product must strictly be administered intratumorally, as other routes of injection are associated with adverse reactions. To reduce local and systemic adverse events, concomitant supportive therapies are advised, consisting of corticosteroids and H1 and H2 receptor blocking agents, both before and after treatment.

Safety and handling: The product is to be administered only by a veterinary surgeon. Personal protective equipment should be worn when handling the product and/or touching the site of injection. People with known hypersensitivity to tigilanol tiglate or to propylene glycol should avoid contact with the product. Irritant and potentially skin sensitizing. Accidental self-injection may result in severe local inflammatory reactions, including pain, swelling, redness and potential wound formation/necrosis, which may take several months to resolve. Caution is required during treatment to avoid self-injection. In case of accidental self-injection, seek medical advice immediately and show the package insert to the physician. Leakage of the product from the site of injection may occur directly after administration. In case of dermal or ocular exposure, repeatedly wash the exposed skin or eye with water. Owners should be informed of the special precautions to be taken at home. Store in a refrigerator (2–8°C).

Contraindications: Do not use in mast cell tumours with a broken surface. Do not administer the product directly into the surgical margins following the surgical removal of a tumour. The effect of this drug is restricted to the location of the injection; do not use in cases of metastatic disease. Treatment does not prevent the development of *de novo* mast cell tumours. Treating tumours in mucocutaneous locations (eyelids, vulva, preputial opening, anus, mouth) and at the extremities (e.g. paws, tail) could impair functionality due to the loss of tissue associated with the treatment. The product is an irritant; therefore, use of the product in the proximity of sensitive tissues, in particular the eye, should be avoided. Safety has not been established during pregnancy or lactation or in dogs <12 months.

Adverse reactions: The most common adverse events described are related to the mode of action at the tumour site: pain, injection site bruising, erythema, oedema, lameness in a treated limb and wound formation. Note that formation of wounds is a secondary intention when using this drug. Other potential adverse events include vomiting and tachycardia, enlargement of the draining lymph node, diarrhoea, anorexia, somnolence, weight loss, tachypnoea, lethargy, pyrexia, cystitis, reduced appetite, new neoplastic mass, personality/behaviour changes, seizures, pruritis, tremor and skin ulceration/other dermatological changes. Changes in clinical pathology parameters include anaemia, neutrophilia, increased band neutrophils, thrombocytopenia, increased alanine aminotransferase, gamma-glutamyl transferase and/or alkaline phosphatase activity, hypoalbuminemia, leucocytosis, monocytosis, increased bilirubin, blood urea nitrogen and triglyceride concentrations, increased creatine kinase activity, hyperkalaemia and proteinuria. Unintentional intravenous administration is expected to cause severe systemic effects.

Drug interactions: No information available.

DOSES

Dogs: Single dose of 0.5 ml Stelfonta per cm^3 of tumour volume determined on the day of dosing as 0.5 × (length (cm) × width (cm) × height (cm)) into the tumour, following initiation of concomitant treatments. Maximum dose is 0.15 ml/kg (corresponding to 0.15 mg tigilanol tiglate/kg), with no more than 4 ml administered per dog, regardless of the number of tumours treated, the tumour volume or the dog's weight. The minimum dose is 0.1 ml, regardless of the tumour volume or the dog's weight.

Cats: No information available.

References

De Ridder TR, Campbell JE, Burke-Schwarz C *et al.* (2021) Randomized controlled clinical study evaluating the efficacy and safety of intratumoral treatment of canine mast cell tumors with tigilanol tiglate (EBC-46). *Journal of Veterinary Internal Medicine* **35**, 415–429

Reddell PW, De Ridder TR, Morton JM *et al.* (2021) Wound formation, wound size and progression of wound healing after intratumoral treatment of mast cell tumors in dogs with tigilanol tiglate. *Journal of Veterinary Internal Medicine* **35**, 430–441

Tigolaner

(Felpreva^c) **POM-V**

Formulations: Topical: Spot-on (3 sizes) containing emodepside + praziquantel + tigolaner.

Action: A potent inhibitor of the neurotransmitter GABA receptor. It exhibits higher functional potency to block insect/acarine receptors compared with mammalian receptors.

Use:
- Tigolaner is active against fleas, ticks, *Notoedres cati* and *Otodectes cynotis*.

The other drugs have action against cestodes and nematodes.

Safety and handling: Children and pregnant people should avoid contact with the newly applied product.

Contraindications: Treatment of kittens <10 weeks or <1 kg is not recommended.

Adverse reactions: Irritation at the application site; avoid contact with eyes.

Drug interactions: No information available.

DOSES

See Appendix for guidelines on responsible parasiticide use.

Dogs: Not applicable.

Cats: 14.4 mg/kg, repeat after 12 weeks (fleas/ticks).

Tiletamine see Zolazepam/Tiletamine

Timolol maleate

(Azarga*, CoSopt*, Timolol*, Timoptol*) **POM**

Formulations: Ophthalmic: 0.25%, 0.5% solutions in 5 ml bottle, single-use vials (0.5% solution most commonly used); 1% brinzolamide + 0.5% timolol (Azarga); 2% dorzolamide + 0.5% timolol (CoSopt) (5 ml bottle, single-use vials).

Action: A topical non-selective beta-blocker that decreases aqueous humour production via beta-adrenoreceptor blockade in the ciliary body. **See also Brinzolamide and Dorzolamide**.

Use:
- Management of canine and feline glaucoma.

Can be used alone or in combination with other topical glaucoma drugs, such as a topical carbonic anhydrase inhibitor. Dorzolamide/timolol or brinzolamide/timolol can be used in the control of most types of glaucoma in dogs; the combination may be more effective than either drug alone. In cats, dorzolamide alone reaches maximal intraocular pressure lowering efficiency. Timolol causes miosis and may therefore not be the drug of choice in uveitis, anterior lens luxation or pupil block.

Safety and handling: Normal precautions should be observed.

Contraindications: Avoid in uncontrolled heart failure and asthma.

Adverse reactions: Ocular adverse effects include miosis, conjunctival hyperaemia and local irritation. Systemic absorption may occur following topical application causing bradycardia and reduced blood pressure.

Drug interactions: Additive adverse effects may develop if given concurrently with oral beta blockers. Prolonged AV conduction times may result if used with calcium antagonists or digoxin.

DOSES

Dogs: One drop per affected eye q8–12h.

Cats: One drop per affected eye q12h.

References

McLellan GJ and Miller PE (2011) Feline glaucoma – a comprehensive review. *Veterinary Ophthalmology* **14**, 15–29

Toceranib

CIL

(Palladia[d]) **POM-V**

Formulations: Oral: 10 mg, 15 mg, 50 mg film-coated tablets.

Action: Selective protein tyrosine kinase inhibitor with particular effects on the split kinase family, which may also have an effect on angiogenesis.

Use:
- Treatment of non-resectable Patnaik grade 2 or 3 recurrent cutaneous mast cell tumours.
- Many studies have now demonstrated variable efficacy in other canine malignancies, including mammary gland carcinomas, anal gland adenocarcinomas, thyroid acrcinomas, neuroendocrine tumours, gastrointestinal stromal tumours (GISTs), multiple myelomas, melanomas, other carcinomas and some sarcomas.

Studies are ongoing to evaluate the combination of toceranib and a number of other chemotherapeutics (vinblastine, cyclophosphamide, carboplatin, lomustine, piroxicam, prednisolone and calcitriol) and use alongside radiotherapy. Dogs should be monitored closely during treatment. As a guideline, blood pressure, urinalysis, haematology and biochemistry should be undertaken before starting therapy, and then at least once a month (some clinicians may also check these parameters 1–2 weeks after drug initiation), reducing to q3months if the patient is clinically stable and tolerating the drug well. Full coagulation profiles and faecal occult blood tests should be undertaken if adverse clinical signs are witnessed. It is good practice to contact owners once a week for the first 6 weeks of therapy to check for potential side effects, so that prompt action can be taken if these occur.

Safety and handling: Cytotoxic drug; see Appendix and specialist texts for further advice on chemotherapeutic agents.

Contraindications: Do not use in pregnant or lactating bitches, in dogs <2 years or <5 kg, if there are any signs of GI haemorrhage or if the patient has shown previous hypersensitivity to toceranib. Wait at least 3 days after stopping the drug before performing any surgery. Use with caution in dogs with pre-existing liver disease.

Adverse reactions: Weight loss, GI signs (diarrhoea, haemorrhage, anorexia, vomiting), lethargy, myelosuppression, lameness/musculoskeletal disorders, skin conditions such as depigmentation, dermatitis and pruritus. Can also cause anaemia, increased alanine aminotransferase activity, coagulation derangements (including pulmonary thromboembolism), decreased albumin and increased blood pressure. Uncommon events that may be related to toceranib administration include pancreatitis, seizures, epistaxis, circulatory shock and death.

Drug interactions: No information available, but use with caution when combining with chemotherapeutic agents and drugs that have the potential to cause GI toxicity (i.e. steroids, NSAIDs) until further information is available.

DOSES

See Appendix for chemotherapy protocols.

Dogs: All uses: 2.2–3.25 mg/kg p.o. q48h or on a Monday, Wednesday, Friday basis. A starting dose of 2.62–2.75 mg/kg is typically recommended.

Cats: 2.5 mg/kg (range 2–4 mg/kg) p.o. on a Monday, Wednesday, Friday basis or q48h (limited information).

References

London CA, Hannah AL, Zadovoskaya R et al. (2003) Phase I dose escalating study of SU11654, a small molecule receptor tyrosine kinase inhibitor, in dogs with spontaneous malignancies. *Clinical Cancer Research* **9**, 2755–2768

London CA, Malpas PB, Wood-Follis SL et al. (2009) Multi-center, placebo-controlled, double-blind, randomized study of oral toceranib phosphate (SU11654), a receptor tyrosine kinase inhibitor, for the treatment of dogs with recurrent (either local or distant) mast cell tumor following surgical excision. *Clinical Cancer Research* **15**, 3856–3865

Toldimphos see Phosphate

Toltrazuril

(Procox [d]) **POM-V**

Formulations: Oral: 18 mg/ml oral suspension with emodepside. Available on a named patient basis in the UK.

Action: Coccidiocidal at all stages of parasite development. It interferes with the enzymes needed to produce energy.

Use:
- Treatment of *Isospora* spp. It stops both the replication of the parasites and also the shedding of oocysts.
- Some efficacy against *Hepatozoon canis*.

Although treatment will reduce the spread of infection, it will not be effective against the clinical signs of infection in animals that are already infected. Not authorized for use in cats but appears to be effective.

Safety and handling: Normal precautions should be observed.

Contraindications: Do not use in animals <2 weeks or <0.4 kg.

Adverse reactions: Occasional mild diarrhoea and/or vomiting.

Drug interactions: None known but see emodepside.

DOSES
See Appendix for guidelines on responsible parasiticide use.

Dogs: 9 mg/kg p.o. once. Further treatment is only indicated if oocyst shedding persists. Higher doses (up to 20 mg/kg q24h for 2–3 days) have also been suggested.

Cats:
- **Coccidiosis:** 30 mg/kg q24h for 2–3 days.
- **Toxoplasmosis:** 5–10 mg/kg q24h for 7–14 days.

References
Altreuther G, Gasda N, Adler K *et al.* (2011) Field evaluations of the efficacy and safety of Emodepside plus toltrazuril (Procox® oral suspension for dogs) against naturally acquired nematode and *Isospora* spp. infections in dogs. *Parasitology Research* **109(S1)**, 21–28
Petry G, Kruedewagen E, Kampkoetter A *et al.* (2011) Efficacy of emodepside/toltrazuril suspension (Procox® oral suspension for dogs) against mixed experimental *Isospora felis/Isospora rivolta* infection in cats. *Parasitology Research* **109(S1)**, 29–36

Topiramate

(Topamax*, Topiramate*) **POM**

Formulations: Oral: 25 mg, 50 mg, 100 mg, 200 mg tablets; 15 mg, 25 mg, 50 mg sprinkle capsules; 15 mg, 25 mg, 50 mg capsules; 50 mg/5 ml, 100 mg/5 ml oral suspension.

Action: The exact antiepileptic mode of action is unknown, but several mechanisms of action include inhibition of voltage-dependent sodium and calcium channels and enhancement of GABA activity at $GABA_A$ receptors. Also inhibits carbonic anhydrase activity.

Use:
- As an adjunctive therapy in animals refractory to standard anticonvulsant therapies and where other adjunctive therapies have been unsuccessful.
- Its use has also been reported in animals with neuropathic pain, although alternative medications should be considered first.

- It has a short half-life (2–4 hours) in dogs but therapeutic activity may persist for longer.

Safety and handling: Normal precautions should be observed.

Contraindications: Avoid rapid withdrawal. Use with caution in patients with impaired hepatic or renal function.

Adverse reactions: Nausea, anorexia, sedation and ataxia.

Drug interactions: Use cautiously with other carbonic anhydrase inhibitors as topiramate also acts as a mild inhibitor. Enzyme induction increases topiramate clearance and an increase in dose is likely if used in conjunction with phenobarbitone.

DOSES
Dogs:
- **Anticonvulsant:** 2–20 mg/kg p.o. q8–12h. Start at lower end of dose range and adjust incrementally.
- **Neuropathic pain:** 10 mg/kg p.o. q8h.

Cats:
- **Anticonvulsant:** no clinical data but experimentally a single dose of 30 mg/kg p.o. has been described; anecdotally, 12.5–25 mg/cat q12h is suggested.
- **Feline idiopathic ulcerative dermatitis:** a single case report used 5 mg/kg p.o. q12h.

References
Kiviranta AM, Laitinen-Vapaavuori O, Hielm-Björkman A et al. (2013) Topiramate as an add-on antiepileptic drug in treating refractory canine idiopathic epilepsy. *Journal of Small Animal Practice* **54**, 512–520

Plessas IN, Volk HA, Rusbridge C et al. (2015) Comparison of gabapentin versus topiramate on clinically affected dogs with Chiari-like malformation and syringomyelia. *Veterinary Record* **177**, 288

Torasemide (Torsemide)
(UpCard[d]) **POM-V**

Formulations: Oral: 0.75 mg, 3 mg, 7.5 mg tablets (UpCard).

Action: Loop diuretic inhibiting the $Na^+/K^+/Cl^-$ co-transporter in the thick ascending limb of the loop of Henle. The net effect is a loss of sodium, potassium, chloride and water in the urine. Potassium excretion is less than with an equivalent dose of furosemide. Torasemide also increases excretion of calcium, magnesium and hydrogen, as well as renal blood flow and glomerular filtration rate. It has an antialdosteronergic effect, which is the result of dose-dependent inhibition of receptor-bound aldosterone. The diuretic effect of torasemide is equivalent to 20 times the effect of furosemide (mg for mg) using current veterinary authorized products (and only 10 times the effect of furosemide based on human generic torasemide products).

Use:
- Authorized to treat the clinical signs of CHF in dogs.

Compared with furosemide at an equivalent dose, torasemide has a higher bioavailability, a longer duration of action (12 hours with a peak effect of 2 hours in dogs and 4 hours in cats) and results in less kaliuresis and calciuresis. Dogs receiving torasemide for 14 days experienced less diuretic resistance and had greater increases in blood urea nitrogen compared with dogs receiving furosemide for 14 days. Long-term therapy should be aimed at lowest effective dose to control CHF signs. Torasemide has also been used to treat oedema associated with hepatic cirrhosis and renal failure in humans. Use with caution in patients with severe electrolyte depletion, hepatic failure, renal failure or diabetes mellitus. In contrast to furosemide, torasemide is not authorized for use in cats.

Safety and handling: Normal precautions should be observed.

Contraindications: Dehydration and anuria.

Adverse reactions: Hypokalaemia, hypochloraemia, hypocalcaemia, hypomagnesaemia, hyponatraemia, dehydration, polyuria/polydipsia and prerenal azotaemia occur readily. A marked reduction in cardiac output can occur in animals with diseases in which cardiac output is already impaired, such as severe pulmonary hypertension, low-output heart failure, hypertrophic cardiomyopathy, pericardial or myocardial disorders and cardiac tamponade. Other adverse effects reported in humans include ototoxicity, blurred vision, GI disturbances, leucopenia, anaemia, weakness and dermatological reactions.

Drug interactions: No information available.

DOSES

Dogs: 0.1–0.6 mg/kg p.o. q24h. Anecdotally, doses are calculated and then divided into q12h intervals. Most dogs will be stabilized at doses ≤0.3 mg/kg p.o. q24h. Dose should be titrated up/down in 0.1 mg/kg p.o. increments.

Cats: Replace furosemide p.o. with torasemide p.o. at a daily dose that is 1/20th of the total daily furosemide dose divided q12–24h.

References
Oyama MA, Peddle GD, Reynolds CA et al. (2011) Use of the loop diuretic torsemide in three dogs with advanced heart failure. *Journal of Veterinary Cardiology* **13**, 287–292
Peddle GD, Singletary GE, Reynolds CA et al. (2012) Effect of torsemide and furosemide on clinical, laboratory, radiographic and quality of life variables in dogs with heart failure secondary to mitral valve disease. *Journal of Veterinary Cardiology* **14**, 253–259

Tramadol

CIL

(Tralieve[d], Tramvetol[d], Tramadol ER*, Ultracet*, Ultram*, Zamadol*) **POM-V, POM CD SCHEDULE 3**

Formulations: Oral: 50 mg tablets; 100 mg, 200 mg, 300 mg immediate-release tablets; 20 mg, 80 mg chewable tablets for dogs; sustained-release tablets are also available in various tablet sizes; smaller tablet sizes (10 mg, 25 mg) are available from some veterinary wholesalers; 5 mg/ml oral liquid. **Injectable:** 50 mg/ml solution.

Action: Some metabolites of tramadol are agonists at all opioid receptors, particularly mu receptors. The parent compound also inhibits the reuptake of noradrenaline and 5-HT and stimulates pre-synaptic 5-HT release, which provides an alternative pathway for analgesia involving the descending inhibitory pathways within the spinal cord. In humans, good and poor metabolizers of tramadol are described, with good metabolizers developing more opioid-like effects following drug administration and improved analgesia. Whether similar individual differences in metabolism of tramadol occur in cats and dogs is currently unknown.

Use:

- Tablets are authorized for use in dogs for the management of mild acute and chronic soft tissue and musculoskeletal pain.
- Perioperatively, injectable tramadol is used instead of opioids to provide analgesia for acute pain.
- Injectable tramadol has also been administered epidurally in dogs but does not appear to confer advantages over systemic administration.

The recommended dose range is currently largely empirical due to a lack of combined pharmacokinetic and pharmacodynamic studies. Plasma concentrations of tramadol and metabolites were low after administration, suggesting that once a day dosing of sustained-release tramadol tablets is unsuitable to provide analgesia in dogs. A recent systematic review and meta-analysis of studies investigating tramadol for postoperative pain management in dogs found a low or very low certainty of evidence for efficacy of analgesia. The main reasons for downgrading the certainty of evidence were risk of bias and imprecision. Tramadol is attractive as an adjunct to manage chronic pain because it can be given orally; however, a larger body of evidence to support dose recommendations is needed and recent studies also show poor efficacy of tramadol to manage osteoarthritic pain. Cats seem to be more susceptible to the dysphoric effects of tramadol, although both dogs and cats can develop nausea and behavioural changes or sedation following repeated dosing. The oral preparations are unpalatable to cats and therefore difficult to administer, even when reformulated in gelatin capsules.

Safety and handling: Normal precautions should be observed.

Contraindications: No information available.

Adverse reactions: Sedation can occur after administration of high doses to dogs. Dysphoria is more likely in cats. Contraindicated in humans with epilepsy; owners should be informed that there may be a slightly increased risk of seizures in treated animals.

Drug interactions: Tramadol can be given in combination with other analgesic drugs such as NSAIDs, amantadine and gabapentin. It has the potential to interact with drugs that inhibit central 5-HT and noradrenaline reuptake, such as tricyclic antidepressants (e.g. amitriptyline), monoamine oxidase inhibitors (e.g. selegiline), selective serotonin reuptake inhibitors and some opioids (e.g. fentanyl, pethidine and buprenorphine), causing serotonin syndrome that can result in seizures and death. Should signs of serotonin syndrome develop (manifest in mild form as hyperthermia, elevated blood pressure and CNS disturbances such as hypervigilance and excitation), these must be managed symptomatically and contributing drug treatments stopped.

DOSES

Dogs: 2–5 mg/kg p.o. q8h, 2 mg/kg i.v.

Cats: 2–4 mg/kg p.o. q8h, 1–2 mg/kg i.v., s.c.

References

Donati P, Tarragona L, Franco J *et al.* (2021) Efficacy of tramadol for postoperative pain management in dogs: systematic review and meta-analysis. *Veterinary Anaesthesia and Analgesia* **48**, 283–296

Giorgi M, Saccomanni G, Lebkowska-Wieruszewska B *et al.* (2009) Pharmacokinetic evaluation of tramadol and its major metabolites after single oral sustained tablet administration in the dog: a pilot study. *Veterinary Journal* **180**, 253–255

Tranexamic acid

(Cyklokapron*) **POM**

`CIL`

Formulations: Injectable: 500 mg/5 ml solution for injection in ampoules. **Oral:** 500 mg tablets.

Action: Tranexamic acid is a synthetic lysine analogue that reversibly binds to the lysine binding sites of plasminogen. This prevents the action of plasmin on fibrin, thereby delaying fibrin dissolution and reducing bleeding. The interruption of fibrinolysis may be beneficial in patients with hyperfibrinolytic conditions and some forms of coagulopathy.

Use:
- To treat bleeding tendencies, particularly if hyperfibrinolysis is believed to be a major contributor to the bleeding.
- The use of tranexamic acid has been suggested as an adjunct treatment in dogs with angiostrongylosis, splenic haemangiosarcoma and trauma.

Safety and handling: Normal precautions should be observed.

Contraindications: Animals with a history of, or at increased risk of, thrombosis (e.g. thromboembolism) should not be treated with tranexamic acid. Disorders involving renal parenchyma resulting in haematuria are a contraindication to tranexamic acid use in humans; use in this setting should be considered carefully.

Adverse reactions: The most common adverse reactions reported in dogs are nausea, vomiting and diarrhoea and these clinical signs appear to be dose-dependent. In dogs and cats, retinal changes have been reported with prolonged treatment at higher doses. Anaphylaxis is also described. Hypersensitivities, dizziness, visual disturbances and thromboses have been reported in humans.

Drug interactions: No studies of interactions between tranexamic acid and other drugs have been conducted. Potential interactions leading to myocardial infarction could occur with coadministration of hormonal contraceptives, hydrochlorothiazide, desmopressin, sulbactam-ampicillin, ranitidine or glyceryl trinitrate.

DOSES

Dogs: 15–20 mg/kg p.o. q8h; 10 mg/kg slow i.v. q8h.

Cats: Limited safety or efficacy data published in this species; a dose of 10–15 mg/kg slow i.v. has been described.

References

Fletcher DJ, Rozanski EA, Brainard BM *et al.* (2016) Assessment of the relationships among coagulopathy, hyperfibrinolysis, plasma lactate, and protein C in dogs with spontaneous hemoperitoneum. *Journal Veterinary Emergency and Critical Care* **26**, 41–51

Kelley M, Sinnott-Stutzman V and Whelan M (2022) Retrospective analysis of the use of tranexamic acid in critically ill dogs and cats (2018–2019): 266 dogs and 28 cats. *Journal of Veterinary Emergency and Critical Care (San Antonio)* **32**, 791–799

Kelmer E, Segev G, Papashvilli V *et al.* (2015) Effects of intravenous administration of tranexamic acid on haematological, hemostatic, and thromboelastographic analytes in healthy adult dogs. *Journal Veterinary Emergency and Critical Care* **25**, 495–501

Travoprost

CIL

(Travatan*) **POM**

Formulations: Ophthalmic: 40 μg (micrograms)/ml (0.004%) solution in 2.5 ml bottle.

Action: Agonist for receptors specific for prostaglandin F. Reduces intraocular pressure by increasing uveoscleral outflow and may have a profound effect on intraocular pressure in the dog.

Use:
- Its main indication is in the management of primary canine glaucoma and it is useful in the emergency management of acute primary glaucoma. Often used in conjunction with other topical antiglaucoma drugs such as carbonic anhydrase inhibitors.
- May be useful in the management of lens subluxation and posterior luxation despite being contraindicated in anterior lens luxation.

Travoprost has comparable activity to latanoprost. There is little published data on its use in the cat; the effect of latanoprost is variable.

Safety and handling: Normal precautions should be observed.

Contraindications: Uveitis and anterior lens luxation. Avoid in pregnant animals.

Adverse reactions: Miosis in dogs; conjunctival hyperaemia and mild irritation may develop. Increased iridal pigmentation has been noted in humans but not in dogs.

Drug interactions: Do not use in conjunction with thiomersal-containing preparations.

DOSES

Dogs: 1 drop per eye once daily (evening) or q8–12h.
Cats: No information available.

Trazodone

CIL

(Desyrel*, Molipaxin*, Oleptro*, Trazodone*) **POM**

Formulations: Oral: 50 mg, 100 mg, 150 mg tablets/capsules; 10 mg/ml liquid.

Action: Trazodone is an atypical antidepressant with mixed serotonergic agonistic (5HT1A) and antagonistic actions (other 5HT receptor sites).

Use:
- Chronic anxiety-related problems in dogs that are unresponsive to other pharmacological interventions. Should be used in conjunction with a behaviour modification plan. Use with caution and carefully monitor patients with renal disease. Less risk in patients with cardiac disease than tricyclic antidepressants such as amitriptyline.
- Reduction of anxiety associated with hospitalization, including postoperative confinement in dogs.
- In cats, may be used for the management of short-term anxiety-related problems, e.g. travel or examination anxiety.

Safety and handling: Normal precautions should be observed.

Contraindications: Glaucoma, history of seizures or urinary retention and severe liver disease.

Adverse reactions: Sedation, vomiting, excitability and dry mouth. Third eyelid protrusion described in some cats.

Drug interactions: Should not be used with monoamine oxidase inhibitors (MAOIs) or drugs metabolized by cytochrome P450 2D6 (e.g. chlorphenamine, cimetidine). There is a risk of serotonin syndrome if combined with other serotonergic substances, but adjunctive therapy is sometimes used (see below). Ketoconazole will inhibit the breakdown of trazodone, leading to increased blood levels, while carbamazepine will have the opposite effect; itraconazole may be similar, although there is no clinical evidence of this.

DOSES
Dogs:
- **Short-term anxiety associated with hospitalization:** 4 mg/kg p.o. q12h titrated upwards to 10–12 mg/kg as needed to a maximum of 300 mg per dose.
- **Chronic anxiety issues:** initial dose for 5–10 kg, 25 mg p.o. q24h; 11–20 kg, 50 mg p.o. q24h; >21 kg, 100 mg p.o. q24h. Doses may be titrated upwards every 10–14 days to a maximum of double the recommended initial dose. Doses for dogs >40 kg may be titrated to a maximum of 300 mg p.o. q24h. Dose may need to be increased if used long term as tolerance over time is common. Lower end doses may be used adjunctively with selective serotonin reuptake inhibitors (e.g. fluoxetine) but not MAOIs, but the risk of serotonin syndrome should be recognized.

Cats: 50–100 mg/cat p.o. q24h; 50 mg/cat administered 1 hour before travel to address transport and examination-related anxiety. For short-term use only.

References
Gruen ME and Sherman BL (2008) Use of trazodone as an adjunctive agent in the treatment of canine anxiety disorders: 56 cases (1995–2007). *Journal of the American Veterinary Medical Association* **233**, 1902–1907
Stevens BJ, Frantz EM, Orlando JM *et al.* (2016). Efficacy of a single dose of trazodone hydrochloride given to cats prior to veterinary visits to reduce signs of transport- and examination-related anxiety. *Journal of the American Veterinary Medical Association* **249**, 202–207

Tretinoin see Vitamin A

Triamcinolone
(Dermanolon [c,d], Recicort [c,d], Kenalog*) **POM**

Formulations: Injectable: 40 mg/ml suspension for deep i.m., intra-articular or intralesional use. **Topical:** 1.77 mg/ml triamcinolone + 17.7 mg/ml salicylic acid solution.

Action: Intermediate-acting glucocorticoid with approximately 1.25 times the anti-inflammatory potency of prednisolone and negligible mineralocorticoid activity.

Use:
- Used topically for otitis externa and for seborrhoeic dermatitis in dogs and cats.
- Adjunctive therapy in the management of strictures (rectal, nasal, oesophageal and others) via intralesional injection.

- Intra-articular injection for treatment of inflammatory arthritides (controversial).
- Treatment of mast cell tumours.

Safety and handling: Normal precautions should be observed. Avoid direct skin contact with products.

Contraindications: Do not use in pregnant animals. Systemic corticosteroids are generally contraindicated in patients with renal disease and diabetes mellitus.

Adverse reactions: Prolonged use of glucocorticoids suppresses the hypothalamic–pituitary–adrenal axis and causes adrenal atrophy. Catabolic effects of glucocorticoids lead to weight loss and cutaneous atrophy. Iatrogenic hypercortisolism may develop with chronic use. Vomiting and diarrhoea may be seen in some patients. GI ulceration may develop. Glucocorticoids may increase urine glucose levels and decrease serum triiodothyronine (T3) and thyroxine (T4) values. Impaired wound healing and delayed recovery from infections may be seen.

Drug interactions: There is an increased risk of GI ulceration if systemic glucocorticoids are used concurrently with NSAIDs. Hypokalaemia may develop if potassium-depleting diuretics (e.g. furosemide, thiazides) are administered with corticosteroids. Insulin requirements may increase in patients taking glucocorticoids. Metabolism of corticosteroids may be enhanced by phenobarbital or phenytoin and decreased by antifungals (e.g. itraconazole).

DOSES
Dogs:
- **Intralesional (e.g. stricture):** 1.2–1.8 mg (total dose) injected intralesionally. Maximum 0.6 mg at any one site; separate injections by 0.5–2.5 cm.
- **Mast cell tumours:** 1 mg per cm of tumour (longest dimension) injected intralesionally.
- **Topical:** 8–10 drops in affected ear q12–24h for a maximum of 14 days. Do not exceed 7 drops per kg total daily dose.
- **Intra-articular:** 1–3 mg per joint (higher doses described by Alves *et al.*, 2021).
- **Systemic anti-inflammatory:** 0.1–0.2 mg/kg i.m., effective for 3–4 weeks.

Cats:
- **Systemic, intralesional:** as for dogs.
- **Intra-articular:** 1–3 mg per joint.

References
Alves JC, Santos A, Jorge P, Lavrador C and Carreira LM (2021) The intra-articular administration of triamcinolone hexacetonide in the treatment of osteoarthritis. Its effects in a naturally occurring canine osteoarthritis model. *PLoS One* **16**, e0245553
Case A and Burgess K (2018) Safety and efficacy of intralesional triamcinolone administration for treatment of mast cell tumors in dogs: 23 cases (2005–2011). *Journal of the American Veterinary Medical Association* **252**, 84–91

L-Tri-iodothyronine see Liothyronine

Trilostane

(Vetoryl[d]) **POM-V**

Formulations: Oral: 10 mg, 30 mg, 60 mg, 120 mg capsules. 5 mg capsules and a liquid formulation are available on a named patient basis. **VSP**

Action: Blocks adrenal synthesis of glucocorticoids by competitively and reversibly inhibiting the adrenocortical enzyme 3-beta-hydroxy-steroid dehydrogenase. Effects on mineralocorticoids are relatively minor.

Use:

- Treatment of canine ACTH-dependent and -independent hypercortisolism.
- Treatment of feline hypercortisolism.
- Canine alopecia X syndrome.

Twice-daily dosing is advocated if clinical signs persist despite an increased dose, when 'escape' polydipsia occurs, or in patients with concurrent diabetes mellitus. Treatment in dogs should be monitored after 10 days, 4 weeks, 12 weeks and then every 3–4 months using a combination of clinical signs ± pre-pill cortisol measurement (aim for pre-pill cortisol of 40–140 nmol/l) or an ACTH response test (start test 3 hours post-dosing, aim for a post-ACTH cortisol of 40–120 nmol/l). Monitor treatment in cats with ACTH response tests. Dosage adjustments may be necessary even after prolonged periods of stability. Trilostane should be given with food as absorption is poor on an empty stomach.

Safety and handling: Normal precautions should be observed. People who are or may become pregnant should not handle this drug.

Contraindications: Do not use in pregnant animals or those with renal or hepatic insufficiency.

Adverse reactions: Reported adverse effects in dogs include vomiting, diarrhoea, lethargy and a reduced appetite. Mild increases in serum potassium, bilirubin and calcium may be seen. Iatrogenic hypoadrenocorticism and adrenal necrosis have been reported and may cause collapse or a hypoadrenocortical crisis. Adrenal hyperplasia may occur with prolonged treatment (clinical significance unknown). Prolonged adrenal suppression after drug withdrawal has been noted.

Drug interactions: Trilostane should not be administered concurrently with other drugs that suppress adrenal function, e.g. mitotane, itraconazole. May have additive aldosterone lowering effects if used with ACE inhibitors. May potentiate hyperkalaemia if used with potassium-sparing diuretics.

DOSES

Dogs: Hypercortisolism: 2 mg/kg p.o. q24h or 1 mg/kg p.o. q12h.

Cats: Hypercortisolism: 10–30 mg/cat p.o. q12–24h.

References

García San José P, Arenas Bermejo C, Alonso-Miguel D et al. (2022) Survival of dogs with pituitary-dependent hyperadrenocorticism treated twice daily with low doses of trilostane. *Veterinary Record* **191**, e1630

Lemetayer J and Blois S (2018) Update on the use of trilostane in dogs. *The Canadian Veterinary Journal* **59**, 397–407

Mellett Keith A, Bruyette D and Stanley S (2013) Trilostane therapy for treatment of spontaneous hyperadrenocorticism in cats: 15 cases (2004–2012). *Journal of Veterinary Internal Medicine* **27**, 1471–1477

Trimethoprim/Sulphonamide
(Potentiated sulphonamides)

(Duphatrim c,d, Norodine c,d, Trimacare, Trimedoxine d, Septrin*) **POM-V, POM**

Formulations: Trimethoprim and sulphonamide are formulated in a ratio of 1:5. **Injectable:** 40 mg/ml trimethoprim + 200 mg/ml sulfadiazine (240 mg/ml total) solution. **Oral:** trimethoprim and sulfadiazine in a variety of tablet sizes designated by the amount of trimethoprim (e.g. 20 mg, 80 mg); 40 mg trimethoprim/5 ml + 200 mg sulfamethoxazole/5 ml paediatric suspension (48 mg/ml); 80 mg trimethoprim + 400 mg sulfamethoxazole tablets. If availability of veterinary formulations is limited, POM products or veterinary specials may be used on a named patient basis. **VSP**

Action: Trimethoprim and sulphonamides block sequential steps in the synthesis of tetrahydrofolate, a cofactor required for the synthesis of many molecules, including nucleic acids. The two-step mechanism ensures that bacterial resistance develops more slowly than to either agent alone. Time-dependent mechanism of action.

Use:
- Many organisms are susceptible, including *Nocardia*, *Brucella*, Gram-negative bacilli, some Gram-positive organisms (*Streptococcus*), plus *Pneumocystis carinii*, *Toxoplasma gondii* and other coccidians. *Pseudomonas* and *Leptospira* are usually resistant.
- Trimethoprim/sulphonamide is useful in the management of urinary, respiratory tract and prostatic infections, but ineffective in the presence of necrotic tissue.
- Trimethoprim alone may be used for urinary, prostatic, systemic salmonellosis and respiratory tract infections (fewer adverse effects anticipated).

Trimethoprim is a weak base which becomes ion-trapped in fluids that are more acidic than plasma (e.g. prostatic fluid and milk). Ensure patients receiving sulphonamides are well hydrated and are not receiving urinary acidifying agents.

Safety and handling: Normal precautions should be observed.

Contraindications: Avoid use in animals with keratoconjunctivitis sicca (KCS) or previous history of adverse reaction to sulphonamides, such as KCS or polyarthritis.

Adverse reactions: Drowsiness, anorexia, leucopenia, anaemia and hypersalivation may be seen in cats. Hepatic necrosis, vomiting, immune-mediated thrombocytopenia and immune-mediated polyarthritis may be seen in dogs. Dobermanns seem to be more susceptible to the development of immune-mediated systemic adverse effects. Acute hypersensitivity reactions are possible with sulphonamide products and may manifest as type III hypersensitivity reactions. Sulphonamides may reversibly suppress thyroid function. KCS has been reported in dogs treated with sulfapyridine and other sulphonamides. Monitor tear production particularly during long-term use and in breeds susceptible to KCS.

Drug interactions: Antacids may decrease the bioavailability of sulphonamides if administered concomitantly. Urinary acidifying agents will increase the tendency for sulphonamide crystals to form within the urinary tract. Concomitant use of drugs containing procaine may inhibit the action of sulphonamides since procaine is a precursor for para-amino benzoic acid.

DOSES

Classified as category D (Prudence) by the EMA.

See Appendix for guidelines on responsible antibiotic use.

Doses of total product (trimethoprim + sulphonamide).

Dogs, Cats: 15–30 mg/kg p.o. q12h; 30 mg/kg s.c. q24h.

References

Weese JS, Blondeau J, Boothe D *et al.* (2019) International Society for Companion Animal Infectious Diseases (ISCAID) guidelines for the diagnosis and management of bacterial urinary tract infections in dogs and cats. *The Veterinary Journal* **247**, 8–25

Yaemsiri S and Sykes J (2018) Successful treatment of disseminated nocardiosis caused by nocardia veterana in a dog. *Journal of Veterinary Internal Medicine* **32**, 418–422

Tropicamide

(Mydriacyl*, Tropicamide*) **POM**

Formulations: Ophthalmic: 0.5%, 1% solution (single-use vials), 1% (5 ml bottle).

Action: Synthetic, short acting anticholinergic. Inhibits acetylcholine at the iris sphincter and ciliary body muscles, causing mydriasis and cycloplegia (paralysis of the ciliary muscle).

Use:
- For mydriasis and cycloplegia.
- Mydriatic of choice for intraocular examination due to its rapid onset (20–30 minutes) and short duration of action (2–12 hours in dogs, 4–9 hours in cats).

Tropicamide is more effective as a mydriatic than as a cycloplegic and is therefore less effective than atropine in relieving ciliary body muscle spasm associated with uveitis. Use with care in patients with lens luxation.

Safety and handling: Normal precautions should be observed.

Contraindications: Avoid in glaucoma.

Adverse reactions: May cause salivation in cats, but less marked than with atropine.

Drug interactions: No information available.

DOSES

Dogs, Cats: 1 drop per eye, repeat after 20–30 min if necessary.

Tylosin

(Bilosin, Tylan, Tyluvet) **POM-V**

Formulations: Injectable: 200 mg/ml solutions (Bilosin, Tylan, Tyluvet). Oral: 100 g/bottle soluble powder (Tylan); 50 mg, 100 mg tablets (veterinary special). **VSP**

Action: A time-dependent macrolide antibiotic that binds to the 50S ribosomal subunit, suppressing bacterial protein synthesis.

Use:
- Tylosin has good activity against mycoplasmas and has the same antibacterial spectrum of activity as erythromycin but is generally less active against bacteria.
- It has been used for the treatment of antibiotic-responsive diarrhoea in dogs and for cryptosporidiosis. However, antibiotics are rarely indicated in the treatment of acute or chronic diarrhoea.

Administration is predominantly by the oral route in dogs and cats.

Safety and handling: Normal precautions should be observed.

Contraindications: No information available.

Adverse reactions: GI disturbances. The activity of tylosin is enhanced in an alkaline pH. Tylosin can cause pain at the site of injection.

Drug interactions: Not well documented in small animals. It does not appear to inhibit the same hepatic enzymes as erythromycin.

DOSES
 Classified as category C (Caution) by the EMA.
See Appendix for guidelines on responsible antibiotic use.
Dogs:
- **Various doses:** 7–15 mg/kg p.o. q12–24h.
- **In colitis:** 12–20 mg/kg q8h with food, gradually increase the dosing interval to q24h.

Cats: 7–15 mg/kg p.o. q12–24h.

References
Westermarck E, Frias R and Skrzypczak T (2005) Effect of diet and tylosin on chronic diarrhoea in Beagles. *Journal of Veterinary Internal Medicine* **19**, 822–827
Westermarck E, Skrzypczak T, Harmoinen J *et al.* (2005) Tylosin-responsive chronic diarrhoea in dogs. *Journal of Veterinary Internal Medicine* **19**, 177–186

Ursodeoxycholic acid (UDCA) `CIL`

(Cholurso*, Destolit*, Ursodeoxycholic acid*, Ursofalk*, Ursogal*) **POM**

Formulations: Oral: 150 mg, 250 mg, 300 mg, 500 mg tablets; 250 mg capsules; 50 mg/ml suspension.

Action: A relatively hydrophilic bile acid used for its choleretic, hepatoprotectant and immunomodulatory properties. It inhibits ileal absorption of hydrophobic bile acids, thereby reducing their concentration in the body pool; hydrophobic bile acids are toxic to hepatobiliary cell membranes and may potentiate cholestasis. It also has an immunomodulatory effect, and may modify apoptosis of hepatocytes. Ursodeoxycholic acid also acts as an antioxidant to prevent mitochondrial oxidative stress.

Use:
- Adjunctive therapy for patients with a variety of liver diseases, particularly where cholestasis is present.

The administration of UDCA does not alter the bile acid stimulation test of normal healthy dogs, but a small but significant increase has been demonstrated in both the pre- and postprandial bile acids in healthy cats.

Safety and handling: Normal precautions should be observed.

Contraindications: Avoid in patients with complete biliary obstruction due to the possibility of increased bile flow leading to rupture. May be contraindicated in cats with hepatic lipidosis.

Adverse reactions: Safety has not been demonstrated in dogs or cats but side effects appear to be rare. Diarrhoea is the more frequently reported adverse effect in human patients. Some human patients have an inability to sulphate lithocholic acid (a natural metabolite of UDCA), which is a known hepatotoxin; the veterinary significance of this is unclear. Ursofalk and ursodiol suspensions (commercial or compounded) contain xylitol as an excipient, so care should be used when administering to dogs and cats.

Drug interactions: Aluminium-containing antacids may bind to UDCA, thereby reducing its efficacy. UDCA can increase the absorption of ciclosporin, leading to raised serum levels.

DOSES

Dogs, Cats: 10–15 mg/kg p.o. q24h or divided daily.

References

Day DG, Meyer DJ, Johnson SE *et al.* (1994) Evaluation of total serum bile-acids concentration and bile-acid profiles in healthy cats after oral administration of ursodeoxycholic acid. *American Journal of Veterinary Research* **55**, 1474–1478

Deitz KL, Makielski KM, Williams JM *et al.* (2015) Effect of 6–8 weeks of oral ursodeoxycholic acid administration on serum concentrations of fasting and postprandial bile acids and biochemical analytes in healthy dogs. *Veterinary Clinical Pathology* **44**, 431–436

Vecuronium

(Norcuron*) **POM**

Formulations: Injectable: 10 mg powder for reconstitution.

Action: Inhibits the actions of acetylcholine at the neuromuscular junction by binding competitively to the alpha subunit of the nicotinic acetylcholine receptor on the postjunctional membrane.

Use:

- Provision of neuromuscular blockade during anaesthesia.
- To improve surgical access through muscle relaxation, to facilitate positive pressure ventilation or for intraocular surgery.

Intermediate dose-dependent duration of action of approximately 20 minutes. Has no cardiovascular effects and does not cause histamine release. Monitoring (using a nerve stimulator) and reversal of the neuromuscular blockade are recommended to ensure complete recovery before the end of anaesthesia. Hypothermia, acidosis and hypokalaemia will prolong the duration of neuromuscular blockade. In healthy animals, repeated doses are relatively non-cumulative and it can be given by i.v. infusion to maintain neuromuscular blockade. It is metabolized by the liver; therefore, in animals with liver dysfunction atracurium is advised rather than vecuronium. The duration of action of vecuronium is shorter in diabetic dogs compared with non-diabetic animals, although the underlying reasons for this difference are unclear. This may be clinically relevant when using vecuronium to provide neuromuscular blockade in diabetic dogs undergoing ocular surgery. Sugammadex, a cyclodextrin developed to reverse neuromuscular blockade induced by rocuronium, can also be used to reverse neuromuscular blockade caused by vecuronium in dogs at a dose of 8 mg/kg i.v.

Safety and handling: Unstable in solution and so is presented as a freeze-dried powder. The prepared solution can be diluted further if required.

Contraindications: Do not administer unless the animal is adequately anaesthetized and facilities to provide positive pressure ventilation are available.

Adverse reactions: No information available.

Drug interactions: Neuromuscular blockade is more prolonged when vecuronium is given in combination with volatile anaesthetics, aminoglycosides, clindamycin and lincomycin.

DOSES

Dogs, Cats: 0.1 mg/kg initially produces neuromuscular blockade for 25–30 min. The block can be maintained by increments of 0.03 mg/kg or a CRI of 0.1–0.2 mg/kg/h. Lower loading doses of 0.05 mg/kg i.v. produce neuromuscular blockade of shorter duration (16–19 min).

References

Clark L, Leece E and Brearley J (2012) Diabetic mellitus affects the duration of vecuronium in dogs. *Veterinary Anaesthesia and Analgesia* **39**, 472–479

Mosing M, Auer U, West E *et al.* (2012) Reversal of profound rocuronium or vecuronium induced neuromuscular block with sugammadex in isoflurane anaesthetised dogs. *The Veterinary Journal* **192**, 467–471

Verapamil

CIL

(Securon*, Verapamil*) **POM**

Formulations: Injectable: 2.5 mg/ml solution. **Oral:** 40 mg, 80 mg, 120 mg, 160 mg tablets; 40 mg/5 ml oral solution.

Action: Inhibits inward movement of calcium ions through slow (L-type) calcium channels in myocardial cells, cardiac conduction tissue and vascular smooth muscle. Verapamil causes a reduction in myocardial contractility (negative inotrope), depressed electrical activity (slows AV conduction) and vasodilation (cardiac vessels and peripheral arteries and arterioles).

Use:

- Primarily used to control supraventricular tachyarrhythmias, such as accessory pathway-mediated supraventricular tachycardia, atrial tachycardia and flutter.

Verapamil is a second-choice calcium channel blocker behind diltiazem as it has a more pronounced negative inotropic effect. Patients with severe hepatic disease may have a reduced ability to metabolize the drug; reduce the dose by 70%.

Safety and handling: Normal precautions should be observed.

Contraindications: Do not use in patients with 2nd or 3rd degree AV block, hypotension, sick sinus syndrome, left ventricular dysfunction or heart failure.

Adverse reactions: Can cause hypotension, bradycardia, dizziness, precipitation or exacerbation of CHF, nausea, constipation and fatigue in humans.

Drug interactions: Do not use concurrently with beta blockers. Both drugs have a negative inotropic and chronotropic effect and the combined effect can be profound. Co-administration with sodium channel blockers may also lead to cardiovascular depression and hypotension. Verapamil activity may be adversely affected by vitamin D or calcium salts. Cimetidine may increase the effects of verapamil. Verapamil may increase the blood levels of digoxin, digitoxin or theophylline, leading to potentially toxic effects from these drugs. Calcium-channel blockers may increase intracellular vincristine. The neuromuscular blocking effects of non-depolarizing muscle relaxants may be enhanced by verapamil.

DOSES

Dogs: 0.5–3 mg/kg p.o. q8h or 0.05 mg/kg slowly i.v. over 5 minutes (with ECG monitoring). Up to 4 repeat i.v. administrations at a reduced dose of 0.025 mg/kg q5min if necessary.

Cats: 0.5–1 mg/kg p.o. q8h or 0.025 mg/kg slowly i.v. over 5 minutes (with ECG monitoring). Up to 3 repeat i.v. administrations q5min if necessary.

Vinblastine

(Velbe*, Vinblastine*) **POM**

Formulations: Injectable: 1 mg/ml solution.

Action: Interferes with microtubule assembly, causing metaphase arrest and ultimately resulting in cell death.

Use:
- Vinblastine is used less frequently than vincristine for treatment of lymphoproliferative disorders
- Used with prednisolone for treatment of canine mast cell tumours.
- Treatment of bladder transitional carcinomas.

Use with care in patients with abnormal liver function; dose reduction recommended. Potentially a neurotoxic substrate of P-glycoprotein, use with caution in herding breeds (e.g. collies) that may have the *ABCB1* gene mutation that causes a non-functional glycoprotein. Drug is locally irritant and must be administered i.v. through a carefully pre-placed catheter.

Safety and handling: Cytotoxic drug; see Appendix and specialist texts for further advice on chemotherapeutic agents. Store under refrigeration.

Contraindications: Bone marrow suppression, a dose reduction is recommended in patients with liver dysfunction.

Adverse reactions: Main dose-limiting toxicity is myelosuppression with neutropenia. Mucositis, stomatitis, ileus, jaw/muscle pain, loss of deep tendon reflexes and GI tract toxicity may also occur. At higher doses, vinblastine can cause neurotoxicity similar to vincristine. Cats may develop neurotoxicity manifesting as constipation and/or ileus.

Drug interactions: Any drugs that inhibit metabolism via hepatic cytochrome P450 system (CYPs) may reduce metabolism and thus increase toxicity of vinblastine, e.g. calcium-channel blockers, cimetidine, ciclosporin, erythromycin, metoclopramide and itraconazole. Drugs that are inhibitors of P-glycoprotein (ciclosporin, verapamil, phenothiazines and itraconazole) may increase the toxicity.

DOSES

See Appendix for chemotherapy protocols and conversion of bodyweight to body surface area.

Dogs: All uses: 1.5–3 mg/m^2 q7–14d, depending on the protocol used.

Cats: Doses of 1.5 mg/m^2 are described as part of a COP regime.

References

Arnold EJ, Childress MO, Fourez LM *et al.* (2011) Clinical trial of vinblastine in dogs with transitional cell carcinoma of the urinary bladder. *Journal of Veterinary Internal Medicine* **25**, 1385–1390

Thamm DH, Turek MM and Vail DM (2006) Outcome and prognostic factors following adjuvant prednisone/vinblastine chemotherapy for high-risk canine mast cell tumour: 61 cases. *Journal of Veterinary Medicine and Science* **68**, 581–587

Vincristine

(Oncovin*, Vincristine*) **POM**

Formulations: Injectable: 1 mg, 2 mg, 5 mg vials.

Action: Interferes with microtubule assembly, causing metaphase arrest and ultimately resulting in cell death. Vincristine can also induce thrombocytosis through an unknown mechanism.

Use:
- With other neoplastic agents in the treatment of canine and feline neoplastic diseases, particularly lymphoproliferative disorders.
- Management of immune-mediated thrombocytopenia to stimulate release of platelets.
- Treatment of transmissible venereal tumour.

Use with caution in patients with hepatic disease, leucopenia, infection, or pre-existing neuromuscular disease. Potentially a neurotoxic substrate of P-glycoprotein, use with caution in herding breeds (e.g. collies) that may have the *ABCB1* gene mutation that causes a non-functional glycoprotein. Solution is locally irritant and must be administered i.v. through a carefully pre-placed catheter.

Safety and handling: Cytotoxic drug; see Appendix and specialist texts for further advice on chemotherapeutic agents. Store under refrigeration.

Contraindications: Pre-exisiting myelosuppression (unless this is a result of the disease under treatment).

Adverse reactions: Include peripheral neuropathy, ileus, GI tract toxicity/constipation and severe local irritation if administered perivascularly. Potentially myelosuppressive.

Drug interactions: Concurrent administration of vincristine with drugs that inhibit cytochromes of the CYP3A family may result in decreased metabolism of vincristine and increased toxicity. If used in combination with asparaginase, vincristine should be given 24 hours before the enzyme to reduce the risk of additive neurotoxicity and myelosuppression.

DOSES

See Appendix for chemotherapy protocols and conversion of bodyweight to body surface area.

Dogs, Cats:
- **Transmissible venereal tumours:** 0.5 mg/m^2 (up to a maximum dose of 1 mg) i.v. q7d for 4–6 weeks.
- **Other neoplastic diseases:** usual doses are 0.5–0.75 mg/m^2 i.v. every 1–3 weeks, dependent upon protocol used.
- **To increase circulating platelet numbers:** 0.02 mg/kg i.v. once (limited reports of the use of vincristine to raise circulating platelet numbers in cats, in three reported cases it provided minimal or no improvement to platelet count).

References

Nakamura RK, Tompkins E, Bianco D (2012) Therapeutic options for immune-mediated thrombocytopenia. *Journal of Veterinary Emergency and Critical Care* **22**, 59–72
Northrup NC, Rassnick KM, Snyder LA et al. (2002) Neutropenia associated with vincristine and L-asparaginase induction chemotherapy for canine lymphoma. *Journal of Veterinary Internal Medicine* **16**, 570–575

Vinorelbine
(Navelbine*) **POM**

Formulations: Injectable: 10 mg, 50 mg vials (usually 10 mg/ml).

Action: Vinorelbine is a semisynthetic derivative of the vinca alkaloid vinblastine. Its main mechanism of action is through the disruption of the structure and function of cellular mitotic spindles.

Use:
• Various malignant neoplasias, including pulmonary carcinoma, histiocytic sarcoma, urothelial cell carcinoma, mast cell tumour, lymphoma and melanoma.

Safety and handling: Cytotoxic drug; see Appendix and specialist texts for further advice on chemotherapeutic agents. Store under refrigeration.

Contraindications: Pre-existing myelosuppression or known previous allergic reaction.

Adverse reactions: The most commonly reported adverse event in dogs is neutropenia (myelosuppression), but other potential adverse events include thrombocytopenia and GI toxicity (inappetence, vomiting and/or diarrhoea). Adverse events described in humans include fatigue, alopecia, mild to moderate peripheral neuropathy, jaw pain, myalgia, arthralgia, haemorrhagic cystitis, thrombophlebitis or moderate tissue necrosis, and inappropriate arginine vasopressin secretion.

Drug interactions: Unknown. Do not use with other myelosuppressive agents.

DOSES
See Appendix for chemotherapy protocols and conversion of bodyweight to body surface area.

Dogs: 10–20 mg/m^2 (most commonly 12–15 mg/m^2 as a starting dose) i.v. as a bolus q1–2wk, depending on tolerance. The dose to be administered should be diluted with sterile 0.9% NaCl; the treatment should be given through a cleanly placed i.v. catheter over approximately 5 minutes.

Cats: 11.5 mg/m^2 i.v. has been recommended as the starting dose in cats (minimal information).

References
Poirier VJ, Burgess KE, Adams WM and Vail DM (2004) Toxicity, dosage, and efficacy of vinorelbine (Navelbine) in dogs with spontaneous neoplasia. *Journal of Veterinary Internal Medicine* **18**, 536–539

Wouda RM, Miller ME, Chon E and Stein TJ (2015) Clinical effects of vinorelbine administration in the management of various malignant tumor types in dogs: 58 cases (1997–2012). *Journal of the American Veterinary Medical Association* **246**, 1230–1237

Vitamin A (Retinol, Isotretinoin, Tretinoin)
(Isotrex*, Isotrexin*, Roaccutane*) **POM**

Formulations: Injectable: vitamin A (retinol) 50,000 IU/ml. **Oral:** 10 mg, 20 mg isotretinoin capsules. **Topical:** 0.05% isotretinoin gel.

Action: An essential nutrient that influences growth, reproduction, epithelial health and gene expression of structural proteins and hormones.

Use:
- Prevention or treatment of hypovitaminosis A.
- Also used in conjunction with other appropriate therapies for sebaceous adenitis, vitamin A responsive dermatosis, primary seborrhoea and other keratinization dirorders.

Animals receiving oral dosing should be monitored for vitamin A toxicity. Avoid concurrent use of oral and topical preparations because of toxicity. Avoid using formulations of vitamins A, D3 and E that are authorized for farm animals or horses as they are too concentrated for small animal use.

Safety and handling: Vitamin A is teratogenic; gloves should be worn when applying topical preparations. Avoid contact with eyes, mouth or mucous membranes. Minimize exposure of the drug to sunlight.

Contraindications: Do not use in pregnant animals.

Adverse reactions: Many adverse effects are reported in humans following the use of oral isotretinoin, predominantly involving the skin, haematological parameters, hepatotoxicity, nervous system and bone changes. Similar abnormalities are reported in dogs and cats receiving high doses. Teratogenic if administered in the first trimester or at high doses. Redness and skin pigmentation may be seen after several days. It changes the lipid content of tears, which can result in kerato-conjunctivitis sicca. It may also cause hyperlipidaemia and can be hepatotoxic at high doses. Prolonged use of vitamin A can promote loss of calcium from bone and lead to hypercalcaemia. Do not use topical preparations simultaneously with other topical drugs.

Drug interactions: Numerous, depending on preparation and route given. Consult specialist texts before using with another drug. Oral vitamin A may alter ciclosporin levels, which should therefore be monitored closely.

DOSES
Dogs:
- **Hypovitaminosis A:** 10,000–100,000 IU/dog i.m. q3d, no more than 2 doses; 10,000 IU/dog p.o. q24h for 3 days.
- **Dermatological lesions:** 10,000 IU/dog p.o. q24h or apply isotretinoin/tretinoin gel/cream to clean skin q12h; 1 mg isotretinoin/kg p.o. q12h for 1 month, reducing the dosage to 1 mg/kg p.o. q24h if improvement is seen.

Cats: Hypovitaminosis A: 10,000–100,000 IU/cat i.m. q3d, no more than 2 doses; 10,000 IU/cat p.o. q24h for 3 days.

References
Lam AT, Affolter VK, Outerbridge CA *et al.* (2011) Oral vitamin A as an adjunct treatment for canine sebaceous adenitis. *Veterinary Dermatology* **22**, 305–311

Vitamin B complex
(Anivit 4BC, Duphafral, Duphafral Extravite, Multivitamin injection, Vitamin B tablets) **POM-VPS, general sale**

Formulations: Various preparations containing varying quantities of vitamins are available, authorized for farm animals only. Most are for parenteral use and all those are POM-VPS.

Action: Cofactors for enzymes of intermediary metabolism and biosynthesis.

Use:
- Multiple deficiencies of B vitamins may occur in patients with renal or hepatic disease or significant anorexia.

Parenteral administration of B vitamins is not a substitute for nutritional support. Dosages and routes vary with individual products. Check manufacturer's recommendations prior to use. Most products are intended for large animal use and some may contain vitamin C and other vitamins or minerals.

Safety and handling: All B vitamins are photosensitive and must be protected from light once reconstituted. Multidose vials require aseptic technique for repeated use.

Contraindications: No information available.

Adverse reactions: Anaphylaxis may be seen when used i.v. and products should be given slowly and/or diluted with i.v. fluids. Use of large animal products which also contain fat-soluble vitamins (A, D, E, K) may lead to toxicity.

Drug interactions: None reported.

DOSES
Dogs: 1 ml/dog (dogs up to 15 kg), 2–4 ml/dog (dogs >15 kg) s.c., i.m., i.v. q24h.
Cats: 1 ml/cat s.c., i.m., i.v. q24h or as required.

Vitamin B1 (Thiamine)
(Vitamin B1) **POM-V, general sale**

Formulations: Injectable: 100 mg/ml solution (authorized for veterinary use, although only in farm animals). **Oral:** various.

Action: Cofactor for enzymes in carbohydrate metabolism, it forms a compound with adenosine triphosphate to form thiamine diphosphate/thiamine pyrophosphate employed in carbohydrate metabolism. Does not affect blood glucose.

Use:
- Thiamine supplementation is required in deficient animals.
- Thiamine may be beneficial in alleviating signs of lead poisoning and ethylene glycol intoxication.

Although uncommon, deficiency may occur in animals fed raw fish diets or uncooked soy products.

Safety and handling: Protect from air and light; multidose vials require aseptic technique for repeated use.

Contraindications: Do not use in pregnant animals unless absolutely necessary.

Adverse reactions: Anaphylaxis can be seen with i.v. use; dilute with fluids and/or give slowly if using i.v. Adverse effects in pregnant animals are documented.

Drug interactions: There are no specific clinical interactions reported, although thiamine may enhance the activity of neuromuscular blocking agents.

DOSES
Dogs:
- **Vitamin B1 deficiency:** 50–250 mg/dog i.m., s.c., p.o. q12–24h for several days until signs resolve.
- **Lead poisoning:** 2 mg/kg i.m., s.c. q12h.
- **Ethylene glycol intoxication:** 100 mg/dog i.m., s.c., p.o. q24h.

Cats:
- **Vitamin B1 deficiency:** 10–25 mg/cat i.m., s.c. q12–24h for several days until signs resolve or 10–20 mg/kg i.m. until signs resolve then 10 rng/kg p.o. for 21 days.
- **Refeeding syndrome:** 25 mg/cat i.m., s.c. q24h until neurological signs resolve.

Vitamin B3 see **Nicotinamide**

Vitamin B12 (Cyanocobalamin, Hydroxocobalamin)

(Anivit B12 250 and 1000, Cobalaplex, Cobalin, Cyanocobalamin PXN-B12, Neo-Cytamen (hydroxocobalamin), Vitbee 250 and 1000) **POM-VPS**

Formulations: Injectable: 0.25 mg/ml, 1 mg/ml solutions. Oral: 0.5 mg capsules (Cyanocobalamin); 0.5 mg vitamin B12 + 0.2 mg vitamin B9 capsules (Cobalin).

Action: Essential cofactor in metabolic processes involving growth, cell reproduction, haematopoiesis and myelin synthesis.

Use:
- Used to treat cobalamin (vitamin B12) deficiency. Such a deficiency may develop in patients with a familial cobalamin deficiency, significant malabsorptive disease of the distal ileum or exocrine pancreatic insufficiency.

Safety and handling: Injectable preparations must be protected from light.

Contraindications: Do not give i.v.

Adverse reactions: Hypersensitivity to the phenol preservative in the injectable solutions can occur; animals should be monitored after injections for rash, fever and urticaria.

Drug interactions: None reported.

DOSES
Dogs:
- **Injectable:** 0.02 mg/kg s.c., i.m. q7d for 4–6 weeks until the seru~~m~~ concentration normalizes. Then as required to maintain normal serum levels.
- **Oral:** <10 kg: ½ capsule per day or 1 capsule every other day 10–20 kg: 1 capsule per day; >20 kg: 2 capsules per day. Th~~e~~ of capsules can be increased or decreased as needed to ~~maintain~~ normal cobalamin.

Cats:
- **Injectable:** 0.02 mg/kg s.c., i.m. q7d for approximatel~~y~~

the serum concentration normalizes. Then as required to maintain normal serum levels.

- **Oral:** <10 kg: ½ capsule per day or 1 capsule every other day The number of capsules can be increased or decreased as needed to maintain normal cobalamin.

References

Toresson L, Steiner JM, Olmedal G et al. (2017) Oral cobalamin supplementation in cats with hypocobalaminaemia: a retrospective study. *Journal of Feline Medicine and Surgery* **19**, 1302–1306

Toresson L, Steiner JM, Suchodolski JS and Spillmann T (2016) Oral cobalamin supplementation in dogs with chronic enteropathies and hypocobalaminemia. *Journal of Veterinary Internal Medicine* **30**, 101–107

Vitamin D (1,25-dihydroxycholecalciferol (active vitamin D3), cholecalciferol (vitamin D3))

(Alfacalcidol*, Calcijex*, Calcitriol*, One-alpha*, Rocaltrol*)
POM-VPS, POM

Formulations: Oral: 2 µg (micrograms)/ml solution (Alfacalcidol, One-alpha), 0.25–1 µg capsules (Alfacalcidol, One-alpha), 0.25 µg capsules (Calcitriol, Rocaltrol). **Injectable:** 1 µg/ml solution (Calcitriol, Calcijex). Vitamin D is a general term used to describe a range of hormones that influence calcium and phosphorus metabolism, including vitamin D2 (ergocalciferol or calciferol), vitamin D3 (cholecalciferol), dihydrotachysterol, alfacalcidol and calcitriol (1,25-dihydroxycholecalciferol, the active form of vitamin D3). These different drugs have differing rates of onset and durations of action.

Action: In conjunction with other hormones (calcitonin and parathyroid hormone), regulates calcium homeostasis through numerous complex mechanisms, including accretion of calcium to bone stores and absorption of calcium from dietary sources.

Use:

- Chronic management of hypocalcaemia when associated with low parathyroid hormone concentrations which are most commonly associated with immune-mediated hypoparathyroidism and iatrogenic hypoparathyroidism following thyroidectomy.
- Calcitriol has also been used in the management of renal secondary hyperparathyroidism; in this circumstance it reduces serum parathyroid hormone concentrations.

Calcitriol and alfacalcidol (1-alpha-hydroxycholecalciferol) have a rapid onset of action (1–2 days) and a short half-life (<1 day), they are the preferred forms for use. Vitamin D2 (ergocalciferol) has a very slow onset of action and has limited use in dogs and cats. Vitamin D requires hydroxylations (one in the liver and the other in the kidney) to become active. Thus, only the active form (calcitriol) should be used in animals with renal failure. Vitamin D has a very narrow therapeutic index and toxic doses are easily achieved. Serum calcium and preferably ionized calcium concentrations need to be monitored closely and adjusted. Avoid using formulations of vitamins A, D3 and E that are intended for farm animals as they are too concentrated for small animal use.

Safe handling: Normal precautions should be observed.

Contraindications: Do not use in patients with hyperphosphataemia or malabsorption syndromes. Do not use in pregnant animals.

Adverse reactions: Hypercalcaemia, hyperphosphataemia.

Drug interactions: Corticosteroids may negate the effect of vitamin D preparations. Sucralfate decreases absorption of vitamin D. Drugs that induce hepatic enzyme systems (e.g. barbiturates) will increase the metabolism of vitamin D and lower its effective dose. Magnesium- or calcium-containing antacids may cause hypermagnesaemia or hypercalcaemia when used with vitamin D. Thiazide diuretics may also cause hypercalcaemia with concurrent use. Hypercalcaemia may potentiate the toxic effects of verapamil or digoxin; monitor carefully.

DOSES
Dogs:
- **Hypocalcaemia/vitamin D deficiency:** calcitriol: 10–15 ng (nanograms)/kg p.o. q12h for 3–4 days then decrease to 2.5–7.5 ng/kg p.o. q12h for maintenance; alfacalcidol: 0.01–0.03 µg (micrograms)/kg p.o. q24h and thereafter titrated to effect.
- **Renal secondary hyperparathyroidism:** calcitriol: 1.5–3.5 ng/kg p.o. q24h; some authors recommend higher doses of up to 6 ng/kg/day if there is refractory hyperparathyroidism and ionized serum calcium concentrations can be assessed. Assess serum calcium and phosphate levels serially and maintain total calcium × phosphate product below 4.2 (calcium and phosphate in mmol/l); do not use if this is not possible.

Cats:
- **Hypocalcaemia:** calcitriol: 10–15 ng (nanograms)/kg/day p.o. q12h for 3–4 days, then decrease to 2.5–7.5 ng/kg p.o. q12h for maintenance; alfacalcidol: 0.01–0.03 µg (micrograms)/kg p.o. q24h and thereafter titrated to effect.
- **Renal secondary hyperparathyroidism:** calcitriol 2.5–3.5 ng/kg/day p.o.

Vitamin E (Alpha tocopheryl acetate)
(Vitamin E suspension*) **POM-VPS**

Formulations: Oral: 20 mg/ml, 100 mg/ml suspension. Several oral preparations for humans and injectable preparations for other veterinary species, some of which also contain selenium, are available. Various nutraceuticals, often also containing SAMe, are available.

Action: Lipid-soluble antioxidant that protects cell membranes and structures from lipid peroxidation, protects red blood cells against haemolysis and protects low-density lipoproteins from oxidation. Inhibits platelet adhesion and aggregation. Affects expression and activities of enzymes in immune and inflammatory cells.

Use:
- Patients with exocrine pancreatic insufficiency and other severe malabsorptive diseases may be at risk of developing deficiency.
- Vitamin E has been used as an antioxidant in dogs with liver disease, especially in patients with copper-associated hepatitis.
- Its use has been suggested for numerous conditions, including discoid lupus, demodicosis and hepatic diseases including fibrosis.

These are, however, only anecdotal suggestions and there may be some significant risks.

Vitamin E supplementation is very rarely required in small animals. Avoid using formulations of vitamins A, D3 and E that are authorized for farm animals as they are too concentrated for small animal use.

Safety and handling: Normal precautions should be observed.

Contraindications: Do not use in patients at high risk for thrombosis. Do not use in neonates.

Adverse reactions: Thrombosis. Anaphylactoid reactions have been reported.

Drug interactions: Vitamin E may enhance vitamin A absorption, utilization and storage. Vitamin E may alter ciclosporin pharmacokinetics and, if used concurrently, ciclosporin therapy should be monitored by checking levels.

DOSES
Dogs: 1.6–8.3 mg/kg p.o. q24h for the first 30 days, then as needed; alternatively, 100–400 IU/dog.
Cats: 1.6–8.3 mg/kg p.o. for the first 30 days, then as needed; alternatively, 30 IU/cat.

Vitamin K1 (Phytomenadione) `CIL`

(Vitamine K1 Laboratoire TVM[d], Konakion*, Phytomenadione*) **POM-V, NFA-VPS, POM**

Formulations: Injectable: 10 mg/ml. Oral: 50 mg tablets. Some nutraceuticals also contain small amounts of vitamin K.

Action: Involved in the formation of active coagulation factors II, VII, IX and X by the liver.

Use:
- Treatment of toxicity due to coumarin and its derivatives.
- Before performing a liver biopsy in patients (primarily cats) with prolonged coagulation times.

Deficient states may also occur in prolonged significant anorexia. Although vitamin K is fat-soluble, its biological behaviour is like that of a water-soluble vitamin; it has a relatively short half-life and there are no significant storage pools. It may still require 6–12 hours for effect. Oral absorption is increased 4–5-fold in dogs if given with tinned food, especially food with increased fat content. Prothrombin time is the best method of monitoring therapy. Use a small gauge needle when injecting s.c. or i.m. in a patient with bleeding tendencies.

Safety and handling: Normal precautions should be observed.

Contraindications: Avoid giving i.v. if possible. For animals with active haemorrhage, p.o. administration is preferred over i.m., i.m., or s.c. routes due to risk of haematoma formation with injections.

Adverse reactions: Anaphylactic reactions have been reported following i.v. administration. Safety not documented in pregnant animals. Haemolytic anaemia occurs in cats when overdosed.

Drug interactions: Many drugs will antagonize the effects of vitamin K, including aspirin, chloramphenicol, allopurinol, diazoxide, cimetidine, metronidazole, erythromycin, itraconazole, propranolol and thyroid drugs as well as coumarin-based anticoagulants. If the animal is receiving other long-term medications it is advisable to check specific literature. The absorption of oral vitamin K is reduced by mineral oil.

DOSES

Dogs, Cats:

*   **Known 1st generation coumarin toxicity or vitamin K1 deficiency:** initially 2.5 mg/kg s.c. in several sites, then 1–2.5 mg/kg in divided doses p.o. q8–12h for 5–7 days. Recheck prothrombin time (PT) 48 hours after last dose. Restart therapy for another week if PT is still prolonged. If not prolonged, therapy can be discontinued. The patient's activity should be restricted for 1 week following full course of treatment.
*   **Known 2nd generation coumarin (brodifacoum) toxicity:** initially 5 mg/kg s.c. in several sites, then 2.5 mg/kg p.o. q12h for 3 weeks (due to longer persistence in body), then re-evaluate PT 48 hours after last dose. Restart therapy for another week if PT is still prolonged. If not prolonged, therapy can be discontinued. The patient's activity should be restricted for 1 week following full course of treatment.
*   **Known inandione (diphacinone) or unknown anticoagulant toxicity:** initially 2.5–5 mg/kg s.c. over several sites, then 2.5 mg/kg p.o. divided q8–12h for 3–4 weeks. Re-evaluate coagulation status 48 hours after last dose. If PT is prolonged, continue therapy for 2 additional weeks. If not prolonged, therapy can be discontinued. The patient's activity should be restricted for 1 week following full course of treatment.
*   **Before performing a liver biopsy, particulary in cats:** 0.5–1.5 mg/kg s.c. q12h. After 24–48 hours, re-evaluate coagulation times and if normal proceed with biopsy. If not, the dose should be increased and the procedure delayed. If there is further minimal improvement in coagulation times, fresh frozen plasma may be required.

References
Kavanagh C, Shaw S and Webster CR (2011) Coagulation in hepatobiliary disease. *Journal of Veterinary Emergency and Critical Care* **21**, 589–604

Xylazine

(Chanazine [c,d], Nerfasin [c,d], Rompun [c,d], Sedaxylan [c,d], Virbaxyl, Xylacare [c,d], Xylapan [c,d]) **POM-V**

Formulations: Injectable: 20 mg/ml solution.

Action: Agonist at peripheral and central alpha-2 adrenoreceptors, producing dose-dependent sedation, muscle relaxation and analgesia.

Use:

- Authorized to provide sedation and premedication when used alone or in combination with opioid analgesics.
- Xylazine combined with ketamine is used to provide a short duration (20–30 min) of surgical anaesthesia.
- Xylazine stimulates growth hormone production and may be used to assess the ability of the pituitary gland to produce this hormone (xylazine stimulation test). Consult specialist texts for protocol.
- Has been used to induce self-limiting emesis in cats where vomiting is desirable (e.g. following the ingestion of toxic, non-caustic foreign material). Emesis generally occurs rapidly within a maximum of 10 min. Further doses depress the vomiting centre and may not result in any further vomiting.

Has been largely superseded by medetomidine or dexmedetomidine and is no longer recommended for sedation. Xylazine causes significant alpha-1 adrenoreceptor effects and is less specific for the alpha-2 adrenoreceptor than are medetomidine and dexmedetomidine. This lack of specificity is likely to be associated with the poorer safety profile of xylazine compared with medetomidine and dexmedetomidine. Xylazine also sensitizes the myocardium to catecholamine arrhythmias, which increases the risk of cardiovascular complications. Xylazine is a potent drug that causes marked changes in the cardiovascular system. Spontaneous arousal from deep sedation following stimulation can occur with all alpha-2 agonists; aggressive animals sedated with xylazine must still be managed with caution.

Safety and handling: Normal precautions should be observed.

Contraindications: Do not use in animals with cardiovascular or other systemic disease. Use of xylazine in geriatric patients is also not advisable. It causes increased uterine motility and should not be used in pregnant animals, nor in animals likely to require or receiving sympathomimetic amines. Due to effects on blood glucose, use in diabetic animals is not recommended. Avoid when vomiting is contraindicated (e.g. foreign body, raised intraocular pressure). Induction of emesis is contraindicated if a strong acid or alkali has been ingested, due to the risk of further damage to the oesophagus. Induction of vomiting is contraindicated if the dog or cat is unconscious, fitting or has a reduced cough reflex, or if the poison has been ingested for >2 hours or if the ingesta contains paraffin, petroleum products or other oily or volatile organic products, due to the risk of inhalation.

Adverse reactions: Xylazine has diverse effects on many organ systems as well as the cardiovascular system. It causes a diuresis by suppressing arginine vasopressin secretion, a transient increase in blood glucose by decreasing endogenous insulin secretion, mydriasis and decreased intraocular pressure. Vomiting after xylazine is common, especially in cats.

Drug interactions: When used for premedication, xylazine will significantly reduce the dose of all other anaesthetic agents required to maintain anaesthesia. Atipamezole is not authorized as a reversal agent for xylazine, but it is effective and can be used to reverse the effects of xylazine if an overdose is given.

DOSES
When used for sedation is generally given as part of a combination. See Appendix for sedation protocols in cats and dogs.

Dogs: Growth hormone response test: 100 μg (micrograms)/kg i.v.

Cats:
- Emesis: 0.6 mg/kg i.m. or 1 mg/kg s.c. once (effective in >75% of cats).
- Growth hormone suppression test: 100 μg (micrograms)/kg i.v.

References
Kolahian S and Jarolmasjed S (2010) Effects of metoclopramide on emesis in cats sedated with xylazine hydrochloride. *Journal of Feline Medicine and Surgery* **12**, 899–903

Zidovudine (Azidothymidine, AZT)

(Azidothymidine*, Retrovir*) **POM**

Formulations: Oral: 100 mg, 250 mg capsules; 50 mg/5 ml syrup. Injectable: 10 mg/ml solution.

Action: Competitive inhibition of reverse transcriptase. Requires activation to the 5'-triphosphate form by cellular kinases.

Use:
- Treatment of feline immunodeficiency virus (FIV)-positive cats:
- Relief of severe stomatitis and FIV-related neurological signs
- In cats not showing clinical signs, it may delay the onset of the clinical phase.

Haematological monitoring is recommended weekly for first month then monthly.

Safety and handling: Normal precautions should be observed.

Contraindications: Animals that are severely anaemic or leucopenic should not be given this drug.

Adverse reactions: Severe non-regenerative anaemia can occur rapidly with high doses. Long-term adverse effects of lower doses have not been ascertained.

Drug interactions: NSAIDs may delay zidovudine metabolism, increasing the risk of nephrotoxicity or neutropenia.

DOSES

Dogs: Not applicable.

Cats: 5 mg/kg daily p.o., s.c. q12h.
- The dose may be increased to 10 mg/kg q12h but incurs increased risk of non-regenerative anaemia.

References

Hartmann K (2015) Efficacy of antiviral chemotherapy for retrovirus-infected cats: what does the current literature tell us? *Journal of Feline Medicine and Surgery* **17**, 925–939
Little S, Levy J, Hartmann K et al. (2020) AAFP Feline Retrovirus Testing and Management Guidelines. *Journal of Feline Medicine and Surgery* **22**, 5–30

Zinc salts

(Various trade names*) **POM, P, general sale**

Formulations: Oral: various zinc sulphate, zinc gluconate, zinc acetate, zinc methionine and chelated zinc preparations.

Action: Primarily involved in DNA and RNA synthesis, although also involved in essential fatty acid synthesis, white blood cell function and numerous reactions in intermediary metabolism. When administered orally, can reduce GI absorption and hepatic uptake of copper.

Use:
- Treatment of zinc-responsive dermatoses.
- Reduction of copper in dogs with copper-associated hepatitis.

Bioavailability of elemental zinc varies depending on formulation. The amount of elemental zinc based on zinc contribution to molecular weight is: zinc acetate 30%; zinc sulphate 23%; zinc methionine 21%; zinc gluconate 14.3%. Higher bioavailability is also associated with improved tolerance. Zinc gluconate is associated with fewer GI side effects. Concurrent supplementation with essential fatty acids is advised for the treatment of skin disorders.

Safety and handling: Normal precautions should be observed.

Contraindications: Copper deficiency.

Adverse reactions: Nausea, vomiting and occasional diarrhoea. Haemolysis may occur with large doses or serum levels >10 mg/ml, particularly if a coexistent copper deficiency exists.

Drug interactions: Significant interactions with other divalent heavy metals such as iron and copper can occur and long-term administration of zinc may lead to decreased hepatic copper or iron stores and functional deficiency. Penicillamine and ursodeoxycholic acid may potentially inhibit zinc absorption; the clinical significance is unclear. Zinc salts may chelate oral tetracycline and reduce its absorption; separate doses by at least 2 hours. Zinc salts may reduce the absorption of fluoroquinolone antibiotics.

DOSES
Dogs:
- **Zinc-responsive dermatosis:** 2–3 mg/kg of elemental zinc p.o. q24h.
- **Management of copper-associated hepatitis:** 5–10 mg/kg of elemental zinc p.o. q12h.

Give with food to minimize vomiting. The amount of zinc-containing supplement to administer depends on the amount of elemental zinc in the supplement. To calculate the amount of zinc-containing supplement to administer:
- **Calculate the patient's dose of elemental zinc:** Multiply the mg/kg dosage of elemental zinc by the patient's bodyweight.
- **Calculate the amount of elemental zinc in the preparation:** Multiply the supplement's amount of zinc salt by the percentage of elemental zinc.

Cats: Not applicable.

References
Dirksen K and Fieten H (2017) Canine copper-associated hepatitis. *Veterinary Clinics of North America: Small Animal Practice* **47**, 631–644
White SD, Bourdeau P, Rosychuk RA *et al.* (2001) Zinc-responsive dermatosis in dogs: 41 cases and literature review. *Veterinary Dermatology* **12**, 101–119

Zolazepam/Tiletamine
(Zoletil [c,d]) **POM-V**

Formulations: Injectable: when reconstituted contains 50 mg/ml zolazepam + 50 mg/ml tiletamine (i.e. 100 mg/ml).

Action: Zolazepam (like diazepam) enhances the activity of GABA, which is the major inhibitory neurotransmitter within the CNS. Tiletamine (like ketamine) antagonizes glutamic acid receptors.

Use:
- Used for general anaesthesia in dogs and cats.

Zolazepam (like diazepam) has a sedative, anxiolytic and muscle-relaxing action. Tiletamine generates a so-called dissociative anaesthesia because it depresses certain cerebral regions such as the thalamus and the cortex while other regions, in particular the limbic system, remain active. The duration of anaesthesia is 20–60 minutes depending on dose. The combined product should not be used as a sole anaesthetic agent for painful operations. For these operations, the product should be combined with an appropriate analgesic. Following anaesthesia, return to normal is progressive and can take 2–6 hours in a calm environment (avoid excessive noise and light). Recovery may be delayed in obese, old or debilitated animals. Remove any antiparasitic collar 24 hours before anaesthesia. Excessive salivation can occur after administration; this can be controlled by the administration of an anticholinergic. Muscle rigidity during recovery is common. Higher doses are more likely to be associated with a prolonged and excitable recovery in dogs. Premedication has been shown to increase the smoothness of recovery after tiletamine/zolazepam. Recovery from anaesthesia after tiletamine/zolazepam is more prolonged in cats than in dogs.

Safety and handling: Normal precautions apply. People who are or may become pregnant should not handle this drug. Store the reconstituted product in the fridge at 4°C and use within 8 days.

Contraindications: Do not use in animals with severe cardiac, respiratory or hypertensive disease, renal, pancreatic or hepatic insufficiency, head trauma or intracranial tumours. The product crosses the placenta and may cause respiratory depression that can be fatal for puppies and kittens.

Adverse reactions: Injection may sometimes cause pain in cats.

Drug interactions: Premedication with phenothiazine tranquilizers (e.g. acepromazine) can cause increased cardiorespiratory depression and an increased hypothermic effect that occurs in the last phase of anaesthesia. Do not use medications containing chloramphenicol during the pre- or intraoperative period, as this slows down elimination of the anaesthetics.

DOSES

Dogs: 5–10 mg/kg i.v.; 7–25 mg/kg i.m., depending on the degree of pain expected and the depth of anaesthesia required. Dose refers to the tiletamine/zolazepam combination (100 mg/ml when properly reconstituted).

Cats: 5–7.5 mg/kg i.v.; 10–15 mg/kg i.m., depending on the degree of pain expected and the depth of anaesthesia required. Dose refers to the tiletamine/zolazepam combination (100 mg/ml when properly reconstituted).

Zoledronate (Zoledronic acid)

(Zometa*) **POM**

Formulations: Injectable: 4 mg/100 ml solution as either a readymade formulation or concentrated (4 mg/5 ml) solution that requires dilution.

Action: Induces osteoclast apoptosis via the formation of adenosine triphosphate analogues that prevent cellular energy metabolism. Also causes osteoclast apoptosis through mevalonate pathway inhibition.

Use:
- To reduce refractory hypercalcaemia.
- To reduce pain associated with osteolytic conditions (for example, bone tumours).

It is recommended that a complete blood cell count and a biochemical profile are checked before each zoledronate infusion. Patients should be closely monitored after the administration of bisphosphonates. Please note that there have been no studies providing long-term follow-up of dogs receiving zoledronate.

Safety and handling: No information available.

Contraindications: Use with caution in patients with renal insufficiency and avoid in patients with renal failure. Ensure that the patient is normovolaemic prior to administration. Avoid in patients with a history of hypersensitivity to bisphosphonates.

Adverse reactions: Hypocalcaemia is possible. Local hypersensitivty was reported in 1 of 4 dogs treated for hypercalcaemia. Dose-dependent and infusion length-dependent nephrotoxicity, specifically acute tubular necrosis, has been described following zoledronate administration in humans although this is uncommon in dogs. A transient increase in gamma-glutamyl transferase is reported as well as a trend towards lower alkaline phosphatase activity. Mildly irritant if administered perivascularly; always place an intravenous catheter for administration. Bone necrosis has been described with other bisphosphonates.

Drug interactions: No information available.

DOSES
Dogs: 0.1–0.25 mg/kg slowly i.v. in 100 ml (50 ml for small dogs) of 0.9% normal saline over 15–30 minutes. Some references recommend a total maximum dose of 4 mg and doses at the low end of the range are usually preferred. Anecdotally, infusing 0.9% normal saline for 30 minutes before and 1 hour after the drug infusion may safeguard against nephrotoxicity. Can be repeated as clinically required but no more frequently than every 4 weeks.

Cats: No information available.

References
Schenk A, Lux C, Lane J and Martin O (2018) Evaluation of zoledronate as treatment for hypercalcemia in four dogs. *Journal of the American Animal Hospital Associatio* **54**, e54604

Zonisamide
(Desizon*, Zonegran*, Zonisamide*) **POM**

Formulations: Oral: 25 mg, 50 mg, 100 mg capsules; 20 mg/ml oral solution.

Action: The exact antiepileptic mode of action is unknown, but it is speculated that zonisamide may exert its effect by blocking repetitive firing of voltage-gated sodium channels, inhibiting low-threshold calcium channels and modulating GABA-ergic and glutamatergic neurotransmission thereby preventing the spread of seizure discharge across cells.

Use:
- Zonisamide is a sulphonamide anticonvulsant, which is usually used in dogs and cats as an adjunctive therapy in animals refractory to standard anticonvulsant therapy (in dogs, phenobarbital, imepitoin and potassium bromide). Response to therapy in idiopathic epilepstic dogs is reported to be 60–70%

It is well absorbed with a half-life of 15–17 hours in the dog. The drug is metabolized by the liver and then mostly excreted by the kidneys.

Safety and handling: Normal precautions should be observed.

Contraindications: Avoid use in patients with severe hepatic impairment. Caution in dogs with renal impairment. Do not use in pregnant animals as toxicity has been demonstrated in experimental studies. Do not discontinue abruptly.

Adverse reactions: Ataxia, sedation, vomiting and anorexia have been reported in a few dogs and, experimentally, in cats. Doses up to 75 mg/kg q24h or divided q12h have been used experimentally for up to 52 weeks in dogs; initially weight loss and, in the longer term, minor hepatic and haematological changes were observed. Recently, severe behavioural changes have been associated with zonisamide similar to aggressive behaviour recognized in humans treated with the drug. Signs resolved on termination of medication.

Drug interactions: Phenobarbital increases clearance of zonisamide up to 10 weeks after phenobarbital discontinuation. If using as an adjunctive to phenobarbital, consider using doses at the higher end of the dose range.

DOSES

Dogs: Starting dose of 3–7 mg/kg p.o. q12h, or 7–10 mg/kg p.o. q12h if coadministered with phenobarbital or other enzyme inducers. Human serum levels 10–40 mg/l can be used to guide effective concentrations, measured at a minimum of 1 week after initiation of treatment.

Cats: Starting dose of 5–10 mg/kg p.o. q24h is suggested.

References

Chung JY, Hwang CY, Chae JS *et al.* (2012) Zonisamide monotherapy for idiopathic epilepsy in dogs. *New Zealand Veterinary Journal* **60**, 357–359
von Klopmann T, Rambeck B and Tipold A (2007) A study of zonisamide therapy for refractory idiopathic epilepsy in dogs. *Journal of Small Animal Practice* **48**, 134–138

Appendix I: general information

Abbreviations

In general, abbreviations should not be used in prescription writing; however, it is recognized that at present some Latin abbreviations are used when prescribing. These should be limited to those listed here.

Abbreviations used in prescription writing

a.c.	Before meals
ad. lib.	At pleasure
amp.	Ampoule
b.i.d.	Twice a day
cap.	Capsule
g	Gram
h	Hour(s)
i.m.	Intramuscular
i.p.	Intraperitoneal
i.v.	Intravenous
m^2	Square metre
mg	Milligram
ml	Millilitre
o.m.	In the morning
o.n.	At night
p.c.	After meals
p.o.	By mouth, orally
prn	As required
q	Every, e.g. q8h = every 8 hours
q.i.d./q.d.s	Four times a day
q.s.	A sufficient quantity
s.c.	Subcutaneous
s.i.d.	Once a day
Sig:	Directions/label
stat.	Immediately
susp.	Suspension
tab.	Tablet
t.i.d./t.d.s.	Three times a day

Other abbreviations used in this Formulary

ACE	Angiotensin converting enzyme
ACTH	Adrenocorticotropic hormone
AV	Atrioventricular
CBC	Complete blood count
CHF	Congestive heart failure
CNS	Central nervous system
COX	Cyclo-oxygenase
CRI	Continuous rate infusion
CSF	Cerebrospinal fluid
d	Day(s)
DNA	Deoxyribonucleic acid
ECG	Electrocardiography
EMA	European Medicines Agency
EPI	Exocrine pancreatic insufficiency
GABA	Gamma aminobutyric acid
GI	Gastrointestinal
Hb	Haemoglobin
MIC	Minimum inhibitory concentration
min	Minute(s)
NSAID	Non-steroidal anti-inflammatory drug
PU/PD	Polyuria/polydipsia
RBC	Red blood cell
STC	Special Treatment Certificate
VMD	Veterinary Medicines Directorate
WBC	White blood cell
wk	Week(s)

APPENDIX I: GENERAL INFORMATION

APPENDIX II: PROTOCOLS

INDEX: THERAPEUTIC CLASS

INDEX: GENERIC AND TRADE NAMES

Writing a prescription

A 'veterinary prescription' is defined by EU law as 'any prescription for a veterinary medicinal product issued by a professional person qualified to do so in accordance with applicable national law'. The word 'veterinary' takes its normal meaning 'of or for animals'. In the UK there are two classes of medicines available only on veterinary prescription, POM-V and POM-VPS, described in the **Introduction**. Only in the case of POM-V medicines does the veterinary prescription have to be issued by a veterinary surgeon. The act of prescribing is taken to mean the decision made by the prescriber as to which product should be supplied, taking into account the circumstances of the animals being treated, the available authorized veterinary medicinal products and the need for responsible use of medicines.

A written prescription for a veterinary medicine must include the following and be printed or written legibly in ink or otherwise so as to be indelible:

- Name, address, and telephone number of the person prescribing the product
- Qualifications of the person prescribing the product (it is good practice to include their RCVS or SQP number)
- Name and address of the owner or keeper of the animal
- Identification (including the species) of the animal or group of animals to be treated
- Premises at which the animal(s) are kept, if this is different from the address of the owner or keeper
- Date
- Signature (or other authentication) of the person prescribing the product - sign in ink with your normal signature
- Name and amount of the product prescribed
    - Use product or approved generic name for drugs in capital letters – do not abbreviate. Ensure the full name is stated, to include the pharmaceutical form and strength
    - Write out microgram/nanogram – do not abbreviate
    - Always put a 0 before an initial decimal point (e.g. 0.5 mg), but avoid the unnecessary use of a decimal point (e.g. 3 mg not 3.0 mg)
    - State duration of treatment where known and the total quantity to be supplied
    - Give precise instructions concerning route/dose/formulation. Directions should preferably be in English without abbreviation. It is recognized that some Latin abbreviations are used (see p. 401)
- Necessary warnings
- Withdrawal period, if relevant
- The directions that the prescriber wishes to appear on the labelled product. It is good practice to include the words 'For animal treatment only'
- A declaration that 'This prescription is for an animal under my care' or words to that effect
- If it is prescribed under the cascade, a statement to that effect. If drugs that are not authorized for veterinary use are going to be used when there is an alternative that is 'higher' in the prescribing cascade, there should be a clear clinical justification made on an individual basis and recorded in the clinical notes or on the prescription.

Written prescriptions for POM-V or POM-VPS medicines:

- Are valid for 6 months unless the prescriber states a shorter period
- May only be used once unless the prescriber specifies that it is repeatable
- If repeatable, the number of repeat supplies that may be made must be specified (if the prescription is not repeatable, it is considered good practice for this to be stated).

In addition to the general prescription requirements above, a written prescription for a Schedule 2 or 3 Controlled Drug (CD) should state an exact dose in words as well as in figures (e.g. not 'as directed'), and it must include the RCVS number of the veterinary surgeon prescribing the drug. A written prescription for Schedule 2 or 3 CDs can only be dispensed once and only within 28 days. Single prescriptions with multiple dispenses (repeatable prescriptions) are not allowed for Schedule 2 and 3 CDs. It is good practice to mark the prescription 'no repeats'.

For all prescriptions, any alterations invalidate the prescription – it must be rewritten.

The following is a standard form of prescription used:

From: *Address of practice*	*Date*
Telephone No.	
Animal's name and identification (species, breed, age and sex)	*Owner's name* *Owner's address*
	Premises where animal(s) are kept if different from above

Rx
• *Print name, strength and formulation of drug*
• *Total quantity to be supplied*
• *Amount to be administered*
• *Frequency of administration*
• *Duration of treatment*
• *Any warnings*
• *If not a POM-V and prescribed under the 'Cascade', this must be stated*
• *For animal treatment only*
• *For an animal under my care*
• *Withdrawal period, if relevant*
Non-repeat/repeat X *1, 2 or 3*
 	
       Name, qualifications, RCVS number and signature
       of veterinary surgeon OR SQP number and signature	

Guidelines for responsible antibiotic use

While antibiotics are essential medicines for treating bacterial infections, it is important to remember that their use leads to selection of resistant strains of bacteria. Resistance may be intrinsic (chromosomal DNA changes) or acquired (by plasmid transfer).

It is important that the veterinary profession uses antibiotics responsibly in order to:

- Minimize the selection of resistant veterinary pathogens (and therefore safeguard animal health)
- Minimize possible resistance transfer to human pathogens
- Retain the right to prescribe certain antibiotics.

Following these guidelines will help to maximize the therapeutic success of antibiotic agents while at the same time minimizing the development of antibiotic resistance, thereby safeguarding antimicrobials for future veterinary and human use. These guidelines should be read in conjunction with the individual drug monographs, updated *BSAVA Guide to the Use of Veterinary Medicines* and the **PROTECT ME** guidance (**www.bsavalibrary.com**). Following the **PROTECT ME** guidance can help reduce resistance:

Prescribe only when necessary

Consider non-bacterial disease (e.g. viral infection), nutritional imbalance or metabolic disorders where antibiotic therapy would be redundant. Remember also that some bacterial disease will self-resolve without antibiotics. Offer a non-prescription form to support a decision not to prescribe antibiotic therapy.

Reduce prophylaxis

Antibiotics are not a substitute for surgical asepsis and the need for prophylactic antibiotics in surgery should be carefully considered. Prophylactic antibiotics are only appropriate in a few medical cases (e.g. immunocompromised patients).

Offer other options

Consider therapeutic alternatives (e.g. lavage and debridement of infected material, analgesia, cough suppressants, fluid therapy or nutritional modification). Use topical preparations as these reduce the selection pressure on resident intestinal flora (the microbiome). Use effective hygiene techniques and antiseptics to prevent infections.

Treat effectively

Before prescribing antibiotics, consider which bacteria are likely to be involved and how effectively the chosen drug will penetrate the target site. Use the shortest effective course and avoid underdosing. Ensure compliance with appropriate formulation and clear instructions.

Employ narrow spectrum

Unnecessarily broad-spectrum antibiotics could promote antibiotic resistance; selecting narrow-spectrum antibiotics limits the effects on commensal bacteria. Use culture results to support de-escalation (switching to a narrower spectrum antibiotic) whenever possible.

Culture appropriately

A sample for culture should be collected **before** starting antibiotic therapy. Culture is essential when prolonged (>1 week) treatment courses are anticipated, when resistance is likely (e.g. hospital-acquired infections) and with life-threatening infections. If first-line treatment fails, do not use another antibiotic without culture and susceptibility results (**avoid cycling antibiotics**).

Tailor practice policy to patients

A customized practice policy can guide antibiotic selection to address the bacterial infections and resistance patterns that you encounter, minimizing inappropriate use.

Monitor culture results

Track and record culture profiles and update your practice policy accordingly. Monitor for preventable infections (e.g. postoperative) and alter practices if needed. Audit your own antibiotic use, particularly of critically important antibiotics (e.g. fluoroquinolones and cefovecin).

Educate others

Share this important message to reduce the threat from multi-resistant strains of bacteria and improve the health of pets and people.

European Medicines Agency categorization of antibiotics

In 2019, the EMA launched a public consultation on its updated scientific advice on the categorization of antibiotics. The scientific advice ranks antibiotics by considering both the risk that their use in animals causes to public health through the possible development of antimicrobial resistance and the need to use them in veterinary medicine. It now addresses all classes of antibiotics, including those classified as critically important antimicrobials for human health by the World Health Organization (**see Useful websites**). Readers are encouraged to check and consider the EMA's updated scientific advice on the categorization of antibiotics when prescribing these medicines for animals in their care. The categorization can also be used as a tool for the preparation of treatment guidelines (**see Useful websites**). The classification comprises four categories:

- **Category A (Avoid)** includes antibiotics that are currently not authorized in veterinary medicine in the European Union (EU). These medicines may not be used in food-producing animals and may be given to individual companion animals only under exceptional circumstances.
- **Category B (Restrict)** refers to quinolones, 3rd- and 4th-generation cephalosporins and polymyxins. Antibiotics in this category are critically important in human medicine and their use in animals should be restricted to mitigate the risk to public health.
- **Category C (Caution)** covers antibiotics for which alternatives in human medicine generally exist in the EU, but only few alternatives are available in certain veterinary indications. These antibiotics should only be used when there are no antibiotic substances in Category D that would be clinically effective.
- **Category D (Prudence)** includes antibiotics that should be used as first line treatments, whenever possible. These antibiotics can be used in animals in a prudent manner. This means that unnecessary use and long treatment periods should be avoided, and group treatment should be restricted to situations where individual treatment is not feasible.

References

Allerton F and Nuttall T (2021) Antimicrobial use: importance of bacterial culture and susceptibility testing. *In Practice* **43**, 500–510
Sykes J and Greene J (2011) *Infectious Diseases of the Dog and Cat, 4th edn.* Saunders, Philadelphia

Antimicrobial susceptibility

		Gram positive			
		Cocci			
		MRSA/MRSP	Staphyloccocus	Enteroccocus	Streptoccocus
Aminoglycosides	Amikacin	◐	◐	◐	◐
	Gentamicin	◐	◐	◐	◐
Beta-lactams	Amoxicillin	●	●	◐	◐
	Ampicillin	●	●	◐	◐
	Amoxicillin-clavulanate	●	◐	◐	◐
Cephalosporins	Cefalexin	●	◐	●	◐
	Cefotaxime (3rd gen)	●	◐	●	◐
	Cefovecin (3rd gen)	●	◐	●	◐
	Ceftazidime (3rd gen)	●	◐	●	◐
	Ceftiofur (3rd gen)	●	◐	●	◐
	Cefuroxime (2nd gen)	●	◐	●	◐
Fluoroquinolones	Enrofloxacin	◐	◐	◐	◐
	Marbofloxacin	◐	◐	◐	◐
	Pradofloxacin	◐	◐	◐	◐
Lincosamides	Clindamycin	◐	◐	●	◐
	Lincomycin	◐	◐	●	◐
Macrolides	Azithromycin	●	◐	●	◐
	Erythromycin	●	◐	●	◐
Nitroimidazoles	Metronidazole	●	●	●	●
Sulphonamides	Trimethoprim sulfamethoxazole	◐	◐	◐	◐
Tetracyclines	Doxycycline	◐	◐	◐	◐
	Oxytetracycline	●	◐	◐	◐

Antimicrobial susceptibility chart listing the most likely susceptibility and resistance patterns to commonly available antibiotics. This chart is a summary and does not predict the susceptibility or resistance of an individual isolate; each case must be verified using up-to-date literature published by drug manufacturers. * = Extended-spectrum beta-lactamases (ESBLs) are normally inhibited by clavulanic acid; however, AmpC is resistant to clavulanic acid.

	Gram negative											
	Bacilli											
	Anaerobes			Enterobacteriacae								
Listeria	Clostridium	Bacteroides	Campylobacter	ESBLS*	Escherichia coli	Klebsiella	Enterobacter	Proteus	Salmonella	Pseudomonas	Pasteurella	Acinetobacter

Reproduced from Allerton and Nuttall (2021), with permission from the publisher. Data from this Formulary, Sykes and Greene (2011), and published Veterinary Committee on Antimicrobial Susceptibility Testing and Clinical and Laboratory Standards Institute breakpoints.

Legend:
- Susceptible
- Caution with interpretation and dosing
- Intrinsic resistance
- Acquired resistance

Guidelines for responsible parasiticide use

Parasiticides are essential medicines for the treatment of animal ectoparasites (e.g. ticks, fleas, mites) and endoparasites (e.g. tapeworms, roundworms, protozoa), and for prophylaxis both in the UK and in travelling pets. These parasites can have direct animal health and welfare impacts, indirect impacts through the transmission of disease and pose zoonotic risks. In some cases, parasiticide treatment is legally mandated (e.g. tapeworm treatment of travelling pets).

Overuse of parasiticides in farm animal and equine practice has led to widespread resistance, particularly within endoparasites. Whilst resistance is not currently a significant concern in UK small animal practice, overuse of these agents may lead to increased prevalence of resistant organisms and reduced efficacy of parasiticide treatments.

Parasiticides are harmful to a wide range of invertebrates. In addition, there is increasing recognition of environmental contamination from products used to treat companion animals, with potentially significant detrimental impact on wildlife ecosystems. Significant declines in terrestrial, including bee, and aquatic invertebrate populations are likely worsened by widespread environmental pesticide contamination, including from companion animal parasiticides. Environmental contamination can occur from topical products (such as seen with bathing after treatment), urine and faecal excretion, wastewater from homes and from incorrect disposal of products. Although significant uncertainty surrounds the proportional impact of companion animal parasiticides, veterinary surgeons should be mindful of these concerns and reduce use where possible.

Recommendations for responsible parasiticide use include:

- Prescribing parasiticide treatments based on risk rather than providing blanket treatment. This should take account of health risks (animal, human and environmental), lifestyle and environmental factors, season, geographical prevalence and the results of parasite testing (e.g. faecal examination)
- Ensuring correct dosing and application, as well as avoiding spillage
- Disposing of unused products, packaging and faeces from treated animals responsibly
- Avoiding bathing or swimming after topical application. Avoiding topical products in animals likely to contaminate water
- Treating parasites as needed for the individual animal, including using narrow spectrum products where appropriate
- Encouraging targeted treatment through laboratory testing (e.g. faecal examination) and owner recognition of parasites (e.g. via regular examination for fleas, and for ticks after walks in high prevalence areas). Early treatment of parasites with a significant domestic environmental lifecycle (e.g. fleas) is likely to result in the use of less parasiticide than if severe infestations are allowed to develop
- Considering non-pharmacological interventions to reduce treatment requirements (such as vacuuming and cleaning of bedding, regular bathing of untreated animals, removing faeces from the environment, and avoiding scavenging, hunting or raw feeding)
- Educating owners about parasites and responsible parasiticide use to ensure adherence to guidance and early recognition of parasites.

Guidelines on prescribing glucocorticoids

Glucocorticoids are among the most effective anti-inflammatory and antipruritic drugs available. Glucocorticoids are also rapidly effective in treating several important immune-mediated diseases (Whitley and Day, 2011) as well as many neoplastic conditions. However, chronic systemic glucocorticoid treatment is accompanied by several common, serious and dose-dependent adverse effects, such as polyuria, polydipsia, alopecia, muscle weakness, panting, lethargy and obesity. Several of these adverse effects appear to be of greater concern to pet owners than to the animals themselves. Systemic glucocorticoid treatment is also associated with less common, non-dose-dependent and unpredictable (stochastic) side effects such as diabetes mellitus or thromboembolic disease, which have significant implications for animal welfare. It is not possible to separate the beneficial effects of glucocorticoids from their adverse effects; however, reducing systemic exposure through topical, local and inhaled delivery may alter the balance between the beneficial and adverse effects.

There are very few objective studies examining the optimal doses or dosing intervals for any glucocorticoids for any conditions in dogs or cats. There are wide inter-subject variations in plasma concentrations after administration, which suggest variable drug absorption. Furthermore, no relationship has been demonstrated between these plasma concentrations (unbound or total concentration) and clinical response. As many glucocorticoid effects are due to alteration of gene transcription, their biological activities exceed the plasma half-lives of the drugs. Different glucocorticoids have varying biological half-lives and are presented in varying formulations, which also affect their duration of action and tissue targeting. For example, a single dose of a long-acting ester of methylprednisolone is capable of altering ACTH stimulation testing in dogs for at least 5 weeks (Kemppainen *et al.*, 1981).

Considerations before using glucocorticoids

Many problems that develop with glucocorticoid use arise when a treatment plan is not discussed with the pet owner at the time these drugs are initially prescribed. It is worthwhile considering the following questions before glucocorticoids are used (adapted from Thorn, 1966):

- How serious is the underlying disorder when compared with the predictable adverse effects of glucocorticoids?
- Is the patient likely to be predisposed to more severe, stochastic complications of glucocorticoid therapy (e.g. diabetes mellitus)?
- What is the starting glucocorticoid dose and the predicted length of treatment; when and how will this be adjusted?
- Which glucocorticoid preparation would minimize the adverse effects while retaining the beneficial effects?
- Are there other types of treatment that could be used to minimize the glucocorticoid dose?

Considerations when using glucocorticoids

- Starting doses: Although doses reported in this Formulary and other texts do provide a useful starting point when choosing an initial dose, given the lack of published evidence for many doses and the individual variability in response, glucocorticoids should ultimately be used to the desired effect. Providing the side effects are acceptable, there is no strict maximum dose for glucocorticoids, but it may be wise to obtain the guidance of a relevant veterinary specialist when

APPENDIX I: GENERAL INFORMATION

APPENDIX II: PROTOCOLS

INDEX: THERAPEUTIC CLASS

INDEX: GENERIC AND TRADE NAMES

using doses above those reported in this Formulary. The duration and magnitude of hypothalamic–pituitary–adrenal axis suppression caused by daily oral administration of a glucocorticoid varies based on species, individual, dose, formulation and specific pharmacokinetics of the glucocorticoid used. Larger individuals within a given species generally need proportionately lower doses on a mg/kg basis to achieve the same biological effect. For this reason, some authors dose on a mg/m^2 basis in some medium to large patients. Pharmacological studies evaluating effects of glucocorticoids in cats are lacking. Currently, recommended dosing regimens for cats vary considerably. The predominant opinion, however, is that the cat requires a higher dose than the dog (on a mg/kg basis) (Lowe *et al.*, 2008). Adverse effects of glucocorticoids are very likely in all treated animals and it is worthwhile warning owners about them. A client information leaflet is available to BSAVA members for this purpose.

- Adjusting doses: As there are few studies comparing protocols for tapering immunosuppressive or anti-inflammatory therapy with glucocorticoids, it is appropriate to adjust the therapy according to laboratory or clinical parameters. For example, cases with immune-mediated haemolytic anaemia should have their therapy adjusted following monitoring of their haematocrit. Most of the beneficial effects of glucocorticoids are seen in the short term. If the expected benefits are not apparent, then either the dose needs to be increased until limited by adverse effects, or alternative drugs and/or treatment modalities added and the dose of glucocorticoids reduced. Doses can be reduced to alternate-day therapy as soon as clinical control of the disease is achieved – regardless of the dose needed to achieve control. Although alternate-day dosing of medium-acting glucocorticoids (such as prednisolone) is accepted clinical practice, it assumes that the beneficial effects of these drugs last longer than the side effects. Evidence for this assumption is very limited and whether alternate-day dosing really avoids suppression of the hypothalamic–pituitary–adrenal axis while retaining beneficial therapeutic effect is debatable. Consideration should also be given to using short-acting glucocorticoids in 'pulse doses' to control acute recurrences of disease. Protracted use of any topical glucocorticoid can lead to thinning of the skin and owners should be advised of this possibility.

When not to use glucocorticoids

Glucocorticoids should not be given to animals with disc disease, hypercalcaemia, cutaneous or subcutaneous masses or large lymph nodes without a specific diagnosis and indication to do so. The use of glucocorticoids in most cases of shock is of no benefit and may be detrimental. Glucocorticoids are not analgesics; if animals are in pain then analgesics are required.

References

Kemppainen RJ, Lorenz MD and Thompson FN (1981) Adrenocortical suppression in the dog after a single dose of methylprednisolone acetate. *American Journal of Veterinary Research* **42**, 822–824

Lowe AD, Campbell KL and Graves T (2008) Glucocorticoids in the cat. *Veterinary Dermatology* **19**, 40–47

Thorn GW (1966) Clinical considerations in the use of corticosteroids. New England *Journal of Medicine* **274**, 775–781

Whitley NT and Day MJ (2011) Immunomodulatory drugs and their application to the management of canine immune-mediated disease. *Journal of Small Animal Practice* **52**, 70–85

Topical polypharmaceuticals for ear disease

The following POM-V preparations contain two or more drugs and are used topically in the ear. For further information see relevant monographs. In addition, there are a number of AVM-GSL preparations used for ear cleaning etc. that are not listed here.

Trade name	Antibacterial	Steroid	Antifungal
Aurizon	Marbofloxacin	Dexamethasone	Clotrimazole
Canaural[a]	Fusidic acid, Framycetin	Prednisolone	Nystatin
Easotic	Gentamicin	Hydrocortisone aceponate	Miconazole
Osurnia	Florfenicol	Betamethasone	Terbinafine
Otomax	Gentamicin	Betamethasone	Clotrimazole
Posatex	Orbifloxacin	Mometasone	Posaconozole
Surolan[a]	Polymyxin B	Prednisolone	Miconazole

[a] Note that there is some evidence from clinical trials that products that do not contain a specific acaricidal compound may nevertheless be effective at treating infestations of ear mites. The mode of action is unclear but the vehicle for these polypharmaceutical products may be involved.

Radiographic contrast agents

Barium and iodinated contrast media

See *BSAVA Guide to Procedures in Small Animal Practice.*

MRI contrast media

Several gadolinium chelates are used for magnetic resonance imaging (MRI) contrast studies. None of them is authorized for veterinary use and all are POM.

Action: Gadolinium is a paramagnetic agent and exerts its effects due to seven unpaired electrons, which cause a shortening of T1 and T2 relaxation times of adjacent tissues. This results in increased signal intensity on T1-weighted MR images. Unbound gadolinium is highly toxic and so is chelated to reduce toxicity. Gadolinium chelates do not cross the normal blood–brain barrier due to their large molecular size.

Use:

- During MRI examination to identify areas of abnormal vascularization or increased interstitial fluid, delineate masses and demonstrate disruption of the blood–brain barrier and areas of inflammation.
- Gadodiamide, gadobutrol, gadoteric acid and gadobenic acid are also used for contrast-enhanced magnetic resonance angiography (MRA).
- The low concentration form of gadopentetic acid (2 mmol/l) is authorized for intra-articular use for MR arthrography in humans.
- Gadobenic acid and gadoxetic acid are also transported across hepatocyte cell membranes (gadoxetic acid via organic anionic-acid transporting peptide 1) and are used in the characterization of liver lesions.

Safety and handling: Contact with skin and eyes may cause mild irritation.

Contraindications: Use with caution in cardiac disease, pre-existing renal disease and neonates. Contraindicated in severe renal impairment.

Adverse reactions: Nephrogenic systemic fibrosis (most commonly associated with gadodiamide but also gadopentetic acid and gadoversetamide) reported in humans but not in animals. Increase in QT interval and other arrhythmias have also been reported, and cardiac monitoring is recommended in the event of accidental overdosage. Transient episodes of shortness of breath following intravenous administration of gadoxetic acid have been reported in humans. Many contrast agents are hyper-osmolar and irritant if extravasation occurs (although studies in animals have shown gadopentetic acid and gadoteridol to be less toxic to subcutaneous tissues than an equal volume of iodinated contrast media), and therefore should be given through an intravenous catheter. Anaphylaxis occurs rarely (0.001%–0.01% in human studies). May cause a transient increase in serum bilirubin if there is pre-existing hepatic disease. Retained gadolinium deposits in certain areas of the brain have been reported recently in human patients, the clinical significance of these deposits is unknown at present. May cause fetal abnormalities in rabbits.

Drug interactions: May have interactions with Class 1a and 3 antiarrhythmics. Gadobenic acid may compete for cannalicular multispecific organic anionic transporter sites. Caution should be used if administering anthracyclines, vinca alkyloids and other drugs using this transporter. Anionic drugs excreted in bile (e.g. rifampicin) may reduce hepatic uptake of gadoxetic acid, reducing contrast enhancement. May affect some laboratory results, e.g. serum iron determination using complexometric methods, transient increase in liver enzymes, some linear non-ionic gadolinium gadolinium-based contrast media (gadodiamide, gadoversetamide) may cause false reduction in serum calcium measurement.

Doses and further advice on use: Should be used routinely for MRI examinations of the brain. Use for MRI of other body regions if abnormal vascularization, inflammation or neoplasia is suspected, for postsurgical evaluation or if MRI study is normal despite significant clinical signs. Post-contrast images should ideally be obtained within 30 minutes of contrast administration. Total doses should not exceed 0.3 mmol/kg (varies with product).

Dogs: 0.1 mmol/kg i.v. (all except gadoxetic acid). Give as bolus if performing MRA, dynamic contrast or liver studies; 0.025 mmol/kg i.v. bolus of gadoxetic acid for liver studies; 0.05 mmol/kg of gadobenic acid for liver studies. Repeat doses (not gadoxetic acid) of up to 0.3 mmol/kg total dose may be helpful in some cases if poor contrast enhancement with standard dose or for detection of metastases and if using low-field scanner. Enhancement visible up to 45–60 minutes post-administration.

Generic name	Trade name	Manufacturer	Authorized indications in humans	Excretion	Properties	Protein binding	Dose	Formulations
Gadopentetic acid	Magnevist	Bayer	CNS; whole body (excluding heart); arthrography	Renal	Linear Ionic 1960 mOsm/kg	0	0.1–0.3 mmol/kg	469 mg/ml, 2 mmol/l 5, 10, 15, 20 ml vials; 10, 15, 20 ml pre-filled syringes; 50, 100 ml pharmacy bulk package
Gadoteric acid	Dotarem	Guerbet Laboratories Ltd	CNS; whole body; MRA	Renal	Cyclic Ionic 1350 mOsm/kg	0	0.1–0.3 mmol/kg	279.3 mg/ml 5, 10, 15, 20 ml vials; 15, 20 ml pre-filled syringes
Gadoteridol	Prohance	Bracco	CNS; whole body	Renal	Cyclic Non-ionic 630 mOsm/kg	0	0.1 mmol/kg	279.3 mg/ml 5, 10, 15, 20 ml vials; 5, 10, 15, 17 ml pre-filled syringes
Gadodiamide	Omniscan	Nycomed Amersham	CNS; whole body	Renal	Linear Non-ionic 789 mOsm/kg	0	0.1–0.3 mmol/kg	287 mg/ml 5, 10, 15, 20, 40, 50 ml vials; 10, 15, 20 ml pre-filled syringes
Gadobutrol	Gadovist	Bayer	CNS	Renal	Cyclic Non-ionic 1603 mOsm/kg	0	0.1 mmol/kg	604.72 mg/ml 7.5, 10, 15 ml vials; 7.5, 10, 15 ml pre-filled syringes; 30, 65 ml bulk packages
Gadoxetic acid	Primovist	Bayer	Liver	50% renal, 50% biliary	Linear Ionic 688 mOsm/kg	<15%	0.025 mmol/kg	181.43 mg/ml 10 ml pre-filled syringes
Gadobenic acid	Multi-Hance	Bracco	CNS; liver; MRA; breast	Renal (biliary up to 4%)	Linear Ionic 1970 mOsm/kg	<5%	CNS: 0.1 mmol/kg; liver: 0.05 mmol/kg	334 mg/ml 5, 10, 15, 20 ml vials
Gado-versetamide	Optimark	Covidien	CNS; liver	Renal	Linear Non-ionic 1110 mOsm/kg	0	0.1 mmol/kg	330 mg/ml 10, 15, 20, 30 ml pre-filled syringes

Composition of intravenous fluids

Fluid	Na⁺ (mmol/l)	K⁺ (mmol/l)	Ca²⁺ (mmol/l)	Cl⁻ (mmol/l)	HCO₃⁻ (mmol/l)	Dext. (g/l)	Osmol. (mosl/l)
0.45% NaCl	77			77			155
0.9% NaCl	154			154			308
5% NaCl	856			856			1722
Ringer's	147	4	2	155			310
Lactated Ringer's (Hartmann's)	131	5	2	111	29 *		280
Darrow's	121	35		103	53 *		312
0.9% NaCl + 5.5% Dext.	154			154		50	560
0.18% NaCl + 4% Dext.	31			31		40	264
Duphalyte **		2.6	1.0	3.6		454	Unknown

Dext. = Dextrose; Osmol. = Osmolality. * Bicarbonate is present as lactate.
** Also contains a mixture of vitamins and small quantities of amino acids and 1.2 mmol/l of $MgSO_4$.

Safety and handling of chemotherapeutic agents

Chemotherapy agents are genotoxic, mutagenic and teratogenic therefore, unsurprisingly, their use is considered an occupational health hazard. The use of these agents appears to be increasing due to demand from clients wishing to treat cancer in their pets, therefore, the number of events carrying an exposure risk is on the rise. In addition to the increased use of 'conventional' chemotherapy, innovative dosing strategies such as metronomic chemotherapy reduce the direct control that practices can exert over safe use (as clients are the primary administrators in this context). There is also increasing availability of novel agents such as small molecular c-kit inhibitors, which are not chemotherapeutic in the conventional sense but may carry similar risks especially in relation to pregnancy and should, therefore, be handled as cytotoxic drugs. Considering these risks together, great care must be taken to provide appropriate education to staff and clients in order that exposure to these drugs can be avoided.

Appropriate indication for the use of chemotherapy

Given the potential risks associated with chemotherapy exposure, both to the patient and those involved in preparing and handling chemotherapy agents, they should only be prescribed when absolutely indicated (i.e. for histologically confirmed diseases when the likelihood of response is considered high). Investigational use should be confined to controlled clinical trials.

Routes to exposure

Exposure can occur during the preparation, handling and administration of the agents, as a result of cleaning spills, and through contact with bodily fluids or excreta of patients treated with chemotherapy. The environment in which the patient is treated and housed after chemotherapy is at risk of contamination (both within the hospital and in the home). Therefore, practice staff, owners and subsequent users of administration spaces are all at risk of exposure in the event of contamination. Exposure may occur via direct skin contact, inhalation of aerosolized drug particles, ingestion or needle stick injuries.

Approaches to mitigate the risk of exposure

Practices should assess the suitability of their environment and staffing (both level and training) for chemotherapy administration. In some cases, the facilities or staffing levels or training may be unsuitable. In these instances, patients should be referred. Similarly, veterinary surgeons should consider the suitability of patients and owners prior to starting treatment. This assessment is particularly relevant for oral medications as administration is not under the direct control of the veterinary surgeon and owners may become too relaxed about safety precautions.

The following guidance is provided to help minimize the risks associated with chemotherapy use.

Personnel and owners:
- The preparation and administration of cytotoxic drugs should only be undertaken by trained staff.
- Practices should develop standard operating procedures (SOPs) for preparing, handling and administering chemotherapeutic agents, for managing potentially contaminated spaces after the administration of chemotherapy or following spills, and for housing treated patients. Staff should be trained in these SOPs with regular refreshers sessions held. Records of staff training should be kept.
- Owners and staff (including cleaners, animal carers and veterinary professionals) involved in the care of animals being treated with cytotoxic drugs must be informed of:
  - The risks of working with cytotoxic agents (to them as well as the patient)
  - The potential methods for preventing aerosol formation and the spread of contamination
  - The proper working practices for a safety cabinet (if available)
  - The instructions to clean contaminated spaces and spills
  - The principles of good personal protection and hygiene practice.
- Pregnant and immunocompromised personnel should not be involved in the process of preparing and/or administering cytotoxic agents, caring for animals that have been treated with cytotoxic drugs or cleaning the areas with which these animals have come into contact. Employees should be made aware that the risk to a fetus may be highest in the first trimester of pregnancy; consequently, employees planning to conceive and/or are in the early stages of pregnancy should be assigned to other duties. It is the responsibility of the employee to warn their employers if they are pregnant, likely to become pregnant or are immunocompromised.

Equipment and facilities:
- All areas where cytotoxic agents are prepared and/or administered, or where animals who have received cytotoxic drugs are being cared for, should be identified by a clear warning sign.
- Access to these areas should be restricted, ideally at all times, but at a minimum during chemotherapy preparation and administration.
- No rest activities or food or drink consumption should be permitted in the preparation, administration or post treatment kennelling areas at any time.

- There must be adequate materials for cleaning spilled cytotoxic agents (cytotoxic spill kit), clearly labelled and with associated use instructions, within the preparation and administration area(s).
- Ideally, a negative pressure pharmaceutical isolator with externally ducted exhaust filters, which has been properly serviced and checked, should be used. If such an isolator is not available, then a suitably modified Class 2B Biological Safety Cabinet (BSC) may be used.
- Regardless of whether a BSC is available, use of a needle-free closed or semi-closed system is mandatory to prevent aerosol formation, reduce the risk of stick injury and control exposure to carcinogenic compounds. Available systems include (but are not limited to): ChemoClave/Chemolock, Equashield, Onguard, PhaSeal and Spiros.

Preparation of cytotoxic drugs:
- Printed copies of preparation SOPs and drug data sheets should be available in the room in which the agents are to be prepared.
- Where available, the ventilated cabinet should be used for all chemotherapy preparation.
- If a BSC is not available, veterinary surgeons should consider acquiring pre-prepared patient specific doses of chemotherapy from a commercial company.
- During preparation and administration, disposable chemoprotective personal protective equipment (PPE) should be worn by all involved staff. The PPE should include:
  - A chemotherapy impermeable full-length gown. The gown should have elasticated cuffs
  - Two pairs of chemotherapy impermeable (often nitrile) gloves. One seated underneath the cuff and one covering it entirely
  - Eye protection in the form of goggles or a face shield
  - Fitted respiratory protection is ideal and should be considered mandatory if chemotherapy is prepared outside of a BSC.
- The dosage of chemotherapy should be calculated, and the calculation checked by at least one colleague.
- All essential supplies should be kept inside the BSC. Absorbent padding should be placed in the BSC under the chemotherapy draw area.
- All administration consumables (tubing, fluid bags) should be prepared and primed outside the BSC prior to adding the chemotherapeutic agents (which should be done within the BSC). Heparinized saline should be avoided as it can interact with some chemotherapeutic drugs (e.g. doxorubicin/epirubicin).
- Chemotherapy injection spikes rather than needles should be used for withdrawing liquid chemotherapy.
- Manual handling of oral or topical medicines containing cytotoxic drugs should be avoided. Oral chemotherapy drugs should never be crushed or split. Several companies (e.g. BOVA, Chemopet, NOVA) supply compounded chemotherapy agents in various sizes suitable for different patients. This may be useful for drugs such as piroxicam, hydroxycarbamide, cyclophosphamide and lomustine. If reformulation is not possible, then adjusting the dosage regimen is often sufficient.
- When drug preparation is complete, the final product should be sealed in a plastic bag or other container for transport before it is taken out of the BSC. It should be clearly labelled with the drug name, patient name and dose.

- All potentially contaminated materials should be discarded in special cytotoxic waste disposal containers, which can be opened without direct contact with hands/gloves (e.g. a foot pedal). Local regulations for the disposal of this waste should be followed.
- The chemotherapy preparation space should be decontaminated and disinfected, and the outer pair of gloves discarded.
- Once drug preparation is complete, the inner pair of gloves can be discarded.
- There should be a clear procedure regarding how to handle cytotoxic drugs following an injection accident.

Administration of cytotoxic drugs:

- Prior to prescribing chemotherapy, the veterinary surgeon should make an assessment of the suitability of the patient to receive treatment (and be hospitalized should there be a significant adverse event).
- Drug administration should take place in a quiet and calm environment with restricted entry during the process. The external side of the door should be labelled to warn other staff. Personnel administering chemotherapy should not be disturbed.
- At the time of administration, the veterinary surgeon should again assess whether the patient is adequately calm and cooperative for safe administration. Anxious patients may benefit from the administration of mild anxiolytics prior to arrival at the clinic (e.g. trazodone, gabapentin). Fractious or exuberant animals should be sedated (with the owner's consent).
- Two suitably trained members of staff should be present with the patient throughout the administration process. This is especially important when using vesicant drugs such as vinca alkaloids (vincristine, vinblastine) or anthracyclines (doxorubicin/epirubicin).
- A pre-administration checklist should be developed to confirm:
  - The correct patient identity
  - The blood results have been checked and are adequate for chemotherapy
  - The correct volume of drug has been accurately prepared
  - The catheter has been placed and is functioning properly
  - The patient is calm and can comfortably be restrained for the expected duration of administration
  - All staff are wearing adequate PPE (as described in the preparation section, although a single pair of gloves is acceptable).
- Drugs should be administered safely using a needle-free system (such as those described above).
- Drug administration should occur over a disposable absorbent pad (e.g. incontinence pad).
- The tubing should never be removed from a fluid bag containing a hazardous drug, nor should it be disconnected at any other point in the system. The intravenous catheter, tubing and bag should be removed from the patient and discarded intact as a single unit when possible. A cytotoxic waste bin should be used.
- The patient should be clearly labelled as a chemotherapy recipient (e.g. different coloured name tag). The chemotherapy injection site should be wrapped in a coloured dressing that identifies this procedure has occurred.

- Hands should be washed with soap and water before leaving the drug administration area.
- Procedures should be in place for dealing with any spillages that occur and for the safe disposal of waste. In the event of contact with skin or eyes, the affected area should be washed with copious amounts of water or normal saline. Medical advice should be sought if the eyes are affected.

Procedures for nursing patients receiving chemotherapy:

- Special wards or designated kennels with clear identification that the patients are being treated with cytotoxic agents is required. As well as kennel notices, different coloured bedding can be a helpful indicator.
- Excreta (saliva, urine, vomit, faeces) are all potentially hazardous after the animal has been treated with cytotoxic drugs and should be handled and disposed of accordingly.
- For hospitalized patients, the period of risk (i.e. the period during which the patient is expected to be excreting chemotherapeutic drugs or metabolites) should be clearly marked on the kennel and chemotherapy impervious PPE (such as disposable gloves and protective clothing) should be worn when carrying out nursing procedures (see the ACVIM small animal consensus statement (Smith *et al.*, 2018) for more information on excretion periods).
- All materials that have come into contact with the animal during the period of risk should be considered as potentially contaminated.
- After the animal has left the ward, the kennel should be cleaned according to the chemotherapy specific cleaning protocol.

Guidelines for owners:

- All owners should be given written information about:
  - The potential hazards of cytotoxic drugs (to humans and treated pets)
  - The excretion period relevant to the drug(s) administered
  - How to deal with the patient's excreta (saliva, urine, vomit, faeces).
- If owners are to administer tablets themselves, then they should receive written information stating:
  - The PPE required
  - That oral chemotherapeutic agents should not be crushed or split.
- Medicine containers should be clearly labelled with 'cytotoxic contents' warning tape.
- Veterinary surgeons should:
  - Offer to provide suitable PPE
  - Confirm owners are using the provided PPE during subsequent consultations.

Cost and chemotherapy safety

Undoubtedly some of the mitigating measures described above will increase the cost of chemotherapy and, unfortunately, in some cases may make chemotherapy unaffordable. However, practices have legal responsibilities to safeguard their employees and the public, and veterinary professionals have a duty of care to their patients. Therefore, cost is not a reason for not following suitable safety procedures.

Further information

The guidance provided here is a summary of current best practice, but is subject to continual re-evaluation and, therefore, practices should review their approach from time to time. For further information, readers are encouraged to review the *ACVIM small animal consensus statement on safe use of cytotoxic chemotherapeutics in veterinary practice* (Smith *et al.*, 2018), *Safe handling of cytotoxic drugs in the workplace* (hse.gov.uk/healthservices/safe-use-cytotoxic-drugs.htm) and the NIOSH guidance on *Safe handling of hazardous drugs for veterinary healthcare workers* (cdc.gov/niosh).

Reference

Smith AN, Klahn S, Phillips B *et al.* (2018) ACVIM small animal consensus statement on safe use of cytotoxic chemotherapeutics in veterinary practice. *Journal of Veterinary Internal Medicine* **32(3)**, 904–913

Bodyweight (BW) to body surface area (BSA) conversion tables

Dogs (Formula: BSA (m^2) = 0.101 x (bodywieght in kg)$^{2/3}$

BW (kg)	BSA (m^2)	BW (kg)	BSA (m^2)	BW (kg)	BSA (m^2)
0.5	0.06	11	0.50	24	0.84
1	0.1	12	0.53	26	0.89
2	0.16	13	0.56	28	0.93
3	0.21	14	0.59	30	0.98
4	0.25	15	0.61	35	1.08
5	0.30	16	0.64	40	1.18
6	0.33	17	0.67	45	1.28
7	0.37	18	0.69	50	1.37
8	0.4	19	0.72	55	1.46
9	0.44	20	0.74	60	1.55
10	0.47	22	0.79		

Cats (Formula: BSA (m^2) = 0.1 x (bodyweight in kg)$^{2/3}$

BW (kg)	BSA (m^2)	BW (kg)	BSA (m^2)	BW (kg)	BSA (m^2)
0.5	0.06	2.5	0.184	4.5	0.273
1	0.1	3	0.208	5	0.292
1.5	0.134	3.5	0.231	5.5	0.316
2	0.163	4	0.252	6	0.33

Percentage solutions

The concentration of a solution may be expressed on the basis of weight per unit volume (w/v) or volume per unit volume (v/v).

% w/v = number of grams of a substance in 100 ml of a liquid

% v/v = number of ml of a substance in 100 ml of liquid

% Solution	g or ml/100 ml	mg/ml	Solution strength
100	100	1000	1:1
10	10	100	1:10
1	1	10	1:100
0.1	0.1	1	1:1000
0.01	0.01	0.1	1:10,000

Drugs usage in renal and hepatic insufficiency

With failure of liver or kidney, the excretion of some drugs may be impaired, leading to increased serum concentrations.

Renal failure

a. Double the dosing interval or halve the dosage in patients with severe renal insufficiency. Use for drugs that are relatively non-toxic.

b. Increase dosing interval 2-fold when creatinine clearance (Ccr) is 0.5–1.0 ml/min/kg, 3-fold when Ccr is 0.3–0.5 ml/min/kg and 4-fold when Ccr is <0.3 ml/min/kg.

c. Precise dose modification is required for some toxic drugs that are excreted solely by glomerular filtration, e.g. aminoglycosides. This is determined by using the dose fraction Kf to amend the drug dose or dosing interval according to the following equations:

- Modified dose reduction = normal dose × K_f
- Modified dose interval = normal dose interval/K_f
- where K_f = patient Ccr/normal Ccr

Where Ccr is unavailable, Ccr may be estimated at 88.4/serum creatinine (μmol (micromoles)/l) (where serum creatinine is <350 μmol/l).

K_f may be estimated at 0.33 if urine is isosthenuric or 0.25 if the patient is azotaemic.

Drug	Nephrotoxic	Dose adjustment in renal failure
Amikacin	Yes	c
Amoxicillin	No	a
Amphotericin B	Yes	c
Ampicillin	No	a
Cefalexin	No	b
Chloramphenicol	No	N, A
Digoxin	No	c
Gentamicin	Yes	c

a, b, c = Refer to section above on dose adjustment; A = Avoid in severe renal failure; CI = Contraindicated; N = normal dose. (continues) ▶

Drug	Nephrotoxic	Dose adjustment in renal failure
Nitrofurantoin	No	CI
Oxytetracycline	Yes	CI
Penicillin	No	a
Tobramycin	Yes	c
Trimethoprim/ sulphonamide	Yes	b, A

(continued) a, b, c = Refer to section above on dose adjustment; A = Avoid in severe renal failure; CI = Contraindicated; N = normal dose.

Hepatic insufficiency

Drug clearance by the liver is affected by many factors and thus it is not possible to apply a simple formula to drug dosing. The table below is adapted from information in the human literature.

Drug	DI	CI
Aspirin		✓
Azathioprine		✓
Cefotaxime	✓	
Chloramphenicol		✓
Clindamycin		✓
Cyclophosphamide	✓	
Diazepam		✓
Doxorubicin	✓	
Doxycycline	✓	
Fluorouracil		✓
Furosemide	✓	
Hydralazine	✓	
Lidocaine	✓	
Metronidazole	✓	
Morphine	✓	
NSAIDs	✓	
Oxytetracycline		✓
Pentobarbital	✓	
Phenobarbital	✓	
Propranolol	✓	
Theophylline	✓	
Vincristine	✓	

CI = Contraindicated; avoid use if at all possible. DI = A change in dose or dosing interval may be required.

Further reading

British National Formulary No. 84 (2022) British Medical Association and the Royal Pharmaceutical Society of Great Britain

Compendium of Data Sheets for Animal Medicines (2022) National Office of Animal Health, Enfield, Middlesex

Giguére S, Prescott JF, Baggot JD and Walker RD (2013) *Antimicrobial Therapy in Veterinary Medicine, 5th edn.* Wiley Blackwell, Iowa

Monthly Index of Medical Specialties (2022) Haymarket Medical Publications, London

Papich MG (2015) *Saunders Handbook of Veterinary Drugs, 4th edn.* Saunders Elsevier, St Louis

Plumb DC (2018) *Plumb's Veterinary Drug Handbook, 9th edn.* Wiley Blackwell, New Jersey (also available from www.plumbsveterinarydrugs.com)

Useful websites

www.bnf.org
British National Formulary – registration required through academic institutions to use BNF online but can order paper copy of BNF from this site.

www.bsava.com
British Small Animal Veterinary Association – links to position statements on responsible use of antibacterials and parasite control.

www.bsavalibrary.com
British Small Animal Veterinary Association online Library – links to *Journal of Small Animal Practice*, and contains the *BSAVA Guide to the Use of Veterinary Medicines* and searchable online Formularies (free access for BSAVA members).

www.bva.co.uk
British Veterinary Association.

cdc.gov/niosh
Centers for Disease Control and Prevention – NIOSH guidance on the safe handling of hazardous drugs.

www.ema.europa.eu/en
European Medicines Agency.

www.gov.uk/government/organisations/veterinary-medicines-directorate
Veterinary Medicines Directorate.

www.hse.gov.uk/healthservices/safe-use-cytotoxic-drugs.htm
Health and Safety Executive – safe handling of cytotoxic drugs in the workplace.

www.medicines.org.uk/emc
Electronic Medicines Compendium.

www.ncbi.nlm.nih.gov/pubmed
PubMed is a widely used free service of the U.S. National Library of Medicine and the National Institutes of Health that allows users to search abstracts in the medical literature. All major veterinary publications covered.

www.noahcompendium.co.uk
NOAH compendium site.

prime.vetmed.wsu.edu
Washington State University College of Veterinary Medicine Program in Individualized Medicine – provides guidance and testing relating to multidrug resistance and the *ABCB1* gene.

www.rcvs.org.uk
Royal College of Veterinary Surgeons.

www.who.int
World Health Organization.

www.wiley.com
Journal of Small Animal Practice – free for BSAVA members, free abstracts and pay per article for others.

Websites relating to the manufacture of extemporaneous products

www.gov.uk/government/publications/human-and-veterinary-medicines-register-of-licensed-manufacturing-sites

Human and veterinary medicines – links to the Register of licensed manufacturing sites – manufacturer specials, human (MS) and the Register of licensed manufacturing sites – manufacturer specials authorisation, veterinary (MANSA).

www.bova.co.uk

Site for a company that will reformulate many drugs into conveniently sized tablets, liquids, pastes and transdermal gels.

www.chemopet.co.uk

Site for a company that will reformulate a wide range of injectable and oral chemotherapy drugs.

https://healthcare.pccarx.co.uk

Site for a company that will reformulate many drugs into conveniently sized tablets.

www.novalabs.co.uk

Site for a company that will reformulate many drugs into conveniently sized tablets or liquids.

www.summitvetpharma.co.uk

Site for a company that will reformulate many drugs into conveniently sized tablets, liquids and transdermal gels.

APPENDIX I: GENERAL INFORMATION

APPENDIX II: PROTOCOLS

INDEX: THERAPEUTIC CLASS

INDEX: GENERIC AND TRADE NAMES

Appendix II: Protocols

Chemotherapy protocols

Four chemotherapy protocols for lymphoma are provided below. The CHOP and COP protocols are first-line chemotherapy protocols. LPP is an all-oral protocol, suitable for dogs, that is generally considered a rescue protocol, but may be considered first-line for treatment of T-cell lymphoma or when injectable chemotherapy cannot be given. There is a vast array of other chemotherapy protocols for lymphoma available in the literature.

The vinblastine and prednisolone protocol is a standard protocol for treatment of mast cell tumour (MCT) in the adjuvant or neoadjuvant setting.

Health and safety considerations

Chemotherapeutic agents are mutagenic, teratogenic and carcinogenic; therefore, great care must be taken to ensure safe use of these agents. The ACVIM small animal consensus statement on safe use of cytotoxic chemotherapeutics in veterinary practice (Smith *et al.*, 2018) is a useful resource when developing safe chemotherapy preparation and administration protocols.

Some general considerations are:

- Chemotherapeutic agents should be stored in secure, clearly labelled containers.
- Chemotherapy should be given in a calm and quiet environment.
- People who are or may become pregnant should not be involved in handling or administering chemotherapeutics or handling treated animals (or their excreta).
- When administering chemotherapy, appropriate personal protective equipment must be worn.
- Oral cytotoxic drugs must not be split or divided and should not be crushed.
- Closed administration systems are recommended.

Dosing considerations

The therapeutic index (the gap between the therapeutic and the toxic dose of a drug) is narrow for chemotherapeutic agents. Consequently, careful calculation of treatment dose is required. Ideally, a compounding/reformulating pharmacy should be used to match patient requirements as closely as possible for oral medications. Veterinary specials manufacturers (e.g. ChemoPet) will prepare single, per patient, doses of chemotherapy to allow accurate dosing. These services have the additional benefit of reducing wastage caused by bulk purchase of medicines. If the ideal dose cannot be formulated, then it is safer to slightly underdose than to overdose. For drugs given on an ongoing basis, extending the dosing frequency or alternating administered dose on different days can average out the required dose over a period of time. Refer to specialist texts or seek advice from a veterinary oncologist for support with individual cases.

In addition to factors under the clinician's control, there is marked variation in chemotherapy tolerance between individual animals. Whilst it can be difficult to predict chemotherapy tolerance, certain breeds (generally collie type) are very sensitive to vinblastine, vincristine, doxorubicin and epirubicin due to the *ABCB1* mutation (a commercial test is available, **see Useful websites**).

Pre-chemotherapy checks

- Haematology. Treatment can be given if the neutrophil count is >3 × 10^9/l and platelet count >100 × 10^9/l. If the neutrophil count is <3 × 10^9/l, withhold treatment and recheck in 3–5 days.
- Biochemistry. Significant organ dysfunction (especially liver) can reduce tolerance to chemotherapy; therefore, biochemistry should be checked prior to commencing chemotherapy and then approximately every 6 months during treatment.
- Urinalysis. Test a free-catch urine sample with a dipstick prior to each cyclophosphamide administration. If blood is noted, suspend cyclophosphamide and culture urine. Chlorambucil can be substituted pending culture result or if the urine culture is negative and therefore consistent with sterile haemorrhagic cystitis.
- Consider pre-treatment sedation or anxiolytic therapy if the patient is too lively or anxious for i.v. chemotherapy to be given safely.
- Catheters should be placed in all cases and only catheters placed by 'first-stick' should be used for chemotherapy. Catheters should be flushed thoroughly with 0.9% NaCl prior to use.

Common adverse events associated with chemotherapy

- All of the chemotherapeutic agents included in the protocols below can induce myelosuppression (usually 7–10 days after treatment) or GI problems (vomiting, diarrhoea and inappetence usually within 4 days of treatment). These are transient and will typically resolve in a few days with appropriate supportive management. It is helpful to prescribe some maropitant for owners to have to hand in case of problems. GI problems can be reduced by fasting the patient prior to treatment.
- Certain breeds (generally collie type, although infrequently Border Collies) are more sensitive to vinblastine, vincristine, doxorubicin and epirubicin due to the *ABCB1* mutation (a commercial test is available, **see Useful websites**). Pending return of genetic test results, commencing chemotherapy for lymphoma with cyclophosphamide is a helpful amendment to standard protocols.
- High doses of prednisolone may induce low-grade GI haemorrhage. GI protectants should be considered when prednisolone doses are 20 mg/m^2 q24h or greater. Omeprazole (1 mg/kg q24h or q12h) is often used by oncologists. Ranitidine with sucralfate is an alternative approach. Cimetidine is avoided due to its effect on the hepatic cytochrome P450 enzyme pathway and the potential for altering metabolism of chemotherapeutics. Famotidine is a good option in cats.
- Cyclophosphamide may induce haemorrhagic cystitis. This risk can be reduced by co-administration of furosemide, enabling free access to water and allowing opportunities for dogs to urinate frequently in the 48 hours after treatment.
- Vincristine and vinblastine are vesicants, and doxorubicin and epirubicin are severe vesicants. Should extravasation occur, contact an oncologist immediately.

APPENDIX I: GENERAL INFORMATION

APPENDIX II: PROTOCOLS

INDEX: THERAPEUTIC CLASS

INDEX: GENERIC AND TRADE NAMES

Chemotherapy protocols for lymphoma

Protocol 1: 25-week CHOP/CEOP protocol

Agent and dose	Week							
	1	2	3	4	6	7	8	9
Vincristine 0.5–0.7 mg/m² i.v.	*		*		*		*	
Cyclophosphamide 250 mg/m² p.o. (or i.v.)		*				*		
Furosemide 1 mg/kg p.o. q12h for 2 days		*				*		
Epirubicin or Doxorubicin 30 mg/m² slow i.v. OR 1 mg/kg if <15 kg				*				*
Prednisolone p.o.	40 mg/m² q24h	30 mg/m² q24h	20 mg/m² q24h	20 mg/m² q48h				

Agent and dose	Week							
	11	13	15	17	19	21	23	25
Vincristine 0.5–0.7 mg/m² i.v.	*		*		*		*	
Cyclophosphamide 250 mg/m² p.o. (or i.v.)		*				*		
Furosemide 1 mg/kg p.o. q12h for 2 days		*				*		
Epirubicin or Doxorubicin 30 mg/m² slow i.v. OR 1 mg/kg if <15 kg				*				*

Week 26 and thereafter: Stop chemotherapy and monitor for relapse (see below for options at recurrence/relapse).

Notes:
- The **Pre-chemotherapy checks** and **Common adverse events associated with chemotherapy** sections above should be reviewed.
- Haematology should be checked prior to each treatment.
- Doxorubicin and epirubicin can cause systolic dysfunction at high cumulative doses (>180 mg/m²). Baseline echocardiography should be considered in all patients, especially those with pre-existing heart

disease. Diagnostic yield of echocardiography in patients with no evidence of heart disease is low. Repeat echocardiography is indicated when the cumulative dose reaches 180 mg/m^2. In cases of cardiac dysfunction, mitoxantrone (5.5 mg/m^2 i.v. over 10 minutes) can be considered as an alternative to doxorubicin or epirubicin.

- 0.9% NaCl, rather than calcium-containing fluids, should be used to dilute doxorubicin or epirubicin.
- Maropitant (1 mg/kg i.v. or p.o) should be given alongside epirubicin or doxorubicin.
- Rapid administration of doxorubicin or epirubicin can induce arrythmia and consequent hypotension. Therefore, these drugs should be administered as a slow infusion over 15–20 minutes.
- Chlorambucil (20 mg/m^2 p.o.) may be given as an alternative to cyclophosphamide if haemorrhagic cystitis develops.
- A nadir neutrophil count should be assessed 7 days after the first doxorubicin or epirubicin treatment. If the neutrophil count is <1 × 10^9/l, decrease dose of the causative chemotherapeutic drug by 10% and prescribe prophylactic antibiotics until the neutrophil count is >1 × 10^9/l. If recurrent, contact an oncologist for advice. If the neutrophil count is <1 × 10^9/l and the patient is pyrexic or unwell, administer i.v. antibiotics and contact an oncologist for advice.

Protocol 2: COP (high dose)
Most oncologists prefer a CHOP protocol, but high-dose COP is a useful and relatively straightforward protocol often used in a general practice setting.

Agent and dose	Week							
	1	2	3	4	5	6	7	
Cyclo-phosphamide 250 mg/m^2 p.o./i.v.	*			*			*	Repeat week 7 every third week
Furosemide 1 mg/kg p.o. q12h for 2 days	*			*			*	After 6 months, repeat week 7 every fourth week
Vincristine 0.5–0.7 mg/ m^2 i.v.	*	*	*	*			*	
Prednisolone p.o.	40 mg/m^2 q24h	30 mg/m^2 q24h	20 mg/m^2 q24h	20 mg/m^2 q48h every week after week 3				

After 12 months: Stop chemotherapy and monitor for relapse (see below for options at recurrence/relapse).

Notes:
- The **Pre-chemotherapy checks** and **Common adverse events associated with chemotherapy** sections above should be reviewed.
- Haematology should be checked prior to each vincristine treatment.
- If the post-treatment neutrophil count is <1 × 10^9/l, decrease dose of the causative chemotherapeutic drug by 10% and prescribe

prophylactic antibiotics until the neutrophil count is $>1 \times 10^9/l$. If recurrent, contact an oncologist for advice. If the neutrophil count is $<1 \times 10^9/l$ and the patient is pyrexic or unwell, administer i.v. antibiotics and contact an oncologist for advice.

- Chlorambucil (20 mg/m^2 p.o.) may be given as an alternative for cyclophosphamide if haemorrhagic cystitis develops.
- Delaying cyclophosphamide until 3 days after vincristine may reduce the frequency of adverse GI events (especially in cats).

Protocol 3: COP (low dose)

The description of this protocol is somewhat misleading in that the summated dose intensity is higher for 'low-dose' COP than for 'high-dose' COP in the induction and early maintenance phases. Anecdotally, there may be a higher risk of adverse events (during these phases) than with high-dose COP, especially in cats. Most oncologists prefer a CHOP type or the high-dose COP protocol.

Induction:

Agent and dose	Day							
	1	2	3	4	5	6	7	
Cyclo-phosphamide 50 mg/m^2 p.o.			*	*	*	*		Repeat every week for 10 weeks
Furosemide 1 mg/kg p.o. q12h			*	*	*	*	*	
Vincristine 0.5 mg/m^2 i.v.	*							
Prednisolone p.o.	Week 1: 40 mg/m^2 q24h Week 2: 30 mg/m^2 q24h Week 3: 20 mg/m^2 q24h Thereafter: 20 mg/m^2 q48h							

Maintenance:

Agent and dose	Day							
	1	2	3	4	5	6	7	
Cyclo-phosphamide 50 mg/m^2 p.o.			*	*	*	*		Repeat every other week until 6 months of treatment (including induction)
Furosemide 1 mg/kg p.o. q12h			*	*	*	*	*	
Vincristine 0.5 mg/m^2 i.v.	*							
Prednisolone p.o.	20 mg/m^2 q48h							

Maintenance after 6 months (if disease in remission):

Agent and dose	Day							Repeat every third week until 12 months of treatment (including induction)
	1	2	3	4	5	6	7	
Cyclo-phosphamide 50 mg/m² p.o.			*	*	*	*		
Furosemide 1 mg/kg p.o. q12h			*	*	*	*	*	
Vincristine 0.5 mg/m² i.v.	*							
Prednisolone p.o.	20 mg/m² q48h							

After 12 months: Stop chemotherapy and monitor for relapse (see below for options at recurrence/relapse).

Notes:
- The **Pre-chemotherapy checks** and **Common adverse events associated with chemotherapy** sections above should be reviewed.
- Haematology should be checked prior to each vincristine treatment.
- If the post-treatment neutrophil count is <1 × 10⁹/l, decrease dose of the causative chemotherapeutic drug by 10% and prescribe prophylactic antibiotics until the neutrophil count is >1 × 10⁹/l. If recurrent, contact an oncologist for advice. If the neutrophil count is <1 × 10⁹/l and the patient is pyrexic or unwell, administer i.v. antibiotics and contact an oncologist for advice.
- Chlorambucil (5 mg/m² p.o. on alternate days) may be given as an alternative for cyclophosphamide if haemorrhagic cystitis develops.

Protocol 4: LPP

LPP is an all-oral protocol suitable for dogs, which is generally considered a rescue protocol but may be considered first-line for treatment of T-cell lymphoma or when injectable chemotherapy cannot be given.

- Day 1: Lomustine 70 mg/m² p.o.
- Days 1–14: Procarbazine 50 mg/m² p.o. q24h.
- Days 1–21: Prednisolone 30 mg/m² p.o. q24h.
- Repeat on a 21-day cycle.

Notes:
- The **Pre-chemotherapy checks** and **Common adverse events associated with chemotherapy** sections above should be reviewed.
- Haematology should be checked prior to each lomustine treatment.
- Alanine aminotransferase (ALT) should be checked prior to each lomustine treatment. An elevation of ALT to >250 IU/l is an indication to stop treatment. Co-administration of S-adenosylmethionine has been shown to reduce the frequency of severe hepatopathies related to lomustine.
- A nadir neutrophil count should be assessed 8–10 days after the first lomustine administration. If the neutrophil count is <1 × 10⁹/l, decrease dose of lomustine by 10% and prescribe prophylactic antibiotics until the neutrophil count is >1 × 10⁹/l. If recurrent,

contact an oncologist for advice. If the neutrophil count is <1 × 10^9/l and the patient is pyrexic or unwell, administer i.v. antibiotics and contact an oncologist for advice.

Disease monitoring and relapse

- **Restaging** – ideally, restaging should be performed at the end of the induction phase (prior to week 6/7 of treatment) and at treatment cessation.
- **Remission** – attaining complete remission is an important prognostic indicator (especially in cats). Complete remission is defined as the lack of identifiable disease (for example, the lymph nodes should be normal on palpation and a cytological assessment should not yield evidence of tumour cells).
- **Relapse** – if a patient completes treatment in remission, they should be monitored monthly for at least 6 months. Most canine multi-centric lymphoma patients relapse after 1–3 months. Many patients that relapse after cessation of treatment can re-attain remission by reintroduction of the original chemotherapy protocol. For patients who relapse during treatment or fail to respond to the reintroduction of treatment, rescue therapy is indicated; commonly used rescue protocols in dogs include asparaginase as a single agent, LOPP and DMAC (or doxorubicin if COP used originally). Rescue therapy in cats is less successful than in dogs.

Chemotherapy protocols for mast cell tumour

Chemotherapy is used in the neoadjuvant setting (to shrink tumours and make excision possible) or as an anti-metastatic treatment for tumours that have metastasized or high-risk tumours (high grade and/or elevated miotic index). Conventional chemotherapy is not recommended for the prevention of recurrence of incompletely resected MCTs as further surgery and radiation are considered more effective; if a medical option is required in this context, a tyrosine kinase inhibitor (toceranib or masitinib) should be used first prior to conventional chemotherapy.

Several protocols have been reported. The most used protocol includes vinblastine and prednisolone as below.

12-week vinblastine and prednisolone protocol

Agent and dose	Week											
	1	2	3	4	5	6	7	8	9	10	11	12
Vinblastine 2 mg/m² i.v. once	*	*	*	*		*		*		*		*
Prednisolone 1 mg/kg p.o. q12h	*	*	*	*	*	*	*	*	*	*	*	*

Notes:
- The **Pre-chemotherapy checks** and **Common adverse events associated with chemotherapy** sections above should be reviewed.
- Haematology should be checked prior to each treatment.
- If the post-treatment neutrophil count is <1 × 10^9/l, decrease dose of vinblastine by 10% and prescribe prophylactic antibiotics until the neutrophil count is >1 × 10^9/l. If recurrent, contact an oncologist for advice. If the neutrophil count is <1 × 10^9/l and the patient is pyrexic or unwell, administer i.v. antibiotics and contact an oncologist for advice.

Disease monitoring and relapse

- **Restaging** – Ideally, restaging should be performed at week 12 for high-risk tumours without known metastasis and after week 4 and at week 12 for tumours with known metastasis. If restaging is clear, further restaging is recommended every 3 months (for a year) for high-risk tumours.
- **Relapse** – If additional metastatic lesions are identified (liver, spleen or lymph nodes) or treatment fails to yield remission, further treatment with lomustine or a tyrosine kinase inhibitor is indicated (contact an oncologist).

References

Smith AN, Klahn S, Phillips B *et al.* (2018) ACVIM small animal consensus statement on safe use of cytotoxic chemotherapeutics in veterinary practice. *Journal of Veterinary Internal Medicine* **32**, 904–913

Immunosuppression protocols

There are many protocols described in the literature for different immune-mediated diseases, but it is essential that the regimen should be individualized with consideration of the animal's weight, body condition, previous exposure/response to glucocorticoids, severity of disease presentation and responsiveness once treatment has started. Three examples are provided here. It is vitally important that the diagnosis of immune-mediated disease is confirmed before undertaking any of these protocols.

Protocol 1: Canine immune-mediated haemolytic anaemia (IMHA) and immune-mediated thrombocytopenia (ITP)

Induction:

Immunosuppression: Prednisolone 40 mg/m^2 (or 2 mg/kg if <15 kg) p.o. q24h, with or without:

- Azathioprine 2 mg/kg p.o. q24h or
- Ciclosporin 5 mg/kg p.o. q12h or
- Mycophenolate mofetil (MMF) 8–12 mg/kg p.o. q12h.

See Appendix I for safety and handling of chemotherapeutic agents. There is no evidence to suggest that the addition of a second immunosuppressive agent from the onset of treatment will produce a better outcome, but it should be considered, particularly in:

- Dogs that experience or are expected to experience severe side effects with prednisolone treatment, so that the prednisolone dose may be decreased more rapidly
- Dogs with features of severe disease, such as marked hyperbilirubinaemia or continued transfusion dependence, because some dogs may not respond adequately to the first agent.

Dexamethasone (0.4 mg/kg i.v. q24h) may be substituted for prednisolone if the patient is unable to tolerate oral medications. Mycophenolate mofetil (7–10 mg/kg i.v. q12h) can be used intravenously if desired when oral medication is not tolerated, but preliminary data suggest this is unlikely to produce a faster onset of action. Once the patient can tolerate oral medications, substitute prednisolone for dexamethasone and switch to oral dosing of MMF if used (8–12 mg/kg p.o. q12h) or, if preferred, azathioprine at the above doses.

A single dose of vincristine (0.02 mg/kg i.v.) may be used in cases of ITP because it may increase platelet numbers, but the extent of its benefits is unclear. Dyserythropoiesis may be observed (on blood smears) in such cases but is clinically insignificant.

Antithrombotics: Clopidogrel (1–2 mg/kg p.o. q24h) is indicated for dogs with IMHA that have a platelet count above 30×10^9/l, with or without low molecular weight heparins (e.g. dalteparin at 150–175 IU/kg s.c. q8h) if there is clinical evidence of thromboembolic disease. Discontinue on remission (or once the prednisolone is discontinued).

Antibiotics: Not required unless there is a documented infection or known risk of infection (e.g. previous endocarditis). Empirical treatment with doxycycline (10 mg/kg p.o. q24h) may be indicated pending tests for tick-borne diseases in dogs with a history of travel or known tick exposure.

Gastrointestinal protection: In general, not required. In cases with known or suspected GI bleeding (melaena, haematemesis), omeprazole (1 mg/kg p.o., i.v. q12h) offers effective suppression of gastric acid secretion. The practice of administering ranitidine, for example, to every animal receiving high doses of steroids is not necessary and likely ineffective.

Relapse and rescue

If a mild relapse (e.g. a fall in packed cell volume (PCV) of <5% without any clinical signs of anaemia) occurs following documented remission, this may be treated by reinstigating the drug dosages used at the last visit when the animal was in remission. Severe relapses should be treated by reinstigation of induction doses of all drugs used initially. If this is ineffective, or if rescue is to be attempted during the initial induction phase of treatment (due to progressive deterioration), then additional immunosuppressants may be added. In cases of poor disease control, three immunosuppressive drugs may be used concurrently, but this carries a risk of opportunistic (fungal) infections. Note that azathioprine and MMF should not be administered concurrently in the same patient.

An infusion of human immunoglobulin (0.5–1.0 g/kg i.v. over 6–8 hours) may be administered in dogs not responding to other forms of treatment, but clinical benefit has not been proven.

In the non-acute setting, or if long-term control is necessary in a patient that has previously failed all other orally administered drugs, then leflunomide (2 mg/kg p.o. q24h) or splenectomy (if it can be tolerated by the patient) should be considered.

Decreasing doses:

Principles for dose reduction: Reduction of the prednisolone dose should be considered as soon as a clinical response is apparent (resolution of agglutination, spherocytosis, hyperbilirubinaemia/ haemolysed plasma, and the PCV is stable or increasing); it is not necessary to wait until the PCV returns to a normal value. The prednisolone dose should be decreased by 25–33% every 2–3 weeks, depending on the severity of the side effects and whether the features of disease are well controlled. Expected overall duration of treatment is approximately 3–5 months provided there is no relapse.

Week	Glucocorticoid	Ciclosporin/MMF/Azathioprine
Remission (0)	1 mg/kg q24h	UC
2	0.75 mg/kg q24h	For azathioprine, reduce to every other day dosing. Otherwise, UC
4	0.5 mg/kg q24h	UC
6	0.5 mg/kg q48h	UC
8	UC	For ciclosporin or MMF, 50% dose reduction (or extension of dosing interval). For azathioprine, UC
10	0.25 mg/kg q48h	UC
12	STOP (or further 4 weeks)	UC
16		STOP

UC = dose unchanged.

Notes: Complete blood count to be rechecked at each visit (including 4 and 8 weeks after cessation of therapy) and remission confirmed prior to each dose reduction. Liver parameters should be rechecked at remission and monthly if using azathioprine.

Protocol 2: Feline immune-mediated haemolytic anaemia

Induction:

Immunosuppression: Prednisolone: 3–4 mg/kg p.o. q24h, with or without:

- Chlorambucil: >4 kg bodyweight, 2 mg p.o. q48h; <4 kg bodyweight, 2 mg p.o. q72h or
- Ciclosporin: 5 mg/kg p.o. q12h or
- Mycophenolic acid (MPA): 10 mg/kg p.o. q12h.

See Appendix I for safety and handling of chemotherapeutic agents. If the patient is unable to tolerate oral medications, then dexamethasone (0.6–1.0 mg/kg i.v. q24h) may be substituted for prednisolone, and MMF (7–10 mg/kg i.v. q12h) may be substituted for MPA. Note that azathioprine should not be used in cats.

Antithrombotics: Avoid in cats as there is no evidence of a risk of thrombosis in cats with IMHA, but there is a risk of side effects.

Antibiotics: Not required unless there is a documented infection or known risk of infection (e.g. previous endocarditis) or known exposure to ticks. Empirical treatment with doxycycline (10 mg/kg p.o. q24h) may be indicated pending tests for *Mycoplasma* spp.

Gastrointestinal protection: Not required unless GI bleeding has been diagnosed, in which case effective suppression of gastric acid production is required. Current evidence suggests that only famotidine (1 mg/kg p.o. q12h) or omeprazole (1 mg/kg p.o., i.v. q12h) will provide this. The practice of administering ranitidine, for example, to every animal receiving high doses of steroids is not necessary and likely ineffective.

Relapse and rescue

See **Protocol 1**, above, for details.

Decreasing doses: See **Protocol 1**, above, for details.
(**NB:** reports of feline ITP are too rare to provide a protocol for treatment, but it is likely that a similar approach should be adopted.)

Protocol 3: Steroid-responsive meningitis–arteritis (SRMA)

Induction:

Immunosuppression: Prednisolone: 2 mg/kg p.o. q24h (as a single dose or divided) for 7–14 days. Dexamethasone (0.4 mg/kg i.v. q24h) may be substituted for prednisolone for the first 2 days if the patient is unable to tolerate oral medications.

Antibiotics: Not required unless there is a documented infection, known risk of infection (e.g. previous endocarditis) or known exposure to ticks.

Gastrointestinal protection: In general, not required.

Remission: If remission is achieved, 1 mg/kg p.o. q24h for 6 weeks, followed by 0.5 mg/kg p.o. q24h for 6 weeks, followed by 0.5 mg/kg p.o. q48h for 6 weeks, followed by 0.5 mg/kg p.o. q72h for 6 weeks, then stop.

Relapse: In the event of a relapse during or after completion of the protocol (or if remission is not achieved), 2 mg/kg p.o. q24h can be reinstigated (or continued if remission not achieved) for a further 2 weeks and then continued as the 24-week remission protocol.

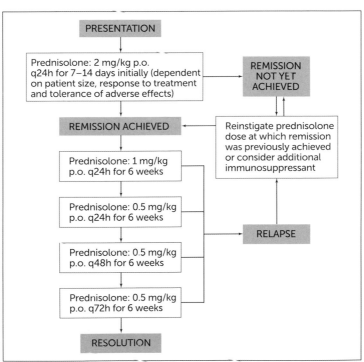

Adapted from Lowrie M, Penderis J, McLaughlin M, Eckersall PD and Anderson TJ (2009) Steroid-responsive meningitis–arteritis: a prospective study of potential disease markers, prednisolone treatment, and long-term outcome in 20 dogs (2006–2008). *Journal of Veterinary Internal Medicine* **23**, 862–870

Mycobacterial protocol for cats

In the UK, the majority of mycobacterial infections in cats are caused by tuberculous mycobacteria. The initial large culture study showed ~35% of infections to be caused by *Mycobacterium microti* (~20%) or *Mycobacterium bovis* (~15%) (Gunn-Moore *et al.*, 2011ab), with ~50% of cases failing to grow. However, further, as yet unpublished work using the more sensitive polymerase chain reaction (PCR) approach found a similar proportion of cases caused by *M. bovis*, but a higher proportion caused by *M. microti* (~35%) (Gunn-Moore and O'Halloran, unpublished data). The most common non-tuberculous mycobacteria (NTM) are in the *M. avium* complex (MAC), and a wide range of NTM can infect cats.

It is important to consider the factors below before undertaking treatment:

- **There is a potential zoonotic risk** – the disease may be caused by a member of the tuberculosis (TB) complex. All members of the affected cat's household must be considered. It is important to determine any potentially immunosuppressed individuals (e.g. people with human immunodeficiency virus or who are undergoing chemotherapy). Treatment is not advised where such individuals may be exposed. Treatment is also not advised if the affected cat has generalized disease, cavitating lesions within the respiratory tract or extensive draining cutaneous lesions as these may increase the risk of transmission
- **Treatment is almost always long term** – this can be difficult to maintain given patient non-compliance, the inherent toxicity of some of the drugs and the financial costs involved. In some cases, the drugs may at best suppress disease and indefinite treatment may be required (Sieber-Ruckstuhl *et al.*, 2007; Greene and Gunn-Moore, 2011). Uncomplicated cutaneous cases with or without diffuse pulmonary changes carry the most favourable prognosis. Placement of a feeding tube may be required to improve compliance
- **Interim management** – pending a definitive diagnosis, interim therapy with a fluoroquinolone is recommended in cases of localized cutaneous infection (Gunn-Moore *et al.*, 2010). Pradofloxacin (or moxifloxacin) is recommended as it is more effective against mycobacteria than the older fluoroquinolones, such as marbofloxacin (Govendir *et al.*, 2011). With more extensive disease, double or triple therapy is advised (Greene and Gunn-Moore, 2011); i.e., start with pradofloxacin and azithromycin, pending confirmation, then add rifampin when TB is confirmed.

Treatment of mycobacterial disease

Previously, anti-tuberculosis treatment was given in an initial and then a continuation phase (Greene and Gunn-Moore, 2011); however, it is now known that it is better to give all three drugs for 4–6 months, depending on the extent of disease, and always for at least 2 months following complete resolution of the lesions. In those cats where triple therapy is not feasible, treatment should still involve two drugs and should be given for a minimum of 6–9 months. Extensive clinical experience supports using rifampin, pradofloxacin and azithromycin as a starting point; however, NTM infections may need different combinations. Potentially useful drugs for the treatment of feline mycobacterial disease are given in the table below.

Drug	Uses	Dose (mg/kg)	Effects of toxicity
Pradofloxacin [a]	First-line treatment for TB, NTM	3–5 p.o. q24h	Reversible neutropenia, seizures in cats with CNS disease
Rifampin [b]	First-line treatment for TB, MAC, NTM	10–15 p.o. q24h	Side effects in ~40% of cases, with severe side effects in ~5%. Poor palatability, nausea, discoloration of body fluids, generalized erythema and pruritus, hyperaesthesia, CNS signs, hepatotoxicity, anaphylaxis Teratogenic
Clarithromycin [c,d]	First-line treatment for TB, MAC, FLS, NTM	7–15 p.o. q12h	Possible pinnal or generalized erythema, hepatotoxicity, possible GI signs
Azithromycin [c]		5–15 p.o. q24h	
Isoniazid [b]	Second-line treatment for TB Prophylaxis for TB	10–20 p.o. q24h 10 p.o. q24h	Hepatotoxicity, peripheral neuritis, seizures, acute renal failure
Ethambutol [b]	Second-line treatment for TB	10–25 p.o. q24h	Optic neuritis
Pyrazinamide [b,e]	Second-line treatment for TB	15–40 p.o. q24h	Hepatotoxicity, GI signs
Dihydro-streptomycin [b]	Second-line treatment for TB	15 i.m. q24h	Ototoxicity
Clofazimine [b,f]	Treatment for FLS, NTM	4–8 p.o. q24–48h Max. 25 total	Hepatotoxicity, GI signs, discoloration of body fluids, photosensitization, pitting corneal lesions
Doxycycline [g]	Second-line treatment for NTM, MAC	5–10 p.o. q12–24h	GI signs, oesophagitis
Amikacin [b]		10–15 i.v., i.m., s.c. q24h	Nephrotoxic, ototoxic
Cefoxitin		20–30 i.v., i.m., s.c. q6–8h	Pain on i.m., s.c. injection

Second-line treatments for tuberculosis should be reserved for resistant infections. Ensure all aspects of cascade prescribing have been considered before using drugs only authorized for human use. Data from Kaufman *et al.*, 1995; Gelatt *et al.*, 2001; Bennett, 2007; Sieber-Ruckstuhl *et al.*, 2007.

FLS = feline leprosy syndrome; MAC = *M. avium-intracellulare* complex; NTM = non-tuberculous mycobacteria; TB = tuberculosis. [a] The authors do not recommend enrofloxacin as it has been associated with retinal degeneration; other than the newer fluoroquinolones (pradofloxacin and moxifloxacin), most others are not effective against MAC infections. [b] These drugs may cause potentially serious side effects (e.g. hepatotoxicity or nephrotoxicity); it is advisable to monitor use closely, including routine haematology and serum biochemistry 2 weeks after starting treatment and again following any change in the cat's demeanour. [c] *M. tuberculosis* and some NTM, potentially including MAC infections, can have inducible resistance genes to macrolides, meaning they appear susceptible *in vitro* but are resistant *in vivo*; where possible (limited by GI signs), use higher doses to reduce the risk of resistance. [d] Particularly useful when treating MAC infections. [e] Not effective against *M. bovis* infection. [f] Can be difficult to obtain. [g] Give with food or give water after the medication to avoid oesophageal injury.

Treatment of NTM

At a minimum, use of a fluoroquinolone is suggested while waiting for PCR or culture results. The new fluoroquinolones (e.g. pradofloxacin or moxifloxacin) are recommended as they have an extended spectrum of activity, which includes some NTM, and they are even effective against MAC infections (Govendir *et al.*, 2011).

MAC infections are particularly difficult to treat (Jordan *et al.*, 1994). Clarithromycin should be included (Piersimoni *et al.*, 1995), ideally in combination with rifampin (Tomioka *et al.*, 2002) ± another antibiotic according to culture and susceptibility testing, such as doxycycline (Baral *et al.*, 2006) or, from human studies, ethambutol (Esteban *et al.*, 2012). Pyogranulomatous panniculitis requires long-term antibiotics and radical well planned surgery: e.g., doxycycline for several weeks, then radical surgical excision and local reconstruction plus parenteral gentamicin perioperatively for 3–5 days, followed by a prolonged course (3–6 months) of a new fluoroquinolone (White *et al.*, 1983; Malik *et al.*, 1994, 2000, 2004). Non-surgical cases may require double or triple therapy.

Feline leprosy-type infections (feline leprosy syndrome; FLS) can usually be treated with surgical removal of small nodules, which may be curative. Where medical management is needed, clarithromycin, pradofloxacin and rifampin or clofazimine are recommended. Doxycycline, fluoroquinolones and aminoglycosides may also be useful (Mundell 1988; Malik *et al.*, 2002, 2006a; Courtin *et al.*, 2007; Malik *et al.*, 2013). Dapsone is considered too toxic for use in cats (Hamanda *et al.*, 1991) and is antagonistic to clofazimine. Treatment should be continued until the lesions have completely resolved, and ideally for a further 2–3 months to reduce the risk of recurrence; however, some cases require life-long clarithromycin to prevent recurrence (Malik *et al.*, 2013).

APPENDIX I: GENERAL INFORMATION

APPENDIX II: PROTOCOLS

INDEX: THERAPEUTIC CLASS

INDEX: GENERIC AND TRADE NAMES

Mycobacterial species	Susceptibility	Generally resistant
M. avium	Clarithromycin, rifampin, doxycycline, ethambutol, pradofloxacin, clofazimine, amikacin **Recommended:** clarithromycin or azithromycin + rifampin + another drug	Older fluoroquinolones, cefovecin Potentially inadvisable to give just a new fluoroquinolone + clarithromycin or azithromycin
M. fortuitum	**Recommended:** pradofloxacin + amikacin (100%), cefoxitin (94%), older fluoroquinolones (75%), clarithromycin (~75%), clofazimine, rifampin, gentamicin or doxycycline (29%[a])	Trimethoprim ± sulphonamide, cefovecin, clarithromycin
M. smegmatis	Fluoroquinolones, tetracyclines, gentamicin, trimethoprim ± sulphonamide, clofazimine **Recommended:** pradofloxacin + doxycycline	Clarithromycin, cefovecin
M. chelonae-abscessus	Amikacin (100%), cefoxitin (94%), ciprofloxacin (75%), clarithromycin (71%[a]), pradofloxacin, clofazimine **Recommended:** azithromycin or clarithromycin + another drug	Many oral medications, including doxycycline + older fluoroquinolones Do not give pradofloxacin or moxifloxacin with azithromycin or clarithromycin
M. xenopi	Fluoroquinolones, clarithromycin, rifampin, clofazimine	
M. simiae	Rifampin, clarithromycin, fluoroquinolones, amikacin, clofazimine	
M. thermoresistible	Rifampin, doxycycline, clarithromycin	
M. terrae	Clarithromycin, azithromycin, ethambutol	
M. genavense	Clarithromycin, fluoroquinolones, ethambutol	

Susceptibility and resistance of mycobacterial species to potential drugs for the treatment of NTM in cats. Data from Studdert and Hughes, 1992; Malik *et al.*, 1994, 2000, 2004, 2006ab; Michaud, 1994; Kiehn *et al.*, 1996; Foster *et al.*, 1999; Smith *et al.*, 2000; Jang and Hirsh, 2002; Tomioka *et al.*, 2002; Dietrich *et al.*, 2003; Govendir *et al.*, 2011; Cho *et al.*, 2012; van Ingen *et al.*, 2012; Bennie *et al.*, 2014. [a] Other studies have shown these drugs to be either more or less effective.

Managing side effects: Cats may suffer side effects while receiving treatment for mycobacterial infections, especially with rifampin. While side effects can be concerning to owners and veterinary professionals, this drug is essential for optimizing the outcome of treating cats with TB and is the only drug in the triple therapy approach with activity against non-replicating bacteria.

To help manage dermatological side effects such as pruritus, oedema and erythema, chlorphenamine is advised (2–4 mg/cat p.o. q8–12h). Focal pruritic lesions can also be managed with topical hydrocortisone aceponate spray.

Hepatotoxicity is another possible side effect of rifampin, which may manifest clinically as hyporexia, nausea or vomiting, or may be identified with increased enzymes on serum biochemistry. *S*-Adenosylmethionine (SAMe) (20 mg/kg p.o. q24h) is one hepatoprotectant agent that is widely used in cases of drug-induced liver toxicity, as well as in cases of liver disease.

An intriguing alternative agent is *N*-acetylcysteine (NAC) (600 mg/cat p.o. q12h); while pharmacological data are lacking for its use in cats, it is safe and well tolerated. NAC has an unpleasant taste and smell, so giving whole capsules is usually advised. Nausea and vomiting are potential side effects, and drooling occurs when the capsule content is mixed with too little food. Since NAC can cause bronchial spasm, it should be used with caution in animals with asthma. NAC helps to restore blood glutathione concentrations, and thus antioxidant capacity. It has also been shown to reduce bacterial counts and the severity of lesions. Restoration of antioxidant capacity helps reduce the toxic side effects of anti-TB drugs such as rifampin and isoniazid, which are mediated by oxidant-driven damage to the liver. Short-term studies have also shown that NAC has some direct anti-mycobacterial activity and can reduce growth of bacteria both *in vitro* and *in vivo*.

References

Baral RM, Metcalfe SS, Krockenberger MB *et al.* (2006) Disseminated *Mycobacterium avium* infection in young cats: overrepresentation of Abyssinian cats. *Journal of Feline Medicine and Surgery* **8**, 23–44

Bennett AD, Lalor S, Schwarz T and Gunn-Moore DA (2011) Radiographic findings in cats with mycobacterial infections. *Journal of Feline Medicine and Surgery* **13**, 718–724

Bennie C, To J, Martin P and Govendir M (2015) *In vitro* interaction of some drug combinations to inhibit rapidly growing mycobacteria isolates from cats and dogs and these isolates' susceptibility to cefovecin and clofazimine. *Australian Veterinary Journal* **93**, 40–45

Cho JH, Yu CH, Jin MK *et al.* (2012) *Mycobacterium kansasii* pericarditis in a kidney transplant recipient: a case report and comprehensive review of the literature. *Transplant Infectious Disease*, E50–E55

Courtin F, Huerre M, Fyfe J, Dumas P and Boschiroli ML (2007) A case of feline leprosy caused by *Mycobacterium lepraemurium* originating from the island of Kythira (Greece): diagnosis and treatment. *Journal of Feline Medicine and Surgery* **9**, 238–241

Dietrich U, Arnold P, Guscetti F, Pfyffer GE and Spiess B (2003) Ocular manifestation of disseminated *Mycobacterium simiae* infection in a cat. *Journal of Small Animal Practice* **44**, 121–125

Esteban J, García-Pedrazuela M, Muñoz-Egea MC and Alcaide F (2012) Current treatment of nontuberculous mycobacteriosis: an update. *Expert Opinion on Pharmacotherapy* **13**, 967–986

Foster SF, Martin P, Davis W *et al.* (1999) Chronic pneumonia caused by *Mycobacterium thermoresistibile* in a cat. *Journal of Small Animal Practice* **40**, 433–438

Gelatt KN, van der Woerdt A, Ketring KL *et al.* (2001) Enrofloxacin-associated retinal degeneration in cats. *Veterinary Ophthalmology* **4**, 99–106

Govendir M, Norris JM, Hansen T *et al.* (2011) Susceptibility of rapidly growing mycobacteria and *Nocardia* isolates from cats and dogs to pradofloxacin. *Veterinary Microbiology* **153**, 240–245

Greene CE and Gunn-Moore DA (2011) Mycobacterial Infections. In: *Infectious Diseases of the Dog and Cat, 4th edn*, ed. J Sykes and CE Greene, pp. 495–510. Saunders, Philadelphia

Gunn-Moore DA (2010) Mycobacterial infections in cats and dogs. In: *Textbook of Veterinary Internal Medicine, 7th edn*, ed SJ Ettinger and EC Feldman, pp. 875–881. Saunders, Philadelphia

Gunn-Moore DA, McFarland SE, Brewer JI *et al.* (2011a) Mycobacterial disease in cats in Great Britain: 1 bacterial species, geographical distribution and clinical presentation of 339 cases. *Journal of Feline Medicine and Surgery* **13**, 934–944

Gunn-Moore DA, McFarland SE, Brewer JI *et al.* (2011b) Mycobacterial disease in cats in Great Britain: 2 histopathology, treatment and outcome of 339 cases. *Journal of Feline Medicine and Surgery* **13**, 945–952

Hamada K, Hiyoshi T, Kobayashi S *et al.* (1991) Anticonvulsive effect of dapsone (4,4'-diaminodiphenyl sulfone) on amygdala-kindled seizures in rats and cats. *Epilepsy Research* **10**, 93–102

Jang SS and Hirsh DC (2002) Rapidly growing members of the genus *Mycobacterium* affecting dogs and cats. *Journal of the American Animal Hospital Association* **38**, 217–220

Jordan HL, Cohn LA and Armstrong PJ (1994) Disseminated *Mycobacterium avium* complex infection in three Siamese cats. *Journal of the American Veterinary Medical Association* **204**, 90–93

Kaufman AC, Green CE, Rakich PM and Weigner DD (1995) Treatment of localized *Mycobacterium avium* complex infection with clofazimine and doxycycline in a cat. *Journal of the American Veterinary Medical Association* **207**, 457–459

Kiehn TE, Hoefer H, Bottger EC *et al.* (1996) *Mycobacterium genavense* infections in pet animals. *Journal of Clinical Microbiology* **34**, 1840–1842

Malik R, Hughes MS, James G *et al.* (2002) Feline leprosy: two different clinical syndromes. *Journal of Feline Medicine and Surgery* **4**, 43–59

Malik R, Hughes MS, Martin P and Wigney D (2006a) Feline leprosy syndromes. In: *Infectious Diseases of the Dog & Cat, 3rd edn*, ed CE Greene, pp. 477–480. Saunders, Philadelphia

Malik R, Hunt GB, Goldsmid SE *et al.* (1994) Diagnosis and treatment of pyogranulomatous panniculitis due to *Mycobacterium smegmatis* in cats. *Journal of Small Animal Practice* **35**, 524–530

Malik R, Martin P, Wigney D and Foster S (2006b) Infections caused by rapidly growing mycobcateria. In: *Infectious Diseases of the Dog & Cat, 3rd edn*, ed. CE Greene, pp. 482–488. Saunders, Philadelphia

Malik R, Shaw SE, Griffin C *et al.* (2004) Infections of the subcutis and skin of dogs caused by rapidly growing mycobacteria. *Journal of Small Animal Practice* **45**, 485–494

Malik R, Smits B, Reppas G *et al.* (2013) Ulcerated and nonulcerated nontuberculous cutaneous mycobacterial granulomas in cats and dogs. Veterinary Dermatology 24, 146–153

Malik R, Wigney DI, Dawson D *et al.* (2000) Infection of the subcutis and skin of cats with rapidly growing mycobacteria: a review of microbiological and clinical findings. *Journal of Feline Medicine and Surgery* **2**, 35–48

Michaud AJ (1994) The use of clofazimine as treatment for *Mycobacterium fortuitum* in a cat. *Feline Practice* **22**, 3

Mundell AC (1995) Mycobacterial skin diseases in small animals. In: *Kirk's Current Veterinary Therapy, XII*, ed. J Bonagura, pp 622–625. Saunders, Philadelphia

Piersimoni C, Tortoli E, Mascellino MT *et al.* (1995) Activity of seven antimicrobial agents, alone and in combination, against AIDS-associated isolates of *Mycobacterium avium* complex. *Journal of Antimicrobial Chemotherapy* **36**, 497–502

Sieber-Ruckstuhl NS, Sessions JK, Sanchez S, Latimer KS and Greene CE (2007) Long-term cure of disseminated *Mycobacterium avium* infection in a cat. *Veterinary Record* **160**, 131–132

Smith DS, Lindholm-Levy P, Huitt GA, Heifets LB and Cook JL (2000) *Mycobacterium terrae*: case reports, literature review, and *in vitro* antibiotic susceptibility testing. *Clinical Infectious Disease* **30**, 444–453

Studdert VP and Hughes KL (1992) Treatment of opportunistic mycobacteria infections with enrofloxacin in cats. *Journal of the American Veterinary Medical Association* **201**, 1388–1390

Tomioka H, Sano C, Sato K and Shimizu T (2002) Antimicrobial activities of clarithromycin, gatifloxacin and sitafloxacin, in combination with various antimycobacterial drugs against extracellular and intramacrophage *Mycobacterium*

avium complex. *International Journal of Antimicrobial Agents* **19**, 139–145
van Ingen J, Totten SE, Helstrom NK *et al.* (2012) *In vitro* synergy between clofazimine and amikacin in treatment of nontuberculous mycobacterial disease. *Antimicrobial Agents and Chemotherapy* **56**, 6324–6327
White SD, Ihrke PJ, Stannard AA *et al.* (1983) Cutaneous atypical mycobacteriosis in cats. *Journal of the American Veterinary Medical Association* **182**, 1218–1222

Sedation/immobilization protocols

Sedative combinations for dogs

Acepromazine as sole agent: Acepromazine alone is not a particularly effective sedative. For further information see monograph. Because larger breeds seem to be more sensitive to acepromazine, it is recommended not to exceed a total dose of 1 mg/patient.

Acepromazine/opioid mixtures (neuroleptanalgesia): Acepromazine used in combination with opioid analgesics reduces the dose requirement of both components and also the incidence of adverse effects. Acepromazine (0.01–0.03 mg/kg, except in Boxers 0.005–0.01 mg/kg, use lower doses i.v.) can be combined with:

- Pethidine (2–10 mg/kg i.m.)
- Methadone (0.1–0.5 mg/kg i.m., i.v.)
- Papaveretum (0.05–0.4 mg/kg i.v., i.m.)
- Buprenorphine (0.02–0.03 mg/kg i.v., i.m)
- Butorphanol (0.1–0.4 mg/kg i.v., i.m.).

Alpha-2 agonists as sole agents: Although authorized for single-agent use, it is generally preferable to use medetomidine or dexmedetomidine in combination with opioids (see below).

Recommended dose in dogs and cats of medetomidine is 5–20 µg (micrograms)/kg i.m. and of dexmedetomidine is 2.5–10 µg/kg i.m. Lower doses of medetomidine (1–10 µg/kg) or dexmedetomidine (1–5 µg/kg) may be given i.v. At higher doses, marked cardiovascular effects (mainly bradyarrhythmias) should be expected.

Adverse effects may be antagonized with i.m. atipamezole at 5 times the agonist dose rate. The (unauthorized) i.v. route is preferable in critical situations.

For information on xylazine, see below.

The use of alpha-2 agonists for sedation is only recommended in healthy animals.

Alpha-2 agonist/opioid mixtures: Including opioids with medetomidine or dexmedetomidine lowers the dose required to achieve a given level of sedation, thereby limiting the marked effects that alpha-2 agonists exert on cardiopulmonary function. If sedation is still inadequate, it is better to proceed to induction of general anaesthesia using an i.v. induction agent, such as alfaxalone or propofol, rather than by giving a repeated or higher dose of alpha-2 agonist.

Medetomidine or dexmedetomidine, at the doses described above, can be combined with:

- Pethidine (2–10 mg/kg i.m.)
- Methadone (0.1–0.5 mg/kg slow i.v., i.m.)
- Buprenorphine (0.02–0.03 mg/kg slow i.v., i.m.)
- Butorphanol (0.1–0.4 mg/kg slow i.v., i.m.).

Although xylazine (1–3 mg/kg) may be used alone or in combinations with opioids, given i.m. or i.v. (unauthorized), its use in dogs and cats has been superseded by use of medetomidine or dexmedetomidine and it is not recommended. Adverse effects may be antagonized with i.m. or i.v. atipamezole, although this use is unauthorized.

Acepromazine/alpha-2 agonist/opioid mixtures: A mixture of acepromazine (up to 0.03 mg/kg) with any of the combinations given for alpha-2 agonists and alpha-2 agonist/opioid mixtures (higher end of dose ranges) is suitable for the chemical restraint of aggressive dogs. Severe depression can be antagonized using naloxone and atipamezole.

Low doses of acepromazine (0.01 mg/kg) and medetomidine (5–10 µg (micrograms)/kg) or dexmedetomidine (2.5–5 µg/kg) combined with opioid agonist drugs provide profound sedation with less cardiovascular depression than with an alpha-2 agonist or acepromazine as the sole agent in combination with the opioid.

Benzodiazepines and benzodiazepine/opioid mixtures:
Benzodiazepines do not reliably sedate healthy dogs when used alone; indeed, stimulation ranging from increased motor activity to gross excitation may be seen. The risk of excitation is proportional to the health of the recipient: the chances of producing sedation are highest (but not guaranteed) in very sick, young or older cases. Diazepam (authorized) or midazolam (unauthorized) (0.2–0.3 mg/kg i.v.) given during anaesthesia can smooth recovery in animals prone to excitability, provided adequate analgesia is present.

Opioid/benzodiazepine mixtures are satisfactory and relatively safe in critically ill animals. These combinations are more effective when given i.v. (with the exception of pethidine). Transient excitation may occur when given by this route. When given i.m., excitation is unlikely although the depth of sedation is also reduced. Midazolam or diazepam at the dose described above can be given with:

- Pethidine (2–10 mg/kg i.m.)
- Methadone (0.1–0.5 mg/kg i.v., i.m.)
- Papaveretum (0.2–0.5 mg/kg i.v., i.m.)
- Buprenorphine (0.02–0.03 mg/kg i.v., i.m.)
- Butorphanol (0.1–0.4 mg/kg i.v., i.m.)
- Fentanyl (0.01 mg/kg slow i.v.).

It is preferable to use midazolam (unauthorized) when choosing the i.m. route, as the absorption of diazepam via this route can be variable.

Alfaxalone: Although not authorized for this use, 2 mg/kg i.m. will provide sedation in dogs that lasts 10–15 minutes. The volume of injectate precludes use of this technique in medium- to large-breed dogs. Alfaxalone can be used in conjunction with opioids and benzodiazepines.

Notes:
- A well managed light level of general (inhalational) anaesthesia is often safer than heavy sedation in sick animals.
- Neuroleptanalgesic combinations are safer than alpha-2 agonist/opioid mixtures, but are less likely to produce adequate conditions for minor operations or investigations involving abnormal body positions. Furthermore, only the opioid component can be antagonized.
- Most of the aforementioned combinations will have a profound sparing effect on i.v. and inhalational anaesthetics, should a general anaesthetic be required after sedation. This is particularly true of combinations containing alpha-2 agonists.

- Any stress induced in the patient may decrease the effectiveness of sedative drugs and higher initial doses may be required.
- Close monitoring of the cardiorespiratory system is recommended during sedation.

Sedative combinations for cats

Acepromazine: Acepromazine alone is not a particularly effective sedative and increasing the dose incurs the same problems as in dogs. Doses of 0.01–0.05 mg/kg may be given i.v., i.m. or s.c. Cats often require higher doses of acepromazine than dogs to achieve comparable sedation. Recumbency is normally not achievable in cats with acepromazine sedation.

Neuroleptanalgesia: Neuroleptanalgesic combinations confer the same advantages in cats as in dogs. Acepromazine (0.01–0.05 mg/kg) can be combined with:

- Pethidine (2–10 mg/kg i.m.)
- Methadone (0.1–0.5 mg/kg i.v., i.m.)
- Buprenorphine (0.02–0.03 mg/kg i.v., i.m.)
- Butorphanol (0.1–0.4 mg/kg i.v., i.m.).

  Use the lower end of the dose ranges i.v.

Alpha-2 agonists as sole agents and alpha-2 agonist/opioid mixtures: See information given for dogs. Adverse effects may be antagonized with i.m. atipamezole at 2.5 times the agonist dose rate; the (unauthorized) i.v. route is preferable in critical situations.

Benzodiazepines: Diazepam (0.2–0.3 mg/kg) or midazolam (0.2–0.3 mg/kg) i.v. can provide satisfactory sedation in very sick cats. The inclusion of opioids at doses given for alpha-2 agonist/opioid mixtures may improve conditions, but benzodiazepine/opioid combinations do not provide reliable sedation in most cats.

Ketamine and ketamine-based techniques: Ketamine is relatively safe in ill animals, but high doses cause prolonged recoveries and are associated with muscle rigidity. Acepromazine (0.05–0.1 mg/kg) with midazolam (0.25 mg/kg) and ketamine (2.5–7.5 mg/kg), mixed and injected i.m., provides good conditions with only modest cardiopulmonary depression. The higher doses of ketamine should be used in excitable animals undergoing more stimulating interventions.

Alternatives: Ketamine (2.5 mg/kg) combined with diazepam or midazolam (0.2–0.3 mg/kg) i.v. provides profound sedation which lasts for about 15–20 minutes. Higher doses of ketamine (5 mg/kg) may be required if given i.m. This combination is preferred over ketamine/acepromazine combinations in sick cats. Diazepam can cause pain on injection, therefore, use of midazolam is preferred.

Ketamine (5 mg/kg) with medetomidine 10–40 μg (micrograms)/kg i.m. produces profound sedation but should only be used in healthy cats. An opioid can be added to this mixture to provide analgesia or further sedation. Atipamezole may be given if severe problems are encountered.

Although ketamine elimination depends heavily on renal function in cats, a full recovery still occurs, albeit more slowly, in cats with renal disease or urinary tract obstruction. However, low doses should be us... in such cases.

Alfaxalone: Although not authorized for this use, 2–3 mg/kg i.m. or s.c. will provide sedation in cats lasting 10–15 minutes. Alfaxalone can be combined with an opioid and/or midazolam to improve sedation.

Notes:
- Careful handling and restraint to achieve injection of sedative is preferred, but a crush cage is useful for restraining fearful aggressive cats. If injection of sedatives proves impossible, anaesthesia can be induced using a large induction chamber into which volatile anaesthetic agents can be delivered via an anaesthetic machine. Most of the aforementioned combinations will have a profound sparing effect on i.v. and inhalational anaesthetics should a general anaesthetic be required after sedation. This is particularly true of combinations containing alpha-2 agonists.
- The high body surface area:volume of cats results in rapid heat loss compared with dogs. Attention to thermoregulation must be diligent.
- A well managed light level of general (inhalational) anaesthesia is frequently safer than heavy sedation in sick animals.
- Any stress induced in the patient may decrease the effectiveness of sedative drugs and higher initial doses may be required.
- Close monitoring of the cardiorespiratory system is recommended during sedation.

Sedation protocol for dogs with the *ABCB1* gene

The *ABCB1* gene, previously known as the *MDR1* gene, codes for P-glycoprotein, which is a transmembrane ATPase that transports small molecules out of the cell in an energy dependent process. This P-glycoprotein is also an important component of the blood–brain barrier where it serves to protect the central nervous system from exposure to some drugs. A mutation in the *ABCB1* gene has been described; dogs that are homozygous or heterozygous for the *ABCB1* gene mutation have an increased sensitivity to certain drugs used for sedation, including acepromazine, morphine, butorphanol and fentanyl.

Collies show the highest frequency of the mutation, with approximately 75% of dogs from this group carrying at least one copy of the mutant gene. Other breeds that frequently carry the mutation include the Australian Shepherd, Shetland Sheepdog and Old English Sheepdog.

Recommendations for sedation

Recommendations are largely empirical because there are limited data on the effect of the mutation on the pharmacodynamics and kinetics of sedative and opioid analgesic drugs.

If appropriate, preferentially use an alpha-2 agonist for sedation. If acepromazine is included in the sedative protocol, use the low end of the dose range (5 µg (micrograms)/kg i.v or 10 µg/kg i.m.).

When selecting an opioid for incorporation in the protocol avoid butorphanol, morphine and fentanyl, and use methadone at the low end of the dose range (0.1–0.2 mg/kg i.v., i.m.).

References

⌐pande D, Hill KE, Mealey KL, Chambers JP and Gieseg MA (2016) The effect of the
e *ABCB-1* D mutation on sedation after intravenous administration of
mazine. *Journal of Veterinary Internal Medicine* **30**, 636–641

Anaesthetics, analgesics and NSAIDs

Anti-infectives

(see also Guidelines for responsible antibiotic use in the Appendix)

APPENDIX I: GENERAL INFORMATION

APPENDIX II: PROTOCOLS

INDEX: THERAPEUTIC CLASS

INDEX: GEM

Anti-infectives *continued*

Cardiovascular

Alpha blockers
  Phenoxybenzamine 289 [CIL]
Antiarrhythmics
  Amiodarone 18 [CIL]
  Digoxin 114 [CIL]
  Esmolol 142
  Mexiletine 244 [CIL]
  Propantheline 311
  Sotalol 347 [CIL]
  Verapamil 383 [CIL]
Antihypertensives
  Amlodipine 21 [CIL]
Antiplatelet aggregators
  Aspirin 29 [CIL]
  Clopidogrel 90 [CIL]
Beta blockers
  Atenolol 30 [CIL]
  Carvedilol 62
  Propranolol 314 [CIL]
Diuretics
  Amiloride 15
  Furosemide 162 [CIL]

  Hydrochlorothiazide 180 [CIL]
  Spironolactone 348
  Torasemide 370
Positive inotropes
  Dobutamine 121
  Dopamine 126
  Pimobendan 296
Vasoconstrictors
  Ephedrine 136
Vasodilators
  Benazepril 39
  Diltiazem 116 [CIL]
  Enalapril 133
  Glyceryl trinitrate 173
  Hydralazine 180
  Imidapril 188
  Prazosin 305 [CIL]
  Ramipril 321
  Sildenafil 340 [CIL]
  Telmisartan 355

Dermatological

Antihistamines
  Cetirizine 70
  Chlorphenamine 76 [CIL]
  Clemastine 85 [CIL]
  Cyproheptadine 97 [CIL]
  Diphenhydramine 120
  Hydroxyzine 184 [CIL]
  Loratadine 218
  Promethazine 311
Anti-inflammatory topical steroids
  Hydrocortisone 181
  Hydrocortisone aceponate 183
Anti-inflammatory - others
  Doxepin 128
  Lokivetmab 216
  Nicotinamide 262
  Oclacitinib 266
  Sodium cromoglicate 345
Anti-oxidants
  Dimethylsulfoxide 118
Cleansers and sebolytics
  Chlorhexidine 75
  Sodium hypochlorite 346
  and endoparasiticides
  Sinomectin 139
  Afoxolaner 142

  Indoxacarb 191
  Milbemycin 247
  Selamectin 336
  Spinosad 348
Ectoparasiticides
  Afoxolaner 6
  Deltamethrin 103
  Dinotefuran 119
  Fipronil 151
  Fluralaner 158
  Imidacloprid 187
  Lotilaner 210
  Lufenuron 220
  Methoprene 238
  Moxidectin 255
  Nitenpyram 262
  Permethrin 285
  Pyriprole 319
  Pyriproxyfen 320
  Sarolaner 334
  Tigolaner 366
Immunosuppressives
  Ciclosporin 78
  Hydrocortisone 181
Vasodilators
  Pentoxifylline 285 [CIL]

Endocrine

Gastrointestinal and hepatic

APPENDIX I: GENERAL INFORMATION

APPENDIX II: PROTOCOLS

INDEX: THERAPEUTIC CLASS

INDEX: GEN...

Gastrointestinal and hepatic *continued*

Emetics
Apomorphine 27
Ropinirole 330

Laxatives
Bisacodyl 43
Bowel cleansing solutions 45
Docusate sodium 123
Ispaghula 198
Lactulose 205 **CIL**
Paraffin 278
Sodium citrate 345
Sterculia 349

Motility modifiers
Cisapride 82 **CIL**
Ispaghula 198
Metoclopramide 242 **CIL**
Sterculia 349

Ulcer-healing drugs
Aluminium antacids 13
Cimetidine 79
Famotidine 145 **CIL**
Misoprostol 251 **CIL**
Omeprazole 268 **CIL**
Ranitidine 323 **CIL**
Sucralfate 350 **CIL**

Genito-urinary tract

Phosphate binders
Aluminium antacids 13
Calcium acetate 53
Chitosan 72
Lanthanum carbonate 206
Sevelamer hydrochloride 339

Urethral relaxants
Diazepam 110 **CIL**
Oxybutynin hydrochloride 272
Phenoxybenzamine 289 **CIL**
Tamsulosin hydrochloride
353 **CIL**

Urinary acidifiers
Methionine 237

Urinary alkalinizers
Potassium citrate 301

Urinary antiseptics
Methenamine 237

Urinary incontinence
Ephedrine 136
Estriol 143
Phenylpropanolamine 291
Propantheline 311

Urinary retention
Bethanecol 42

Urolithiasis
Allopurinol 11 **CIL**
Penicillamine 280
Potassium citrate 301

Metabolic

Antidotes
Acetylcysteine 2 **CIL**
Antivenom 26
Charcoal 71
Colestyramine 94
Deferoxamine 102
Dexrazoxane 109
Dimercaprol 117
Edetate calcium disodium 131
Ethanol 144
Fomepizole 160
Methylthioninium chloride 241

Penicillamine 280
Pralidoxime 304
Protamine sulphate 316
Tetanus antitoxin 358

Anti-hypercalcaemics
Alendronate 8 **CIL**
Pamidronate 275
Zoledronate 398

Antitoxins
Tetanus antitoxin 358

Others
Bezafibrate 42

APPENDIX I: GENERAL INFORMATION

APPENDIX II: PROTOCOLS

INDEX: THERAPEUTIC CLASS

APPENDIX I: GENERAL INFORMATION

APPENDIX II: PROTOCOLS

INDEX: THERAPEUTIC CLASS

IND⌐